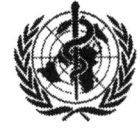

WORLD HEALTH ORGANIZATION

INTERNATIONAL AGENCY FOR RESEARCH ON CANCER

IARC MONOGRAPHS

ON THE

EVALUATION OF CARCINOGENIC RISKS TO HUMANS

Coffee, Tea, Mate, Methylxanthines and Methylglyoxal

VOLUME 51

This publication represents the views and expert opinions
of an IARC Working Group on the
Evaluation of Carcinogenic Risks to Humans,
which met in Lyon,

27 February to 6 March 1990

1991

IARC MONOGRAPHS

In 1969, the International Agency for Research on Cancer (IARC) initiated a programme on the evaluation of the carcinogenic risk of chemicals to humans involving the production of critically evaluated monographs on individual chemicals. In 1980, the programme was expanded to include the evaluation of the carcinogenic risk associated with exposures to complex mixtures.

The objective of the programme is to elaborate and publish in the form of monographs critical reviews of data on carcinogenicity for chemicals and complex mixtures to which humans are known to be exposed, and on specific exposures, to evaluate these data in terms of human risk with the help of international working groups of experts in chemical carcinogenesis and related fields, and to indicate where additional research efforts are needed.

This project is supported by PHS Grant No. 5-UO1 CA33193-08 awarded by the US National Cancer Institute, Department of Health and Human Services. Additional support has been provided by the Commission of the European Communities since 1986.

©International Agency for Research on Cancer 1991

ISBN 92 832 1251 7

ISSN 0250-9555

All rights reserved. Application for rights of reproduction or translation, in part or *in toto*, should be made to the International Agency for Research on Cancer.

Distributed for the International Agency for Research on Cancer
by the Secretariat of the World Health Organization

PRINTED IN THE UK

CONTENTS

NOTE TO THE READER 5

LIST OF PARTICIPANTS 7

PREAMBLE

    Background 13
    Objective and Scope 13
    Selection of Topics for Monographs 14
    Data for Monographs 15
    The Working Group 15
    Working Procedures 16
    Exposure Data 16
    Biological Data Relevant to the Evaluation of Carcinogenicity to
        Humans 18
    Evidence for Carcinogenicity in Experimental Animals 19
    Other Relevant Data in Experimental Systems and Humans 21
    Evidence for Carcinogenicity in Humans 23
    Summary of Data Reported 26
    Evaluation 27
    References 31

GENERAL REMARKS ON THE SUBSTANCES CONSIDERED 35

THE MONOGRAPHS

    Coffee

        Production and use 41
        Chemical composition 61
        Biological data relevant to the evaluation of carcinogenic risk to
            humans 90
        Summary of data reported and evaluation 167
        Appendix 1. Main compounds found in coffee 199

CONTENTS

Tea

Production and use 207
Chemical composition 217
Biological data relevant to the evaluation of carcinogenic risk to humans 233
Summary of data reported and evaluation 259

Mate

Production and use 273
Chemical composition 276
Biological data relevant to the evaluation of carcinogenic risk to humans 278
Summary of data reported and evaluation 282

Methylxanthines

Caffeine 291
Theophylline 391
Theobromine 421

Methylglyoxal 443

GLOSSARY 459

SUMMARY OF FINAL EVALUATIONS 461

APPENDIX 2. SUMMARY TABLE OF GENETIC AND RELATED EFFECTS 463

APPENDIX 3. ACTIVITY PROFILES FOR GENETIC AND RELATED EFFECTS 465

SUPPLEMENTARY CORRIGENDA TO VOLUMES 1-50 483

CUMULATIVE INDEX TO THE *MONOGRAPHS* SERIES 485

NOTE TO THE READER

The term 'carcinogenic risk' in the *IARC Monographs* series is taken to mean the probability that exposure to an agent will lead to cancer in humans.

Inclusion of an agent in the *Monographs* does not imply that it is a carcinogen, only that the published data have been examined. Equally, the fact that an agent has not yet been evaluated in a monograph does not mean that it is not carcinogenic.

The evaluations of carcinogenic risk are made by international working groups of independent scientists and are qualitative in nature. No recommendation is given for regulation or legislation.

Anyone who is aware of published data that may alter the evaluation of the carcinogenic risk of an agent to humans is encouraged to make this information available to the Unit of Carcinogen Identification and Evaluation, International Agency for Research on Cancer, 150 cours Albert Thomas, 69372 Lyon Cedex 08, France, in order that the agent may be considered for re-evaluation by a future working group.

Although every effort is made to prepare the monographs as accurately as possible, mistakes may occur. Readers are requested to communicate any errors to the Unit of Carcinogen Identification and Evaluation, so that corrections can be reported in future volumes.

IARC WORKING GROUP ON THE EVALUATION OF CARCINOGENIC RISKS TO HUMANS: COFFEE, TEA, MATE, METHYLXANTHINES AND METHYLGLYOXAL

Lyon, 27 February – 6 March 1990

LIST OF PARTICIPANTS

Members

M.J. Arnaud, Nestlé Research Centre, Nestec Ltd-Labior, 1350 Orbe, Switzerland

G.A. Bannikov, Laboratory of the Mechanisms of Carcinogenesis, Cancer Research Centre, Kashirskoye Shosse 24, 115478 Moscow, USSR

R.J. Clarke, Ashby Cottage, Donnington, Chichester PO20 7PW, UK

J. Cusick, Department of Mathematics, Statistics and Epidemiology, Imperial Cancer Research Fund Laboratories, PO Box 123, Lincoln's Inn Fields, London WC2A 3PX, UK

L. Fishbein, International Life Sciences Institute, Risk Science Institute, 1126 Sixteenth Street NW, Suite 111, Washington DC 20007, USA

K. Hemminki, Institute of Occupational Health, Topeliuksenkatu 41 a A, 00250 Helsinki, Finland

J. Hiller, Community Medicine Department, University of Adelaide, GPO Box 498, Adelaide, SA 5001, Australia

C. Hsieh, Harvard School of Public Health, Department of Epidemiology, 677 Huntington Avenue, Boston, MA 02115, USA

J. Huttunen, Director-General, National Public Health Institute, Mannerheimintie 166, 00300 Helsinki, Finland

N. Ito, Department of Pathology, Nagoya City University, Medical School, Nagoya 467, Japan

R. Kroes, National Institute of Public Health and Environmental Protection, PO Box 1, 3720 BA Bilthoven, The Netherlands (*Chairman*)

C. La Vecchia, Mario Negri Institute, Department of Clinical Pharmacology, Unit of Epidemiology, via Eritrea 62, 20157 Milan, Italy

J. Lewtas, Genetic Bioassay Branch (MD 68), Health Effects Research Laboratory, US Environmental Protection Branch, Research Triangle Park, NC 27711, USA

O. Møller Jensen, The Danish Cancer Registry, Rosenvængets Hovedvej 35, Box 839, 2100 Copenhagen Ø, Denmark (*Vice-Chairman*)

E. Ron[1], National Cancer Institute, Division of Cancer Etiology, EPN 408, 9000 Rockville Pike, Bethesda, MD 20892, USA

B. Schwetz, National Institute of Environmental Health Sciences, PO Box 12233, Research Triangle Park, NC 27709, USA

A. Sivak, Health Effects Institute, 215 First Street, Cambridge, MA 02142, USA

B. Stavric, Food Research Division, Bureau of Chemical Safety, Health Protection Branch, Ottawa, Ontario K1A 012, Canada

D. Trichopoulos[2], Department of Hygiene and Epidemiology, University of Athens, Athens 115 27, Greece

C. Victora, Department of Social Medicine, Faculty of Medicine, Federal University of Pelotas, PO Box 464, 96100 Pelotas RS, Brazil

R.A. Woutersen, TNO-CIVO, Toxicology and Nutrition Institute, PO Box 360, 3700 AJ Zeist, The Netherlands

F.E. Würgler, Institute of Toxicology, Swiss Federal Institute of Technology, 8603 Schwerzenbach, Switzerland

F. Zajdela, Unit of Cellular Physiology, INSERM, Radium Institute, Bâtiment 110, 91405 Orsay, France

Representatives/Observers

Representatives of the Commission of the European Communities

A.M. Halsberghe & N. van Larebeke-Arschodt, Commission of the European Communities, Health and Safety Directorate, Bâtiment Jean Monnet, BP 1907, 2920 Luxembourg, Grand Duchy of Luxembourg

Representative of the International Programme on Chemical Safety

B.H. Chen, International Programme on Chemical Safety, World Health Organization, 1211 Geneva 27, Switzerland

---

[1]Present address: Radiation Effects Research Institute, 5-2 Hijiyama Park, Minami-ku, Hiroshima 732, Japan

[2]Present address: Department of Epidemiology, Harvard University, School of Public Health, 677 Huntington Avenue, Boston, MA 02115, USA

PARTICIPANTS

American Cocoa Research Institute

S.M. Tarka, Jr, Food Science and Nutrition, Hershey Foods Corporation, Technical Center, PO Box 805, Hershey, PA 17033-0805, USA

Association of Soluble Coffee Manufacturers of the European Community

R. Viani, Nestec Ltd, Avenue Nestlé 55, 1800 Vevey, Switzerland

National Federation of Coffee Growers of Colombia

M. Quijano, National Federation of Coffee Growers, Research Laboratory, Calle 26A No. 37-28, Bogotá, Colombia

Tea Association of the USA

H.V. Graham, 256 Broad Avenue, Englewood, NJ 07631, USA

US National Soft Drink Association

J.L. Emerson, External Technical Affairs Department, The Coca-Cola Company, Coca-Cola Plaza, PO Drawer 1734, Atlanta, GA 30301, USA

Secretariat

H. Bartsch, Unit of Environmental Carcinogenesis and Host Factors
P. Boyle, SEARCH Programme
J. Cheney, Editorial, Translation and Publications Services
D. English, Unit of Biostatics Research and Informatics
J. Fitzgerald, Unit of Mechanisms of Carcinogenesis
M. Friesen, Unit of Environmental Carcinogenesis and Host Factors
M.-J. Ghess, Unit of Carcinogen Identification and Evaluation
E. Heseltine, Lajarthe, Montignac, France
V. Krutovskikh, Unit of Mechanisms of Carcinogenesis
M. Marselos, Unit of Carcinogen Identification and Evaluation
D. McGregor, Unit of Carcinogen Identification and Evaluation
D. Mietton, Unit of Carcinogen Identification and Evaluation
R. Montesano, Unit of Mechanisms of Carcinogenesis
N. Muñoz, Unit of Field and Intervention Studies
S. Narod, Programme of Viral and Hereditary Factors in Carcinogenesis
G. Nordberg, Unit of Carcinogen Identification and Evaluation
C. Partensky, Unit of Carcinogen Identification and Evaluation
I. Peterschmitt, Unit of Carcinogen Identification and Evaluation, Geneva Switzerland

S. San Jose Llongueras, Unit of Field and Intervention Studies
R. Saracci, Unit of Analytical Epidemiology
D. Shuker, Unit of Environmental Carcinogenesis and Host Factors
L. Tomatis, Director
H. Vainio, Unit of Carcinogen Identification and Evaluation
J. Wilbourn, Unit of Carcinogen Identification and Evaluation

Secretarial assistance

J. Cazeaux
M. Lézère
M. Mainaud
S. Reynaud

PREAMBLE

IARC MONOGRAPHS PROGRAMME ON THE EVALUATION OF CARCINOGENIC RISKS TO HUMANS[1]

PREAMBLE

1. BACKGROUND

In 1969, the International Agency for Research on Cancer (IARC) initiated a programme to evaluate the carcinogenic risk of chemicals to humans and to produce monographs on individual chemicals. The *Monographs* programme has since been expanded to include consideration of exposures to complex mixtures of chemicals (which occur, for example, in some occupations and as a result of human habits) and of exposures to other agents, such as radiation and viruses. With Supplement 6(1), the title of the series was modified from *IARC Monographs on the Evaluation of the Carcinogenic Risk of Chemicals to Humans* to *IARC Monographs on the Evaluation of Carcinogenic Risks to Humans*, in order to reflect the widened scope of the programme.

The criteria established in 1971 to evaluate carcinogenic risk to humans were adopted by the working groups whose deliberations resulted in the first 16 volumes of the *IARC Monographs* series. Those criteria were subsequently re-evaluated by working groups which met in 1977(2), 1978(3), 1979(4), 1982(5) and 1983(6). The present preamble was prepared by two working groups which met in September 1986 and January 1987, prior to the preparation of Supplement 7(7) to the *Monographs* and was modified by a working group which met in November 1988(8).

2. OBJECTIVE AND SCOPE

The objective of the programme is to prepare, with the help of international working groups of experts, and to publish in the form of monographs, critical

---

[1]This project is supported by PHS Grant No. 5 UO1 CA33193-08 awarded by the US National Cancer Institute, Department of Health and Human Services, and with a subcontract to Tracor Technology Resources, Inc. Since 1986, this programme has also been supported by the Commission of the European Communities.

reviews and evaluations of evidence on the carcinogenicity of a wide range of human exposures. The *Monographs* may also indicate where additional research efforts are needed.

The *Monographs* represent the first step in carcinogenic risk assessment, which involves examination of all relevant information in order to assess the strength of the available evidence that certain exposures could alter the incidence of cancer in humans. The second step is quantitative risk estimation, which is not usually attempted in the *Monographs*. Detailed, quantitative evaluations of epidemiological data may be made in the *Monographs*, but without extrapolation beyond the range of the data available. Quantitative extrapolation from experimental data to the human situation is not undertaken.

These monographs may assist national and international authorities in making risk assessments and in formulating decisions concerning any necessary preventive measures. The evaluations of IARC working groups are scientific, qualitative judgements about the degree of evidence for carcinogenicity provided by the available data on an agent. These evaluations represent only one part of the body of information on which regulatory measures may be based. Other components of regulatory decisions may vary from one situation to another and from country to country, responding to different socioeconomic and national priorities. *Therefore, no recommendation is given with regard to regulation or legislation, which are the responsibility of individual governments and/or other international organizations.*

The *IARC Monographs* are recognized as an authoritative source of information on the carcinogenicity of chemicals and complex exposures. A users' survey, made in 1988, indicated that the *Monographs* are consulted by various agencies in 57 countries. Each volume is generally printed in 4000 copies for distribution to governments, regulatory bodies and interested scientists. The *Monographs* are also available *via* the Distribution and Sales Service of the World Health Organization.

3. SELECTION OF TOPICS FOR MONOGRAPHS

Topics are selected on the basis of two main criteria: (a) that they concern agents and complex exposures for which there is evidence of human exposure, and (b) that there is some evidence or suspicion of carcinogenicity. The term agent is used to include individual chemical compounds, groups of chemical compounds, physical agents (such as radiation) and biological factors (such as viruses) and mixtures of agents such as occur in occupational exposures and as a result of personal and cultural habits (like smoking and dietary practices). Chemical analogues and compounds with biological or physical characteristics similar to those of suspected carcinogens may also be considered, even in the absence of data on carcinogenicity.

The scientific literature is surveyed for published data relevant to an assessment of carcinogenicity; the IARC surveys of chemicals being tested for carcinogenicity(9) and directories of on-going research in cancer epidemiology(10) often indicate those exposures that may be scheduled for future meetings. Ad-hoc working groups convened by IARC in 1984 and 1989 gave recommendations as to which chemicals and exposures to complex mixtures should be evaluated in the *IARC Monographs* series(11,12).

As significant new data on subjects on which monographs have already been prepared become available, re-evaluations are made at subsequent meetings, and revised monographs are published.

4. DATA FOR MONOGRAPHS

The *Monographs* do not necessarily cite all the literature concerning the subject of an evaluation. Only those data considered by the Working Group to be relevant to making the evaluation are included.

With regard to biological and epidemiological data, only reports that have been published or accepted for publication in the openly available scientific literature are reviewed by the working groups. In certain instances, government agency reports that have undergone peer review and are widely available are considered. Exceptions may be made on an ad-hoc basis to include unpublished reports that are in their final form and publicly available, if their inclusion is considered pertinent to making a final evaluation (see pp. 27 *et seq.*). In the sections on chemical and physical properties and on production, use, occurrence and analysis, unpublished sources of information may be used.

5. THE WORKING GROUP

Reviews and evaluations are formulated by a working group of experts. The tasks of this group are five-fold: (i) to ascertain that all appropriate data have been collected; (ii) to select the data relevant for the evaluation on the basis of scientific merit; (iii) to prepare accurate summaries of the data to enable the reader to follow the reasoning of the Working Group; (iv) to evaluate the results of experimental and epidemiological studies; and (v) to make an overall evaluation of the carcinogenicity of the exposure to humans.

Working Group participants who contributed to the considerations and evaluations within a particular volume are listed, with their addresses, at the beginning of each publication. Each participant who is a member of a working group serves as an individual scientist and not as a representative of any organization, government or industry. In addition, representatives from national and international agencies and industrial associations are invited as observers.

6. WORKING PROCEDURES

Approximately one year in advance of a meeting of a working group, the topics of the monographs are announced and participants are selected by IARC staff in consultation with other experts. Subsequently, relevant biological and epidemiological data are collected by IARC from recognized sources of information on carcinogenesis, including data storage and retrieval systems such as CHEMICAL ABSTRACTS, MEDLINE and TOXLINE — including EMIC and ETIC for data on genetic and related effects and teratogenicity, respectively.

The major collection of data and the preparation of first drafts of the sections on chemical and physical properties, on production and use, on occurrence, and on analysis are carried out under a separate contract funded by the US National Cancer Institute. Efforts are made to supplement this information with data from other national and international sources. Representatives from industrial associations may assist in the preparation of sections on production and use.

Production and trade data are obtained from governmental and trade publications and, in some cases, by direct contact with industries. Separate production data on some agents may not be available because their publication could disclose confidential information. Information on uses is usually obtained from published sources but is often complemented by direct contact with manufacturers.

Six months before the meeting, reference material is sent to experts, or is used by IARC staff, to prepare sections for the first drafts of monographs. The complete first drafts are compiled by IARC staff and sent, prior to the meeting, to all participants of the Working Group for review.

The Working Group meets in Lyon for seven to eight days to discuss and finalize the texts of the monographs and to formulate the evaluations. After the meeting, the master copy of each monograph is verified by consulting the original literature, edited and prepared for publication. The aim is to publish monographs within nine months of the Working Group meeting.

7. EXPOSURE DATA

Sections that indicate the extent of past and present human exposure, the sources of exposure, the persons most likely to be exposed and the factors that contribute to exposure to the agent, mixture or exposure circumstance are included at the beginning of each monograph.

Most monographs on individual chemicals or complex mixtures include sections on chemical and physical data, and production, use, occurrence and analysis. In other monographs, for example on physical agents, biological factors, occupational exposures and cultural habits, other sections may be included, such as: historical perspectives, description of an industry or habit, exposures in the work place or chemistry of the complex mixture.

The Chemical Abstracts Services Registry Number and the latest Chemical Abstracts Primary Name are recorded. Other synonyms and trade names are given, but the list is not necessarily comprehensive. Some of the trade names may be those of mixtures in which the agent being evaluated is only one of the ingredients.

Information on chemical and physical properties and, in particular, data relevant to identification, occurrence and biological activity are included. A separate description of technical products gives relevant specifications and includes available information on composition and impurities.

The dates of first synthesis and of first commercial production of an agent or mixture are provided; for agents which do not occur naturally, this information may allow a reasonable estimate to be made of the date before which no human exposure to the agent could have occurred. The dates of first reported occurrence of an exposure are also provided. In addition, methods of synthesis used in past and present commercial production and different methods of production which may give rise to different impurities are described.

Data on production, foreign trade and uses are obtained for representative regions, which usually include Europe, Japan and the USA. It should not, however, be inferred that those areas or nations are necessarily the sole or major sources or users of the agent being evaluated.

Some identified uses may not be current or major applications, and the coverage is not necessarily comprehensive. In the case of drugs, mention of their therapeutic uses does not necessarily represent current practice nor does it imply judgement as to their clinical efficacy.

Information on the occurrence of an agent or mixture in the environment is obtained from data derived from the monitoring and surveillance of levels in occupational environments, air, water, soil, foods and animal and human tissues. When available, data on the generation, persistence and bioaccumulation are also included. In the case of mixtures, industries, occupations or processes, information is given about all agents present. For processes, industries and occupations, a historical description is also given, noting variations in chemical composition, physical properties or levels of occupational exposure with time.

Statements concerning regulations and guidelines (e.g., pesticide registrations, maximal levels permitted in foods, occupational exposure limits) are included for some countries as indications of potential exposures, but they may not reflect the most recent situation, since such limits are continuously reviewed and modified. The absence of information on regulatory status for a country should not be taken to imply that that country does not have regulations with regard to the exposure.

The purpose of the section on analysis is to give the reader an overview of current methods cited in the literature, with emphasis on those widely used for regulatory purposes. No critical evaluation or recommendation of any of the methods is meant or implied. Methods for monitoring human exposure are also given, when available. The IARC publishes a series of volumes, *Environmental Carcinogens: Methods of Analysis and Exposure Measurement(13)*, that describe validated methods for analysing a wide variety of agents and mixtures.

8. BIOLOGICAL DATA RELEVANT TO THE EVALUATION OF CARCINOGENICITY TO HUMANS

The term 'carcinogen' is used in these monographs to denote an agent or mixture that is capable of increasing the incidence of malignant neoplasms; the induction of benign neoplasms may in some circumstances (see p. 20) contribute to the judgement that the exposure is carcinogenic. The terms 'neoplasm' and 'tumour' are used interchangeably.

Some epidemiological and experimental studies indicate that different agents may act at different stages in the carcinogenic process, probably by fundamentally different mechanisms. In the present state of knowledge, the aim of the *Monographs* is to evaluate evidence of carcinogenicity at any stage in the carcinogenic process independently of the underlying mechanism involved. There is as yet insufficient information to implement classification according to mechanisms of action(6).

Definitive evidence of carcinogenicity in humans can be provided only by epidemiological studies. Evidence relevant to human carcinogenicity may also be provided by experimental studies of carcinogenicity in animals and by other biological data, particularly those relating to humans.

The available studies are summarized by the Working Group, with particular regard to the qualitative aspects discussed below. In general, numerical findings are indicated as they appear in the original report; units are converted when necessary for easier comparison. The Working Group may conduct additional analyses of the published data and use them in their assessment of the evidence and may include them in their summary of a study; the results of such supplementary analyses are given in square brackets. Any comments are also made in square brackets; however, these are kept to a minimum, being restricted to those instances in which it is felt that an important aspect of a study, directly impinging on its interpretation, should be brought to the attention of the reader.

For experimental studies with mixtures, consideration is given to the possibility of changes in the physicochemical properties of the test substance during collection, storage, extraction, concentration and delivery. Either chemical or toxicological interactions of the components of mixtures may result in nonlinear dose-response relationships.

An assessment is made as to the relevance to human exposure of samples tested in experimental systems, which may involve consideration of: (i) physical and chemical characteristics, (ii) constituent substances that indicate the presence of a class of substances, (iii) tests for genetic and related effects, including genetic activity profiles, (iv) DNA adduct profiles, (v) oncogene expression and mutation, suppressor gene inactivation.

9. EVIDENCE FOR CARCINOGENICITY IN EXPERIMENTAL ANIMALS

For several agents (e.g., 4-aminobiphenyl, bis(chloromethyl)ether, diethylstilboestrol, melphalan, 8-methoxypsoralen (methoxsalen) plus ultra-violet radiation, mustard gas and vinyl chloride), evidence of carcinogenicity in experimental animals preceded evidence obtained from epidemiological studies or case reports. Information compiled from the first 41 volumes of the *IARC Monographs*(14) shows that, of the 44 agents and mixtures for which there is *sufficient* or *limited evidence* of carcinogenicity to humans (see p. 28), all 37 that have been tested adequately experimentally produce cancer in at least one animal species. Although this association cannot establish that all agents and mixtures that cause cancer in experimental animals also cause cancer in humans, nevertheless, *in the absence of adequate data on humans, it is biologically plausible and prudent to regard agents and mixtures for which there is sufficient evidence (see p. 29) of carcinogenicity in experimental animals as if they presented a carcinogenic risk to humans*.

The monographs are not intended to summarize all published studies. Those that are inadequate (e.g., too short a duration, too few animals, poor survival; see below) or are judged irrelevant to the evaluation are generally omitted. They may be mentioned briefly, particularly when the information is considered to be a useful supplement to that of other reports or when they provide the only data available. Their inclusion does not, however, imply acceptance of the adequacy of the experimental design or of the analysis and interpretation of their results. Guidelines for adequate long-term carcinogenicity experiments have been outlined (e.g., 15).

The nature and extent of impurities or contaminants present in the agent or mixture being evaluated are given when available. Mention is made of all routes of exposure that have been adequately studied and of all species in which relevant experiments have been performed. Animal strain, sex, numbers per group, age at start of treatment and survival are reported.

Experiments in which the agent or mixture was administered in conjunction with known carcinogens or factors that modify carcinogenic effects are also reported. Experiments on the carcinogenicity of known metabolites and derivatives may be included.

(a) Qualitative aspects

An assessment of carcinogenicity involves several considerations of qualitative importance, including (i) the experimental conditions under which the test was performed, including route and schedule of exposure, species, strain, sex, age, duration of follow-up; (ii) the consistency of the results, for example, across species and target organ(s); (iii) the spectrum of neoplastic response, from benign tumours to malignant neoplasms; and (iv) the possible role of modifying factors.

Considerations of importance to the Working Group in the interpretation and evaluation of a particular study include: (i) how clearly the agent was defined and, in the case of mixtures, how adequately the sample characterization was reported; (ii) whether the dose was adequately monitored, particularly in inhalation experiments; (iii) whether the doses used were appropriate and whether the survival of treated animals was similar to that of controls; (iv) whether there were adequate numbers of animals per group; (v) whether animals of both sexes were used; (vi) whether animals were allocated randomly to groups; (vii) whether the duration of observation was adequate; and (viii) whether the data were adequately reported. If available, recent data on the incidence of specific tumours in historical controls, as well as in concurrent controls, should be taken into account in the evaluation of tumour response.

When benign tumours occur together with and originate from the same cell type in an organ or tissue as malignant tumours in a particular study and appear to represent a stage in the progression to malignancy, it may be valid to combine them in assessing tumour incidence. The occurrence of lesions presumed to be preneoplastic may in certain instances aid in assessing the biological plausibility of any neoplastic response observed.

Of the many agents and mixtures that have been studied extensively, few induce only benign neoplasms. Benign tumours in experimental animals frequently represent a stage in the evolution of a malignant neoplasm, but they may be 'endpoints' that do not readily undergo transition to malignancy. However, if an agent or mixture is found to induce only benign neoplasms, it should be suspected of being a carcinogen and it requires further investigation.

(b) Quantitative aspects

The probability that tumours will occur may depend on the species and strain, the dose of the carcinogen and the route and period of exposure. Evidence of an increased incidence of neoplasms with increased level of exposure strengthens the inference of a causal association between the exposure and the development of neoplasms.

The form of the dose-response relationship can vary widely, depending on the particular agent under study and the target organ. Since many chemicals require metabolic activation before being converted into their reactive intermediates, both metabolic and pharmacokinetic aspects are important in determining the dose-response pattern. Saturation of steps such as absorption, activation, inactivation and elimination of the carcinogen may produce nonlinearity in the dose-response relationship, as could saturation of processes such as DNA repair(16,17).

(c) *Statistical analysis of long-term experiments in animals*

Factors considered by the Working Group include the adequacy of the information given for each treatment group: (i) the number of animals studied and the number examined histologically, (ii) the number of animals with a given tumour type and (iii) length of survival. The statistical methods used should be clearly stated and should be the generally accepted techniques refined for this purpose(17,18). When there is no difference in survival between control and treatment groups, the Working Group usually compares the proportions of animals developing each tumour type in each of the groups. Otherwise, consideration is given as to whether or not appropriate adjustments have been made for differences in survival. These adjustments can include: comparisons of the proportions of tumour-bearing animals among the 'effective number' of animals alive at the time the first tumour is discovered, in the case where most differences in survival occur before tumours appear; life-table methods, when tumours are visible or when they may be considered 'fatal' because mortality rapidly follows tumour development; and the Mantel-Haenszel test or logistic regression, when occult tumours do not affect the animals' risk of dying but are 'incidental' findings at autopsy.

In practice, classifying tumours as fatal or incidental may be difficult. Several survival-adjusted methods have been developed that do not require this distinction(17), although they have not been fully evaluated.

10. OTHER RELEVANT DATA IN EXPERIMENTAL SYSTEMS AND HUMANS

(a) *Structure-activity considerations*

This section describes structure-activity correlations that are relevant to an evaluation of the carcinogenicity of an agent.

(b) *Absorption, distribution, excretion and metabolism*

Concise information is given on absorption, distribution (including placental transfer) and excretion. Kinetic factors that may affect the dose-reponse relationship, such as saturation of uptake, protein binding, metabolic activation, detoxification and DNA repair processes, are mentioned. Studies that indicate the metabolic fate of the agent in experimental animals and humans are summarized briefly, and comparisons of data from animals and humans are made when possible. Comparative information on the relationship between exposure and the dose that reaches the target site may be of particular importance for extrapolation between species.

(c) *Toxicity*

Data are given on acute and chronic toxic effects (other than cancer), such as organ toxicity, immunotoxicity, endocrine effects and preneoplastic lesions. Effects on reproduction, teratogenicity, feto- and embryotoxicity are also summarized briefly.

(d) *Genetic and related effects*

Tests of genetic and related effects may indicate possible carcinogenic activity. They can also be used in detecting active metabolites of known carcinogens in human or animal body fluids, in detecting active components in complex mixtures and in the elucidation of possible mechanisms of carcinogenesis.

The adequacy of the reporting of sample characterization is considered and, where necessary, commented upon. The available data are interpreted critically by phylogenetic group according to the endpoints detected, which may include DNA damage, gene mutation, sister chromatid exchange, micronuclei, chromosomal aberrations, aneuploidy and cell transformation. The concentrations (doses) employed are given and mention is made of whether an exogenous metabolic system was required. When appropriate, these data may be represented by bar graphs (activity profiles), with corresponding summary tables and listings of test systems, data and references. Detailed information on the preparation of these profiles is given in an appendix to those volumes in which they are used.

Positive results in tests using prokaryotes, lower eukaryotes, plants, insects and cultured mammalian cells suggest that genetic and related effects (and therefore possibly carcinogenic effects) could occur in mammals. Results from such tests may also give information about the types of genetic effect produced and about the involvement of metabolic activation. Some endpoints described are clearly genetic in nature (e.g., gene mutations and chromosomal aberrations); others are to a greater or lesser degree associated with genetic effects (e.g., unscheduled DNA synthesis). In-vitro tests for tumour-promoting activity and for cell transformation may detect changes that are not necessarily the result of genetic alterations but that may have specific relevance to the process of carcinogenesis. A critical appraisal of these tests has been published(15).

Genetic or other activity detected in the systems mentioned above is not always manifest in whole mammals. Positive indications of genetic effects in experimental mammals and in humans are regarded as being of greater relevance than those in other organisms. The demonstration that an agent or mixture can induce gene and chromosomal mutations in whole mammals indicates that it may have the potential for carcinogenic activity, although this activity may not be detectably expressed in any or all species tested. Relative potency in tests for mutagenicity and related effects is not a reliable indicator of carcinogenic potency. Negative results in tests for mutagenicity in selected tissues from animals treated *in vivo* provide less weight, partly because they do not exclude the possibility of an effect in tissues other than those examined. Moreover, negative results in short-term tests with genetic endpoints cannot be considered to provide evidence to rule out carcinogenicity of agents or mixtures that act through other mechanisms. Factors may arise in many tests that could give misleading results; these have been discussed in detail elsewhere(15).

The adequacy of epidemiological studies of reproductive outcomes and genetic and related effects in humans is evaluated by the same criteria as are applied to epidemiological studies of cancer.

11. EVIDENCE FOR CARCINOGENICITY IN HUMANS

(a) *Types of studies considered*

Three types of epidemiological studies of cancer contribute data to the assessment of carcinogenicity in humans — cohort studies, case-control studies and correlation studies. Rarely, results from randomized trials may be available. Case reports of cancer in humans are also reviewed.

Cohort and case-control studies relate individual exposures under study to the occurrence of cancer in individuals and provide an estimate of relative risk (ratio of incidence in those exposed to incidence in those not exposed) as the main measure of association.

In correlation studies, the units of investigation are usually whole populations (e.g., in particular geographical areas or at particular times), and cancer frequency is related to a summary measure of the exposure of the population to the agent, mixture or exposure circumstance under study. Because individual exposure is not documented, however, a causal relationship is less easy to infer from correlation studies than from cohort and case-control studies.

Case reports generally arise from a suspicion, based on clinical experience, that the concurrence of two events — that is, a particular exposure and occurrence of a cancer — has happened rather more frequently than would be expected by chance. Case reports usually lack complete ascertainment of cases in any population, definition or enumeration of the population at risk and estimation of the expected number of cases in the absence of exposure.

The uncertainties surrounding interpretation of case reports and correlation studies make them inadequate, except in rare instances, to form the sole basis for inferring a causal relationship. When taken together with case-control and cohort studies, however, relevant case reports or correlation studies may add materially to the judgement that a causal relationship is present.

Epidemiological studies of benign neoplasms and presumed preneoplastic lesions are also reviewed by working groups. They may, in some instances, strengthen inferences drawn from studies of cancer itself.

(b) Quality of studies considered

It is necessary to take into account the possible roles of bias, confounding and chance in the interpretation of epidemiological studies. By 'bias' is meant the operation of factors in study design or execution that lead erroneously to a stronger or weaker association than in fact exists between disease and an agent, mixture or exposure circumstance. By 'confounding' is meant a situation in which the relationship with disease is made to appear stronger or to appear weaker than it truly is as a result of an association between the apparent causal factor and another factor that is associated with either an increase or decrease in the incidence of the disease. In evaluating the extent to which these factors have been minimized in an individual study, working groups consider a number of aspects of design and analysis as described in the report of the study. Most of these considerations apply equally to case-control, cohort and correlation studies. Lack of clarity of any of these aspects in the reporting of a study can decrease its credibility and its consequent weighting in the final evaluation of the exposure.

Firstly, the study population, disease (or diseases) and exposure should have been well defined by the authors. Cases in the study population should have been identified in a way that was independent of the exposure of interest, and exposure should have been assessed in a way that was not related to disease status.

Secondly, the authors should have taken account in the study design and analysis of other variables that can influence the risk of disease and may have been related to the exposure of interest. Potential confounding by such variables should have been dealt with either in the design of the study, such as by matching, or in the analysis, by statistical adjustment. In cohort studies, comparisons with local rates of disease may be more appropriate than those with national rates. Internal comparisons of disease frequency among individuals at different levels of exposure should also have been made in the study.

Thirdly, the authors should have reported the basic data on which the conclusions are founded, even if sophisticated statistical analyses were employed. At the very least, they should have given the numbers of exposed and unexposed cases and controls in a case-control study and the numbers of cases observed and expected in a cohort study. Further tabulations by time since exposure began and other temporal factors are also important. In a cohort study, data on all cancer sites and all causes of death should have been given, to avoid the possibility of reporting bias. In a case-control study, the effects of investigated factors other than the exposure of interest should have been reported.

Finally, the statistical methods used to obtain estimates of relative risk, absolute cancer rates, confidence intervals and significance tests, and to adjust for confounding should have been clearly stated by the authors. The methods used should preferably have been the generally accepted techniques that have been refined since the mid-1970s. These methods have been reviewed for case-control studies(19) and for cohort studies(20).

(c) Quantitative considerations

Detailed analyses of both relative and absolute risks in relation to age at first exposure and to temporal variables, such as time since first exposure, duration of exposure and time since exposure ceased, are reviewed and summarized when available. The analysis of temporal relationships can provide a useful guide in formulating models of carcinogenesis. In particular, such analyses may suggest whether a carcinogen acts early or late in the process of carcinogenesis(6), although such speculative inferences cannot be used to draw firm conclusions concerning the mechanism of action and hence the shape (linear or otherwise) of the dose-response relationship below the range of observation.

(d) Criteria for causality

After the quality of individual epidemiological studies has been summarized and assessed, a judgement is made concerning the strength of evidence that the agent, mixture or exposure circumstance in question is carcinogenic for humans. In making their judgement, the Working Group considers several criteria for causality. A strong association (i.e., a large relative risk) is more likely to indicate causality than a weak association, although it is recognized that relative risks of small magnitude do not imply lack of causality and may be important if the disease is common. Associations that are replicated in several studies of the same design or using different epidemiological approaches or under different circumstances of exposure are more likely to represent a causal relationship than isolated observations from single studies. If there are inconsistent results among investigations, possible reasons are sought (such as differences in amount of exposure), and results of studies judged to be of high quality are given more weight than those from studies judged to be methodologically less sound. When suspicion of carcinogenicity arises largely from a single study, these data are not combined with those from later studies in any subsequent reassessment of the strength of the evidence.

If the risk of the disease in question increases with the amount of exposure, this is considered to be a strong indication of causality, although absence of a graded response is not necessarily evidence against a causal relationship. Demonstration of a decline in risk after cessation of or reduction in exposure in individuals or in whole populations also supports a causal interpretation of the findings.

Although a carcinogen may act upon more than one target, the specificity of an association (i.e., an increased occurrence of cancer at one anatomical site or of one morphological type) adds plausibility to a causal relationship, particularly when excess cancer occurrence is limited to one morphological type within the same organ.

Although rarely available, results from randomized trials showing different rates among exposed and unexposed individuals provide particularly strong evidence for causality.

When several epidemiological studies show little or no indication of an association between an exposure and cancer, the judgement may be made that, in the aggregate, they show evidence of lack of carcinogenicity. Such a judgement requires first of all that the studies giving rise to it meet, to a sufficient degree, the standards of design and analysis described above. Specifically, the possibility that bias, confounding or misclassification of exposure or outcome could explain the observed results should be considered and excluded with reasonable certainty. In addition, all studies that are judged to be methodologically sound should be consistent with a relative risk of unity for any observed level of exposure and, when considered together, should provide a pooled estimate of relative risk which is at or near unity and has a narrow confidence interval, due to sufficient population size. Moreover, no individual study nor the pooled results of all the studies should show any consistent tendency for relative risk of cancer to increase with increasing level of exposure. It is important to note that evidence of lack of carcinogenicity obtained in this way from several epidemiological studies can apply only to the type(s) of cancer studied and to dose levels and intervals between first exposure and observation of disease that are the same as or less than those observed in all the studies. Experience with human cancer indicates that, in some cases, the period from first exposure to the development of clinical cancer is seldom less than 20 years; latent periods substantially shorter than 30 years cannot provide evidence for lack of carcinogenicity.

12. SUMMARY OF DATA REPORTED

In this section, the relevant experimental and epidemiological data are summarized. Only reports, other than in abstract form, that meet the criteria outlined on p. 15 are considered for evaluating carcinogenicity. Inadequate studies are generally not summarized: such studies are usually identified by a square-bracketed comment in the text.

(a) Exposures

Human exposure is summarized on the basis of elements such as production, use, occurrence in the environment and determinations in human tissues and body fluids. Quantitative data are given when available.

(b) Experimental carcinogenicity data

Data relevant to the evaluation of carcinogenicity in animals are summarized. For each animal species and route of administration, it is stated whether an increased incidence of neoplasms was observed, and the tumour sites are indicated. If the agent or mixture produced tumours after prenatal exposure or in single-dose experiments, this is also indicated. Dose-response and other quantitative data may be given when available. Negative findings are also summarized.

(c) Human carcinogenicity data

Results of epidemiological studies that are considered to be pertinent to an assessment of human carcinogenicity are summarized. When relevant, case reports and correlation studies are also considered.

(d) Other relevant data

Structure-activity correlations are mentioned when relevant.

Toxicological information and data on kinetics and metabolism in experimental animals are given when considered relevant. The results of tests for genetic and related effects are summarized for whole mammals, cultured mammalian cells and nonmammalian systems.

Data on other biological effects in humans of particular relevance are summarized. These may include kinetic and metabolic considerations and evidence of DNA binding, persistence of DNA lesions or genetic damage in exposed humans.

When available, comparisons of such data for humans and for animals, and particularly animals that have developed cancer, are described.

13. EVALUATION

Evaluations of the strength of the evidence for carcinogenicity arising from human and experimental animal data are made, using standard terms.

It is recognized that the criteria for these evaluations, described below, cannot encompass all of the factors that may be relevant to an evaluation of carcinogenicity. In considering all of the relevant data, the Working Group may assign the agent, mixture or exposure circumstance to a higher or lower category than a strict interpretation of these criteria would indicate.

(a) *Degrees of evidence for carcinogenicity in humans and in experimental animals and supporting evidence*

It should be noted that these categories refer only to the strength of the evidence that an exposure is carcinogenic and not to the extent of its carcinogenic activity (potency) nor to the mechanism involved. A classification may change as new information becomes available.

An evaluation of degree of evidence, whether for a single substance or a mixture, is limited to the materials tested, and these are chemically and physically defined. When the materials evaluated are considered by the Working Group to be sufficiently closely related, they may be grouped for the purpose of a single evaluation of degree of evidence.

(i) *Human carcinogenicity data*

The applicability of an evaluation of the carcinogenicity of a mixture, process, occupation or industry on the basis of evidence from epidemiological studies depends on the variability over time and place of the mixtures, processes, occupations and industries. The Working Group seeks to identify the specific exposure, process or activity which is considered most likely to be responsible for any excess risk. The evaluation is focused as narrowly as the available data on exposure and other aspects permit.

The evidence relevant to carcinogenicity from studies in humans is classified into one of the following categories:

Sufficient evidence of carcinogenicity: The Working Group considers that a causal relationship has been established between exposure to the agent, mixture or exposure circumstance and human cancer. That is, a positive relationship has been observed between the exposure and cancer in studies in which chance, bias and confounding could be ruled out with reasonable confidence.

Limited evidence of carcinogenicity: A positive association has been observed between exposure to the agent, mixture or exposure circumstance and cancer for which a causal interpretation is considered by the Working Group to be credible, but chance, bias or confounding could not be ruled out with reasonable confidence.

Inadequate evidence of carcinogenicity: The available studies are of insufficient quality, consistency or statistical power to permit a conclusion regarding the presence or absence of a causal association.

Evidence suggesting lack of carcinogenicity: There are several adequate studies covering the full range of levels of exposure that human beings are known to encounter, which are mutually consistent in not showing a positive association between exposure to the agent, mixture or exposure circumstance and any studied cancer at any observed level of exposure. A conclusion of 'evidence suggesting lack of carcinogenicity' is inevitably limited to the cancer sites, conditions and levels of exposure and length of observation covered by the available studies. In addition, the possibility of a very small risk at the levels of exposure studied can never be excluded.

In some instances, the above categories may be used to classify the degree of evidence for carcinogenicity for specific organs or tissues.

(ii) *Experimental carcinogenicity data*

The evidence relevant to carcinogenicity in experimental animals is classified into one of the following categories:

Sufficient evidence of carcinogenicity: The Working Group considers that a causal relationship has been established between the agent or mixture and an increased incidence of malignant neoplasms or of an appropriate combination of benign and malignant neoplasms (as described on p. 20) in (a) two or more species of animals or (b) in two or more independent studies in one species carried out at different times or in different laboratories or under different protocols.

Exceptionally, a single study in one species might be considered to provide sufficient evidence of carcinogenicity when malignant neoplasms occur to an unusual degree with regard to incidence, site, type of tumour or age at onset.

In the absence of adequate data on humans, it is biologically plausible and prudent to regard agents and mixtures for which there is *sufficient evidence* of carcinogenicity in experimental animals as if they presented a carcinogenic risk to humans.

Limited evidence of carcinogenicity: The data suggest a carcinogenic effect but are limited for making a definitive evaluation because, e.g., (a) the evidence of carcinogenicity is restricted to a single experiment; or (b) there are unresolved questions regarding the adequacy of the design, conduct or interpretation of the study; or (c) the agent or mixture increases the incidence only of benign neoplasms or lesions of uncertain neoplastic potential, or of certain neoplasms which may occur spontaneously in high incidences in certain strains.

Inadequate evidence of carcinogenicity: The studies cannot be interpreted as showing either the presence or absence of a carcinogenic effect because of major qualitative or quantitative limitations.

Evidence suggesting lack of carcinogenicity: Adequate studies involving at least two species are available which show that, within the limits of the tests used, the agent or mixture is not carcinogenic. A conclusion of evidence suggesting lack of carcinogenicity is inevitably limited to the species, tumour sites and levels of exposure studied.

(iii) *Supporting evidence of carcinogenicity*

Other evidence judged to be relevant to an evaluation of carcinogenicity and of sufficient importance to affect the overall evaluation is then described. This may include data on tumour pathology, genetic and related effects, structure-activity relationships, metabolism and pharmacokinetics, physicochemical parameters, chemical composition and possible mechanisms of action. For complex exposures, including occupational and industrial exposures, the potential contribution of carcinogens known to be present as well as the relevance of materials tested are considered by the Working Group in its overall evaluation of human carcinogenicity. The Working Group also determines to what extent the materials tested in experimental systems are relevant to those to which humans are exposed. The available experimental evidence may help to specify more precisely the causal factor(s).

(b) Overall evaluation

Finally, the body of evidence is considered as a whole, in order to reach an overall evaluation of the carcinogenicity to humans of an agent, mixture or circumstance of exposure.

An evaluation may be made for a group of chemical compounds that have been evaluated by the Working Group. In addition, when supporting data indicate that other, related compounds for which there is no direct evidence of capacity to induce cancer in animals or in humans may also be carcinogenic, a statement describing the rationale for this conclusion is added to the evaluation narrative; an additional evaluation may be made for this broader group of compounds if the strength of the evidence warrants it.

The agent, mixture or exposure circumstance is described according to the wording of one of the following categories, and the designated group is given. The categorization of an agent, mixture or exposure circumstance is a matter of scientific judgement, reflecting the strength of the evidence derived from studies in humans and in experimental animals and from other relevant data.

Group 1 — The agent (mixture) is carcinogenic to humans.

The exposure circumstance entails exposures that are carcinogenic to humans.

This category is used only when there is *sufficient evidence* of carcinogenicity in humans.

Group 2

This category includes agents, mixtures and exposure circumstances for which, at one extreme, the degree of evidence of carcinogenicity in humans is almost sufficient, as well as those for which, at the other extreme, there are no human data but for which there is experimental evidence of carcinogenicity. Agents, mixtures and exposure circumstances are assigned to either 2A (probably carcinogenic) or 2B (possibly carcinogenic) on the basis of epidemiological, experimental and other relevant data.

Group 2A — The agent (mixture) is probably carcinogenic to humans.
The exposure circumstance entails exposures that are probably carcinogenic to humans.

This category is used when there is *limited evidence* of carcinogenicity in humans and *sufficient evidence* of carcinogenicity in experimental animals. Exceptionally, an agent, mixture or exposure circumstance may be classified into this category solely on the basis of *limited evidence* of carcinogenicity in humans or of *sufficient evidence* of carcinogenicity in experimental animals strengthened by supporting evidence from other relevant data.

Group 2B — The agent (mixture) is possibly carcinogenic to humans.
The exposure circumstance entails exposures that are possibly carcinogenic to humans.

This category is generally used for agents, mixtures and exposure circumstances for which there is *limited evidence* of carcinogenicity in humans in the absence of *sufficient evidence* of carcinogenicity in experimental animals. It may also be used when there is *inadequate evidence* of carcinogenicity in humans or when human data are nonexistent but there is *sufficient evidence* of carcinogenicity in experimental animals. In some instances, an agent, mixture or exposure circumstance for which there is *inadequate evidence* of or no data on carcinogenicity in humans but *limited evidence* of carcinogenicity in experimental animals together with supporting evidence from other relevant data may be placed in this group.

Group 3 — The agent (mixture, exposure circumstance) is not classifiable as to its carcinogenicity to humans.

Agents, mixtures and exposure circumstances are placed in this category when they do not fall into any other group.

Group 4 — The agent (mixture, exposure circumstance) is probably not carcinogenic to humans.

This category is used for agents, mixtures and exposure circumstances for which there is *evidence suggesting lack of carcinogenicity* in humans together with *evidence suggesting lack of carcinogenicity* in experimental animals. In some instances, agents, mixtures or exposure circumstances for which there is *inadequate evidence* of or no data on carcinogenicity in humans but *evidence suggesting lack of carcinogenicity* in experimental animals, consistently and strongly supported by a broad range of other relevant data, may be classified in this group.

References

1. IARC (1987) *IARC Monographs on the Evaluation of Carcinogenic Risks to Humans*, Supplement 6, *Genetic and Related Effects: An Updating of Selected* IARC Monographs *from Volumes 1 to 42*, Lyon
2. IARC (1977) *IARC Monographs Programme on the Evaluation of the Carcinogenic Risk of Chemicals to Humans. Preamble* (IARC intern. tech. Rep. No. 77/002), Lyon

3. IARC (1978) *Chemicals with Sufficient Evidence of Carcinogenicity in Experimental Animals* — IARC Monographs *Volumes 1-17* (IARC intern. tech. Rep. No. 78/003), Lyon
4. IARC (1979) *Criteria to Select Chemicals for* IARC Monographs (IARC intern. tech. Rep. No. 79/003), Lyon
5. IARC (1982) *IARC Monographs on the Evaluation of the Carcinogenic Risk of Chemicals to Humans*, Supplement 4, *Chemicals, Industrial Processes and Industries Associated with Cancer in Humans (IARC Monographs, Volumes 1 to 29)*, Lyon
6. IARC (1983) *Approaches to Classifying Chemical Carcinogens According to Mechanism of Action* (IARC intern. tech. Rep. No. 83/001), Lyon
7. IARC (1987) *IARC Monographs on the Evaluation of Carcinogenic Risks to Humans*, Supplement 7, *Overall Evaluations of Carcinogenicity: An Updating of* IARC Monographs *Volumes 1 to 42*, Lyon
8. IARC (1988) *Report of an IARC Working Group to Review the Approaches and Processes Used to Evaluate the Carcinogenicity of Mixtures and Groups of Chemicals* (IARC intern. tech. Rep. No. 88/002), Lyon
9. IARC (1973-1988) *Information Bulletin on the Survey of Chemicals Being Tested for Carcinogenicity*, Numbers 1-13, Lyon
   Number 1 (1973)   52 pages
   Number 2 (1973)   77 pages
   Number 3 (1974)   67 pages
   Number 4 (1974)   97 pages
   Number 5 (1975)   88 pages
   Number 6 (1976)   360 pages
   Number 7 (1978)   460 pages
   Number 8 (1979)   604 pages
   Number 9 (1981)   294 pages
   Number 10 (1983)   326 pages
   Number 11 (1984)   370 pages
   Number 12 (1986)   385 pages
   Number 13 (1988)   404 pages
10. Coleman, M. & Wahrendorf, J., eds (1989) *Directory of On-going Research in Cancer Epidemiology 1989/90* (IARC Scientific Publications No. 101), Lyon, IARC [and previous annual volumes]
11. IARC (1984) *Chemicals and Exposures to Complex Mixtures Recommended for Evaluation in* IARC Monographs *and Chemicals and Complex Mixtures Recommended for Long-term Carcinogenicity Testing* (IARC intern. tech. Rep. No. 84/002), Lyon
12. IARC (1989) *Chemicals, Groups of Chemicals, Mixtures and Exposure Circumstances to be Evaluated in Future* IARC Monographs, *Report of an ad-hoc Working Group* (IARC intern. tech. Rep. No. 89/004), Lyon
13. *Environmental Carcinogens. Methods of Analysis and Exposure Measurement*:
    Vol. 1. *Analysis of Volatile Nitrosamines in Food* (IARC Scientific Publications No. 18). Edited by R. Preussmann, M. Castegnaro, E.A. Walker & A.E. Wasserman (1978)

Vol. 2. *Methods for the Measurement of Vinyl Chloride in Poly(vinyl chloride), Air, Water and Foodstuffs* (IARC Scientific Publications No. 22). Edited by D.C.M. Squirrell & W. Thain (1978)

Vol. 3. *Analysis of Polycyclic Aromatic Hydrocarbons in Environmental Samples* (IARC Scientific Publications No. 29). Edited by M. Castegnaro, P. Bogovski, H. Kunte & E.A. Walker (1979)

Vol. 4. *Some Aromatic Amines and Azo Dyes in the General and Industrial Environment* (IARC Scientific Publications No. 40). Edited by L. Fishbein, M. Castegnaro, I.K. O'Neill & H. Bartsch (1981)

Vol. 5. *Some Mycotoxins* (IARC Scientific Publications No. 44). Edited by L. Stoloff, M. Castegnaro, P. Scott, I.K. O'Neill & H. Bartsch (1983)

Vol. 6. N-*Nitroso Compounds* (IARC Scientific Publications No. 45). Edited by R. Preussmann, I.K. O'Neill, G. Eisenbrand, B. Spiegelhalder & H. Bartsch (1983)

Vol. 7. *Some Volatile Halogenated Hydrocarbons* (IARC Scientific Publications No. 68). Edited by L. Fishbein & I.K. O'Neill (1985)

Vol. 8. *Some Metals: As, Be, Cd, Cr, Ni, Pb, Se, Zn* (IARC Scientific Publications No. 71). Edited by I.K. O'Neill, P. Schuller & L. Fishbein (1986)

Vol. 9. *Passive Smoking* (IARC Scientific Publications No. 81). Edited by I.K. O'Neill, K.D. Brunnemann, B. Dodet & D. Hoffmann (1987)

Vol. 10. *Benzene and Alkylated Benzenes* (IARC Scientific Publications No. 85). Edited by L. Fishbein & I.K. O'Neill (1988)

14. Wilbourn, J., Haroun, L., Heseltine, E., Kaldor, J., Partensky, C. & Vainio, H. (1986) Response of experimental animals to human carcinogens: an analysis based upon the IARC Monographs Programme. *Carcinogenesis, 7*, 1853-1863

15. Montesano, R., Bartsch, H., Vainio, H., Wilbourn, J. & Yamasaki, H., eds (1986) *Long-term and Short-term Assays for Carcinogenesis — A Critical Appraisal* (IARC Scientific Publications No. 83), Lyon, IARC

16. Hoel, D.G., Kaplan, N.L. & Anderson, M.W. (1983) Implication of nonlinear kinetics on risk estimation in carcinogenesis. *Science, 219*, 1032-1037

17. Gart, J.J., Krewski, D., Lee, P.N., Tarone, R.E. & Wahrendorf, J. (1986) *Statistical Methods in Cancer Research*, Vol.3, *The Design and Analysis of Long-term Animal Experiments* (IARC Scientific Publications No. 79), Lyon, IARC

18. Peto, R., Pike, M.C., Day, N.E., Gray, R.G., Lee, P.N., Parish, S., Peto, J., Richards, S. & Wahrendorf, J. (1980) Guidelines for simple, sensitive significance tests for carcinogenic effects in long-term animal experiments. In: *IARC Monographs on the Evaluation of the Carcinogenic Risk of Chemicals to Humans*, Supplement 2, *Long-term and Short-term Screening Assays for Carcinogens: A Critical Appraisal*, Lyon, pp. 311-426

19. Breslow, N.E. & Day, N.E. (1980) *Statistical Methods in Cancer Research*, Vol. 1, *The Analysis of Case-control Studies* (IARC Scientific Publications No. 32), Lyon, IARC

20. Breslow, N.E. & Day, N.E. (1987) *Statistical Methods in Cancer Research*, Vol. 2, *The Design and Analysis of Cohort Studies* (IARC Scientific Publications No. 82), Lyon, IARC

GENERAL REMARKS ON THE SUBSTANCES CONSIDERED

This fifty-first volume of *IARC Monographs* describes the evidence for possible carcinogenic effects of coffee, tea, mate, three methylated xanthines (caffeine, theophylline and theobromine) and methylglyoxal. Caffeine, other methylated xanthines and coffee drinking were recommended in June 1984 for evaluation in the *IARC Monographs* by an ad-hoc Working Group of scientists from many countries engaged in the study of human health problems (IARC, 1984). The topics for consideration were broadened by the IARC to include tea and mate because these are also methylxanthine-containing beverages which are consumed in large quantities. Serious consideration was also given to the inclusion of caffeinated soft drinks and chocolate, which are widely consumed thoughout the world, but these products have not been the specific object of any epidemiological or experimental studies.

Green coffee beans are one of the major commodities of world trade. More than five million tonnes are produced annually in some 50 coffee-growing nations, and coffee is second only to oil in international commerce. Green coffee is the second most important food commodity in the world after wheat (Viani, 1986). Approximately 1.5 billion cups of coffee are drunk every day throughout the world (Anon., 1987). The highest per-caput consumption of coffee prevails in the Scandinavian countries and amounts to four to five cups per person per day. Therefore, the safety of this product has major consequences for international public health as well as for the world economy.

Tea is presently the most popular beverage in the world. In parts of Asia and North Africa, green tea is the principal type consumed, whereas black tea is preferred elsewhere in the world. Mate, prepared from the dried leaves of a local tree, is a popular beverage in parts of South America.

The basis for preparing the monograph on coffee was the results of early case-control studies in which an association between bladder cancer and coffee consumption was suggested. In many parts of the world, an individual may drink coffee, tea and caffeine-containing soft drinks; therefore, the health effects of these beverages are difficult to isolate and assess. Some of the case-control studies that have been undertaken examined both tea and coffee consumption or estimated total methylxanthine intake. Furthermore, coffee and tea are complex mixtures of hundreds of compounds of widely different chemical classes. Some components of these beverages have been the subject of long-term experiments in animals to study their potential carcinogenicity. Compounds that have been reported to occur in coffee and tea and which have been evaluated previously in the *IARC Monographs* series are listed in Table 1. Various strains of beans and of tea are grown under different conditions and are processed for consumption in a variety of ways. The beverages are then prepared according to different local customs, which may include boiling, filtration and the addition of other plant materials (e.g., lemon juice) or milk. A third problem is that it is difficult to quantify individual consumption of coffee and tea, as there is no standardized measure for a cup of either beverage. Lastly, the use of these beverages is associated with other widespread concomitant behaviours, such as cigarette smoking and certain dietary habits, and these associations may vary even within regions.

Table 1. Compounds that have been reported to occur in coffee and tea and which have been evaluated previously in the *IARC Monographs* series[a]

Compound	*IARC Monographs* (volume, year)	Evaluation		
		Humans	Animals	Overall
Coffee beverage				
Acetaldehyde	36, 1985[b]	I	S	2B
Catechol	15, 1977	ND	I	3
Formaldehyde	29, 1982[b]	L	S	2A
Hydrogen peroxide	36, 1985	ND	L	3
Hydroquinone	15, 1977	ND	I	3
Phenol	47, 1989	I	I	3
Black tea				
Hydrogen peroxide	36, 1985	ND	L	3
Kampferol	31, 1983	ND	I	3
Phenol	47, 1989	I	I	3
Quercetin	31, 1983	ND	L	3
Green tea				
Phenol	47, 1989	I	I	3
Additives in tea				
Bergamot oil (containing 5-methoxypsoralen)	40, 1986[b]	I	S	2A

[a] Possible contaminants are discusssed in the respective monographs.
[b] Also considered in Supplement 7

An important component of coffee is caffeine; its stimulatory action is considered to be one of the reasons for the popularity of coffee and other caffeine-containing beverages (Viani, 1986), although consumption of decaffeinated coffee is increasing in some parts of the world. Quantification of caffeine intake is difficult not only because of the lack of standardization of cups of tea or coffee but also because of the multiplicity of sources containing it; it is the dominant pharmacologically active constituent of coffee and tea and is also present in many nonprescription pharmaceutical preparations.

It has been suggested that excessive use of caffeine-containing beverages, particularly coffee, influences the risk for coronary heart disease. The question is still open, despite a vast body of research, reviewed only in part in this volume. Concern over the past 10-15 years about the potential of caffeine and caffeine-containing foods and beverages to cause adverse reproductive effects or birth defects in humans stemmed from a series of studies in laboratory animals, dating back to 1960. These showed that caffeine was teratogenic in animals at doses far in excess of the levels of consumption of caffeine by humans. Recent studies in which human exposure was mimicked more appropriately have been used to assess the potential reproductive and developmental toxicity from the use of caffeinated products by humans. The large number of animal studies in which reproductive and developmental toxicity was evaluated compared to other manifestations of toxicity, including cancer, reflects the concern over potential adverse reproductive effects.

Mate had been reported to be associated with increased risks of oesophageal cancer.

Carcinogenicity studies in experimental animals were available on coffee, tea (or tea fractions) and caffeine. With regard to theophylline and theobromine, experimental studies were available only on their modifying effects on carcinogenesis. Methylglyoxal, which is present in brewed and instant coffee, was the subject of a carcinogenicity study in animals which had been reported at the time the substances were selected. No monograph was prepared on glyoxal, which is also present in brewed and instant coffee and in many foods, because no carcinogenicity data were available. A recent study by Takahashi *et al.* (1989) examined only the potential modifying effects of glyoxal on carcinogenesis in the rat stomach and was not designed to investigate its carcinogenic potential in an adequate manner.

It is noteworthy that all these beverages, which have been consumed worldwide in large quantities for centuries, have been tested for carcinogenicity in experimental animals only recently. No proper carcinogenicity testing has been done for tea, the world's most commonly consumed beverage, or for mate.

References

Anon. (1987) *Coffee (Retail Business No.356; Market Report No. 4)*, London, Economist Publications

IARC (1984) *Chemicals and Exposures to Complex Mixtures Recommended for Evaluation in IARC Monographs and Chemicals and Complex Mixtures Recommended for Long-term Carcinogenicity Testing* (IARC intern. tech. Rep. No. 84/002), Lyon

Takahashi, M., Okamiya, H., Furukawa, F., Toyoda, K., Sato, H., Imaida, K. & Hayashi, Y. (1989) Effects of glyoxal and methylglyoxal administration on gastric carcinogenesis in Wistar rats after inhalation with N-methyl-N'-nitro-N-nitrosoguanidine. *Carcinogenesis*, *10*, 1925-1927

Viani, R. (1986) Coffee. In: *Ullmann's Encyclopaedia of Industrial Chemistry*, 5th ed., Weinheim, VCH Verlagsgesellschaft mbH, pp. 315-339

THE MONOGRAPHS

COFFEE[1]

1. Production and Use

1.1 Introduction

'Coffee has never been a mere beverage. Some three centuries have passed since it became the overnight rage among the fashionable and witty in cities throughout Europe. Even in the late twentieth century, however, it has yet to be relegated to the rank of the more pedestrian potions with which we quench our thirst or warm our insides. Little of coffee's original mystique has been worn off by centuries of familiarity.' (Hattox, 1988).

The year 575 is often cited as the date of the arrival of coffee on the Arabian peninsula from Ethiopia. Commercial and political links were at that time becoming quite strong across the Red Sea. Coffee cherries (*bun* or *bon*) were then probably only dried and chewed as a stimulant against fatigue. It is only by the middle of the fifteenth century that coffee as a beverage (*kahwah* in Arabic), an infusion of roasted and ground coffee beans that had been cultivated in the Yemen, near the harbour of Mocha, came into general use throughout the Ottoman empire. By the end of the sixteenth century, it had crossed the Mediterranean Sea, and in less than a century it had spread throughout Europe and to the British settlements in North America (Wellman, 1961).

During the seventeenth century, the cultivation of coffee spread to the Malabar coast of India and to Ceylon; and, from the beginning of the eighteenth century, seedlings of *Coffea arabica* L. cultivated in European glasshouses, as first described by Linnaeus in 1737 (Debry, 1989), were introduced into the Dutch West Indies and to the Portuguese, French and Spanish colonies of Asia and America (Wellman, 1961).

Low-altitude coffee cultures in Asia were destroyed during the last part of the nineteenth century by the coffee rust, *Hemileia vastatrix*. A rust-resistant species,

---

[1]Unless otherwise specified, the term 'coffee' is used to mean brewed, caffeinated coffee.

Coffea canephora, var. *robusta*, was introduced during the twentieth century in Asia, Africa and, more recently, Brazil (Viani, 1986).

1.2 Production processes

(a) Green coffee

(i) *Botany and culture* (Wrigley, 1988; Viani, 1989)

Approximately 60 species of the genus *Coffea* L. (Rubiaceae family) have been described. The commercially important varieties are *C. arabica* L., arabica coffee, which accounts for 85-90% of world production, and *C. canephora* (Pierre ex Froehner), robusta coffee, which contributes 10-15% of world production. Two other species, which contribute less than 1% of world production, are also grown: *C. liberica* (Bull ex Hiern), liberica coffee, and *C. dewevrei* (de Wild.), excelsa coffee.

The main characteristics of arabica and robusta coffees are given in Table 1.

Table 1. Main botanical and physical characteristics of arabica and robusta coffee plants[a]

Parameter	Arabica species	Robusta species
Botanical varieties, mutants and cultivars	Arabica or typica bourbon, Caturra, Maragogipe, etc.	Robusta (upright), nganda (spreading), Kouilouensis (various spellings: kouilou, quillou, conilon), etc.
Optimal growth		
Climate	Temperate, equable	Warm, humid
Altitude (m)	700–1700	0–800
Average temperature (°C)	15–23	18–27
Maximal temperature (°C)	25	30
Rain/year (mm)	1500–2200	2200–3000
Plant	Self-fertilizing	Sterile
Chromosomes (2n)	44	22
Root system	Deep	Shallow
Leaf	Small, glossy, oval	Large, broad, corrugated
Flower (white to pink)	After rain, small	Irregular, large
Fruit, cherry or berry (crimson), 60–65% water	Oblong ellipsoid, 15 mm long, 8–9 months to ripen	Ellipsoid, 12-mm long, 10–11 months to ripen
Seed, bean (blue-green to yellow-green), 10–12% water	Round to oval, flat, deeply grooved, 5–13-mm long	Oval to round, grooved, 4–8-mm long
Caffeine content of seed (% dry basis)	0.8–1.4, average 1.2	1.7–4.0, average 2.0
Weight of clean beans from fully ripened cherries (%)	12–20 (usually 16–18)	17–22 (usually >20)

Table 1 (contd)

Parameter	Arabica species	Robusta species
Density of beans (g/l)	550–700	550–700
Pests (diseases)[b]		
Hemileia vastatrix (rust)	Susceptible	Resistant
Colletotrichum coffeanum (coffee berry disease)	Susceptible	Resistant
Stephanodores coffeae (*Hypothenemus hampei*) (coffee berry borer)	Susceptible	Susceptible

[a] From Viani (1986, 1989)
[b] From Clarke & Macrae (1988a)

The seeds of arabica and cuttings of robusta coffee plants are propagated in nurseries and are cultivated on sheltered slopes, protected from wind and frost on porous, well-drained soil rich in organic matter and slightly acidic.

Natural and botanical interspecific hybrids have been described: 'Hibrido de Timor' is a natural cross between arabica and robusta, while arabusta and *Icatu* were created artificially (Wrigley, 1988).

(ii) *Harvesting and processing of coffee cherries* (Viani, 1986, 1989)

The operations necessary to transform harvested cherries into green beans vary depending upon ecological conditions. Where water is scarce or labour unskilled, the 'dry' process is applied; such is the case in Brazil and Ethiopia, the main producers of 'natural' unwashed arabicas and most robustas. Where all cherries can be picked at the optimal degree of ripeness, where water is abundant and equipment is available, coffee is treated by the 'wet' process, resulting in 'washed' arabicas. The two processes are shown schematically in Table 2.

In the 'dry' or 'natural' process, cherries of different degrees of ripeness are strip-picked and handled simultaneously. They are spread in a thin layer on the ground, where they are sun-dried for up to three weeks. Husks (skin and pulp) are removed in centrifugal hulling machines.

In the 'wet' or 'washed' process, freshly picked berries are separated in water channels into 'floaters' (overripe and one-bean cherries) and 'sinkers' (ripe cherries), which are pulped mechanically; floaters are usually dry-processed and consumed locally. Enzymatic fermentation of the mucilage which still adheres to the bean solubilizes the mass so that it can be removed by stirring with water. Some pulpers remove skin, pulp and mucilage mechanically in a single operation. The beans, which are still surrounded by parchment, are then washed and either sun-dried for four to eight days or dried in a hot-air dryer for 24-30 h. The parchment is removed in centrifugal hulling machines, and the beans are cleaned by density, sorted electronically by colour, graded by size through screens and bagged in 60- or 70-kg jute bags.

Table 2. Dry and wet processes for processing coffee cherries[a]

Operation	Dry	Wet
Harvesting of cherries	strip	selective
Floating in water	no	yes
Pulping of 'sinkers'	no	yes
Fermenting	no	yes
Washing	no	yes
Drying	yes	yes
Hulling	yes	yes
Polishing	no	usually
Cleaning	yes	yes
Sorting/grading	usually	yes
Bagging	yes	yes

[a] From Viani (1989)

(b) *Decaffeination* (Viani, 1986, 1989)

The presence of water is essential in decaffeination in order to open the cellular structure of the bean and to ensure diffusion of caffeine out of the bean by solubilizing the caffeine-potassium chlorogenate complex. Decaffeination is usually performed on green beans before aromatic substances are formed by roasting; however, a process for decaffeinating roasted coffee extract is also used. The techniques applied can be divided approximately into two types: 'bean decaffeination' at moisture levels below 40% and 'extract decaffeination' at moisture levels above 60%.

(i) *Solvents/adsorbents*

The solvents and adsorbents currently employed during decaffeination are: dichloromethane (see IARC, 1986a, 1987), ethyl acetate, edible fats and oils, supercritical carbon dioxide and acid-activated carbon. Formerly trichloroethylene (see IARC, 1979, 1987) was used.

(ii) *Bean decaffeination*

This technique was patented in 1905 by Roselius (Meyer, 1906; Meyer *et al.*, 1908; Katz, 1987) and is still the most commonly used. Green coffee beans are swollen to contain 30-40% moisture with water and steam at temperatures of 20-100°C for up to 5 h and decaffeinated in static or rotating drums with a water-saturated solvent, such as dichloromethane (Patel & Wolfson, 1972), ethyl acetate (Morrison & Phillips, 1983) or edible fats and oils (Malizia & Trumbetas, 1984; Pagliaro *et al.*, 1984), at temperatures ranging from 60 to 105°C for 2-12 h, depending upon the level of residual caffeine permitted. Most countries require that the content be reduced to less than 0.1% on a dry weight basis. The beans are then freed from residual volatile solvent (deodorized) by steam stripping at 100-110°C for 1-4 h to levels usually well below those required by local regulations (<5-15 ppm according to country and solvent), and dried to their initial moisture content (approximately 10%) at 40-48°C for 0.5-10 h with hot air or under vacuum.

The solvent is recovered by batch or continuous evaporation or by steam stripping of the caffeine under vacuum, and the caffeine is purified by repeated crystallization for further use in, e.g., cola-type drinks.

Green coffee beans can also be decaffeinated using supercritical carbon dioxide at temperatures and pressures above its critical point (31.06°C, 73.8 bar), usually at 40-80°C and 200-300 bar for 5-30 h (Zosel, 1981; Martin, 1982). Supercritical carbon dioxide is circulated in a pressurized vessel through moist coffee, where it dissolves the caffeine selectively; the caffeine solution is then passed through a second pressurized vessel containing activated carbon or water which retains the caffeine.

(iii) *Extract decaffeination*

Green (or roasted) coffee beans are extracted with water (Berry & Walters, 1943), and the extract is decaffeinated either by liquid-liquid extraction with dichloromethane (Katz, 1980) followed by steam deodorization or by selective adsorption of caffeine on acid-activated carbon. Processes that do not employ an organic solvent are known as 'water decaffeination'.

The decaffeinated extract is concentrated and reincorporated on the predried decaffeinated beans (Fischer & Kummer, 1979; Green & Blanc, 1981). Alternatively, the decaffeinated extract can be used to decaffeinate new beans (Katz & Proscia, 1981). The beans are then dried to their initial moisture level.

(c) *Roasted coffee* (Rothfos, 1986)

(i) *Process*

During the roasting process, hard green coffee beans which are stone-hard increase in volume and develop a brittle structure, a dark-brown colour and a characteristic flavour rich in volatile constituents. During the first phase of roasting, the beans are dried at temperatures of up to 120-150°C, after which pyrolysis starts. The release of carbon dioxide and volatile aroma increases at temperatures above 150°C. In the last phase of roasting, when the temperature reaches approximately 190°C, the reaction becomes exothermic and the beans puff, doubling in size.

The chemical constituents of green beans can change dramatically with roasting. For example, the total chlorogenic acid content of green arabica coffee beans is typically 6.9%; following light roasting, the concentration decreases to about 2.7%, and after dark roasting is only about 0.2% (Trugo & Macrae, 1984a).

After cooling, which can be accelerated by quenching with water, residual carbon dioxide trapped in the bean is released slowly over a period of days.

The main operations used in the manufacture of roasted coffee are shown in Table 3.

Table 3. Main operations in the manufacture of roasted coffee

Operation	Means
Reception	Green coffee arrives at the plant either loose in containers or in bags.
Emptying	Manually or mechanically
Weighing	In hoppers of 250- or 500-kg capacity
Cleaning	Through vibrating screens (removal of small stones and large, heavy bodies); by air levitation (removal of dust); with magnets (removal of iron scrap)
Conveying	Pneumatically, to storage silos
Storage	In bins of 1- to 100-tonnes capacity
Weighing	Manually or automatically for blending
Blending	Manually (1-2 bags max.) or mechanically (up to 10 different coffee types)
Roasting	In batch or continuous roasters (a few to 5000 kg/h)
Weighing	To determine the roast weight loss
Conveying	With bucket (vertically) or belt conveyors (horizontally) or with dense-phase air conveyors to avoid breakage
Sorting	Electronically by colour
Degassing	Freshly roasted coffee releases carbon dioxide: the gas must be allowed to escape before whole coffee beans are packaged in gas-tight wrappings
Grinding	In stainless-steel mills
Packaging	Under vacuum or inert gas to maintain freshness
or Processing	In instant coffee plants

(ii) *Roasters*

Many models of roasters exist, which operate both by batch and continuously, with capacities ranging from a few kilograms to over 5000 kg/h, and range from manually operated to fully automated. They can be divided into conduction roasters with direct-flame heating and convection roasters employing preheated gas. Modern gas-heated roasters are equipped with gas recirculation units and catalysts to reduce emissions. Some models are also equipped with automatic cleaning cycles to avoid a build-up of tars (Viani, 1986).

In some of the more recent models, so-called 'high yield' or 'fast roasted' coffee can be prepared by heating green coffee beans by convection to temperatures of up to 300°C for 2-3 min and by increasing the ratio of hot air to beans. This type of roasted coffee can yield up to 20% more extractable matter with a sharper taste when brewed.

(iii) *Grinders*

Roasted beans are ground in mills that vary in capacity from a few grams to 4 tonnes/h. The average particle size of the ground coffee depends on the extraction equipment to be used; indicative sizes are given in Table 4.

Table 4. Particle sizes of roasted coffees[a]

Use	Particle size (mm)
Instant coffee manufacture	1.5 to whole beans
US drip, percolator	0.7–1.0
Filter	0.4–0.6
Espresso	0.3–0.4
Middle East	<0.1

[a] From Viani (1986)

(iv) *Packaging*

Unlike green beans, roasted coffee spoils relatively quickly if unprotected from oxygen and moisture; at ambient temperature, whole beans become stale after four to six weeks and ground coffee after two weeks.

Since coffee beans release carbon dioxide for up to 48 h after roasting, they cannot be packed in airtight containers immediately. Whole beans are therefore either placed in non-airtight packs or allowed to degas and then packed under vacuum or in an inert atmosphere in metal cans or impermeable plastic containers. Coffee is now sold pre-ground and packed in brick packs or cans after short degassing (2-4 h) or under an initial slight vacuum in flexible bags with a one-way degassing valve (Viani, 1986).

(d) Instant coffee (Viani, 1986)

The first commercially acceptable instant (or soluble) coffee was produced in Switzerland in 1938 as 50% coffee solids and 50% corn syrup solids; 100% pure instant coffee became available from the 1950s.

Instant coffee is the dried water extract of roast and ground coffee, which readily dissolves in both cold and hot water and eliminates the need for brewing equipment. The unit operations performed during the manufacture of instant coffee are: storing, blending, decaffeination and roasting of green beans; grinding, recovery of volatile aroma and extraction of roasted beans; stripping of aroma; concentrating and drying of the extract; and agglomeration, aromatization and packaging of the powder. The operations performed on the beans up to and including roasting have already been described. The steps described below are specific to instant coffee technology.

(i) Extraction

Whole roasted coffee beans or coffee ground to a particle size of 1.5 mm are extracted with softened water in a battery of five to eight percolation columns called 'cells', with a capacity of a few kilograms to one tonne. The process is semi-continuous; water at 160-180°C enters the most completely extracted cell and circulates through to the most recently filled cell (see Figure 1). The cells are divided into 'hot' cells at a temperature of 140-180°C under a pressure of 14-16 bar and 'cold' cells at a temperature of approximately 100°C. In the hot cells, high-molecular-weight material (in particular carbohydrates) is extracted. In the cold cells, the material with the most flavour is extracted. The extract is withdrawn from the fresh cell, cooled to 4-5°C and sent into a scale in amounts that depend on the desired yield (33-55% based on roasted coffee) and on the concentration of the extract (10-30%). At the end of the 'draw-off' period, a new cell enters the circuit, which may have been steam-stripped to recover volatile aroma, and the spent grounds are evacuated from the most completely extracted cell.

(ii) Concentration

Extracts with a concentration of 25-30% (w/w) soluble solids can be dried directly but with loss of volatile components. The volatile constituents present in extracts coming from the hot section are, however, unimportant from the point of view of aroma or flavour. The hot extract can then be evaporated to a concentration of 50-60% (w/w) and mixed with cold extract; if both hot and cold extracts are collected together, the dilute extract is stripped prior to concentration and the volatile components added back ('standardization') before drying. A technique that preserves most of the volatile aroma is freeze concentration, in which pure ice is

Figure 1. Battery for instant coffee extraction[a]

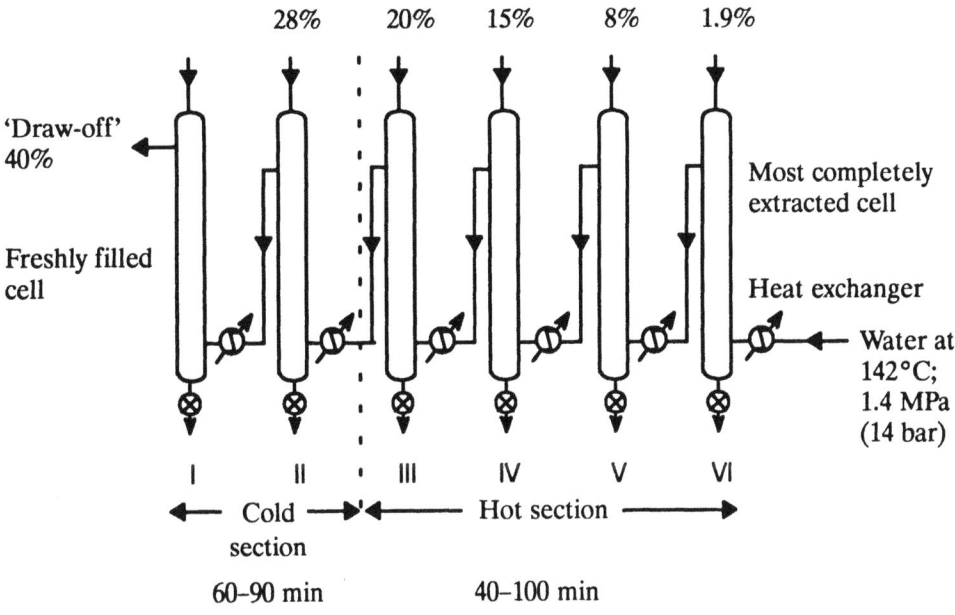

[a] From Viani (1986)

separated from the frozen extract in gradient columns at a concentration of up to 35-40%. The extract is then cooled to 4-5°C and clarified.

(iii) Spray-drying

The extract is sprayed through a pressure nozzle into the top of a tower and dried by a concurrent flow of hot air at approximately 250°C; the dry powder is collected at the bottom of the tower. Powder with a bulk density of 230-300 g/l can thus be obtained. For the convenience of consumers, the powder can be agglomerated to a coarse structure by rewetting and redrying.

(iv) Freeze-drying

The extract is gradually frozen to –40 to –50°C; ice crystals are separated and sublimed under vacuum.

(v) Aromatization

The volatile aroma fractions collected during stripping of the fresh cell can be emulsified with oil from pressed roasted coffee or spent grounds and sprayed or injected onto the powder at levels of 0.3-1.0% (w/v) during packaging.

(vi) *Packaging*

The powder, which should contain less than 5% moisture (Commission of the European Communities, 1985), is packed under vacuum or in an inert atmosphere in jars or flexible bags and is stable for more than two years if unopened.

1.3 Worldwide production, trade and consumption

(a) *Production and export*

Coffee is one of the major commodities of world trade; it is often the main source of foreign exchange for the producing countries in the belt between the tropics. World coffee supply and distribution in 1984-88 are given in Table 5.

Table 5. World production and distribution of coffee in 1984-88 (millions of 60-kg bags [millions of tonnes])[a]

Year	Total production	Domestic consumption	Total exports
1984	83.8 (5.03)	19.4 (1.16)	64.4 (3.86)
1985	90.0 (5.40)	19.2 (1.15)	70.8 (4.25)
1986	81.1 (4.87)	19.8 (1.19)	61.3 (3.68)
1987	107.7 (6.46)	18.6 (1.12)	89.1 (5.35)
1988	87.1 (5.23)	19.7 (1.18)	67.5 (4.05)
Average	89.9 (5.39)	19.3 (1.16)	70.6 (4.24)

[a]From International Coffee Organization (1989a)

International coffee trade is regulated by the International Coffee Organization, which administers the International Coffee Agreement. The current 1983 (International Coffee Organization, 1982) agreement expired in September 1989 but was extended for a further two years as of October 1989. It has been signed by 74 members — 50 exporting and 24 importing countries comprising 99% of world production and 85% of world consumption (International Coffee Organization, 1989b,c). The producing countries are divided into three main categories, according to botanical origin (arabica or robusta) and method of preparation (dry or wet processing). The majority of the coffee produced is traded as milds (wet-processed arabica), Brazilian and other arabicas (dry-processed arabicas) and robustas (dry-processed) (Viani, 1989).

The production, exports and consumption of green coffee by the main producing countries are given in Table 6. The consumption figures are only indicative, as they were calculated by dividing the amount of coffee that disappeared (produced but not exported, 1984-87 average) by the 1987 population of the country concerned (Anon., 1989).

Table 6. Production, exports (millions of 60-kg bags) and consumption of green coffee (kg *per caput* per year) of the main producing countries[a]

Country	Production[a] (1984–88 average)	Exports[b] (1983–88 average)	Consumption[c]
Wet-processed arabicas	42.16	29.93	
Colombia	14.25	10.49	3.64
Mexico	4.93	3.25	1.36
Guatemala	2.85	2.46	1.29
India	2.78	1.41	0.07
Costa Rica	2.24	1.94	5.06
El Salvador	2.19	2.61	1.66
Kenya	1.88	1.65	0.08[d]
Ecuador	1.82	1.59	2.13
Honduras	1.41	1.31	2.37
Peru	1.20	1.03	0.60
Venezuela	1.06	0.18	2.60
Dominican Republic	0.85	0.52	2.88
Tanzania, United Republic of	0.78	0.79	0.01[d]
Nicaragua	0.72	0.70	1.88
Others	3.20	–	
Dry-processed arabicas	28.93	18.46	
Brazil	26.13	17.14	3.10
Ethiopia	2.80	1.32	2.09
Robustas	16.23	16.27	
Indonesia	6.01	4.76	0.41
Ivory Coast	4.35	3.84	1.24
Zaire	1.86	1.52	0.38
Madagascar	1.11	0.81	1.31
Philippines	1.02	0.49	0.51
Others	1.88	4.85	
Total	87.32	64.66	

[a] From International Coffee Organization (1989b,d)
[b] From International Coffee Organization (1989e)
[c] Calculated by the Working Group
[d] From Viani (1989)
–, not available

(b) Imports and consumption

The disappearance (industry term: net imports adjusted for changes in visible inventories; in millions of 60-kg bags) and consumption (disappearance divided by the population of the country in 1987; in kg *per caput* per year) of green coffee in the main importing members of the International Coffee Organization are given in Table 7.

Per-caput disappearance of coffee in importing member countries of the International Coffee Organization in 1981-86 is given in Table 8. Annual per-caput consumption of coffee in major consuming countries in 1970-81 is given in Table 9.

Imports (in millions of 60-kg bags) and estimated consumption (in kg *per caput* per year) of green coffee by non-International Coffee Organization member consuming countries importing more than 100 000 bags per year are given in Table 10.

(c) Brewing techniques (Pictet, 1987)

The most common brewing techniques are indicated below. Extraction yields of 16-30% (w/w) for the so-called 'super-high-yield' coffees are usual, depending on the type of roasting, contact time and pressure and fineness of grind. Brewing techniques encompass a wide range of procedures used in different parts of the world, which are based on the types of coffee and roasting procedures traditionally used. Local cultural practices associated with the preparation and use of coffee result in a wide range of individual consumption patterns.

(i) Decoction/boiling

To prepare northern Scandinavian 'boiled' coffee, roasted ground arabica coffee is brewed in continuously boiling water. The brew is made by boiling about 70 g coffee grounds in 1 l boiling water for 10-30 min (1 cup $\sim$ 150 ml). The decoction usually lasts upwards of 10 min. Sometimes, fresh coffee and water are added to a boiling kettle during the day.

Very finely ground Turkish coffee (less than 0.1 mm particle size) is brewed by gentle boiling of proportions of 5 g coffee grounds, 10 g sugar, 60 ml water until a foam is formed (1 cup $\sim$ 60 ml).

(ii) Infusion

Light-to-medium roasted, coarsely ground coffee (particle size, 0.7-1.0 mm) is infused with boiling water in a pot for a few minutes, stirred and separated from the grounds by pouring through a metal strainer. In the 'plunger' system, the metal strainer is pushed down the coffee pot to separate the grounds from the coffee. This system is used in northern Europe and Australia with a concentration of grounds to

Table 7. Disappearance (millions of 60-kg bags) and consumption [calculated by the Working Group] of green coffee in main importing countries by order of consumption (average, 1984–1988)

Country	Disappearance[a]		Consumption (kg *per caput* per year)	Coffee used in 1988 (%)[b]		
	1984–88 average	1989		Arabica	Robusta	Other
Finland	1.00	1.01	12.24 stable (10–11 in 1988)[b]	99	1	
Sweden	1.60	1.47	11.57 down	99	1	
Denmark	0.92	0.89	10.83 down (10–11 in 1988)[b]	80	17	3
Norway	0.71	0.69	10.12 stable (10 in the 1980s)[b]	97	2	1
Netherlands	2.38	2.34	9.65 stable (8.13 in 1988)[b]	68	27	5
Austria	0.98	1.31	7.88 up (8.7 in 1988)[b]	87	12	1
Germany, Federal Republic of	7.68	9.02	7.60 up (7.92 in 1988)[b]	89	10	1
Belgium/Luxembourg	1.23	1.11	7.52 stable	NA		
Switzerland	0.73	0.87	6.46 down	81	17	2
France	5.16	5.18	5.63 up	45	54	1
USA	18.09	18.69	4.48 down	81	15	4
Italy	4.22	4.30	4.41 up	52	48	
Canada	1.82	1.83	3.33 down	NA		
Spain	2.06	2.50	3.17 stable (2.7)[b]	58	41	1
Cyprus	0.03	0.04	2.77 NA	NA		
Greece	0.45	0.56	2.77 stable (2.75 in 1987)[b]	94	5	1
UK	2.33	2.24	2.49 up	57	42	1
Australia	0.64	0.65	2.39 up	NA		
Japan	4.57	4.80	2.25 up	NA		
Portugal	0.40	0.45	2.04 up (2.2)[b]	30	62	8
Yugoslavia	0.65	0.74	1.67 NA	NA		
Ireland	0.10	0.10	1.46 stable	NA		
Total	57.75	60.79				

[a] From International Coffee Organization (1989f, 1990)
[b] According to Müller–Henniges & Rothfos (1989)
NA, not available

water of up to 65 g/l. In North America, this method is used with high-yield, lightly roasted coffee with grounds concentrations of 28–40 g/l. One cup equals 150–190 ml.

Table 8. Derived per–caput disappearance of coffee in importing member countries of the International Coffee Organization, 1981–86[a]

Importing member	Kilograms green coffee equivalent for total population					
	1981	1982	1983	1984	1985	1986
USA[b]	4.80	4.77	4.63	4.71	4.65	4.41
EEC						
Denmark	11.79	11.46	11.15	11.05	11.04	11.00
Netherlands	9.09	8.97	9.58	9.46	9.41	9.65
Germany, Federal Republic of	7.06	7.34	7.29	7.03	6.84	7.38
Belgium/Luxembourg	8.58	7.15	8.84	7.25	7.60	7.14
France	6.05	5.91	5.94	5.39	5.47	5.49
Italy	3.98	4.33	4.34	3.89	4.93	4.37
Spain	2.75	2.76	3.19	2.92	2.74	3.44
UK	2.55	2.43	2.41	2.51	2.44	2.42
Greece	2.63	2.65	2.81	3.00	2.96	2.18
Ireland	1.10	1.00	1.16	1.47	1.59	1.81
Portugal	1.48	1.42	1.90	1.96	2.19	1.64
Other importing members						
Finland	13.52	12.78	12.93	14.59	10.09	12.09
Sweden	12.91	11.73	12.14	11.29	11.55	11.64
Norway	10.26	10.51	11.36	10.39	10.47	10.09
Austria	6.55	7.92	8.53	7.73	7.34	7.75
Switzerland	6.57	5.58	6.00	6.04	6.17	6.59
Canada	4.79	4.33	4.25	4.27	4.41	4.15
Singapore	[c]	[c]	[c]	2.36	[c]	[c]
Yugoslavia	2.01	1.05	1.51	0.89	0.58	2.31
Australia	2.51	2.62	2.31	2.44	2.11	2.24
Japan	1.68	1.85	1.94	2.01	2.14	2.23
New Zealand	2.09	1.96	2.25	2.01	1.94	1.88
Cyprus	2.95	2.63	6.55	[c]	2.87	1.34
Fiji	0.37	0.18	0.18	0.17	0.09	0.09

[a] From Clarke & Macrae (1988b)
[b] Based on estimates of civilian population by the US Department of Commerce
[c] Re–exports exceeded imports in these years.

Table 9. Per-caput coffee consumption per year in major consuming countries[a]

Country	Per-caput consumption in green bean equivalents (kg)								Ratios to 1970	
	1970	1975	1976	1977	1978	1978–79	1979–80	1980–81	1977	1980–81
Finland	14.13	13.72	15.18	10.54	11.72	13.22	12.46	12.41	0.75	0.88
Sweden	13.15	14.10	14.03	8.59	12.13	11.92	12.10	11.92	0.65	0.91
Denmark	12.88	13.02	12.14	10.75	11.00	10.50	11.03	11.59	0.83	0.90
Norway	10.10	9.74	10.33	7.20	11.14	10.02	9.80	10.11	0.71	1.00
Belgium	6.61	6.96	8.74	5.67	7.12	8.33	7.17	8.91	0.86	1.35
Netherlands	6.97	9.41	9.63	5.53	7.38	8.51	7.84	8.36	0.79	1.20
Germany, Federal Republic of	4.86	5.65	5.87	5.73	5.94	6.47	6.45	7.04	1.18	1.45
Austria	3.73	4.88	4.99	4.15	4.82	5.66	6.54	6.54	1.11	1.75
Switzerland	5.58	6.93	6.47	5.25	5.28	5.30	5.91	6.50	0.94	1.17
France	4.71	5.65	5.47	5.01	5.58	5.75	5.67	6.24	1.06	1.32
Canada	4.27	4.33	4.38	3.52	4.23	4.54	4.28	4.86	0.82	1.14
USA	6.23	5.62	5.82	4.34	4.94	5.13	4.59	4.68	0.70	0.75

[a]From Gilbert (1984)

Table 10. Imports and consumption of green coffee in main non-International Coffee Organization member consuming countries, by order of consumption (average, 1982–86)[a]

Country	Imports (millions of 60-kg bags)	Consumption[b] (kg *per caput* per year)
German Democratic Republic	1.08	3.94
Hungary	0.65	3.83
Lebanon	0.18	3.38
Algeria	1.10	2.31
Czechoslovakia	0.44	2.09
Saudi Arabia	0.39	1.93
New Zealand	0.11	1.91
Argentina	0.60	1.08
Poland	0.52	0.99
Bulgaria	0.13	0.83
Syria	0.12	0.61
Korea, Republic of	0.28	0.55
South Africa	0.27	0.49
Chile	0.10	0.43
Morocco	0.22	0.40
Hong Kong	0.06	0.33
Korea, Democratic People's Republic of	0.13	0.32
USSR	0.84	0.23
China	0.03	–
Others	0.67	–
Total	7.92	

[a] From International Coffee Organization (1989g)
[b] Estimated by the Working Group by dividing the quantity of green coffee imported by the country during the 'coffee year' 1987–88, less the average re-exports of 1985–87, by the population of the country in 1984
–, not available

(iii) *Filtration*

Filtered coffee, generally known as 'drip coffee' in North America, is made by pouring boiling water over finely ground, light-to-dark roasted coffee (average particle size, 0.5-0.7 mm) in a filter paper set in a funnel. The brew drips into a warmed pot within about 2-5 min. Automatic coffee makers are now used in most central and northern European, North American and Japanese households; the system is also widely adopted for food-service coffee-making equipment. Brew strengths vary according to the degree of roasting, the process and local habits;

concentrations as high as 75-80 g/l (dark roast; 1 cup ~ 60-150 ml) are common in France and Brazil. For automatic coffee makers, concentrations of 28-65 g/l are used.

(iv) *Percolation*

Coarsely ground coffee (average particle size, 0.7-1.0 mm) is extracted by recirculating boiling water until the desired brew strength is reached. In more modern equipment, continuous recirculation and filtration by gravity (under pressure) improve extraction and shorten brewing time to under 2 min. The use of percolators has declined significantly in favour of automatic drip coffee makers. Ground coffee concentrations normally used range from 40 g/l (light roast) in North America to 60 g/l (medium roast) in the UK.

(v) *Vaporization under pressure* (espresso)

Water heated to just above boiling-point is forced by slight excess pressure through a bed of medium-to-dark roasted coffee ground to an average particle size of 0.3-0.4 mm ('mocca' or 'Neapolitan' coffee machines). This method is used in most Italian and Spanish households. In Italian 'espresso' machines, the addition of a high-pressure pump working at 8-12 bar allows rapid extraction of grounds during 15-35 sec at a water temperature of 92-95°C. For 5-8 g of roasted coffee, one 25-60 ml cup is obtained with an extraction yield of coffee soluble solids from the roasted coffee of 18-26% and a soluble solids concentration in the cup of 20-60 g/l brew; 70-85% caffeine is recovered (Petracco, 1990).

(vi) *Instant coffee*

Average concentrations used in most countries are 1.5-2.5 g/150 ml cup, although in Latin countries, 2 g/60 ml cup are common. Consumption in the ten countries where the most instant coffee was drunk in 1987 is given in Table 11.

(d) *Consumption in selected countries*

Worldwide consumption of green coffee (1983-87 average) can be estimated at 1 million tonnes of arabica and 200 000 tonnes of robusta in producer countries and 2.9 million tonnes of arabica and 1 million tonnes of robusta in consumer countries, giving a total of 5.1 million tonnes per year. Using a conversion factor of 1.19 kg green coffee for each kilogram of roasted coffee (International Coffee Organization, 1982), the total quantity of roasted coffee consumed per year is thus 4.29 million tonnes.

Table 11. Consumption of instant coffee in the ten countries where the most was drunk in 1987[a]

Country	Retail sales (tonnes)	Share of total coffee market (%)
USA	55 090	33
UK	37 500	94
Japan	34 200	86
France	19 850	32
Mexico	19 380	71
South Africa	16 970	91
Australia	9 820	96
Canada	8 540	52
Germany, Federal Republic of	8 400	10
Spain	7 600	37

[a] From Viani (1989)

On the basis of a caffeine content of 1.1% for green arabica and 2.2% for green robusta, with no loss due to either decaffeination or processing, worldwide consumption of caffeine from coffee can be estimated to be 65 500 tonnes per year (1983-87 average), which is equivalent to 40 mg per day *per caput*. This figure corresponds to just over half of the caffeine consumed from all sources (Roberts & Barone, 1983; Gilbert, 1984; Simpson, 1988).

Data on actual coffee or caffeine consumption are often based on the reported number of cups per day; but the wide variability in volume and strength of a 'cup' of brewed coffee renders such data difficult to interpret. The actual variation of 'cups' has been reported in several studies in North America. According to a study in Canada (Stavric *et al.*, 1988), one household cup equals approximately 225 ml but can vary between 25 and 330 ml, with mean caffeine contents of 84, 71 and 82 mg/cup for drip, instant and percolated coffee, respectively. In another study in Canada (Gilbert *et al.*, 1976), cup size varied between 140 and 285 ml, with a caffeine content of 29-176 mg/cup for brewed and instant coffees. In the USA, mean caffeine contents were 115 mg (range, 60-180 mg)/150-ml cup of drip coffee, 80 mg (40-170 mg) of percolated coffee and 65 mg (30-120 mg) of instant coffee (Lecos, 1984).

Coffee consumption by different populations also varies widely, depending on the type of coffee used and brewing practices. In any single region, coffee brews differ widely in terms of the concentration of soluble solids and chemical constitution, as in urban areas of Scandinavia where boiled, filtered and espresso types are likely to be consumed. Data on consumption of coffee and caffeine are thus available for only a few countries.

(i) *Australia*

Tea consumption is still greater than that of coffee, which is, however, increasing at a rate of approximately 2% per year (94 l per person in 1986). Instant coffee constitutes 85% of total consumption, but brewed coffee usage is increasing slowly. Consumption of decaffeinated coffee is static and contributes only a few percent to the total.

(ii) *Germany (western)*

Coffee is the most popular beverage (170 l per person in 1986), and consumption, which is still increasing (+6% in 1987), is slightly higher than that of fruit juice, mineral water, soft drinks and beer; 90% of the coffee consumed is arabica. Tea consumption is estimated to be 27 l *per caput*. The market shares of various coffee preparations are: brewed coffee, approximately 90%; instant coffee, 10% (down and still decreasing); 'treated' coffees (health coffees), 8.9% (in 1987; decreasing slowly); 'natural mild taste' coffees, 20.8% (in 1987; increasing fast); and decaffeinated coffee, 13.8% (increasing slowly). Approximately 90% of the population drink coffee (*versus* 16% tea and 14% cola drinks), and 80% of it is consumed at home (Hudler, 1988). The number of cups drunk is slowly increasing (4.18 cups per person aged 15 years or more per day in 1987; International Coffee Organization, 1988a).

(iii) *France*

Consumption of coffee is decreasing slightly, while the percentage of arabica coffee compared to robusta consumed is increasing, leading to a decrease in caffeine intake from coffee. Levels of consumption are: brewed coffee, 75%; instant coffee, 15%; coffee-chicory mixtures, 10%; and decaffeinated coffee, approximately 8% of all types drunk. The number of cups consumed per day is 1.47 per person; 80% of the total population drink coffee (44 million persons drinking 1.83 cups per day): 40% of children aged 0-14 years (4.4 million children) drink 0.87 cup per day, and 90% of people aged 15 years or more (39.6 million people) drink 1.88 cups per day (Debry, 1989).

(iv) *Italy*

Consumption of coffee is still increasing slowly. The market shares of the various coffees are: brewed, 95.4% (in 1986); instant, 2.4% (increasing); and decaffeinated, 2.2%. Approximately 70% of coffee is drunk at home (brewed in a 'mocca' machine), 27% in bars (espresso machine) and 3% in vending machines (mostly instant coffee) (Anon., 1988).

(v) *Japan*

Consumption of coffee is increasing rapidly, although it is still much lower than that of tea. In 1983, 83.9% of the population drank coffee (*versus* 93% green tea, 63% black tea and approximately 50% cola drinks), with instant accounting for 58%, brewed, 32%, and canned, 10%. In 1987, total consumption was 1.38 cups per day (brewed, 0.44; instant, 0.73; canned, 0.19), was higher among men than among women and was highest among people aged 18-39 years (International Coffee Organization, 1988b).

(vi) *Netherlands*

Consumption of coffee is increasing slowly, and per-caput consumption is the highest in Europe outside the northern European countries (Anon., 1987). Practically all of the coffee consumed is brewed, 70% of which is drunk at home (Douwe-Egberts, 1989).

(vii) *Nordic countries* (Denmark, Finland, Iceland, Norway and Sweden) (Kraft General Foods, 1989)

Consumption of brewed coffee is relatively stable (approximately 10 kg *per caput* per year), with small declines in Sweden and Iceland and a marked decline in Denmark. Nearly all of the caffeine consumed is from coffee (Gilbert, 1984). More than 95% of all coffee consumed is brewed arabica, and the rest is instant (ranging from 2% in Finland to 10% in Denmark); hardly any decaffeinated coffee is drunk. Estimated ratios of coffee to water used are 55-65 g/l in Finland, 50-60 g/l in Norway and Sweden, 45-55 g/l in Iceland and 40-50 g/l in Denmark, with extraction yields of soluble coffee solids of 18-25%. Filtration is the most common brewing method, followed by boiling (Table 12).

Table 12. Brewing methods used in Nordic countries

Country	Filtered (%)	Boiled (%)
Norway	65	35
Finland	65	35
Sweden	75	25
Denmark	95	5
Iceland	95	5

(viii) *Switzerland*

Per-caput consumption of coffee is estimated at 2.58 cups per day. It is the most popular beverage, followed by milk, mineral water and soft drinks. Brewed coffee is most commonly drunk, but instant coffee is consumed frequently (Nestlé, 1989).

(ix) *UK*

In 1985, tea (mostly black tea) was still the most popular beverage, accounting for 65% of the total hot drink intake *versus* 26% for coffee, but coffee consumption is increasing. Instant coffee accounts for 85-90% of total consumption; 70-75% of brewed coffee is filtered, 20% is percolated and 5% is espresso coffee. In one report, decaffeinated coffee accounted for 20% of instant and 9% of brewed coffee and for 6% of retail consumption at home (Anon., 1987).

(x) *USA*

In 1989, 52.5% of the population over 10 years of age drank coffee (40.2% brewed, 15% instant), and 29.4% drank tea and 58.8% drank soft drinks. The number of cups of coffee consumed per person per day was 3.12 in 1962, decreased to 1.67 in 1988 and increased to 1.75 in 1989. Consumption per coffee drinker has been stable since 1985 at 3.34 cups per day, but this value had decreased from 4.17 cups per day in 1962. Consumption of decaffeinated coffee has increased from 4% in 1962 to 16.7% in 1989, at 2.40 cups per drinker per day (International Coffee Organization, 1989f,h).

Trends in coffee consumption over 1957-89 in the USA by type of coffee, region, age group, sex, location and time of day are given in Table 13. Consumption of brewed and instant coffee declined by an average of about 46% between 1962 (the year of highest average consumption) and 1989. The proportion of cups prepared from decaffeinated coffee (ground and soluble) increased from 3% to 19% during 1962-89, and the proportion of the total population drinking coffee has declined sharply, from 74.7% to 52.5% (Gilbert, 1984; International Coffee Organization, 1989f,h). Consumption of decaffeinated coffee in the USA in 1985-88 and in 1962 is given in Table 14 (International Coffee Organization, 1989h), which shows an increase of nearly four times. The decrease in the proportion of the population drinking coffee in 1988 from that in 1985 was seen across all age groups, with a large decrease in drinkers aged 30-59 years. Almost twice as many people aged 30 years and over drink coffee than do those younger than 30.

2. Chemical Composition

2.1 General aspects

Roasted, ground and decaffeinated coffee, in their dry form, consist of a soluble and an insoluble portion; the proportions of each in the beverage depends upon the brewing conditions and the appliance used. While it is possible by exhaustive extraction in the laboratory to obtain 30-32% w/w soluble substances from roasted coffee, the more usual yield in household brews is 15-25% w/w. As mentioned above, the ratio of weight of dry product to volume of water used for brewing also varies according to national and local tastes; variations also occur in

Table 13. Coffee consumption trends in the USA in people aged 10 years and over, 1957–89[a]

	Cups per person per day													Difference 1962–89	Change (%)
	1957	1962	1967	1972	1977	1982	1983	1984	1985	1986	1987	1988	1989		
Type															
Brewed	2.32	2.45	2.19	1.67	1.30	1.33	1.31	1.44	1.39	1.37	1.37	1.31	1.43	-1.02	-42
Instant	0.50	0.67	0.65	0.68	0.64	0.56	0.53	0.54	0.42	0.36	0.37	0.34	0.32	-0.35	-52
Decaffeinated	NA	0.10	0.16	0.17	0.27	0.38	0.39	0.44	0.42	0.41	0.43	0.38	0.40	+0.30	+200
All	2.82	3.12	2.84	2.35	1.94	1.90	1.87	1.99	1.83	1.74	1.76	1.67	1.75	-1.37	-44
Region															
North-east	2.72	2.91	2.63	2.10	1.79	1.85	1.90	1.90	1.84	1.86	1.75	1.58	1.79	-1.12	-38
North-central	2.99	3.34	3.18	2.66	2.34	2.18	2.06	2.27	2.04	1.92	1.90	1.96	1.98	-1.36	-41
South	2.48	2.78	2.39	1.97	1.99	1.68	1.66	1.84	1.57	1.53	1.58	1.45	1.52	-1.26	-45
West	3.25	3.52	3.19	2.74	1.98	1.96	1.86	2.00	2.01	1.70	1.91	1.77	1.81	-1.71	-49
All	2.82	3.12	2.84	2.35	1.94	1.90	1.87	1.99	1.83	1.74	1.76	1.67	1.75	-1.37	-44
Age group															
10–14	0.19	0.18	0.19	0.12	0.07	0.03	0.04	0.04	0.03	0.02	0.03	0.04	0.02	-0.16	-89
15–19	1.11	1.09	0.82	0.55	0.45	0.33	0.26	0.30	0.21	0.16	0.19	0.23	0.20	-0.89	-82
20–24	2.60	2.99	2.22	1.48	1.36	0.92	0.88	0.92	1.00	0.79	0.55	0.63	0.72	-2.27	-76
25–29	3.65	3.88	3.21	2.47	1.89	1.75	1.60	1.64	1.48	1.32	1.39	1.22	1.23	-2.65	-68
30–39	3.67	4.50	3.99	3.51	2.62	2.37	2.39	2.42	2.24	2.11	2.19	1.91	2.03	-2.47	-55
40–49	3.74	4.44	4.48	3.72	3.49	3.11	2.85	3.15	3.02	2.62	2.75	2.57	2.57	-1.79	-40
50–59	3.16	3.83	3.70	3.35	3.22	3.09	3.27	3.33	2.93	2.77	2.95	2.85	2.97	-0.86	-22
60–69	2.75	3.01	3.16	2.85	2.72	2.65	2.49	2.87	2.51	2.70	2.49	2.49	2.64	-0.37	-12
≥70	2.29	2.39	2.50	2.49	2.00	2.03	1.95	2.18	1.87	2.04	1.85	1.83	1.93	-0.46	-19
Sex															
Male	2.91	3.28	2.93	2.48	2.12	2.06	1.90	2.10	1.91	1.80	1.89	1.86	1.85	-1.43	-44
Female	2.73	2.98	2.77	2.23	1.95	1.75	1.81	1.89	1.76	1.68	1.64	1.50	1.66	-1.32	-44

Table 13 (contd)

	Cups per person per day												Difference 1962–89	Change (%)
	1957	1962	1967	1972	1977	1982	1983	1984	1985	1986	1987	1988	1989		
Location															
Home	2.35	2.57	2.29	1.86	1.62	1.36	1.37	1.40	1.29	1.24	1.23	1.19	1.23	-1.34	-52
Work	0.21	0.26	0.30	0.28	0.16	0.38	0.33	0.38	0.35	0.31	0.33	0.32	0.34	+0.08	+131
Eating places	0.26	0.29	0.25	0.21	0.25	0.14	0.13	0.17	0.14	0.14	0.14	0.12	0.18	-0.11	-38
Time of day															
Breakfast	1.14	1.17	1.13	1.00	0.91	0.88	0.89	0.92	0.88	0.84	0.85	0.83	0.90	-0.27	-23
Other meals	0.96	0.98	0.77	0.59	0.46	0.36	0.36	0.35	0.30	0.27	0.30	0.25	0.22	-0.76	-78
Between meals	0.72	0.97	0.94	0.76	0.66	0.66	0.62	0.71	0.65	0.65	0.61	0.59	0.63	-0.34	-35
% of US population drinking coffee	77.3	74.7	71.4	65.0	57.9	56.3	55.2	57.3	54.9	52.4	52.0	50.0	52.5	-22.2	-30
Cups per drinker per day	3.65	4.17	3.98	3.62	3.51	3.38	3.36	3.48	3.33	3.32	3.38	3.34	3.34	-0.83	-20

[a]From Gilbert (1984); International Coffee Organization (1989f,h)
NA, not available

Table 14. Consumption of decaffeinated coffee in the USA in 1985–88 and in 1962[a]

Year	% of US population drinking coffee	No. of cups per day	
		per person	per drinker
1962	4.0	0.10	2.61
1985	17.3	0.42	2.42
1986	17.1	0.41	2.37
1987	17.5	0.43	2.48
1988	15.8	0.38	2.40
% change:			
1962–88	+11.8	+0.28	−0.21
1985–88	−1.5	−0.04	−0.02

[a] Adapted from International Coffee Organization (1989h)

the nature and origin of the coffee, the appliance and the amount of additives (e.g., milk) used subsequently. All of these factors influence the concentration of soluble substances in the resultant brews and their chemical compositions. Generally, 42, 48 and 57 g roasted, ground coffee are used typically per litre of water in the USA, UK and Europe, respectively, and some 150 ml of the water are retained in the spent coffee grounds.

Soluble substances have already been extracted from instant coffee at the point of manufacture. The percentage removed varies according to brand and may be up to 50%, so that more of the normally insoluble substances are rendered soluble at 100°C. About 12 g/l is a typically used average concentration of product in water for UK and US tastes; it is higher and lower in other countries. Clearly, the composition of different instant coffees varies considerably, especially in the relative proportions of the various constituents.

The main component of the beverages consumed is therefore water. Caffeine has particularly important stimulatory properties, but all three preparations contain other nonvolatile soluble compounds. Compounds of known physiological importance in roasted coffee and instant coffee have been reviewed by Viani (1988). Volatile compounds occur in the dry product, and their presence in the brews is again dependent on the amount and type of product and on the brewing conditions: 40-100% is extracted in practice (Pictet, 1987). The content of volatile substances in instant coffees is particularly dependent upon the sophistication of the method for extracting and retaining such substances on drying. The influence of nonvolatile and volatile components on the flavour of coffee has been described in detail (Clarke, 1986).

Tables 15 and 16 give a broad tabulation of all components of green and roasted arabica and robusta coffees (Clarke, 1987). It should be noted that considerable variation may occur, depending on factors such as the exact source and storage conditions, especially with regard to the concentrations of compounds that occur at low levels, such as aliphatic acids, reducing sugars and free amino acids. The values for polysaccharides, lignin and pectin are considered to be less reliable than others, as they are derived by indirect analysis from data on hydrolysis; however, they are indicative. For roasted coffee, further differences depend on the degree of roasting. Roasted coffee may also contain roasted seeds, tubers and other parts of vegetable plants, such as chicory. Instant coffee may similarly contain the soluble parts of these materials (Clarke & Macrae, 1987a).

Table 15. Composition of green coffee[a]

Component	Typical average content (dry basis, %)	
	Arabica	Robusta
Alkaloids (caffeine)	1.2	2.2
Trigonelline	1.0	0.7
Minerals (as oxide ash)		
41% potassium and 4% phosphorus	4.2	4.4
Acids		
Total chlorogenic	6.5	10.0
Aliphatic	1.0	1.0
Quinic	0.4	0.4
Sugars		
Sucrose	8.0	4.0
Reducing	0.1	0.4
Polysaccharides ('mannan', 'galactan', 'glucan' and 'araban')	45.0	50.0
Lignin	2.0	2.0
Pectins	3.0	3.0
Proteinaceous compounds		
Protein	11.0	11.0
Free amino acids	0.5	0.8
Lipids		
Coffee oil (triglyceride with unsaponifiable fat)	16.0	10.0

[a] From Clarke (1987)

Table 16. Composition of a medium-roasted coffee[a]

Component	Typical average content (dry basis, %)		% extractable with water at 100°C[b]
	Arabica	Robusta	
Alkaloids (caffeine)	1.3	2.4	75–100
Trigonelline (including roasted by-products)	1.0	0.7	85–100
Minerals (as oxide ash)	4.5	4.7	90
Acids			
Residual chlorogenic	2.5	3.8	100
Quinic	0.8	1.0	100
Aliphatic	1.6	1.6	100
Sugars			
Sucrose	0.0	0.0	–
Reducing	0.3	0.3	100
Polysaccharides (unchanged from green)	33	37	10
Lignin	2.0	2.0	0
Pectins	3.0	3.0	–
Proteinaceous compounds			
Protein	10	10	15–20
Free amino acids	0.0	0.0	–
Lipids (coffee oil)	17	11	1
Caramelized or condensation products (e.g., melanoidins) by difference	23	22.5	20–25
Volatile substances other than acids	0.1	0.1	40–80

[a] From Clarke (1987)
[b] From Maier (1981), for normal household brewing

A general and detailed description of all aspects of the chemistry of coffee has been published (Clarke & Macrae, 1985).

2.2 Compounds present in green, roasted, brewed, instant and decaffeinated coffees

The formulae of some of the compounds described below are given in Appendix 1 to this monograph (p. 199).

The quantitative data presented are generally for dry roasted coffee. To calculate representative values for the content in the beverage consumed, an average usage of 10 g roasted coffee per cup of filtered coffee (150 ml), equivalent to 57 g roasted coffee brewed with 1 l of water, can be assumed. Approximately 86% of the water is in the brew and the remainder left with the grounds. At an extraction yield of 20% total soluble solids, a concentration of 1.3% w/w would therefore be consumed. Assuming 100% extraction of particulate substances, their content in a cup can be estimated by dividing the content in roasted coffee (mg/kg) by 100.

With some filter devices and using finer grinds (as in the UK), smaller quantities of roasted coffee are used, e.g., 48 g/l of water or 8.3 g/cup. Spiller (1984b) assumed 7.5 g/150-ml cup from US experience; however, Clinton (1985) analysed data from 3000 respondents across the USA and found an average strength of 1.38 g coffee solubles per cup, equivalent to only 6.9 g roasted, ground coffee at 20% yield. Weaker coffee was drunk in the west than in the east.

Another form of expression is that 10 g per cup is equivalent to 100 cups/kg roasted, ground coffee, 8.3 g is equivalent to 122 cups/kg and 6.9 g to 147 cups/kg.

Table 16 gave an indication of the percentages of various components that are extracted. The level may be 75-100% for components such as caffeine and chlorogenic and other acids, but is rather less for volatile components.

(a) Nonvolatile substances

(i) Caffeine and other purines

Extensive determinations of caffeine in green coffees have been reported (Macrae, 1985). These indicate an average of 1.2% on a dry basis (commercial range, 0.9-1.4%) for arabica coffee and 2.2% (commercial range, 1.5-2.6%) for robusta coffee. (Analytical methods are reported in the monograph on caffeine.) The content in roasted coffee is usually somewhat higher than in the corresponding green — by up to 10% in darker roasts — due to physical loss in weight of other components; 0-5% of the caffeine is lost by sublimation. Few reliable direct determinations have been made on roasted coffee, but several have been done on brewed coffee (Table 17; Bunker & McWilliams, 1979; Clinton, 1985). Minute amounts of related alkaloids have been identified and quantified in roasted coffee, e.g., theobromine at 0.009-0.037% and theophylline at 0.00-0.013% (Kazi, 1985; Macrae, 1985); traces of paraxanthine, theacrine and liberine have been detected in unripe green coffees (Viani, 1988).

(ii) Chlorogenic acids and related substances

A number of different chlorogenic acids are present; the amount of each depends largely on the degree and type of roasting to which the green coffee has been subjected (Clifford, 1985). 5-Caffeoylquinic acid is present in the largest amounts, in both green and roasted coffees. Dicaffeoyl and feruloyl quinic acids are also present, together with the 3- and 4-isomers of monocaffeoylquinic acid. The total percentage of chlorogenic acids in eight commercial roasted coffee samples ranged from 0.2-3.5% (very dark to light roasting) (Trugo, 1984), and that in 19 samples was 1.6-3.8% (Maier, 1987a). On the basis of 10 g coffee per cup of brew and 85% recovery, this would indicate a level of 15-325 mg/cup (Viani, 1988). Actual data (Clinton, 1985) from the USA give an average value of 190 mg total chlorogenic acids per cup of brewed coffee. Pyrolysis products of chlorogenic acid, in particular quinic acid and caffeic acid (see p. 69), are also found, depending upon the origin and degree of roasting, as are phenols (see p. 76).

Table 17. Caffeine content per cup of brewed coffee

Reference and location	Type of brew	No. of samples	Cup size (ml)	Caffeine (mg/cup)	
				Average	Range
Estimated by the Working Group[a]	10 g/cup				
	Arabica	-	150 ml	-	102-120
	Robusta	-	150 ml	-	187-220
	7 g/cup				
	Arabica	-	150 ml	-	71-84
	Robusta	-	150 ml	-	131-154
Burg (1975)[b] USA	Percolated	2000	150 ml	83	64-124
Gilbert et al. (1976) Canada	Percolated	-	150 ml	74	39-168
	Drip	-	150 ml	112	56-176
Bunker & McWilliams (1979) USA	Percolated	-	150 ml	104	89-122
	Drip	-	150 ml	142	137-149
Lecos (1984) USA	Percolated	-	150 ml	80	40-170
	Drip	-	150 ml	115	60-180
Clinton (1985) USA	Percolated/Drip	3000	197 ml	85	-

[a]On the basis of 1.2% caffeine in roasted dry arabica and 2.2% in roasted dry robusta, and range given for 85% and 100% efficiencies of extraction of caffeine
[b]Cited by Roberts & Barone (1983)
-, not given

(iii) *Glycosides*

Atractyligenin (a nor-diterpenoid substance of the (-)-kaurane series) has been found in coffee, both as the free compound and as the aglycone of three glycosides (Mätzel & Maier, 1983). The content of atractyligenin has been estimated at 2.9-11.5 mg/cup of brewed arabica and 0-0.2 mg/cup of brewed robusta (Viani, 1988).

(iv) *Lipids*

Roasted coffee has a very high lipid content — approximately 16% w/w in arabica and 11% in robusta — associated with two diterpenes specific to coffee, kahweol and cafestol, mostly combined as glycerides. The total diterpene content is typically reported at 1.3% in green arabica (ratio of cafestol:kahweol, 40:60 to 70:30) and at only 0.2% in green robusta (predominately cafestol) (Viani, 1988).

There appears to be little destruction on roasting; but of greater importance is the fact that little of the oil (lipids) and of these terpenes occurs in brewed coffee, e.g., 0.9 mg lipid (coffee oil) per cup and 0.005 mg diterpenes in filter brews, with rather more in espresso brews (40 and 3.2 mg, respectively) (Viani, 1988).

Various sterols (and their esters with fatty acids) and tocopherols are also present in the lipids, but there is no evidence of their presence in brewed coffee. The presence of various alkanoylated 5-hydroxytryptamines (high C_n fatty acids plus 5-hydroxytryptamine) in the wax on the outer surface of green coffee beans has been examined extensively by Folstar (1985); they are present at 500-1000 ppm (mg/kg), but they are partly destroyed on roasting and very little passes into the brew (van der Stegen, 1979).

(v) *Trigonelline and nicotinic acid*

Trigonelline is present typically at 1.1% in dry arabica green coffee (range, 0.6-1.3) and 0.65% in dry robusta green coffee (range, 0.3-0.9) (Macrae, 1985). The amount destroyed during roasting depends on the degree of roast, e.g., an original 1.1% level will decline to around 0.2% in dark roasts (Trugo, 1984), corresponding to 110 and 20 mg/cup assuming 10 g of roasted coffed per cup. An average content of 53 mg/cup has been reported by Clinton (1985) in the USA. Trigonelline is transformed into several volatile products but also into nicotinic acid (niacin; vitamin PP), of which roasted and brewed coffee can be important sources (100-400 mg/kg) (Macrae, 1985). A content of 0.03-0.05 mg nicotinic acid per cup was reported from six samples (Viani, 1988); Macrae (1985) reported 1 mg/cup and 2-3 mg from a dark roast. Residual trigonelline has been reported at a level of 40-55 mg/cup (Viani, 1988).

(vi) *Acids*

The nature and amount of nonvolatile acids in roasted coffee has been examined extensively, since they can contribute significantly to its flavour (Woodman, 1985; Maier, 1987a; van der Stegen & van Duijn, 1987). Apart from residual chlorogenic acids, the main acids present in significant quantities are quinic, malic, citric, lactic, pyruvic, succinic and glycolic acids (Table 18).

The amount of each acid is strongly dependent upon the degree of roasting, sometimes peaking in medium roasts, such as citric acid in Kenya arabica with 'fine' acidity (van der Stegen & Duijn, 1987).

Table 18. Content of selected nonvolatile acids in roasted coffee

Acid	Content (%, dry weight)[a]					
	Arabica (during roasting)[b]		Arabica (4 samples)[c]	Robusta (4 samples)[c]	Commercial (17 samples)[d]	
	Tanzania	Kenya			Average	Range
Citric	0.87 to 0.55	0.70 to 0.18	[0.67]	[0.48]	0.59	0.43–0.70
Malic	0.39 to 0.24	0.30 to 0.19	[0.33]	[0.13]	0.27	0.10–0.39
Lactic	0.08 to 0.10	0.09 to 0.16	–	–	0.10	0.00–0.18
Pyruvic	0.17 to 0.14	0.09 to 0.09	–	–	–	–
Glycolic	–	–	[0.26]	[0.19]	0.26	0.17–0.49
Succinic	–	–	–	–	0.40	0.19–0.80
Quinic	–	0.56 to 0.87	[0.96]	[1.15]	1.04	0.89–1.50

[a]To convert to milligrams per kilogram, multiply by 10 000; to convert to milligrams per cup multiply by 100.
[b]From Blanc (1977); in samples roasted in the laboratory, with 9–20% loss (i.e., from very light to dark)
[c]From Maier (1987a); in samples roasted in the laboratory, with 17% loss for arabica and 19% for robusta (medium to dark roast); graphic data in millimoles per kilogram, converted by the Working Group
[d]From van der Stegen & van Duijn (1987)

Maier (1987a) also found phosphoric acid [estimated from a graph by the Working Group at 0.19%] in roasted arabica and [0.29%] in roasted robusta; he also found significant amounts of an unspecified high-molecular-weight acid. Other acids have been identified (Spiller, 1984b) but in minor quantities. Maier (1987a) quantified these as citraconic at 0.048-0.070%, 2-furoic at 0.009-0.0250%, itaconic at 0.013-0.020%, pyrrolidone carboxylic (pyroglutamic acid) at 0.06-0.10%, mesaconic at 0.005-0.013%, fumaric at 0.010-0.016% and maleic at 0.006-0.016%; a number of others were found at even lower levels, all in commercial roasted coffees. Tressl *et al.* (1978a) reported 2-furoic acid at 0.008% in an arabica roasted coffee.

The total content of major nonvolatile acids estimated by the Working Group from the data of van der Stegen and van Duijn (1987) is 276 mg/cup (assuming use of 10 g roasted coffee per cup), ranging from 246 to 300; the content estimated from the data of Maier (1987a), including phosphoric acid, averages 231 mg in arabica and 224 mg in robusta. These figures are somewhat higher than the average of 178 mg, including formic/acetic acids, given by Clinton (1985) on the basis of use of 7 g/cup.

Maier (1987a) regarded the combination of citric and acetic acids as the reason for the higher acidity of arabica than robusta coffee. Also significant for flavour is the relatively high amount of quinic acid lactone, which, like quinic acid itself, increases and decreases again with increasing severity of roasting, peaking at 0.7% on a dry basis (Clifford, 1985). Brews containing this compound and standing at elevated temperatures show increasing acidity, partly because this lactone is transformed into more quinic acid but also because the concentrations of some other acids increase (van der Stegen & van Duijn, 1987).

(vii) *Maillard reaction products (melanoidins)*

Products of the Maillard reaction are important constituents of roasted coffee; in a dry medium roast, they can comprise some 15-20%, of which 20-25% are hot water-soluble. At present, they are poorly characterized as caramelized products of sucrose and condensation products of polysaccharides with 'proteins' and other compounds (Trugo, 1985).

(viii) *Other compounds*

Clinton (1985) found reducing sugars at an average content per cup of 15 mg, other carbohydrates at 205 mg and peptides/'protein' at 62 mg.

(b) *Volatile substances*

The volatile compounds in coffee include carbonyl compounds, alcohols, acids, esters, terpenoid compounds, nitrogen- and sulfur-containing compounds, hydrocarbons, heterocyclic and aromatic compounds. The quantity (apart from the volatile aliphatic acids) obtained by distillation of roasted coffee is about 0.1% or 1000 mg/kg (Silwar *et al.*, 1986a). Volatile compounds are present in smaller amounts than in most other foods, but the range of types is greater.

The number of volatile components that have been identified has risen sharply over the last 20 years (Flament, 1987). The most up-to-date, complete listing of all identified components is that of Maarse and Visscher (1986) — now comprising over 700. An earlier listing by Vitzthum (1976) gave 550 volatile compounds (an English version is provided by Spiller, 1984a). Listings by Silwar *et al.* (1986a) and Flament (1987) give numbers only for categories of compounds. The systems of chemical grouping used differ somewhat in these lists, particularly with regard to sulfur-containing and furan-based compounds. The numbers of volatile compounds identified in roasted coffee are listed by group in Tables 19-22.

Those compounds that have been quantified have been listed by van Straten *et al.* (1983) and Silwar *et al.* (1986a,b). Only those detected by modern gas chromatography (GC)/mass spectrometry methods (i.e., published since about 1970) can be regarded as reliably identified, however. Contents are usefully given per cup of brew (standardized at 150 ml) or per litre, and suitable bases for calculation were given above.

Table 19. Classification of volatile compounds in roasted coffee: aliphatic benzenoid and alicyclic compounds[a]

Group/subgroup	Number identified			
	Total	Aliphatic	Benzenoid	Alicyclic
Hydrocarbons	73			
Saturated		24	9	1
Unsaturated		16	2 (in side chain)	1
Condensed polynuclear		-	20	-
Alcohols	20			
Saturated		12	2	1
Unsaturated		4	0	1
Aldehydes	29			
Saturated		11	5	0
Unsaturated		7	1	0
Hydroxy-		0	4	0
Alkoxy-		0	1	0
Ketones	69			
Mono-				
Saturated		23	2	2
Unsaturated		5	0	8
Hydroxy		6	3	0
Acyl-		0	0	1
Di-				
Saturated		13	1	5
Unsaturated		0	0	0
Acids	22			
Saturated		15	1	2
Unsaturated		4	0	0
Esters	29	23	6	0
Ethers	2	2	0	0
Acetal	1	1	0	0
Nitrogen-containing	21			
Amines		12	5	0
Nitriles		3	0	0
Oxime		1	0	0
Sulfur-containing	18			
Thiols		3	0	0
Thioethers (sulfides)				
Mono-		2	1	0
Di-		3	0	0
Tri-		2	0	0

Table 19 (contd)

Group/subgroup	Number identified			
	Total	Aliphatic	Benzenoid	Alicyclic
Sulfur-containing (contd)				
Thioester		1	0	0
Thioketone		1	0	0
Thiophenol		-	1	-
Miscellaneous (CS_2 etc.)		4	0	0
Phenols	40			
Mono-			1	
Alkylated		-	22	-
Alkoxy-		-	8	-
Dihydroxy benzenes		-	7	-
Trihydroxy benzenes		-	2	-
Total	324	198	104	22

"From Maarse & Visscher (1986)
-, not applicable

Silwar et al. (1986a,b) stated that steam distillation of a medium-roasted arabica coffee released 700-800 ppm (mg/kg) by weight of 'aromatics', which corresponds to the 0.1% generally previously believed to be present, if acetic and formic acids are excluded. By GC analysis, they were able to account for 85-95% of this amount by summation of individually determined amounts: 170 compounds were found in the parts per million (milligrams per kilogram) range (1-150 ppm) and 70 in the parts per billion range (1-500 ppb); however, actual data were given for only 157 compounds. The greatest amount of the steam volatile complex by weight was contributed by heterocyclic compounds (80-85%), comprising furans of all kinds (at 38-45%), pyrazines (25-30%), pyridines (3-7%), pyrroles (2-3%), sulfur-substituted furans (0.4%), thiophenes (0.4%), thiazoles (0.15%) and oxazoles (< 0.01%). Only 3-5% by weight were aliphatic compounds, 3-5% were aromatic compounds and < 0.5% were alicyclic compounds.

A compilation of the data of Silwar et al. (1986a,b) is given in Table 23 to illustrate the expected content of volatile compounds per cup of brewed coffee. It is assumed that the extraction efficiency of home brewing is 100%, although in practice it is substantially less. Maarse and Visschler (1986) identified 715 compounds (see Tables 19-22).

Table 20. Classification of volatile compounds in roasted coffee: heterocyclic (oxygen ring-containing compounds)[a]

Group/subgroup	Number identified						
	Total	Furans	Benzo-furans	Pyrones	Pyrans	Lactones (maleic)	Anhydrides
Simple	5	1	1	0	0	3	0
Hydrogenated	8	5	1	0	2	0	0
Alkyl-	42	29	1	3	0	6	3
Alkoxy-	1	1	0	0	0	-	-
Aryl-	1	1	0	0	0	-	-
Difuryl	8	8	0	-	-	-	-
Aldehydes	6	6	0	-	-	-	-
Ketones (including hydrogenated)	15						
Mono-		10	0	-	-	-	-
Di-		5	0	-	-	-	-
Acyl-	9	9	0	-	-	-	-
Alcohols	2	2	0	-	-	-	-
Acid	1	1	0	-	-	-	-
Esters	11	11	0	-	-	-	-
Ethers	4	4	0	-	-	-	-
Sulfur-containing	18						
Thiols		2	0	-	-	-	-
Thioethers		14	0	-	-	-	-
Thioester		1	0	-	-	-	-
Thioketone		1	0	-	-	-	-
Total	131	111	3	3	2	9	3

[a] From Maarse & Visscher (1986)
-, not applicable

Table 21. Classification of volatile compounds in roasted coffee: heterocyclic (nitrogen ring-containing compounds)[a]

Group/subgroup	Number identified						
	Total	Pyrroles	Benzopyrroles (indoles)	Pyrazines	Benzo[a]pyrazines (quinoxalines)	Pyridines	Benzo[b]pyridines (quinolines)
Simple	6	1	1	1	1	1	1
Hydrogenated	9	2	1	0	5	1	0
Alkyl-	77	28	2	34	4	6	3
Furfuryl-	27	14	0	13	0	0	0
Aryl-	1	1	0	0	0	0	0
Acyl-	30	20	0	7	0	3	0
Alkoxy-	4	0	0	4	0	0	0
Ketones (mono- and di-)	3	2	1	0	0	0	0
Alicyclic	12	0	0	12	0	0	0
Other	2	0	0	0	1	1	0
Total	171	68	5	71	11	12	4

[a]From Maarse & Visscher (1986)

(i) *Carbonyl compounds* (Table 24)

Maarse and Visscher (1986) listed 18 aliphatic aldehydes in freshly roasted coffee, in a saturated series up to heptanal, including seven unsaturated but no alicyclic compounds. *trans*-2-Nonenal is believed to be present in a very small amount. Glyoxal, methylglyoxal and ethylglyoxal are not listed as being present in roasted coffee by Maarse and Visscher (1986) and were not quantified by Silwar *et al.* (1986a) using a direct, non-derivative GC method; however, methylglyoxal has been detected by indirect GC methods (Kasai *et al.*, 1982; Hayashi & Shibamoto, 1985; Nagao *et al.*, 1986a; Shane *et al.*, 1988; Aeschbacher *et al.*, 1989) (Table 25; see also the monograph on methylglyoxal, p. 446).

Table 22. Classification of volatile compounds in roasted coffee: heterocyclic (sulfur, sulfur/nitrogen and nitrogen/oxygen ring–containing compounds)[a]

Group/subgroup	Number identified						
	Total	Thiophenes	Benzothiophenes	Thiazoles	Benzothiazoles	Oxazoles	Benzoxazoles
Simple	4	1	1	1	1	0	0
Hydrogenated	1	0	0	0	0	1	0
Alkyl-	56	7	0	23	0	20	5
Di-		1	0	0	0	0	0
Aryl-	2	1	0	0	0	1	0
Ketones	5	5	0	0	0	0	0
Acyl-	13	9	0	2	0	2	0
Alcohols	1	1	0	0	0	0	0
Esters	3	3	0	0	0	0	0
Other	4	4	0	0	0	0	0
Total	89	32	1	26	1	24	5

[a] From Maarse & Visscher (1986)

Table 23. Volatile compounds in coffee brewed from 10 g medium-roasted arabica coffee[a]

Group	Number identified	Number quantified	Total (mg/cup)[b]
Carbonyls	≥97 26 furanoid	≥12 18 furanoid	0.10–0.20 1.30–1.91
Volatile acids	≥21 1 furanoid	≥2 1 furanoid	65 (mainly acetic acid)
Alcohols	≥20 2 furanoid	≥5 2 furanoid	0.9–1.35 (mainly furfuryl alcohol)
Esters, lactones and ethers	≥40 15 furanoid	≥0 7 furanoid	<0.07
Pyrroles	≥66 4 indoles	≥14 2 indoles	0.13–0.16
Pyrazines	71	28	} 1.7–2.2
Pyridines	10	2	
Furans (not already included)	45	21	<0.04
Phenols and phenol ethers	40	9	0.12–0.29

Table 23 (contd)

Group	Number identified	Number quantified	Total (mg/cup)[b]
Sulfur compounds	95	21	0.1
Others	139	14	Very small
Total	≥692	158	<4.46–6.11 (excluding acids)

[a] Adapted from Silwar et al. (1986a,b)
[b] Calculated by the Working Group

Table 24. Contents of carbonyls in roasted coffee (mg/kg)

Compound	Content[a] (ppm; mg/kg)	Reference
Aldehydes		
Aliphatic		
3-Methyl butanal	6.7	van Straten et al. (1983)
n-Hexanal	0.3–0.7	Silwar (1982)
Benzenoid		
Benzaldehyde	1.8, 0.7–1.10	Silwar (1982); Silwar et al. (1986a)
3,4-Dihydroxybenzaldehyde	8–20	Tressl et al. (1978a)
4-Hydroxy-3-methoxybenzaldehyde (vanillin)	2–3	Tressl et al. (1978a)
3,4-Dihydroxycinnamaldehyde	5–12	Tressl et al. (1978a)
2-Phenylbut-2-enal	0.6, 0.1–0.20	Silwar (1982); Silwar et al. (1986a)
2-Phenylacetaldehyde	3.7, 1.5–2.0	Silwar (1982); Silwar et al. (1986a)
Furanoid		
Furfural	5.2–232, 55–80	Silwar (1982); Silwar et al. (1986a)
5-Methylfurfural	216, 50–70	Silwar (1982); Silwar et al. (1986a)
5-(Hydroxymethyl)-2-furfural	10–35	Tressl et al. (1978a)
(2-Furyl)acetaldehyde	0.5	Silwar (1982)
Ketones and diketones		
Aliphatic		
1-Hydroxypropan-2-one	4, 0.25–0.30	Silwar (1982); Silwar et al. (1986a)
3-Hydroxybutan-2-one	4.9, 0.25–0.35	Silwar et al. (1986a)
2,3-Butanedione (diacetyl)	2.7, 0.05–0.15	Silwar et al. (1986a)
2-Pentanone	0.4–4.3	Silwar (1982)
4-Methylpentan-2-one	6.5	Silwar (1982)
2-Hydroxypentan-3-one	5.2, 0.05–0.15	Silwar (1982); Silwar et al. (1986a)

Table 24 (contd)

Compound	Content[a] (ppm; mg/kg)	Reference
Ketones and diketones (contd)		
Aliphatic (contd)		
2,3-Pentanedione	1.0–3.0	Silwar et al. (1986a)
5-Methylhexan-2-one	0.5	Silwar (1982)
2,3-Hexanedione	3.2, 0.3–0.5	Silwar (1982); Silwar et al. (1986a)
3-Heptanone	0.4	Silwar (1982)
4-Heptanone	0.5	Silwar (1982)
2-Pentadecanone	2.9, 0.10–0.15	Silwar (1982); Silwar et al. (1986a)
1-Acetoxy-2-propanone	2.0–5.0	Silwar et al. (1986a)
1-Acetoxy-3-butanone	2.0–4.0	Silwar et al. (1986a)
1-Acetoxy-2-butanone	2.0–3.0	Silwar et al. (1986a)
Benzenoid		
2-Hydroxyacetophenone	1.6	Silwar (1982)
Alicyclic		
3-Methylcyclopentane-1,2 dione (3-Methyl-2-hydroxycyclopent-2-ene-1-one) (cyclotene)	17–40	Tressl et al. (1978a)
Furanoid		
2-Methyltetrahydrofuran-3-one	10.0–16.0	Silwar et al. (1986a)
2,4-Dimethyl-2H-furan-3-one	0.50–0.60	Silwar et al. (1986a)
2,5-Dimethyl-2H-furan-3-one	10.7	Silwar (1982)
2,5-Dimethyl-4-hydroxy-2H-furan-3-one (furaneol)	25–50	Tressl et al. (1978a)
2,5-Dimethyl-4-ethoxy-2H-furan-3-one	2–8	Tressl et al. (1978a)
2-Acetylfuran	24.1–31.4	Silwar (1982)
	6.0–12.00	Silwar et al. (1986a)
2-Acetonylfuran	2.2	Silwar (1982)
2-Propionylfuran	0.5, 1.10–1.50	Silwar (1982); Silwar et al. (1986a)
1-(2-Furyl)butan-2-one	1.4, 0.10–0.20	Silwar (1982); Silwar et al. (1986a)
4-(2-Furyl)butan-2-one	4.6, 0.10–0.15	Silwar (1982); Silwar et al. (1986a)
1-(5-Methyl-2-furyl)butan-2-one	0.8, 0.25–0.35	Silwar (1982); Silwar et al. (1986a)
4-(5-Methyl-2-furyl)butan-2-one	0.25–0.30	Silwar et al. (1986a)
1-(2-Furyl)pentan-1,2-dione	1.0, 0.05–0.10	Silwar (1982); Silwar et al. (1986a)
2-Acetyl-5-methylfuran	0.5–1.0	Silwar et al. (1986a)
2-Methyl-5-propionylfuran	4.2	Silwar (1982)
1-(2-Furyl)-propane-1,2-dione	3.9, 0.10–0.15	Silwar (1982); Silwar et al. (1986a)
1-(5-Methyl-2-furyl)propane-1,2-dione	3.4, 0.25–0.30	Silwar (1982); Silwar et al. (1986a)

Table 24 (contd)

Compound	Content[a] (ppm; mg/kg)	Reference
Ketones and diketones (contd)		
Furanoid (contd)		
1-(2-Furyl)butane-1,2-dione	3.3, 0.10–0.15	Silwar (1982); Silwar et al. (1986a)
1-(5-Methyl-2-furyl)butane-1,2-dione	1.4, 0.05–0.10	Silwar (1982); Silwar et al. (1986a)

[a] One figure is given for one sample; Silwar et al. (1986a) tested five commercial samples of roasted arabica coffee, while Silwar (1982) and Tressl et al. (1978a) tested numerous samples of arabica and robusta coffee.

Table 25. Contents of methylglyoxal in coffee

Content			Reference
Roasted coffee (mg/kg)	Brewed coffee		
	Amount	Conditions	
[58–75]	470–730 µg/cup	8 g/100 ml	Kasai et al. (1982)
25	76 µg	3 g/180 ml	Hayashi & Shibamoto (1985)
–	7 µg/ml	10 g/150 ml	Nagao et al. (1986a)
–	273–341 µg/g (filtered coffee)	25 g/250 ml	Shane et al. (1988)
[21–39][a]	106–197 µg/g dried product	1 g/10 ml	Aeschbacher et al. (1989)

[a] Calculated assuming extraction yield of 20% dry soluble solids in the brew

van Straten et al. (1983) reported quantitative data on only two of the 18 aldehydes. While acetaldehyde has been reported repeatedly as being present, no reliable quantitative data appear to be available. Hayashi et al. (1986) reported a level of 3.4-4.5 ppm (mg/l) formaldehyde (see IARC, 1982, 1987) in brewed coffee.

Maarse and Visscher (1986) listed 11 benzenoid aldehydes; van Straten et al. (1983) reported quantitative data on five of them, including 3,4-dihydroxybenzaldehyde at 8-20 ppm (mg/kg) and benzaldehyde at 1.8 ppm (mg/kg). The later work of Silwar et al. (1986a), which was not in this listing, generally reported lower levels of all carbonyls quantified in a medium-roasted arabica coffee and a lower level of benzaldehyde, and included 2-phenylacetaldehyde (1.5-2 mg/kg).

Other important aldehydes present are furanoid (six quantified by van Straten et al., 1983); in particular, furfural has been found at up to 255 ppm (mg/kg) [equivalent to 2.6 mg/cup] and 5-methylfurfural at up to 216 ppm (mg/kg; Silwar, 1982). However, Silwar et al. (1986a) reported much lower quantities (up to 80 and 70 ppm (mg/kg), respectively).

Maarse and Visscher (1986) list 47 aliphatic and 16 alicyclic ketones, including diketones, three acetophenones, two benzenoid ketones and one benzenoid diketone. van Straten et al. (1983) reported quantitative data on 14 of these, although only 3-methylcyclopentane-1,2-dione (cyclotene) is present at significant amounts of 17-40 ppm (mg/kg; Tressl et al. (1978a). This compound was not reported by Silwar et al. (1986a). Diacetyl (2,3-butadione) was present at 2.7 ppm (mg/kg; Silwar, 1982), but Silwar et al. (1986a) reported only 0.05-0.15 ppm (mg/kg) diacetyl [equivalent to 0.5-15 µg/cup]. They also gave data on 10 aliphatic ketones, three benzenoid aldehydes and 14 furanoid ketones.

Strictly speaking, a number of other pyrrole-based carbonyls could be included; but these are described with nitrogen compounds, and the quantities involved are small. Isomaltol (2-acetyl-3-hydroxyfuran) has been found in arabica and robusta coffees at levels of 8 and 1.5 ppm (mg/kg), respectively (Tressl et al., 1978a).

(ii) *Alcohols*

Maarse and Visscher (1986) listed 18 basic aliphatic and alicyclic alcohols and two aromatic alcohols; van Straten et al. (1983) quoted quantitative amounts for only four of them.

Furfuryl alcohol (grouped by Maarse & Visscher (1986) in the furan group) is the most prevalent volatile compound in roasted coffee (except acetic acid), with reported levels of 300 ppm (mg/kg) in arabica and 520 ppm (mg/kg) in robusta (Tressl et al., 1978a), up to 881 ppm (mg/kg; van Straten et al., 1983) and 678 ppm (mg/kg; Silwar, 1982). 5-Methylfurfuryl alcohol was reported at 25 ppm (mg/kg; Silwar, 1982). Silwar et al. (1986a) later reported levels of 90-135 ppm (mg/kg) furfuryl alcohol and 1.2-1.8 ppm (mg/kg) 5-methylfurfuryl alcohol. Furfuryl alcohol is regarded as detrimental to the flavour of coffee.

(iii) *Acids*

Maarse and Visscher (1986) listed 19 volatile acids in an aliphatic series up to decanoic, one benzoic and two alicyclic. The quantitative data quoted by van Straten et al. (1983) are derived from Kung et al. (1967), but the later data of Blanc (1977), Maier (1987a) and van der Stegen and van Duijn (1987) are more reliable (Table 26). The total content of formic and acetic acids found by van der Stegen and van Duijn (1987) would be 6500 ppm [which amount to about 65 mg per cup].

Table 26. Volatile acid content of dry roasted coffees

Coffee	Content (%)		Reference
	Formic acid	Acetic acid	
Colombian and Santos robusta	0.066–0.140	0.25–0.33	Kung et al. (1967)
Kenya arabica (very dark to very light)	–	0.4–0.09	Blanc (1977)
Arabica (average of 4 samples, peak value)[a]	0.23	0.60	Maier (1987a)
Robusta medium roast (average of 4 samples)[a]	0.23	0.54	Maier (1987a)
17 commercial coffees (average and range)	0.22 (0.18–0.25)	0.43 (0.36–0.55)	van der Stegen & van Duijn (1987)

[a]Calculated by the Working Group
–, not tested

Kung et al. (1967) reported the presence of nine other acids in relatively low quantities. Silwar et al. (1986a) gave levels only for 2-methylbutanoic acid, at 25.0-40.0 ppm (mg/kg).

(iv) *Esters, ethers and lactones*

Maarse and Visscher (1986) reported the presence of 23 aliphatic, six benzenoid esters and 11 furanoid-based esters. None of these is reported to be present in any substantial amount; methyl salicylate is reported at 1.4 ppm (mg/kg) and furfuryl acetate at 16.3 ppm (mg/kg; Silwar, 1982) or 3.5-5.5 ppm (mg/kg; Silwar et al., 1986a), but there are few other quantitative data. Six ethers and nine lactones are listed by Maarse and Visscher (1986), and are reported in relatively small amounts by Silwar et al. (1986a).

(v) *Nitrogen compounds*

Amines and amides: Maarse and Visscher (1986) listed the presence of 12 aliphatic amines; van Straten et al. (1983) reported quantitatively only on dimethylamine at 2 ppm (mg/kg) and on five aromatic amines. One imide, N-α-dimethylsuccinimide (Maarse & Visscher, 1986), and the secondary amine, pyrrolidine (Singer & Lijinsky, 1976), have been reported.

N-N/S- *and* N/O-*Heterocyclic compounds*: This is an important group of compounds with regard to the flavour of roasted coffee. Maarse and Visscher (1986) listed the presence of 71 pyrazines, 12 pyridines, four quinolines, 11 quinoxalines, 26 thiazoles, 24 oxazoles, 68 pyrroles and five indoles.

A considerable amount of quantitative data was reported by Tressl et al. (1981) and van Straten et al. (1983) on 44 of the pyrroles and 25 of the pyrazines. The quantities of individual pyrroles are quite low (in general < 1 ppm), although levels of 1.1-2.7 ppm (mg/kg) pyrrole itself and 17 ppm (mg/kg) 2-formyl-1-methylpyrrole were reported. Some pyrazines occur at higher levels (104 ppm (mg/kg) methyl pyrazine), but most are found at lower levels (acetyl pyrazine, 1.3 ppm (mg/kg)). Pyridine was reported to be present at up to 49 ppm (mg/kg; van Straten et al., 1983). Quantitative data on 18 pyrroles (including 13 carbonylic) give a total of 79 ppm (mg/kg); 2 ppm (mg/kg) were found for two indoles and 395 ppm for 28 pyrazines (Silwar, 1982). Silwar et al. (1986a) provided quantitative data on 28 pyrazines (170-218 mg/kg), two pyridines, 14 pyrroles (mainly carbonylic, 12.6-15.0 mg/kg) and two indoles.

2-Amino-3,4-dimethylimidazo[4,5-f]quinoline (MeIQ) (see IARC, 1986b) has been detected in coffee beans at 16 ng/kg (hot-air-roasted), 32 ng/kg (charcoal-roasted) and 150 ng/kg (high-temperature-roasted) only after alkaline hydrolysis (Kikugawa et al., 1989; Takahashi et al., 1989).

S- and O/S-Heterocyclic compounds: Maarse and Visscher (1986) reported the presence of 28 thiophenes and two dithiolanes and provided some quantitative data; none occurs in apparently significant amounts. Silwar (1982) found six thiophenes at a total content of 8.9 ppm (mg/kg) and one dithiolane at 3.7 ppm (mg/kg). Silwar et al. (1986b) reported the total content of six thiophenes at 4.7 ppm (mg/kg) in roasted Colombian arabica and 3.2 in roasted robusta coffee.

(vi) *Furan-based compounds*

Maarse and Visscher (1986) reported the presence of 92 furan compounds and a further 18 sulfur-containing furan compounds, many of which have been mentioned previously (as aldehydes, ketones and esters). Furfurylthiols (furfuryl mercaptans) and sulfides appear to be especially important with regard to flavour but are present in only small absolute quantities, e.g., furfurylthiol at 2.2 ppm (mg/kg) in roasted robusta, at 1.1 ppm (mg/kg) in arabica (Tressl & Silwar, 1981), at 1.65 ppm (mg/kg) in roasted Ivory Coast robusta and at 0.9 ppm (mg/kg) in roasted Colombias (Silwar et al., 1986b). The total content of ten sulfur-containing furans was only 2.5-6.4 ppm (mg/kg; van Straten et al., 1983). The total content of 17 furans was 41 ppm (mg/kg), with 2-acetylfuran contributing 31.4 ppm (Silwar, 1982; van Straten et al., 1983). Kahweofuran (2-methyl-3-oxa-8-thiabicyclo(3.3.0)-1,4-octadiene), of particular importance in flavour, has been reported at 1.75 ppm (mg/kg) in roasted Colombian arabicas, at 2.0 ppm (mg/kg) in Kenyan coffees and at 0.45 ppm (mg/kg) in roasted Ivory Coast robustas (Silwar et al., 1986b).

(vii) *Other sulfur compounds*

A number of other aliphatic and aromatic sulfides, including di- and trisulfides, are especially important in the aroma of dry roasted coffee. Maarse and

Visscher (1986) listed 14 aliphatic and two aromatic sulfides. The quantities involved are very small; e.g., dimethyldisulfide was found at 0.01 ppm (mg/kg) in roasted Colombian arabica and at 0.1 ppm in roasted Ivory Coast robustas (Tressl & Silwar, 1981; Silwar et al., 1986b).

(viii) *Phenols*

Phenols are another important group of flavour compounds; 39 were listed by van Straten et al. (1983). Quantitative determinations were reported by Tressl (1977), Tressl et al. (1978a,b), van Straten et al. (1983) and Silwar et al. (1986a). Silwar et al. (1986a) reported on the contents of 13 phenols (excluding dihydroxy- and trihydroxybenzenes) in a medium-roasted arabica. The actual quantities present are again small; the differences between roasted robusta and arabica are shown in Table 27. When arabica coffee is roasted very darkly, greater quantities of some phenols have been found, e.g., the phenol content increased from 13 to 63 ppm (mg/kg) and that of guaiacol from 2.7 to 10.6 ppm (Tressl et al., 1978b).

(ix) *Pyrones*

Three pyrones have been identified and quantified by Tressl et al. (1978a) and reported by van Straten et al. (1983; Table 28).

(x) *Hydrocarbons*

Seventy-three hydrocarbons have been identified in roasted coffee (Maarse & Visscher, 1986); 11 have been quantified at the parts per billion (micrograms/kilogram) level and four at the parts per million (milligrams/kilogram) level (van Straten et al., 1983).

As both roasted and instant coffee are derived by roasting procedures (at temperatures of the order of 210°C, with higher air temperatures), polycyclic aromatic hydrocarbons (PAH), and in particular benzo[a]pyrene, can be expected to be present. Numerous studies have been conducted on their actual occurrence (e.g., Ruschenburg, 1985; de Kruijf et al., 1987; reviewed by Strobel, 1988a). Determinations in roasted coffee, best done by high-performance liquid chromatography (HPLC) and fluorimetric techniques, suggest a range of <0.1-1.2 µg/kg, with an average of 0.3 µg/kg; however, PAH are largely removed in the spent grounds (e.g., on filter papers), leading to contents in the brews of <0.01 µg/l (Ruschenburg, 1985) or 0.0003-0.0008 µg/l (de Kruijf et al., 1987). Darker roasts produce slightly higher values. It has been shown that the chaff produced during roasting contains much higher levels (2-23 µg/kg) (de Kruijf et al., 1987); although this material is usually discarded, it is sometimes mixed in with subsequently ground roasted coffee. Strobel (1988a) calculated that coffee consumption contributes <0.1% (or 0.25 µg per year per person) of the total PAH inhaled or ingested from all sources.

Table 27. Phenol content of roasted coffees[a]

Phenolic compound	Content (mg/kg)		
	Arabica	Robusta	Not stated
Phenol	13, 1.20–2.20[b]	17	60
2-Methylphenol (ortho-cresol)	1.2, 0.70–1.10[b]	1.1	12.4
3-Methylphenol (meta-cresol)	0.7, 0.15–0.50[b]	1.2	7.4
4-Methylphenol (para-cresol)	1.3, 0.30–0.60[b]	1.0	13.2
2-Ethylphenol			1.7
3-Ethylphenol			1.3
4-Vinylphenol	0.2	0.2	0.6
2,3-Dimethylphenol			2.1
2,4-Dimethylphenol			2.0
2,5-Dimethylphenol			1.5
2,6-Dimethylphenol			0.2
3,4-Dimethylphenol			0.8
2-Ethyl-4-methylphenol			1.0
4-Ethyl-2-methylphenol			0.9
Ethylmethylphenol			0.4
2-Propyl-4-methylphenol			0.2
Methylpropylphenol			0.2
2,3,5-Trimethylphenol			0.3
2,4,5-Trimethylphenol			0.3
2,3,6-Trimethylphenol			0.2
1,2-Dihydroxybenzene (pyrocatechol)	80	120	
1,4-Dihydroxybenzene (hydroquinone)	40	30	
1,2-Dihydroxy-3-methylbenzene		9[c]	
1,2-Dihydroxy-4-methylbenzene	16	13	
1,2-Dihydroxy-4-ethylbenzene	37	80	
1,2-Dihydroxy-4-vinylbenzene	25	25	
2-Methoxyphenol (guaiacol)	2.7, 2–3[b]	8.4	10.6
4-Methyl-2-methoxyphenol	0.01–0.02[b]		0.1
4-Ethyl-2-methoxyphenol	0.8–1.50[b]		2.2
4-Vinyl-2-methoxyphenol	9.5, 8–20.0[b]	19.5	7.9
4-Propenyl-2-methoxyphenol (isoeugenol)			0.1
1,2-Dimethoxy-4-vinylbenzene	0.40–0.80[b]		3[d]
1,2,4-Trihydroxybenzene	20	13	
1,2,3-Trihydroxybenzene (pyrogallol)	45	55	

[a] Data from Tressl et al. (1978a,b) unless noted otherwise
[b] From Silwar et al. (1986a)
[c] From van Straten et al. (1983)
[d] From Silwar (1982)

Table 28. Pyrone content of roasted coffees[a]

Pyrone	Content (mg/kg)	
	Arabica	Robusta
3-Hydroxy-2-methyl-4-pyrone (maltol)	39	45
5,6-Dihydro-3,5-dihydroxy-2-methyl-4-pyrone (or 5,6-dihydro-5-hydroxymaltol)	13	10
3,5-Dihydroxy-2-methyl-4-pyrone (5-hydroxymaltol)	15	6

[a] From Tressl et al. (1978a)

(xi) *Other compounds*

Hydrogen peroxide has been found in roasted coffee (Fujita et al., 1985a).

(c) *Compounds in instant coffee*

The quantitative data presented refer generally to dry instant coffee (powder or granules). To obtain representative values for the content in the beverage, it is convenient and realistic to assume use of 2 g instant coffee per 150-ml cup. With 100% solubility, the content in milligrams per kilogram for a given component of instant coffee should be divided by 500 to give the content in milligrams per cup.

(i) *Nonvolatile substances*

Caffeine and other purines: Caffeine levels have been determined directly in 12 commercial samples using HPLC methods (Trugo et al., 1983); the range was 28-48 g/kg [which would correspond to 56-92 mg/cup]. The higher level resulted from higher levels of robusta in the blend. The caffeine contents of instant coffees manufactured in Brazil are somewhat lower: Angelucci et al. (1973), using a spectrophotometric method on 15 arabica samples, reported levels of 1.63-3.86%, with one robusta containing 4.64%. Minute amounts of the other alkaloids that occur in roasted and green coffees also appear in instant coffee, at approximately half the amount.

Chlorogenic acids and related substances: Trugo and Macrae (1984b) determined by HPLC the chlorogenic acid content of 13 commercial instant coffees bought in the UK. Total chlorogenic acids ranged from 3.61 to 10.73%; the levels were 2.55-7.64% for total caffeoylquinic acids, 0.16-0.58% for total dicaffeoylquinic acids and 0.74-1.93% for total feruloyl quinic acids. The levels found depended on the extraction conditions and on differences between varieties. Data from other workers (summarized by Clifford, 1985) showed a similar range for total chlorogenic acids; Maier (1987a) found [2.7-8.9%] in five samples. The lower figures resulted from use of darkly roasted coffees. The Working Group estimated that these values correspond to 54-215 mg/cup.

Glycosides: Viani (1988) estimated the content of atractyligenin at 0.8-0.9 mg/cup of arabica instant coffee and negligible for robusta.

Lipids: Instant coffees are generally free of lipids (and therefore the diterpenes, kahweol and cafestol), but many commercial brands are plated with about 0.3-0.5% coffee oil obtained by expression from roasted coffee or other methods to provide headspace aroma. Viani (1988) reported 0.02% oil and 0.0002% diterpenes in nonaromatized powder and 0.3% and 0.02%, respectively, in aromatized powder, corresponding to 0.4 mg/cup oil and 0.004 mg/cup diterpenes in nonaromatized powder and 7 mg/cup oil and 0.4 mg/cup diterpenes in aromatized powder. Certain commercial brands of instant coffee contain up to 10% by weight of very finely ground roasted coffee; this will increase these figures by 1.6% oil and 0.12% diterpenes in the powder, or 32 and 2.4 mg/cup, respectively, making this brew comparable with an espresso-type brew.

Trigonelline and nicotinic acid: Trigonelline has been determined in 12 UK commercial dry instant coffees by HPLC; an average of 1.37% (range, 0.94-1.69%) was found (Trugo *et al.*, 1983), [corresponding to 20-35 mg/cup, although the data on roasted coffee would suggest figures of 8-44 mg/cup]. Viani (1988) reported trigonelline at 5-15 mg/cup in 22 samples, which were therefore probably darkly roasted. In the same samples, nicotinic acid was found at 0.2-1.2 mg/cup; the data for roasted coffee suggest similar levels [0.4-1.6 mg/cup].

Acids: Of the nonvolatile acids, quinic, citric, malic and pyruvic acids are known to be present in fairly large quantities. Blanc (1977) reported on the total quantity of citric, malic, lactic and pyruvic acids and of the volatile acetic acid in instant coffees from four different countries. A range of 1.5-4.9% was found, which suggests that the acid content is increased only slightly as a consequence of industrial processing from roasted to dried extracts. Any increase occurring during extraction is balanced by loss during drying. Schormüller *et al.* (1961) reported average values of 2.20% citric acid, 0.50% malic acid, 0.45% lactic acid, 0.95% acetic acid and 0.08% pyruvic acid in dry instant coffee, to give a total of 4.18%, suggesting a marked increase in the level of acetic acid. Instant coffees derived from medium-roasted arabica coffee tend to have higher acid contents than darkly roasted robusta. Average levels of 3.8% (German instant coffees) and 2.3% (French instant coffee) result in [76 and 46 mg/cup], respectively.

Trace elements: The main mineral element in roasted and instant coffee is potassium, and levels can range from 3.6 to 5.9% in dry instant coffee (Clarke, 1985). Maier (1981) compiled data on all other elements present or likely to be present. In instant coffee, trace elements can originate both from the roasted coffee and from the water used for extraction: the content in the water can be at least tripled during evaporation and drying of the extracts to the final product. Instant coffee is manufactured almost entirely in stainless-steel equipment, from which contamination is minimal (Clarke, 1985).

Other components: As a consequence of industrial extraction, higher percentages of melanoidins (see p. 71), polysaccharides and 'proteins' are found in instant coffee than in the soluble part of brewed coffee. Dissolution of a greater amount of polysaccharides is accompanied by some cleavage into constituent monoses, indicated by the presence of small quantitites of arabinose, galactose and mannose (Trugo, 1985).

(ii) *Volatile compounds*

Little quantitative information and few comprehensive listings are available of the volatile compounds present in commercial instant coffee. Certain volatile compounds, particularly sulfides and other non-polar substances, that occur preferentially in the oil of roasted coffee rather than in the carbohydrate matrix will be present as a result of 'aromatization' with coffee oil. Over 80 volatile compounds were identified in a commercial freeze-dried brew, including thiazoles, thiophenes, pyridines, pyrroles, pyrazines and furfurals (Dart & Nursten, 1985); the preparation was relatively rich in the latter two groups of compounds. In general, the volatile compounds found in brewed coffee can be expected to occur, to a greater or lesser extent.

Carbonyls: Methylglyoxal has been quantified in instant coffee by derivative GC (see also the monograph on methylglyoxal, p. 445), at levels of 23 ppm (μg/g; Hayashi & Shibamoto, 1985), 404-994 ppm (Shane *et al.*, 1988) and 70-217 ppm (Aeschbacher *et al.*, 1989). Kasai *et al.* (1982) found 100-150 μg/cup assuming 1.5 g of instant coffee for 100 ml water. Aeschbacher *et al.* (1989) also reported the presence of 13-42 μg/g diacetyl and 5-25 μg/g glyoxal in dry product.

Acids: The volatile and nonvolatile acid content of instant coffee is discussed above (pp. 80 and 86).

Esters: Methyl salicylate was found at 0-8.4 mg/l in nine samples of instant coffee (2 g powder/100 ml water; Swain *et al.*, 1985).

Furan- and sulfur-based compounds: Some compounds containing sulfur were quantified in instant coffee: furfuryl thiol, 3.90 ppm (mg/kg); 5-methyl furfuryl methyl disulfide, 0.015 mg/kg; and kahweofuran, 0.60 mg/kg. Three other furans have also been quantified (Tressl & Silwar, 1981). In general, these figures are comparable with those for roasted coffee, but when they are calculated as milligrams per cup they are quite low [e.g., kahweofuran, 1.2 μg/cup].

Pyrones: Tressl (1980) found more maltol (60-120 ppm (mg/kg)) than was expected.

Other compounds: Hydrogen peroxide has been detected at 180 ppm (mg/kg) in instant coffee (Aeschbacher *et al.*, 1989), and formaldehyde was found at 10-16.3 ppm (Hayashi *et al.*, 1986). Cyclotene, found at 70-110 mg/kg, occurred at a higher level than would have been expected from roasted coffees (Tressl, 1980).

No data were available to the Working Group on alcohols, nitrogen compounds, other sulfur compounds or phenols.

(d) Compounds in decaffeinated coffee

Under the Directives of the Commission of the European Communities (1977, 1985), dry decaffeinated instant coffees must contain no more than 0.3% caffeine; in practice, they contain less. This figure corresponds to 0-6 mg/cup of instant coffee brew, which also corresponds to that found (Barone & Roberts, 1984).

The solvents used in decaffeination may remove small quantities of aroma precursors, e.g., trigonelline, or increase their levels, e.g., amino acids and reducing sugars.

(e) Additives and contaminants

(i) Flavouring additives

Both roasted and instant coffees are largely marketed throughout the world as 100% pure coffee products, and are clearly labelled as such in developed countries (Commission of the European Communities, 1985). Blends are also available with many different kinds of roasted plant products, including chicory and malted and unmalted barley. Worldwide consumption in 1985 of dried chicory roots was estimated at 128 000 tonnes per annum, of which 32% was consumed in France, 55% in other European countries and 12% in South Africa. After roasting, chicory is mixed with both roasted and instant coffee, but no information was available on the quantities used. The quantities consumed annually of mixtures with barley vary considerably, in relation to the cost of coffee (Maier, 1987b).

(ii) Other additives

Preservatives are not used. Occasionally, roasted and instant coffees have been used as vehicles for vitamins and minerals. Flow agents (sodium aluminium silicates) may be incorporated in instant coffees used in vending machines (by national derogation in the Directive of the Commission of the European Communities).

(iii) Contaminants

For the purpose of this section of the monograph, the term 'contaminants' is used to mean those constituents sometimes present in the products, and therefore in the beverages derived from them, which are not essential to the flavour and properties of the beverage. Some of these potential contaminants have known toxicological and, in some cases, carcinogenic effects.

Mycotoxins: Numerous studies, especially since 1965, have been conducted on the occurrence of mycotoxins in green coffee, and therefore in roasted and brewed coffee, due to the presence of mouldy beans. These studies were reviewed comprehensively by Strobel (1988b) and more briefly by Viani (1988). In particular, aflatoxin B_1 (see IARC, 1976a, 1987), ochratoxin A (see IARC, 1983, 1987) and, less often, sterigmatocystin (see IARC, 1976b) have been found in consignments of green coffees containing mouldy beans, although regulations seek to prevent such importation. Levels of aflatoxin B_1 at 3-12 ppb (μg/kg) in 2% of samples analysed, of ochratoxin A at 0.5-360 ppb in 3.5% of samples, and of sterigmatocystin at 1140 and 12 000 ppb in two very mouldy samples have been measured in some 2000 consignments examined. Decaffeinated green coffee beans that have been allowed to go mouldy show a greater tendency to develop toxins than nondecaffeinated coffee on account of the absence of the inhibitory action of caffeine. Ochratoxin A was found to be largely destroyed (80-99%) on roasting, as was aflatoxin B_1, to a slightly lesser extent.

Pesticides: Coffee beans are protected from pests within the cherry by direct application of pesticides, details of which have been reported (Mitchell, 1988; Snoeck, 1988). Coffee itself is consumed in the producing countries only after further processing, including roasting and brewing or extracting, which eliminate these contaminants almost quantitatively. Viani (1988) compiled available data on α- and β-hexachlorocyclohexanes, lindane, the DDT group, aldrin, dieldrin and others. Of six instant coffee samples, one contained 1.2 ng/g total hexachlorocyclohexanes and one contained 3 ng/g lindane, but no other pesticide was found. In contrast, 15 of 150 samples of green coffee had traces up to 290 ng/g lindane.

Nitrosamines: *N*-Nitrosopyrrolidine (see IARC, 1978) was found in five of ten instant coffees at 0.3-1.4 ppb (μg/kg) by Sen and Seaman (1981). The presence of this nitrosamine has been confirmed in two of seven samples of instant coffee by mass spectrometry as well as by liquid chromatography-thermal energy analysis at levels of 1.5 and 2.8 ppb (μg/kg). In one of six samples of roasted, ground coffee, *N*-nitrosopyrrolidine was found at a level of 0.4 ppb (μg/kg) (Sen *et al.*, 1990).

3. Biological Data Relevant to the Evaluation of Carcinogenic Risk to Humans

3.1 Carcinogenicity studies in animals

(a) Perinatal exposure/oral administration

Mouse: In a study available only as a preliminary report, groups of 150 male and 150 female Swiss mice (CRL:COBS, CD-1) were mated at 12 weeks of age, and mothers of mice to be allocated to treated groups received 1% instant coffee in the diet throughout gestation and lactation. After weaning, offspring were housed singly and received diets containing 0, 1, 2.5 or 5% (w/w) instant coffee [origin unspecified] until the end of the experiment at 720 days. Increasing levels of coffee in the diet impaired the growth of animals, but better survival was noted in animals that received the higher doses: at 24 months, the survival rate in the group receiving 5% instant coffee was 50% compared with about 25% in controls. Tumours of the liver, lung and lymphatic tissue were observed frequently. The incidences of benign liver-cell tumours in males were 42/150 controls, 38/150 receiving 1%, 20/150 receiving 2.5% and 16/150 receiving 5%; those in females were 2/150 controls, 2/150 receiving 1%, 1/150 receiving 2.5% and 1/150 receiving 5%. Two hepatocellular carcinomas were observed in one male mouse treated with 1% instant coffee and in one male mouse treated with 2.5%, but none was seen in mice receiving 5% or in controls. [The Working Group noted that hepatocellular tumours are common in Swiss mice.] No increase in the incidence of benign or malignant lung tumours was observed. Lymphosarcomas (all histological types) were observed in male and female control and treated animals. In males, the incidence of these tumours decreased from 32% in controls to 12% in the high-dose group. In females, no clear dose-dependent decrease was observed, although the incidence of lymphosarcomas was 46% in controls and 18% in the high-dose group (Stalder *et al.*, 1984). [The Working Group noted that the reduced numbers of liver adenomas in males and of lymphosarcomas in animals of each sex in the higher-dose groups might have been due to impaired growth; these animals also had longer survival. Neither of these factors was taken into account in the analysis.]

Rat: Groups of 55 male and 55 female F_1 Sprague-Dawley rats, five to six weeks old, were given 25, 50 or 100% freshly brewed coffee as drinking fluid *ad libitum* for two years, at which time all survivors were killed. The animals were derived from females given 50% coffee as drinking fluid for about five weeks before mating and throughout gestation and lactation. Parent males, parent control females and two groups of F_1 control rats received tap-water only. Ten rats of each sex per group were killed at one year and were submitted to blood sampling and necropsy. Lower mean body weights were observed in males that received 100% coffee, and significantly increased mortality was seen in females given 50 and 100% coffee. Two statistical methods were used to adjust the incidence data for survival differences: In the first, which assumes that tumours are non-fatal (i.e., incidental), a significant increase in the number of tumour-bearing males was seen in the low-dose group (relative risk (RR), 1.26; $p < 0.05$) but in no other group. In the second analysis, which assumes that tumours are lethal, increased numbers of tumour-bearing animals were seen among males in the low- and mid-dose groups (RR, 1.71, $p < 0.01$ and 1.43, $p < 0.05$, respectively) and among females in the mid- and high-dose groups (RR, 1.47, $p < 0.05$ and 1.45, $p < 0.05$, respectively) (Palm *et al.*, 1984). [The Working Group noted that the first statistical analysis was more appropriate, since the tumours were not the cause of death.]

(b) *Oral administration*

Rat: In a study reported as a letter to the Editor of *The Lancet*, 144 male and 144 female Sprague-Dawley rats, 21 days of age, were administered 5% instant coffee in the diet for two years, at which time the survivors were killed. An untreated control group of 41 males and 41 females was available. The urinary bladders of 94 male and 99 female treated and 29 male and 29 female control animals were examined histologically. No hyperplasia or tumour of the urinary bladder was observed (Zeitlin, 1972). [The Working Group noted the incomplete reporting of the study: no information on survival was given, and only the bladder was examined histologically.]

Groups of 40 male and 40 female Sprague-Dawley rats, weighing approximately 100 g, were fed diets containing 6% of 13 different samples of instant coffee; caffeine had been removed by extraction with dichloromethane from seven of the samples, but in three of these the caffeine had been put back. Treatment was for two years, at which time all survivors were killed. A control group of 40 males and 40 females was available. Survival was similar in all groups, although males given the decaffeinated coffees had slightly lower death rates, but the body weights of treated males were lower than those of controls. No increase in the incidence of any type of tumour was noted. In males in two of the six groups given instant coffee and in one of the three groups given decaffeinated coffee plus caffeine (see also the monograph on caffeine p. 310), the incidence of benign and malignant tumours was significantly lowered (all $p < 0.05$); in females, the decrease was not statistically significant. A logistic regression analysis showed that the level of caffeine significantly lowered the incidence of tumours (Würzner *et al.*, 1977a,b). [The Working Group noted that only one control group was used for the 13 treatment groups and that the reduced numbers of tumours might have been due to impaired growth.]

(c) *Administration with known carcinogens*

The Working Group was aware of various other experiments (e.g., Mori & Hirono, 1977; Fujii *et al.*, 1980; Wattenberg & Lam, 1984; Nishikawa *et al.*, 1986) that were part of studies on the modifying effects of coffee on the activity of known carcinogens, which are not included here since their design was inadequate to reveal any effect of coffee on tumour production (short duration of exposure and/or limited numbers of animals).

(i) *Azaserine*

Rat: Groups of 40 male SPF Wistar rats, 19 days of age, were given a single intraperitoneal injection of azaserine, a pancreatic carcinogen, at 30 mg/kg bw and were then fed a low-fat diet, a high-fat diet or a high-fat diet plus coffee solution as the drinking fluid. The concentration of coffee was increased gradually from 25% during the first two weeks to 100% within four weeks, which was continued for the life span of the animals. Animals were autopsied 15 months after the end of azaserine treatment. The mean body weight of rats given the high-fat diet and coffee was significantly lower than that of the high-fat controls. The number of pancreatic tumours was significantly smaller in the group maintained on the high-fat diet and coffee than in the group on a high-fat diet only (44 adenomas *versus* 176 [$p < 0.001$] and 28 carcinomas *versus* 57 [$p < 0.05$]) (Woutersen *et al.*, 1989). [The Working Group noted that the decrease could have been due, at least partly, to the impaired growth of the animals.]

(ii) *7,12-Dimethylbenz[a]anthracene*

Rat: Groups of 40-41 female Sprague-Dawley rats, 53-55 days of age, were given a single intravenous injection of 7,12-dimethylbenz[*a*]anthracene (DMBA) at 20 mg/kg bw. Coffee (moderate or full strength) and decaffeinated (97% caffeine-free) coffee were given instead of drinking-water 29 days before up to three days after DMBA treatment; the experiment was terminated 12-18 weeks after DMBA treatment. Further groups of 80 or 84 female rats received a single dose of DMBA at 5 mg by gavage at 54 or 55 days of age and three days later were given coffee in the drinking fluid until 18-21 weeks after DMBA treatment. After DMBA treatment, all rats were palpated at two-week intervals for the presence of mammary tumours. When tumours reached 2 cm in diameter, they were excised surgically, and the rat was placed back in the experiment. In rats treated by intravenous administration of DMBA, moderate and high doses of coffee significantly ($p < 0.05$) reduced the number of mammary carcinomas per rat. Consumption of high and moderate doses of decaffeinated coffee did not have this effect, but addition of caffeine at 860 mg to decaffeinated coffee resulted in a significant reduction ($p < 0.05$) in the number of mammary carcinomas per animal. Coffee consumption did not significantly affect the percentage of rats with mammary tumours. Administration of coffee to rats treated with DMBA by gavage did not significantly affect the number of mammary carcinomas per animal (Welsch et al., 1988).

In a subsequent study with the same experimental protocol (intravenous and gastric administration of DMBA) but with administration of a chemically defined diet containing 5% unsaturated fat (corn oil) *ad libitum*, similar results with coffee were obtained, i.e., a reduction in the number of mammary tumours per rat but no effect on the percentage of rats with tumours (Welsch & DeHoog, 1988).

Hamster. Groups of 20 female Syrian golden hamsters, weighing approximately 70 g, were fed powdered chow or chow supplemented with 20% powdered green coffee beans. Two weeks later, the right buccal pouch of 16 animals from each group was painted three times with a 0.5% solution of DMBA in heavy mineral oil; the remaining four animals per group were treated three times weekly with heavy mineral oil alone and served as controls. The experiment was terminated after a total of 50 treatments (16.5 weeks). At the end of the experiment, 12/16 animals given chow alone and 9/16 also given green coffee beans were still alive; most of the losses were due to respiratory infections or ether anaesthesia. Tumours of the buccal pouch were seen in 9/12 animals receiving chow (eight had multiple tumours) and 2/9 also receiving green coffee beans. Two hamsters receiving chow had mild to moderate dysplasia of the right buccal pouch and one had dysplasia, including carcinoma *in situ*; the buccal pouches of the nine remaining animals had various grades of dysplasia, including carcinoma *in situ* and papillary carcinomas. Of the animals receiving green coffee beans, only two had carcinomas of the right buccal pouch; the remaining seven showed dysplasia. A statistically significant reduction in average tumour mass was observed in the latter group (Miller et al., 1988). [The Working Group noted that survival was low.]

(iii) *N-Nitrosobis(2-oxypropyl)amine*

Hamster. Groups of 40 male Syrian golden hamsters, six weeks old, received two weekly subcutaneous injections of 20 mg/kg bw *N*-nitrosobis(2-oxypropyl)-amine and were then fed a low-fat diet, a high-fat diet or a high-fat diet plus daily preparations of coffee as the drinking fluid. The concentration of coffee was gradually increased from 25% during the first two weeks to 100% within four weeks, which was continued for the life span of the animals. The hamsters were killed 12 months after the second injection of nitrosamine, and autopsied. Mean body weights of animals on high-fat diet alone were significantly greater than those of animals on low-fat diet; those of hamsters fed high-fat diets with caffeine did not differ significantly from those of animals on the high-fat diet alone. The total number of ductal/ductular adenocarcinomas of the pancreas was significantly increased in the high-fat group (eight; $p < 0.05$) as compared to the low-fat group (two). The total number of adenocarcinomas in the group receiving high-fat diet plus coffee (five) was slightly but not significantly smaller than that in the group on high-fat diet alone (Woutersen *et al.*, 1989).

3.2 Other relevant data

(a) *Experimental systems*

(i) *Absorption, distribution, metabolism and excretion*

No data were available to the Working Group (see the monograph on caffeine p. 321).

(ii) *Toxic effects*

Groups of male Wistar rats were given 4 or 8% brewed or decaffeinated coffee in the drinking-water for six to eight months. Body weights of coffee-treated rats were 6-7% lower than those of controls receiving water only. Coffee induced 'no untoward effect' on the liver (Strubelt *et al.*, 1973).

Weanling male Sprague-Dawley rats were fed starch-based diets supplemented with either brewed coffee, decaffeinated coffee, tea, caffeine or nothing (controls). Compared with controls, rats consuming coffee or caffeine had elevated concentrations of cholesterol and phospholipids. In addition, both groups had lower levels of triglycerides, although the difference was significant only for the group receiving caffeine (Naismith *et al.*, 1969).

Six male and nine female adult rhesus monkeys were fed an atherogenic diet *ad libitum* for 12 months. Major changes in the profiles of total plasma lipids and lipoproteins occurred within three to six months and remained at the higher level thereafter. Four females and three males were then given 50% coffee as drinking fluid for 12 months, while the remaining animals were given water. The authors reported no significant difference in total plasma protein or lipids between coffee-treated and control animals after 15 and 18 months (Callahan *et al.*, 1979).

In a study reported as an abstract, coffee did not enhance the number or size of pancreatic atypical acinar-cell foci induced in rats by azaserine (Roebuck *et al.*, 1985).

(iii) *Effects on reproduction and prenatal toxicity*

Brewed coffee: In a combined subchronic, reproductive and developmental toxicity study, Sprague-Dawley rats were given 12.5, 25 or 50% freshly percolated coffee as the drinking fluid (daily caffeine intake, 9, 19 or 38 mg/kg bw) for five weeks before mating, throughout gestation and until 27 days after parturition. No effect on fertility, litter size, neonatal growth or survival was observed with any dose level. Among the offspring, underdevelopment of the renal pelvis was observed in the mid- and high-dose groups; cleft palate and delayed ossification were also observed in the offspring, but these were not clearly dose-related (Palm *et al.*, 1978).

In a similarly designed study, Sprague-Dawley rats received 25, 50 or 100% percolated coffee as the drinking fluid (approximate daily caffeine intake, 20, 40 or 80 mg/kg bw) for 91 days, after which they were mated to produce F_{1a} litters, while the administration of coffee continued. Female rats were mated again ten days after their first litters had been weaned to produce F_{1b} litters, which were used for teratological examination. Parent rats treated with 50 and 100% coffee had enlarged livers and kidneys, but no significant effect on reproduction or lactation was observed. Body weights of F_{1a} offspring of the high-dose rats were comparable to those of controls at four days of age but had decreased significantly by weaning at 21 days of age. No teratogenic effect or decrease in neonatal body weight was observed in F_{1b} pups delivered by caesarean section, although offspring of rats given the mid- and high doses showed a significantly increased incidence of delayed ossification of the sternebrae (Nolen, 1981).

In a behavioural teratology study, Sprague-Dawley rats were given either drinking-water or fresh drip coffee as drinking fluid from the time of mating until parturition. The average daily dose of caffeine was 122 mg/kg bw. Significant decreases in body, liver and brain weights were observed in the offspring of the coffee-treated group at birth but not at 30 days of age. In addition, a significant increase in motor activity and a decrease in grooming time and time spent with a novel object were observed in this group at 30 days of age (Groisser *et al.*, 1982).

In another behavioural study, Sprague-Dawley rats received 0, 25 or 100% brewed coffee as the drinking fluid from 60 days before mating until weaning of the F_1 offspring. No effect on reproduction was observed. Among the offspring of treated rats, there were delays in the eruption of incisor teeth and maturation of swimming skills. A significant decrease in running wheel and preweaning open-field activities was also observed, but no effect was seen on learning, memory or motor function. On the basis of post-weaning measurements, the authors concluded that the treatment did not result in a significant risk for irreversible damage in the offspring (Butcher *et al.*, 1984).

Instant coffee: In a combined subchronic, reproductive and developmental toxicity study of instant coffee (Nolen, 1981), described above, the body weights of F_{1a} offspring of high-dose dams were comparable to those of controls at four days of age but had decreased significantly by weaning at 21 days of age. No teratogenic effect or decrease in fetal body weight was observed in F_{1b} pups delivered by caesarean section, although offspring of the high-dose group had a significantly increased incidence of delayed ossification of the sternebrae.

Groups of white mice [strain unspecified] were fed instant coffee crystals in the diet, at doses equivalent to human consumption of 0, 4, 8, 12, 16 or 20 cups of coffee per day, from the time of mating to parturition. No abnormality or gross malformation of the alimentary tract was observed in the offspring, but pup body weight and length were significantly decreased at doses equivalent to eight cups of coffee or more (Murphy & Benjamin, 1981).

Sprague-Dawley rats were given 1.5% (w/v) solvent-free, freeze-dried coffee solution as the drinking fluid from the time of mating until gestation day 21 or postnatal day 14. When treatment was continued until postnatal day 14, offspring of coffee-treated and control groups were cross-fostered. No gross malformation, difference in organ or fetal body weights, or change in iron, zinc or copper levels in maternal plasma, liver or kidney or in fetal liver were observed. Offspring of dams treated with coffee prenatally had significantly decreased birth weights; no change in body weight was observed three or four days after birth (Muñoz et al., 1986).

Decaffeinated coffee: In a combined subchronic, reproductive and developmental toxicity study, Sprague-Dawley rats received 25, 50 or 100% decaffeinated brewed and instant coffee as the drinking fluid (equivalent to 12, 25 or 50 cups of coffee per day) with the same study design as described previously (Nolen, 1981). No effect on reproduction, litter size or postnatal viability of the F_{1a} litters was observed. Body weights of offspring of mid- and high-dose dams were comparable to those of controls at four days of age but were significantly decreased at weaning. No malformation or variation was observed in F_{1b} offspring, and no delay in ossification was seen (Nolen, 1982).

In a behavioural teratology study, Sprague-Dawley rats received freshly brewed decaffeinated coffee (average daily caffeine intake, 4.5 mg/kg bw) as the drinking fluid from the time of mating until parturition. A significant decrease in the liver weights of the offspring was observed at birth, and a significant increase in motor activity and a decrease in time spent grooming or with a novel object were seen (Groisser et al., 1982).

(iv) *Genetic and related effects*

The genetic and related effects of various types of coffee have been reviewed (Sugimura, 1982; Sugimura & Sato, 1983; Aeschbacher et al., 1984a; Nagao et al., 1984; Sugimura et al., 1984; Nagao et al., 1986b; Aeschbacher, 1990). In bacteria, there is evidence that dicarbonyls (e.g., methylglyoxal) and hydrogen peroxide acting together contribute to the mutagenic activity of roasted coffee (Nagao et al., 1984; Fujita et al., 1985a,b). Both the dicarbonyls and hydrogen peroxide may be deactivated by enzymes present in cells and tissue, such as glyoxalase, glutathione (for methylglyoxal), catalase and peroxidase (for hydrogen peroxide) (Nagao *et al.*, 1984; Friederich *et al.*, 1985; Fujita *et al.*, 1985b; Tucker *et al.*, 1989). In mammalian cells, coffee aroma stripped from roasted coffee and the dicarbonyls contained therein may contribute to the genetic effects (Aeschbacher *et al.*, 1985; Tucker *et al.*, 1989). There is substantial evidence in various genetic test systems, with one exception (Graf & Würgler, 1986), that caffeine is not involved in the genetic activity observed (Nagao *et al.*, 1979; Aeschbacher, 1990).

Coffee has been studied in experimental genetic and related systems as both instant coffee powders and as finely ground roasted coffee beans prepared with water in the normal way for drinking and then lyophilized. The doses are expressed as mass of coffee powder used in the treatment, which generally required the powder to be dissolved in the treatment solvent. Sterilization of preparations to be tested for bacterial mutagenicity, by filtration or autoclaving, did not influence the results significantly (Aeschbacher *et al.*, 1980). Time between sample preparation and test may affect the genetic response. In several studies, where specifically noted, the coffee was solvent-extracted or chemically fractionated. Studies in bacteria of green coffee beans indicate a lack of mutagenic activity (Kosugi *et al.*, 1983; Albertini *et al.*, 1985; Dorado *et al.*, 1987); similar comparisons of roasted and unroasted beans have not been made with other systems.

The results of the studies on genetic and related effects are listed at the end of this section in Table 29, with the evaluation of the Working Group, as positive, negative or inconclusive, as defined in the footnotes. The results are tabulated separately for the presence and absence of an exogenous metabolic activation system. The lowest effective dose (LED), in the case of positive results, and the highest ineffective dose (HID), in the case of negative results, are shown together with the appropriate reference. The studies are summarized briefly below.

Brewed coffee: Freshly brewed coffee induced prophage lambda in lysogenic *Escherichia coli* K12.

A number of studies have been conducted on the mutagenicity of coffees to *Salmonella typhimurium* under different conditions. Brewed coffee consistently induced mutations in *S. typhimurium* TA100, and mutations were also induced in TA102 and TA104, which are more sensitive to oxidative mutagens, and in *E. coli* WP2 *uvrA*/pKM101. There are conflicting reports on the mutagenicity of coffee to *S. typhimurium* TA98. [The Working Group noted the inadequate reporting of several of the studies with TA98.] Coffee gave negative results in standard strains of *S. typhimurium*, which do not contain the pKM101 plasmid. Brewed coffee was also mutagenic in the *S. typhimurium* L-arabinose-resistance forward mutation assay in strain BA13.

There was no significant response in tests for sex-linked recessive lethal mutation, dominant lethal mutation or chromosome loss in *Drosophila melanogaster*, but weak activity was observed in the somatic cell (wing imaginal disc) mutation and mitotic recombination tests following larval feeding. These effects were attributed to caffeine.

Treatment of cultured human lymphocytes with brewed coffee induced sister chromatid exchange, gaps, breaks and total chromosomal aberrations. Endoreduplicated cells were induced in Chinese hamster ovary AUXB1 cells. Bisulfite, which complexes carbonyls, reduced the frequency of sister chromatid exchange and endoreduplicated cells, while catalase and peroxidase treatment had no effect (Tucker *et al.*, 1989). Coffee aroma stripped from roasted coffee beans also induced gaps, breaks and total chromosomal aberrations in human peripheral lymphocytes.

Instant coffee: Instant coffee induced prophage lambda in lysogenic *E. coli* K12, strain GY5027 but did not induce SOS activity in *S. typhimurium* TA1535/pSK1002.

Instant coffee induced mutations in *S. typhimurium* TA100 but not in TA98, TA1535, TA1537 or TA1538. Instant coffees were mutagenic to *S. typhimurium* strains TA102 and TA104, which are more sensitive to oxidative mutagens. Instant coffee was also active in the *S. typhimurium* L-arabinose-resistance forward mutation assay in strain BA13. The mutagens in coffee are inactivated by the cytosolic fraction of exogenous metabolic systems from rat liver, by heat in the presence of oxygen (Friederich *et al.*, 1985), by sodium sulfite (Suwa *et al.*, 1982) and by catalase (Fujita *et al.*, 1985b). This evidence, together with that from other studies, led to the conclusion that an interaction of methylglyoxal with hydrogen peroxide accounts for most of the mutagenicity of instant coffee (Fujita *et al.*, 1985a,b).

Negative results were obtained in host-mediated assays in which coffee was administered to male Swiss mice by gavage after intraperitoneal injection of *S. typhimurium* TA1530. Similarly, negative results were obtained in the intrasanguinous test following intravenous injection of *E. coli* K12 into male Swiss mice and assaying for reverse and forward mutation at the nia^+ and gal^+ loci, respectively.

Treatment of Chinese hamster lung cells with instant coffee increased the frequency of mutations in the diphtheria toxin resistance assay. Most of the mutagenicity was suppressed by sodium bisulfite. Methylglyoxal was shown to account for less than 3% of the mutagenicity (Nakasato *et al.*, 1984).

There was no significant response in tests for sex-linked recessive lethal mutation, dominant lethal mutation or chromosome loss in *Drosophila melanogaster*, but weak activity was observed in the somatic cell (wing imaginal disc) mutation and mitotic recombination tests following larval feeding. These effects were attributed to caffeine.

Treatment of cultured human lymphocytes with instant coffee induced gaps, breaks and total chromosomal aberrations. Sister chromatid exchange and endoreduplicated cells were induced in Chinese hamster ovary AUXB1 cells (Tucker et al., 1989).

Instant coffee administered to Chinese hamsters as a single oral dose did not increase the frequency of sister chromatid exchange. In a micronucleus test, Swiss mice were given five consecutive daily oral doses of instant coffee; no significant induction of micronuclei above spontaneous levels was observed. Two oral doses to Swiss mice of coffee aroma (up to 50 ml/kg bw) also gave negative results (Aeschbacher et al., 1984b). In another study, no significant increase in the frequency of micronuclei was induced by single or multiple administrations of instant coffee by gavage (Shimizu & Yano, 1987). [The Working Group noted that the authors reported a tendency for the number of micronuclei to increase in a dose-related fashion.]

Decaffeinated coffee: Decaffeinated coffee induced prophage lambda in lysogenic *E. coli* K12, strain GY5027. It induced mutation in *S. typhimurium* TA98, TA100, TA102 and TA104, which are sensitive to oxidative mutagens. No effect was observed in *Drosophila melanogaster* when decaffeinated coffee was assayed for the induction of somatic cell (wing imaginal disc) mutation and mitotic recombination. Treatment of cultured human lymphocytes with decaffeinated coffee induced gaps, breaks and total chromosomal aberrations. Sister chromatid exchange and endoreduplicated cells were induced in Chinese hamster ovary AUXB1 cells (Tucker et al., 1989).

Coffee in combination with known mutagens: Brewed coffee, instant coffee and decaffeinated coffee suppressed SOS induction by ultra-violet light, 2-(2-furyl)-3-(5-nitro-2-furyl)acrylamide, 4-nitroquinoline-N-oxide and N-methyl-N'-nitro-N-nitrosoguanidine in *S. typhimurium* TA1535/pSK1002 (Obana et al., 1986). Instant, decaffeinated and brewed coffee inhibited mutagenesis resulting from the nitrosation of methylurea in *S. typhimurium* TA1535 (Stich et al., 1982).

In mouse bone-marrow micronucleus tests, positive responses to mitomycin C, cyclophosphamide and procarbazine (but not adriamycin) were significantly reduced by administration of instant coffee 2 h before the clastogens. Similar effects were observed with decaffeinated and brewed coffee on the micronucleating effect of mitomycin C, and with brewed coffee on the effect of procarbazine (Abraham, 1989). In contrast, it has been reported that instant coffee caused no significant alteration in the incidence of micronuclei induced by N-nitrosodimethylamine (Shimizu & Yano, 1987).

Table 29. Genetic and related effects of brewed, instant and decaffeinated coffee

Test system	Results without exogenous metabolic activation	Results with exogenous metabolic activation	Dose[a] LED/HID	Reference
Brewed coffee				
PRB, λ Prophage induction in E. coli K12, strain GY5027	+	0	5700.0000	Kosugi et al. (1983)
PRB, λ Prophage induction in E. coli, strain GY5022	–	0	21400.0000	Kosugi et al. (1983)
SAF, Salmonella typhimurium BA13, forward mutation to AraR	+	0	1000.0000	Dorado et al. (1987)
SAF, Salmonella typhimurium BA13, forward mutation to AraR	–	0	500.0000	Ariza et al. (1988)
SA0, Salmonella typhimurium TA100, reverse mutation	+	–	7000.0000	Nagao et al. (1979)
SA0, Salmonella typhimurium TA100, reverse mutation	+	(+)	12500.0000	Aeschbacher & Würzner (1980)
SA0, Salmonella typhimurium TA100, reverse mutation	+	(+)	5000.0000	Shane et al. (1988)
SA0, Salmonella typhimurium TA100, reverse mutation	+	0	6000.0000	Kosugi et al. (1983)
SA0, Salmonella typhimurium TA100, reverse mutation	+	–	50000.0000	Kam (1980)
SA2, Salmonella typhimurium TA102, reverse mutation	+	(+)	2500.0000	Shane et al. (1988)
SA4, Salmonella typhimurium TA104, reverse mutation	+	(+)	5000.0000	Shane et al. (1988)
SA5, Salmonella typhimurium TA1535, reverse mutation	–	–	25000.0000	Aeschbacher & Würzner (1980)
SA7, Salmonella typhimurium TA1537, reverse mutation	–	–	25000.0000	Aeschbacher & Würzner (1980)
SA8, Salmonella typhimurium TA1538, reverse mutation	–	–	25000.0000	Aeschbacher & Würzner (1980)
SA9, Salmonella typhimurium TA98, reverse mutation	–	–	0.0000	Nagao et al. (1979)
SA9, Salmonella typhimurium TA98, reverse mutation	–	–	25000.0000	Aeschbacher & Würzner (1980)
SA9, Salmonella typhimurium TA98, reverse mutation	+	–	50000.0000	Kam (1980)
ECR, E. coli WP2 uvrA/pKM101, reverse mutation	+	0	7500.0000	Kosugi et al. (1983)
DMN, Drosophila melanogaster, sex chromosome losses	(+)	0	30000.0000	Graf & Würgler (1986)
DMM, Drosophila melanogaster, somatic mutation (larval feeding)	(+)	0	30000.0000	Graf & Würgler (1986)
DMM, Drosophila melanogaster, mitotic recombination	–	0	30000.0000	Graf & Würgler (1986)
DMX, Drosophila melanogaster, sex-linked recessive lethal mutation	–	0	30000.0000	Graf & Würgler (1986)
DML, Drosophila melanogaster, dominant lethal test	+	0	30000.0000	Graf & Würgler (1986)
SIC, Chinese hamster ovary AUXB1, sister chromatid exchange	+	0	200.0000	Tucker et al. (1989)
CHL, Chromosomal aberrations, human lymphocytes in vitro	+	+	2500.0000	Aeschbacher et al. (1985)
SHL, Human peripheral lymphocytes, sister chromatid exchange, in vitro	+	0	300.0000	Tucker et al. (1989)
MVH, Micronuclei, human (splenectomised) erythrocytes/reticulocytes in vivo	+	0	0.0000	Smith et al. (1990)

Table 29 (contd)

Test system	Results		Dose[a] LED/HID	Reference
	Without exogenous metabolic activation	With exogenous metabolic activation		

Instant coffee

Test system	Without	With	Dose	Reference
PRB, λ Prophage induction in E. coli K12, strain GY5027	+	0	5700.0000	Kosugi et al. (1983)
PRB, SOS repair	–	0	9000.0000	Obana et al. (1986)
PRB, λ Prophage induction in E. coli GY5022	+	0	21400.0000	Kosugi et al. (1983)
SAF, Salmonella typhimurium BA13, forward mutation	–	0	500.0000	Dorado et al. (1987)
SAF, Salmonella typhimurium BA13, forward mutation	+	0	500.0000	Ariza et al. (1988)
SA0, Salmonella typhimurium TA100, reverse mutation	+	–	1500.0000	Nagao et al. (1979)
SA0, Salmonella typhimurium TA100, reverse mutation	+	–	17500.0000	Aeschbacher & Würzner (1980)
SA0, Salmonella typhimurium TA100, reverse mutation	+	(+)	12500.0000	Shane et al. (1988)
SA0, Salmonella typhimurium TA100, reverse mutation	+	0	5000.0000	Aeschbacher et al. (1989)
SA2, Salmonella typhimurium TA102, reverse mutation	+	0	10000.0000	Aeschbacher et al. (1989)
SA2, Salmonella typhimurium TA102, reverse mutation	+	+	5000.0000	Shane et al. (1988)
SA4, Salmonella typhimurium TA104, reverse mutation	+	+	10000.0000	Shane et al. (1988)
SA5, Salmonella typhimurium TA1535, reverse mutation	–	–	25000.0000	Aeschbacher & Würzner (1980)
SA7, Salmonella typhimurium TA1537, reverse mutation	–	–	25000.0000	Aeschbacher & Würzner (1980)
SA8, Salmonella typhimurium TA1538, reverse mutation	–	–	25000.0000	Aeschbacher & Würzner (1980)
SA9, Salmonella typhimurium TA98, reverse mutation	–	–	0.0000	Nagao et al. (1979)
SA9, Salmonella typhimurium TA98, reverse mutation	–	–	25000.0000	Aeschbacher & Würzner (1980)
DMN, Drosophila melanogaster, sex chromosome losses	(+)	0	40000.0000	Graf & Würgler (1986)
DMM, Drosophila melanogaster, somatic mutation	(+)	0	40000.0000	Graf & Würgler (1986)
DMM, Drosophila melanogaster, mitotic recombination	–	0	40000.0000	Graf & Würgler (1986)
DMX, Drosophila melanogaster, sex-linked recessive lethal mutation	–	0	40000.0000	Graf & Würgler (1986)
DML, Drosophila melanogaster, dominant lethal test	–	0	40000.0000	Graf & Würgler (1986)
GCL, Chinese hamster lung (CHL) cells, diphtheria toxin resistance	+	0	4000.0000	Nakasato et al. (1984)
CHL, Chromosomal aberrations, human lymphocytes in vitro	+	+	25000.0000	Aeschbacher et al. (1985)
HMM, Host mediated assay, Salmonella typhimurium TA1530 in Swiss mice	–	0	6000.0000	Aeschbacher & Würzner (1980)
HMM, Intrasanguinous test, E. coli, Swiss mice	–	0	6000.0000	Aeschbacher & Würzner (1980)
SIC, Chinese hamster ovary AUXB1, sister chromatid exchange	+	0	200.0000	Tucker et al. (1989)
SVA, Sister chromatid exchange, Chinese hamsters in vivo	–	0	2500.0000	Aeschbacher et al. (1984b)
MVM, Micronucleus test, Swiss mice in vivo	–	0	3000.0000	Aeschbacher et al. (1984b)
MVM, Micronucleus test, ddy mice in vivo	–	0	2500.0000	Shimizu & Yano (1987)
MVM, Micronucleus test, ddy mice in vivo	–	0	1000.0000	Shimizu & Yano (1987)

Table 29 (contd)

Test system	Results		Dose[a] LED/HID	Reference
	Without exogenous metabolic activation	With exogenous metabolic activation		
Decaffeinated coffee				
PRB, λ Prophage induction in E. coli K12, strain GY5027	+	0	5700.0000	Kosugi et al. (1983)
SA0, Salmonella typhimurium TA100, reverse mutation	+	–	1500.0000	Nagao et al. (1979)
SA0, Salmonella typhimurium TA100, reverse mutation	+	(+)	2500.0000	Shane et al. (1988)
SA0, Salmonella typhimurium TA100, reverse mutation	+	–	50000.0000	Kam (1980)
SA2, Salmonella typhimurium TA102, reverse mutation	+	(+)	5000.0000	Shane et al. (1988)
SA4, Salmonella typhimurium TA104, reverse mutation	+	(+)	5000.0000	Shane et al. (1988)
SA9, Salmonella typhimurium TA98, reverse mutation	–	–	0.0000	Nagao et al. (1979)
SA9, Salmonella typhimurium TA98, reverse mutation	+	–	50000.0000	Kam (1980)
DMM, Drosophila melanogaster, somatic mutation	–	0	200000.0000	Graf & Würgler (1986)
DMM, Drosophila melanogaster, mitotic recombination	–	0	200000.0000	Graf & Würgler (1986)
SIC, Chinese hamster ovary AUXB1 cells, sister chromatid exchange	+	0	300.0000	Tucker et al. (1989)
CHL, Chromosomal aberrations, human lymphocytes in vitro	+	+	2500.0000	Aeschbacher et al. (1985)

[a]Expressed as dry weight of extract

(b) Humans

(i) *Toxic effects*

Coffee drinking has been associated with a number of adverse effects (Goldman, 1984; Spiller, 1984c; Stone, 1987). Many of the undesirable effects of coffee have been ascribed to caffeine, and they are dealt with in the respective monograph; at least some of the effects of coffee on plasma cholesterol and lipids, however, can be attributed to ingredients other than caffeine.

A weak association was seen between coffee drinking and total mortality among men in a 25-year follow-up from the Netherlands. No cause-specific mortality was reported (Vandenbroucke *et al.*, 1986).

Plasma cholesterol and lipoproteins: A series of epidemiological studies have investigated possible associations between coffee drinking and serum cholesterol levels; these have been reviewed (Thelle *et al.*, 1987). Many of the studies found that coffee consumption was positively associated, to variable degrees, with levels of total serum cholesterol in people of each sex (Thelle *et al.*, 1983; Kark *et al.*, 1985; Klatsky *et al.*, 1985; Tuomilehto *et al.*, 1987; Aro *et al.*, 1989). Other investigators found some association in men or women (Nichols *et al.*, 1976; Shirlow & Mathers, 1984; Mathias *et al.*, 1985; Curb *et al.*, 1986; Pietinen *et al.*, 1988) or in only some segments of the general population, e.g., individuals with coronary heart disease (Little *et al.*, 1966) or hypertension (Davis *et al.*, 1988). There are also a number of studies in which no association was observed (Phillips *et al.*, 1981; Hofman *et al.*, 1983; Kovar *et al.*, 1983; Aro *et al.*, 1985; Donahue *et al.*, 1987; Paoletti *et al.*, 1989).

Only a few scientists have investigated the relationship between coffee consumption and the concentration of individual serum lipoproteins. A positive association was observed between the level of low-density lipoproteins and coffee intake, whereas no such relation was seen with high-density lipoproteins or triglycerides (Førde *et al.*, 1985; Aro *et al.*, 1987; Bak & Grobbee, 1989; Paoletti *et al.*, 1989).

The conflicting data on the effects of coffee on serum cholesterol may be due to the use of different methods in the preparation of coffee. Thus, boiled coffee, but not filtered coffee, raised serum cholesterol (0.5-1.0 mmol/l) in three separate clinical trials conducted in Norway, Finland and the Netherlands (Førde *et al.*, 1985; Aro *et al.*, 1987; Bak & Grobbee, 1989). Epidemiological observations agree with the results of these clinical trials (Stensvold *et al.*, 1989; Pietinen *et al.*, 1990). Zock *et al.* (1990) suggest that a nonsaponifiable lipid fraction, isolated from boiled coffee by ultracentrifugation, raised serum cholesterol in healthy volunteers.

Coronary heart disease: The results of the Boston Collaborative Drug Surveillance Program (1972) suggest that consumption of more than five cups of coffee per day doubles the risk for myocardial infarction, as compared to no consumption at all. Similar results were reported by other investigators (Jick *et al.*, 1973; Mann & Thorogood, 1975; LaCroix *et al.*, 1986; LeGrady *et al.*, 1987; Rosenberg *et al.*, 1988). Some established only a modest association between myocardial infarction and heavy coffee consumption and for only some segments of the population (Rosenberg *et al.*, 1980, 1987; La Vecchia *et al.*, 1989a). Several other epidemiological studies found no association (Klatsky *et al.*, 1973; Dawber *et al.*, 1974; Hennekens *et al.*, 1976).

In some studies, the apparent association between coffee drinking and ischaemic heart disease can be accounted for by cigarette smoking (Hennekens *et al.*, 1976; Wilhelmsen *et al.*, 1977; La Vecchia *et al.*, 1989a).

[The Working Group was not aware of any longitudinal study on the association between coffee intake and the risk of coronary heart disease from populations with high consumption of boiled coffee.]

(ii) *Effects on reproduction and prenatal toxicity*

The reproductive effects of coffee on humans have been reviewed (Ernster, 1984; Leviton, 1984; James & Paull, 1985; Pieters, 1985; Heller, 1987; Schneider, 1987; Leviton, 1988). Most epidemiological studies have been affected by a number of methodological issues, including (i) inadequate measurement of intake: almost all studies relied on reported intakes; some studies were limited to coffee consumption and ignored other sources of caffeine; and most studies ignored distinctions between different types of preparation and different strengths of coffee; (ii) inadequate control for the possible confounding effects of variables such as smoking, alcohol consumption, age, nutrition and life-style factors in some studies; (iii) low response rates in several studies; (iv) biased selection of adequate controls because of self-selection into groups of drinkers and nondrinkers of coffee; (v) recall bias in retrospective studies, particularly those of malformations; and (vi) insufficient statistical power in some of the studies. Despite these limitations, epidemiological studies are the single source of information on human reproductive effects of coffee.

Malformations: Borlée *et al.* (1978) identified 202 infants with congenital malformations of any type among 17 970 births in eight Belgian hospitals between 1972 and 1974. A group of 175 control infants was also selected. The parents of cases and controls were interviewed about consumption of coffee and other possible risk factors. Compared to women who did not drink coffee, the relative risks (RR) were calculated by the Working Group to be [0.7] for women drinking one to four cups per day, [0.8] for those drinking five to seven cups and [1.5] for those drinking eight or more cups. In a chi-square test, the linear trend was barely significant [(p = 0.05)]. No significant association was found between coffee drinking and smoking or use of medicines. [The Working Group noted that no information was given on refusals or other losses, that the possibility of recall bias was not considered, and that there was no proper control of confounding variables.]

Jacobson et al. (1981) reported three cases of infants with ectrodactyly born to women who drank eight to 25 cups of percolated coffee per day. The women were selected from among those who contacted the authors after reading press accounts of the relationship between coffee drinking and malformations. [The Working Group noted that this letter to the Editor constitutes only anecdotal information.]

Linn et al. (1982) studied the association between coffee consumption and several outcomes of pregnancy in 12 205 women in Boston, MA, USA, in 1977-80, who represented 71% of women giving birth in one hospital. Women were interviewed one to two days after delivery about their previous medical and obstetric history and habits, including coffee and tea consumption during the first trimester. Diabetic and asthmatic women and those with multiple pregnancies were excluded. The analysis was controlled for a number of confounding factors. No association was found between coffee drinking and the frequency of malformations.

The association between drinking caffeine-containing beverages and six types of malformation (inguinal hernia, oral clefts, cardiac defects, pyloric stenosis and neural tube defects) was studied in a case-control study of 2030 children from a number of hospitals in Boston, MA, Philadelphia, PA, and Toronto, Canada, between 1976 and 1980 (Rosenberg et al., 1982). Controls were 712 children with other malformations, mainly of the gastrointestinal, musculoskeletal and central nervous systems. Mothers were interviewed in their homes within six months of delivery about consumption of a number of caffeine-containing beverages, including coffee, tea and cola. Consumption of coffee was 0, occasional, 1-2 or >3 cups per day. No association was found between coffee consumption and any of the six malformations [all RRs, ≤1.4]. Adjustment for a large number of potentially confounding variables — but not for alcohol consumption — in the analysis did not change these estimates. [The Working Group noted that the use of malformed infants as controls helps reduce recall bias, but it might be inadequate if caffeine were a teratogen that affects many sites.]

A monitoring system identified 755 children with birth defects in Finland between 1980 and 1982 (Kurppa et al., 1983) including 112 with central nervous system defects, 241 with orofacial clefts, 210 with musculoskeletal defects and 143 with cardiovascular malformations. Thirty-five pairs that included habitual tea drinkers and 14 pairs with incomplete data were excluded. One control infant matched to each case was an infant whose birth immediately preceded that of the case in the same maternity district. Information on coffee drinking was collected through interviews; cola drinking was infrequent. No important difference was seen between mothers of cases and of controls regarding the consumption of coffee during pregnancy. After adjustment for maternal age, smoking and alcohol consumption, the RR for coffee drinkers relative to those who did not drink coffee was 1.1 (95% confidence interval [CI], 0.8-1.3). Separate analyses of the four diagnostic categories showed no significant association.

As reported in an abstract, a case-control study of risk factors for cleft palate was carried out in five areas of Japan from 1978 to 1981. One control was matched to each of 194 cases for residence, sex, birth order and maternal age. Questionnaires answered by mothers included information on dietary habits. Frequent intake of coffee was associated with a RR of 2.3 ($p < 0.05$) (Tohnai et al., 1984).

Furuhashi et al. (1985) carried out a prospective study in Japan in which 9921 women at 24 weeks' gestation or more were interviewed about coffee and tea drinking. Women were divided into five consumption groups: those who drank neither tea nor coffee, drinkers of fewer than five cups of coffee per day, five or more cups of coffee per day, coffee (any quantity) plus green tea, and green tea only. The rates of congenital anomalies of any type were 3.7% among coffee and/or tea drinkers and 1.7% among women who drank neither beverage. [The Working Group calculated that this difference was highly significant ($p < 0.001$), although the authors stated the opposite.] The association with coffee drinking was particularly strong for multiple anomalies. [The Working Group noted that no data are given on how the women were selected, or on when and where the study was carried out. Data on refusals and losses to follow-up are not given. Confounding variables were not adjusted for. It was surprising that the excess risk was seen for a wide variety of congenital malformations, including those associated with chromosomal anomalies.]

Tikkanen and Heinonen (1988) carried out a case-control study of maternal exposure to organic solvents and cardiovascular malformations in Finland in 1982-84. The 569 cases were identified from a population-based registry of congenital malformations; all diagnoses were confirmed by a cardiologist with experience in teratology. Controls were selected randomly from 52 hospitals in the country, and of 1200 controls selected, 1052 (88%) were included in the study. Mothers were interviewed at maternity welfare centres concerning exposures during the first trimester of pregnancy. Coffee drinkers were equally distributed among cases and controls: 82.3% and 81.8%, respectively.

Low birthweight and/or preterm delivery: The three best-designed studies are summarized in Table 30.

Table 30. Summary of selected[a] studies that provide relative risks (RR) for low birthweight in relation to coffee or caffeine intake of mothers

Reference, location and design	No. of women	Coffee or caffeine consumption	RR (95% CI[b])	Comments
van den Berg (1977) California, USA Prospective	8 514	≤1 cup/day 2-6 cups/day ≥7 cups/day	1.0 [1.4][c] [2.2][c]	Coffee intake
		≤6 cups/day ≥7 cups/day	1.0 1.2	RR adjusted for smoking $p = 0.01$, calculated by Hogue (1981)
Linn et al. (1982) Boston, USA Cross-sectional	12 205	<4 cups/day ≥4 cups/day	1.0 1.2 (0.9-1.6)	Adjusted for smoking and other confounding variables Coffee intake
Martin & Bracken (1987) New Haven, USA Prospective	3 891	Nondrinkers 1-150 mg/day 151-300 mg/day >300 mg/day	1.0 1.4 (0.7-3.0) 2.3 (1.1-5.2) 4.6 (2.0-10.5)	Term deliveries only; RR adjusted for race, parity, smoking and gestational age Caffeine intake

[a] Selected on the basis of design and quality
[b] CI, confidence interval
[c] Crude RR calculated by the Working Group

Mau and Netter (1974) carried out a prospective study of over 5200 pregnant women from 20 maternity departments in the Federal Republic of Germany. The women were interviewed during the first trimester of pregnancy, but little information was provided on how coffee drinking was quantified. Compared to nondrinkers, women who occasionally drank coffee had a RR of [1.4]; frequent drinkers had a RR of [1.6] for delivering a low birthweight (<2500 g) baby [($p < 0.01$)]. The risk among drinkers remained unchanged after stratification for smoking (as reanalysed by Hogue, 1981).

van den Berg (1977) studied the effect of coffee consumption on birthweight and preterm delivery in a prospective study carried out in California, USA, between 1960 and 1967. Approximately 15 000 pregnant women receiving antenatal care under a prepaid medical plan were enrolled. Data were obtained from their medical records as well as from interviews covering reproductive history, socioeconomic factors, smoking habits and beverage consumption. A dose-response effect of coffee drinking was seen on low birthweight (see Table 30). A similar effect was noted on prematurity (gestational age under 37 weeks at birth), with RRs of [1.3] for women drinking two to six cups per day and [1.8] for those drinking seven or more cups, compared to women drinking up to one cup per day. Hogue (1981) examined the data on low birthweight after adjustment for smoking and length of gestation: a smaller but still significant RR of 1.2 was found for women who drank seven or more cups per day as compared to women who drank fewer than seven cups per day.

Arnandova and Kaculov (1978) reported a study of the pregnancy outcomes of 600 women in the USSR in 1976. Coffee consumption was not associated with prematurity, but the mean birthweight of infants born to coffee drinkers (usually one to two cups per day) was 115 g less than that of babies of women who did not drink coffee. The authors commented that this difference was probably due to greater consumption of alcohol and tobacco among coffee drinkers.

Kuzma and Sokol (1982) carried out a study of pregnant women who gave birth at four hospitals in California, USA, in 1974-78. About three-quarters of the women receiving antenatal care in these hospitals answered a self-administered questionnaire on their first visit, which included information on demographic and socioeconomic variables and on the use of coffee, alcohol, tobacco and other substances. If a mother had not sought antenatal care or had been missed in the enrollment procedure, the same data were obtained shortly after delivery; 37% of the study sample was recruited in this way. No important difference was found between information collected prospectively and retrospectively. Complete data were available for 5093 mother-infant pairs. After adjustment for gestational age, pre-pregnancy weight, weight gain, ethnicity and smoking, caffeine use was significantly ($p < 0.01$) associated with lower birthweight. [The Working Group noted that it is not clear what percentage of eligible women were included in the study and that no information was given on how caffeine intake was calculated, particularly as to whether sources other than coffee were accounted for.]

In the study of Linn *et al.* (1982), described on p. 105, coffee drinking during the first trimester was associated in the crude analysis with a greater proportion of low birthweight. After adjustment for smoking, with or without other confounding variables, no significant effect of coffee drinking was seen: the RR for women drinking four or more cups a day was 1.2 (95% CI, 0.9-1.6) (see Table 30). No dose-response effect was present, and the association between coffee drinking and duration of gestation was nonsignificant.

In a case-control study, Berkowitz *et al.* (1982) compared 175 preterm infants and 313 term infants delivered at a Connecticut, USA, hospital in 1977. Preterm infants (cases) were defined as those born before 37 weeks of gestation, as determined by the Dubowitz criteria, and controls were a random sample of term infants. Interviews were completed with the mothers of 86% of potential cases and 95% of potential controls and included data on alcohol, smoking and on the average daily number of cups of coffee or tea taken during each trimester. Cases were of lower socioeconomic status than controls. Coffee drinking was not associated with shortened gestation period.

Watkinson and Fried (1985) investigated the possible association between coffee consumption during pregnancy and perinatal outcomes among women in the Ottawa area, Canada. From 1978, 371 women were studied for a range of perinatal outcomes. Five years later, in 1983, those women whose offspring were at least one year of age by that date were mailed a questionnaire concerning their consumption of coffee, tea, cola and other sources of caffeine throughout their pregnancies; 284 women (77%) responded. Coffee and tea samples were collected from 53 mothers and were used to estimate the caffeine content of these drinks. Caffeine consumption was greater among smokers and among women of low educational level. Caffeine intake, expressed as a continuous variable, was not significantly associated with birthweight or gestational age; however, the mean weight of babies born to 12 heavy users (> 300 mg caffeine/day) was 3158 g, compared to 3537 g for the remaining sample ($p < 0.05$). This association was still significant after adjustment for nicotine use but not quite significant ($p = 0.06$) after controlling for maternal education. No association was found between heavy use and gestational age. [The Working Group noted that women had been asked to recall the intake of a number of caffeine-containing substances several years after a pregnancy. No dose-response effect was present.]

In the study of Furuhashi *et al* (1985), described on p. 106, no significant difference in mean birthweight was seen between the five categories. Infants born to 53 women who drank five or more cups of coffee per day, however, were on average about 70 g lighter than the other infants. The incidence of infants who were small for gestational age was approximately three times greater [$p < 0.05$; Poisson test] in the women who drank more than five cups of coffee per day. [The Working Group noted that no information on smoking was available, and no definition was given of 'small for gestational age'.]

Martin and Bracken (1987) carried out a prospective study of 3891 pregnant women receiving antenatal care in greater New Haven, Connecticut, USA, between 1980 and 1982. A total of 6219 women were considered for the study but only 5331 agreed to be contacted. Of these, 4926 fulfilled the entry criteria, and 85% were interviewed at home within a few weeks of the first prenatal visit. Caffeine consumption during pregnancy was estimated from data on the consumption of coffee, tea, colas and drugs. Data on pregnancy outcomes were obtained from hospital records and were analysed using logistic regression. Caffeine consumption was associated with lower socioeconomic status, smoking and alcohol intake. The effect of caffeine on birthweight was restricted to term infants. After adjustment for gestational age, race, parity and smoking, intake of caffeine at > 300 mg/day was associated with a RR of 4.6 (95% CI, 2.0-10.5) for low birthweight compared with that of women who did not consume caffeine-containing beverages or drugs. A dose-response pattern was present (see Table 30). No association was seen between caffeine intake and gestational age.

Brooke *et al.* (1989) studied the effects on birthweight of smoking, alcohol, caffeine, socioeconomic factors and psychosocial stress among 1860 white women in London, UK, of whom 1513 were included in the study and interviewed prenatally. Birthweight was corrected for gestational age, maternal height, parity and baby's sex (adjusted to a standard population). Smoking was found to be the most important single factor, inducing a 5% reduction in birthweight, which was statistically significant even when corrected for consumption of alcohol, tea, coffee or caffeine. Total caffeine consumption (milligrams per week) was calculated for the entire pregnancy and was found to be related to birthweight (adjusted to 40 weeks): with an intake of 0-200 mg/day, birth weight was 3664 g; with 200-400 mg/day, birthweight was 3609 g; and with a daily intake of more than 400 mg/day, the average birthweight was 3556 g. The corresponding birthweight ratios were 1.050, 1.034 and 1.019. In a crude analysis (not corrected for smoking), the difference across groups gives $p = 0.005$; however, when corrected for smoking, the adjusted birthweight ratios did not differ with caffeine consumption categories, being 1.051 (95% CI, 1.039-1.062) for 0-200 mg/day, 1.055 (95% CI, 1.043-1.068) for 200-400 mg/day and 1.054 (95% CI, 1.033-1.075) for > 400 mg/day. The authors concluded that smoking was the main environmental cause of variations in birthweight (corrected for gestational age). [The Working Group noted that the study was not designed to detect a possible effect on birthweight mediated through prematurity.]

In Costa Rica, women of low socioeconomic status were contacted at an antenatal care service before they were six months' pregnant (Muñoz *et al.*, 1988). Of 378 women contacted, 301 fulfilled the entry criteria, which included being aged between 17 and 30 years, uncomplicated pregnancy and delivery, term delivery, avoidance of smoking and alcohol, and initiation of breastfeeding. The study was restricted to non-coffee drinkers and to women who drank 450 ml or more coffee per day. Of 110 eligible women, 62 (56%) dropped out, so that the study was limited to 22 coffee drinkers and 26 who did not drink coffee. Dropouts had had less education and higher parity than the women studied. Birthweight was 121 g lower for the children of coffee drinkers than those of non-coffee drinkers ($p < 0.001$). This difference was still significant after adjustment for potential confounding factors through multiple linear regression. Iron deficiency anaemia was found in 23% of the coffee consumers and in none of the non-consumers. The haematocrit levels of infants of coffee-drinking mothers at one week and one month of age were lower than those of the controls. This association persisted after adjustment for confounding factors. [The Working Group noted the high rate of dropouts.]

The effect of first-trimester maternal caffeine consumption on birthweight was examined in a case-control study of 131 cases and 136 controls (Caan & Goldhaber, 1989). Heavy consumption of caffeine (300 mg/day or three servings) from coffee, tea or cola drinks was associated with a high prevalence of low birthweight. For women who had drunk three or more cups of coffee per day, the crude odds ratio was 2.1; when adjusted for ethnicity, alcohol, cigarettes, pre-pregnancy weight, weight gain and parity, the odds ratio increased to 2.8 (95% CI; 0.89-8.7).

Spontaneous abortions and stillbirths: In the study of Arnandova and Kaculov (1978), described on p. 108, no difference was reported in the rates of spontaneous abortions and stillbirths in relation to coffee drinking.

In the study of Furuhashi *et al.* (1985), described on p. 106, 2% of pregnant women who had drunk coffee and 1.2% of controls had spontaneous abortions ($p < 0.001$). [Reservations regarding this study are given on p. 106. The Working Group noted further that most abortions are likely to have been missed in this study, since women were recruited at 24 weeks' gestation or more. It is unclear whether stillbirths were included among abortions since there was no mention of stillbirths in the report. No confounding variable was adjusted for.]

Srisuphan and Bracken (1986) carried out a prospective study of 3135 pregnant women who had sought antenatal care in the New Haven, Connecticut, area, USA, between 1980 and 1982. Details of the study design are given on p. 110 in the description of the study by Martin and Bracken (1987). The abortion rates were 1.8% for non-caffeine users, 1.8% for light users (1-150 mg/day) and 3.1% for moderate-to-heavy users (> 150 mg/day) (trend not significant). Comparing moderate-to-heavy users with the remainder, the RR was 1.7 (95% CI, 1.0-2.7; $p = 0.03$). This estimate was unchanged (RR, 1.7; $p = 0.03$) after adjustment for maternal age, gestational age, Jewish religion, prior gynaecological surgery and previous spontaneous abortions. Women who received caffeine only from coffee appeared to have a higher risk of miscarriage (RR, 2) than those who drank only tea (1.1) or colas (1.3), but the numbers were small and the differences not significant.

Kršnjavi and Mimica (1987) studied 308 pregnant women in Zagreb, Yugoslavia, in 1982-83, of whom 246 (80%) responded to a questionnaire on alcohol, tobacco and coffee consumption. No association was found between coffee drinking and the frequency of spontaneous abortions.

Effects on fertility: Information on caffeine consumption before trying to conceive was obtained for 221 women. The adjusted mean fecundability ratio for higher caffeine users compared to non-users was 0.80 (Wilcox *et al.*, 1988). An association between reduced fertility and caffeine intake received further support from data presented in a letter to the Editor of *The Lancet* (Christianson *et al.*, 1989). In a further study, however, no association was found between time to conceive and coffee consumption among 2817 women who had recently had a liveborn child, while there was a suggested effect of tea and also of age and tobacco smoking (Joesoef *et al.*, 1990).

(iii) *Genetic and related effects*

The nonpolar fractions of urine from humans who had ingested 12 g of instant coffee per day for four days or 12 g within 2 h were not mutagenic to *S. typhimurium* TA98 or TA100 in the presence or absence of an exogenous metabolic system, with or without β-glucuronidase treatment of the urine (Aeschbacher & Chappuis, 1981).

Organic fractions isolated from the urine of drinkers of at least five cups of coffee per day induced chromosomal aberrations in cultured Chinese hamster ovary cells. This clastogenic effect was abolished in two of the organic fractions by the addition of either catalase or superoxide dismutase to the cell system, suggesting that active oxygen species are involved (Dunn & Curtis, 1985).

In a population of 30 smokers and 30 nonsmokers, a positive, statistically significant linear relationship between the square-root transformed frequency of sister chromatid exchange in cultured peripheral blood lymphocytes and coffee consumption was reported (Reidy *et al.*, 1988). In the same population, a positive linear relationship was observed between the average number of cups of coffee consumed per day and the proportion of low-folate cultured blood lymphocytes with chromosomal aberrations. Only about 5% of the variance was attributable to coffee consumption. In comparison, smoking contributed about 10% and the use of two different slide scorers contributed about 15% (Chen *et al.*, 1989). [The Working Group noted that this study of smokers and nonsmokers was not designed to evaluate coffee consumption.]

In a study on 44 otherwise healthy splenectomized persons, drinking coffee (and occasionally tea) was associated with a significant, dose-dependent increase in the frequency of micronuclei in both reticulocytes and mature erythrocytes (Smith *et al.*, 1990).

3.3 Epidemiological studies of carcinogenicity to humans[1]

(a) Descriptive epidemiology

These studies are of four main types. Ecological studies examining geographic variation in coffee consumption and either cancer incidence or mortality rates (Takahashi, 1964; Stocks, 1970; Shennan, 1973; Armstrong & Doll, 1975; Binstock *et al.*, 1983; Decarli & La Vecchia, 1986; Phelps & Phelps, 1988) are the most common. A second type of study examines time trends in cancer rates and coffee consumption within a given country or countries (Morrison, 1978; Pannelli *et al.*, 1989). A hybrid design combines an examination of time trends (Cuckle & Kinlen, 1981; Benarde & Weiss, 1982) and geographic differences among countries. The final type of descriptive studies examines cancer rates among special population groups such as Mormons, a cultural group one of whose practices is abstension from tea and coffee drinking (Enstrom, 1975; Lyon *et al.*, 1976; Enstrom, 1978, 1980; Lyon *et al.*, 1980), in which incidence and mortality rates for different cancer sites were compared either with the general population or with non-practising Mormons. It is not possible in these studies, however, to distinguish between the effect of reduced coffee and tea consumption, reduced cigarette smoking and alcohol drinking and the other prohibited behaviours of this sect; they do not contribute to our knowledge of the association between coffee drinking and cancer risk and are not discussed further in this monograph.

(i) Bladder cancer

In an examination of time trends in incidence rates and per-caput coffee imports in the USA and Denmark, coffee consumption was adjusted for cigarette consumption. No association was noted between changes in bladder cancer rates

---

[1]The Working Group was aware of a large multicentre case-control study on pancreatic cancer which has been completed, but the results were not available.

and coffee imports in Denmark or among women in the USA; a weak positive association was noted for US men (Morrison, 1978). Cohort and period variation in bladder cancer mortality in Italy between 1950-54 and 1980-81 was compared with changes in coffee, cocoa, tea and cigarette consumption. The authors stated that changes in coffee intake do not explain the cohort changes (Pannelli *et al.*, 1989). No association was noted in the study of either Armstrong and Doll (1975) or Stocks (1970).

(ii) *Breast cancer*

Weak positive correlations were reported between incidence ($r = 0.42$) and mortality ($r = 0.37$) from breast cancer and coffee consumption in a geographical study (Armstrong & Doll, 1975). Phelps and Phelps (1988) conducted an ecological study, which did not distinguish between tea and coffee consumption, and reported a correlation of 0.004 with breast cancer mortality ratios after adjusting for dietary fat intake.

(iii) *Endometrial cancer*

A positive correlation was reported between the incidence of corpus uterine cancer ($r = 0.43$) and international variation in coffee consumption (Armstrong & Doll, 1975).

(iv) *Kidney cancer*

The correlation between age-adjusted mortality rates from kidney cancer in 1964 and per-caput coffee consumption was 0.79 ($p < 0.001$) (Shennan, 1973). A reported correlation between coffee consumption and the incidence of kidney cancer (men, 0.62; women, 0.40) was explained by the stronger association with consumption of animal protein (Armstrong & Doll, 1975), which is also correlated with coffee consumption.

(v) *Leukaemia*

A positive correlation was reported between mean, age-adjusted mortality rates for leukaemia in 1964-65 and annual coffee consumption (males, $p = 0.001$; females, $p = 0.03$) (Stocks, 1970).

(vi) *Ovarian cancer*

A positive correlation was reported between mean, age-adjusted mortality rates in 1964-65 and annual coffee consumption ($p = 0.006$) (Stocks, 1970). A weak correlation was reported between incidence ($r = 0.50$) and mortality ($r = 0.50$) and coffee consumption in the study of Armstrong and Doll (1975).

(vii) *Pancreatic cancer*

An association was reported between mean, age-adjusted death rates for males in 1964-65 and annual coffee consumption ($p = 0.008$) (Stocks, 1970). An examination of international time trends in mortality rates and coffee consumption, in which adjustment was made for changes in lung cancer mortality as a proxy for smoking, showed correlations of 0.58 (males) and 0.66 (females) (Cuckle & Kinlen, 1981). An additional correlation study in the USA, which used lag periods to examine trends in mortality ratios and coffee consumption, reported correlation coefficients ranging from 0.39 to 0.68 over the period of the study (Benarde & Weiss, 1982). A simple correlation coefficient of 0.59 ($p = 0.001$) between coffee consumption in 1957-65 and mortality in 1971-74 was found to be significant after controlling for confounding variables (Binstock *et al.*, 1983). Positive but nonsignificant correlation coefficients have been reported between age-standardized, sex-specific mortality rates and per-caput coffee consumption in 20 regions of Italy (Decarli & La Vecchia, 1986).

(viii) *Prostatic cancer*

The correlation between age-adjusted mortality ratios for 1956-59 and per-caput coffee consumption for 1955-59 was 0.7 ($p < 0.001$) (Takahashi, 1964). This association was confirmed using mortality data for 1964-65 ($p < 0.001$) (Stocks, 1970).

(b) *Cohort studies*

The association between coffee consumption and subsequent cancer incidence or mortality has been investigated in a number of prospective studies. In the following text, the most recent publication on cancer outcomes has been summarized when a number of papers have been generated from a single cohort study. The studies are summarized in Table 31 on p. 119.

(i) *All sites combined*

Heyden *et al.* (1979) conducted a nine-year follow-up of 2530 US men and women interviewed about their daily coffee consumption in 1967-69. Seventy-four cancer deaths with biopsy or hospital data were analysed. Two sets of controls consisted of age-, race- and sex-matched deaths from cardiovascular disease and live study participants. Coffee consumption was more common among each set of controls than among the cancer cases (odds ratio, 0.67; $p > 0.05$). The matched-pairs odds ratios were based on 6:9 discordant pairs for each set of controls.

The association between coffee consumption and mortality from all causes, coronary heart disease and noncoronary causes over 19 years was examined among 1910 white men, aged 40-56 at the time of the baseline examination, who took part in a study of the Chicago Western Electric Company (LeGrady *et al.*, 1987). Intake was measured in terms of 6-oz (178-ml) cups over 28 days. Since only 97 men consumed two or more cups of decaffeinated coffee per day, intake of caffeinated and decaffeinated coffee was combined. The Cox proportional hazards model was used to analyse the association between coffee intake and mortality after adjustment for age, diastolic blood pressure, serum cholesterol and smoking. The adjusted RR for cancers at all sites comparing none to one cup per day with all other levels of intake was 1.6 (95% CI, 0.95-2.6). [The Working Group noted that no analysis of site-specific cancer risks was undertaken.]

(ii) *Site-specific analyses*

A case-control analysis of a cohort study investigated pancreatic cancer mortality in a 16-50-year follow up of 50 000 male former college students (Whittemore *et al.*, 1983). There were 126 deaths from pancreatic cancer. Data on coffee and tea consumption and other variables had been collected during a physical examination at college. No significant association was noted with coffee consumption.

A series of letters to the Editor of *The Lancet* (Nomura *et al.*, 1981; Kinlen *et al.*, 1984; Nomura *et al.*, 1984) report pancreatic cancer incidence in cohort studies. Since Nomura *et al.* (1986) reported on pancreatic cancer and coffee consumption in the same cohort, no additional data from these letters are reported here. Kinlen *et al.* (1984) carried out a cohort study of 14 085 men in London, UK. There were 47 deaths from pancreatic cancer, identified from death certificates, in the 13 years of follow-up to 1982. The mean daily consumption of coffee, adjusted for age and smoking, was 0.83 cup for cases and 1.00 cup for controls.

In a Hawaiian cohort study of the association between cancer incidence and coffee consumption, 7355 Japanese men were followed for a minimum of 14 years from the time of collection of 24-h consumption data in 1965-68 (Nomura *et al.*, 1986). There were 672 incident cancers in the cohort as of July 1983. Incidence rates were adjusted for age or both age and smoking, using the entire cohort as the standard population. The reference category for all analyses included the 1173 men who reported drinking no coffee. Coffee intake was analysed according to none, one to two, three to four and five or more cups per day. No significant association was reported between coffee drinking and age- and smoking-adjusted RRs for pancreatic cancer (p for trend, 0.41), lung cancer (p for trend, 0.19) or bladder cancer (p for trend, 0.25). No association was noted with colon cancer risk. [The Working Group noted that dietary information was based on a single 24-h recall.]

A series of papers has examined the association between coffee intake and 21-year mortality among Seventh-day Adventists in the USA (Phillips & Snowdon, 1983; Snowdon & Phillips, 1984; Phillips & Snowdon, 1985).

The final analysis in the series was based on a cohort of 25 493 subjects (Phillips & Snowdon, 1985). Univariate analyses indicated a consistent positive relationship between colon and rectal cancer death rates and increased coffee consumption for both men and women. Drinking two or more cups of coffee per day was associated with a crude RR for colon cancer of 2.0 (95% CI, 1.1-3.6) for men and 1.5 (0.8-2.6) for women. Different multivariate analyses were completed for the first 10 and the last 11 years of follow-up since the association between coffee drinking and colorectal cancer varied across this period. The excess risk associated with drinking two or more cups of coffee per day in the latter follow-up period was 3.0 ($p > 0.05$) for men following adjustment for age, egg consumption, excess weight and meat consumption. The equivalent adjusted risk for women was 2.4 ($p < 0.05$). [The Working Group noted that the distribution of coffee drinking in this population is unusual because there are few heavy coffee drinkers: 17-18% of the population drank two or more cups per day. There may be residual confounding by other factors associated with non-adherence to dietary restrictions.]

Two papers have been published from a prospective study conducted in Norway examining the relationship between coffee drinking and cancer incidence and mortality among approximately 16 000 men and women (Heuch et al., 1983; Jacobsen et al., 1986). Site-specific incidence and mortality were determined among three groups of people: a probability sample of adult males selected from the 1960 census, Norwegian brothers of migrants to the USA, and spouses and siblings of people interviewed for a case-control study of gastrointestinal cancer. Average daily coffee consumption was determined by questionnaire in 1967-69. No data are presented on the completeness of the 11.5-year follow-up, during which time there were 602 cancer deaths and 1498 incident cancers (including 207 nonmelanomatous skin cancers). Incidence data that were presented for approximately 20 cancer sites were adjusted for sex, age and residence; some additional analyses among males were also adjusted for smoking. In the calculation of RRs, comparisons were made between the consumption of two or fewer and seven or more cups per day. The RR for mortality from cancers at all sites was 1.3 (p for trend = 0.09). Raised RRs were reported for the incidence of cervical (10.6; p for trend = 0.07) and lung cancer (1.8; p for trend = 0.02); the smoking-adjusted RR for lung cancer incidence among males was 1.1 (p for trend = 0.84). Heavy coffee drinking was associated with reduced risks for the incidence of colon (RR, 0.6; p for trend = 0.10) and kidney cancer (RR, 0.3; p for trend = 0.01). The RR for the incidence of pancreatic cancer was 0.7 (p for trend = 0.37) and that for bladder cancer was 0.99 (p for trend = 0.99). [The Working Group noted that odds ratios were in fact calculated and presented as RRs.]

A cohort study investigated a six-year follow-up of pancreatic cancer incidence among 122 894 men and women who had completed a questionnaire collecting data on coffee, tea, smoking and alcohol use in 1978-84 (Hiatt et al., 1988). There were 49 cases of pancreatic cancer. A multivariate analysis (adjusting for age, sex, ethnicity, blood glucose level, smoking, alcohol and diabetes) identified no increased risk associated with increasing coffee consumption.

A cohort study (Mills *et al.*, 1988) of approximately 34 000 non-Hispanic, white Californian Seventh-day Adventists followed participants for six years after their completion of a questionnaire determining their exposures in 1976. Forty deaths from pancreatic cancer were reported. In the analyses of age- and sex-adjusted RRs for pancreatic cancer, current consumption of coffee at least once a day relative to no consumption was associated with a RR of 2.0 (95% CI, 0.9-4.4). Past consumption showed an inconsistent, nonsignificant protective relationship with mortality from pancreatic cancer. Multivariate analyses, using the Cox proportional hazards model, give a RR for current coffee consumption, adjusted for age, sex and smoking of 2.2 (95% CI, 0.6-8.0).

A cohort study of colorectal cancer incidence in a retirement community (Wu *et al.*, 1987) identified 58 male and 68 female cases among 11 888 people in a 4.5-year follow up. Questionnaires were completed between 1981 and 1982 by 62% of community members. In an analysis that adjusted only for age, there was no effect of increased coffee intake on cancer risk in women and a nonsignificant increase in men.

Paffenbarger *et al.* (1978) examined the association between coffee drinking and mortality from six cancers in a nested case-control analysis of a cohort study in the USA of 50 000 male former college students (the same population as used by Whittemore *et al.*, 1983, p. 116). Each case was matched with four controls chosen randomly from among classmates born in the same year and known to have survived the decedent. Information on risk factors was obtained from medical records completed at the time of college entry. Coffee drinking at that time was associated with a two- to three-fold higher risk for Hodgkin's disease, lymphatic and myeloid leukaemia, but no significant association was found with non-Hodgkin's lymphoma, with malignant melanoma or with other and unspecified leukaemias.

(c) *Case-control studies*

(i) *Bladder and urinary tract*

Bladder cancer. More than two dozen case-control studies have been published on the association between coffee and bladder cancer. Their main results are summarized in Tables 32 (users *versus* non-users) and 33 (dose-response relationships and significance of the linear trend in risk) on pp. 129 and 132. Whenever possible, combined RRs are derived from data presented in strata of sex, age, race and other possible covariates.

Cole (1971) reported a population-based case-control study of 445 cases of cancer of the lower urinary tract (renal pelvis, ureter, bladder (90% of cases) and

Table 31. Summary of results of cohort studies on cancer and coffee consumption

Reference, location and site	Subjects	Events (deaths or cases)	Coffee consumption (cups/day)	RR (95% CI)	Comments
Heyden et al. (1979) USA All sites	2530 men and women	74	<5 ≥5	1.0 0.7	$p > 0.05$; same RR with each control group
LeGrady et al. (1987) USA All sites	1910 white men	117	0–1 ≥2	1.0 1.6 (0.95–2.6)	Adjusted for age, diastolic blood pressure, serum cholesterol and smoking
Whittemore et al. (1983) USA Pancreas	50 000 men	126	0 Any	1.0 1.1 (0.7–1.9)	Past coffee consumption Adjusted for age, college and class year
Kinlen et al. (1984) UK Pancreas	14 085 men	47	Mean: cases, 0.83 controls, 1.00		Adjusted for age and smoking
Nomura et al. (1986) Hawaii Pancreas	7355 Japanese men	21	0 1–2 3–4 ≥5	1.0 [1.2] [2.1] [1.6]	$p = 0.41$, adjusted for age and smoking
Lung		110	0 1–2 3–4 ≥5	1.0 1.1 1.1 1.4	$p = 0.19$, adjusted for age and smoking
Bladder		39	0 1–2 3–4 ≥5	1.0 1.0 1.4 1.6	$p = 0.25$, adjusted for age and smoking

Table 31 (contd)

Reference, location and site	Subjects	Events (deaths or cases)	Coffee consumption (cups/day)	RR (95% CI)	Comments
Phillips & Snowdon (1985) USA	Seventh-day Adventists				
Colon	9 175 men	53	<1 1 ≥2	1 1.3 (0.5–3.4) 2.0 (1.1–3.6)	$p = 0.04$, adjusted for age
	16 336 women	83	<1 1 ≥2	1 1.2 (0.6–2.4) 1.5 (0.8–2.6)	$p = 0.20$, adjusted for age
Rectum	25 493 men and women	28	<1 1 ≥2 }	1.0 1.4 (0.6–3.1)	$p = 0.38$, adjusted for age and sex
Wu et al. (1987) USA Colon and rectum	11 888 men and women	58 men	0–1 2–3 ≥4	1.0 1.3 (0.7–2.5) 1.5 (0.6–3.7)	Adjusted for age
		68 women	0–1 2–3 ≥4	1.0 1.5 (0.8–2.7) 1.2 (0.4–3.1)	
Hiatt et al. (1988) USA Pancreas	122 894 men and women	49	0 <1 1–3 ≥4	1.0 0.8 (0.3–2.6) 0.9 (0.4–2.1) 0.7 (0.2–1.9)	Adjusted for age, sex, ethnic group, blood glucose, smoking, alcohol and diabetes
Mills et al. (1988) USA Pancreas	34 198 white male and female Seventh-day Adventists	40	Current use Never <Daily Daily	1.0 1.4 (0.6–3.6) 2.0 (0.9–4.4)	p for trend = 0.087, adjusted for age and sex

Table 31 (contd)

Reference, location and site	Subjects	Events (deaths or cases)	Coffee consumption (cups/day)	RR (95% CI)	Comments
Mills et al. (1988) USA Pancreas (contd)			Past use Never <Daily Daily	1.0 0.7 (0.2-1.9) 0.7 (0.3-1.5)	$p = 0.254$, adjusted for age and sex
Paffenbarger et al. (1978) USA	50 000 men				
Hodgkin's disease		45	Never Ever	1.0 2.5	$p = 0.07$; RR based on matched analysis
Non-Hodgkin's lymphoma		89	Never Ever	1.0 1.6	Nonsignificant
Malignant melanoma		45	Never Ever	1.0 1.3	Nonsignificant
Lymphatic leukaemia		27	Never Ever	1.0 2.7	$p = 0.06$
Myeloid leukaemia		41	Never Ever	1.0 3.2	$p = 0.02$
Other/unspecified leukaemias		30	Never Ever	1.0 0.8	Nonsignificant

urethra) and 451 controls from Massachusetts, USA. The study, in which 90% of cases and controls participated, found a RR of 1.2 for men and 2.6 for women among coffee drinkers *versus* non-coffee drinkers, after adjustment for age and smoking at three levels (non-smokers, ≤1/2 pack, > 1/2 pack per day). The RR was significant for women, and was 1.6 for one, 3.8 for two to three and 2.2 for four or more cups per day. The association was apparently stronger among the 90 cases who neither smoked nor had a high-risk occupation.

In a study conducted in Louisiana, USA, Dunham *et al*. (1968) obtained information on 493 patients with bladder cancer and 527 controls admitted to hospital for a wide spectrum of other conditions. The data were stratified for type of coffee, sex and race, and reanalysed by Fraumeni *et al*. (1971), in a study reported as a letter to the Editor of *The Lancet*. Some association was found for blacks (significant in females) but not for whites. After adjustment for age and smoking, the overall RR was 1.5 (nonsignificant). There was no consistent dose-response relationship.

In a Canadian case-control study of 158 men and 74 women with bladder cancer and similar numbers of controls with benign prostatic hypertrophy (men) or stress incontinence (women), data were collected using a postal questionnaire on previous health, employment, beverage and artificial sweetener intake (Morgan & Jain, 1974). The overall response rate was 69% among the cases and 57% among the controls, but the numbers of subjects included in the final analysis were further reduced by matching for age. The mean number of cups of coffee drunk per day was 1.8 for cases and 2.0 for controls among females, and 2.1 for both cases and controls among males. The RR (calculated by the Working Group) for coffee drinkers *versus* non-drinkers was [0.7] for males and [1.3] for females. None of these estimates, nor the corresponding trends in risk with dose was significant.

A study by Simon *et al*. (1975) was based on 216 white female cases of cancer of the lower urinary tract (renal pelvis, ureter, bladder (95% of cases) and urethra) identified at 10 hospitals in urban areas in Massachussets, USA. Among them, 40 had died and 41 did not respond. The remaining 135 cases were compared with 390 respondent controls out of a total of 648 selected from the discharge lists of the same hospitals. Postal questionnaires were used for data collection. Ninety-three percent of cases drank coffee *versus* 85% of the controls, with an unadjusted RR of 2.1 (95% CI, 1.1-4.3). The unadjusted RRs were 2.2 for one or two cups per day, 1.9 for three to four and 2.3 for five or more. [Adjustment for smoking by the Working Group was possible according to two categories only (nonsmokers and light smokers *versus* moderate to heavy smokers); the RR declined to [1.9] and was no longer significant.]

Wynder and Goldsmith (1977) utilized data collected between 1969 and 1974 on patients interviewed in 17 hospitals in six areas of the USA (46% from Memorial

Hospital in New York City). A total of 574 male and 158 female bladder cancer patients and equal numbers of hospital controls were considered. The refusal or nonparticipation rate was less than 4%. The RRs for whether coffee was ever drunk or not, adjusted for smoking at four levels, were above unity [RR, 1.5 for males, 1.3 for females]. Trends in risk with dose were not significant.

Miller *et al.* (1978) published data from a study originally planned to consider the possible association between isonicotinic acid hydrazide, a drug used in the treatment and prophylaxis of tuberculosis, and bladder cancer. Patients admitted to a hospital in Ottawa for bladder cancer (255 cases) and other urological conditions (510 controls) completed a questionnaire including, among other items, information on coffee and tea consumption. In relation to coffee, a matched, unadjusted analysis provided a RR of 1.3 for males and of 1.6 for females. [The Working Group noted that no information was provided on the confounding or modifying effect of covariates, including smoking.]

Mettlin and Graham (1979) studied the role of dietary factors in the risk for bladder cancer using data from the Roswell Park Memorial Institute, NY, USA, collected between 1957 and 1965 (Bross & Tidings, 1973). A total of 429 white male and 140 white female patients with primary bladder cancer were compared with 1025 controls admitted for non-neoplastic conditions. After adjustment for smoking in two categories (less than half a pack *versus* half a pack or more per day), the RR for five subsequent levels of coffee drinking was around unity in women, but above unity in men, in the absence, however, of any trend in risk (RRs, 1 (referent), 1.4, 1.2, 2.1 and 1.6). Consequently, in the two sexes combined, there was a small, inconsistent increase in smoking-adjusted RRs for bladder cancer risk with increasing coffee consumption: 1 (referent), [1.2, 1.1, 1.8 and 1.3].

Howe *et al.* (1980) reconsidered the relation between coffee and bladder cancer in a Canadian population-based case-control study of 480 male and 152 female case-control pairs (Miller, 1977). The overall response rate was 77% for the cases and 86% for the controls. For users *versus* non-users of any coffee preparation, the RR was 1.4 for men and 1.0 for women, neither estimate being significant. The unadjusted RRs were 1.5 (95% CI, 1.0-2.2) for men consuming brewed coffee and 1.5 (1.1-2.0) for those drinking instant coffee, and 1.4 (0.8-2.6) for women consuming instant coffee, but no dose-response relationship was found.

Cartwright *et al.* (1981) conducted a case-control study of bladder cancer in West Yorkshire, UK, a high incidence area for the disease. The study population included 841 cases (631 male, 210 female; 622 prevalent, 219 incident) and 1060 hospital patients of similar age and same sex. In this preliminary report, no information was given on participation rate. Questions were asked on coffee drinking habits and various types of coffee, besides other known and potential bladder cancer risk factors (smoking, saccharin use, occupational history, past medical history). No relation was found between any type of coffee consumption and bladder cancer risk after adjustment for smoking. The RRs for drinking all types of coffee, adjusted for age, type of case (incident/prevalent) and cigarette smoking, were 1.1 for males and 0.8 for females (corresponding estimates not adjusted for smoking were 1.3 and 1.1, respectively). Similarly, no heterogeneity in risk was observed between instant and ground coffee. The authors concluded that the correlation between cigarette and coffee consumption can explain the moderate association observed in the unadjusted analysis.

Morrison *et al.* (1982) published data from a population-based case-control study from Boston, MA, USA (587 cases, 528 controls), Manchester, UK (541 cases, 725 controls) and Nagoya, Japan (289 cases, 586 controls). A further report of a section of this study was made by Ohno *et al.* (1985). Controls were selected from electoral rolls or other population registries. Participation rates in various centres were over 80% for both cases and controls. The overall RR for coffee drinkers *versus* non-drinkers, adjusted for age, sex, centre and smoking was 1.0 (95% CI, 0.8-1.2), and in none of the centres was there consistent evidence of a dose-response relationship.

Najem *et al.* (1982) considered several risk factors for bladder carcinogenesis in a case-control study in New Jersey, USA, of 75 histologically confirmed cases among white people and 142 matched controls derived from the same clinic and hospital populations from which bladder cancer cases were obtained. Only five cases and 16 controls did not consume coffee. The RR (not adjusted) was 1.8, with a very wide 95% CI (0.1-10.0). [The Working Group noted the small number of cases and the limited information provided.]

Sullivan (1982) analysed 82 bladder cancer cases (out of 101 diagnosed) and 169 controls selected through random digit dialling in the area of greater New Orleans, LA, USA. In relation to coffee drinking, a number of inconsistent relationships was observed. White male cases, for instance, reported significantly greater consumption of brewed ground coffee than controls, and white women consumed more decaffeinated ground coffee than controls. No relationship was found with duration of use. [The Working Group noted that no RR was given, and there was no indication that adjustment was made for covariates.]

The largest case-control study on bladder cancer was that published by Hartge *et al.* (1983), based on 2982 cases and 5782 general population controls interviewed in a collaborative, population-based study conducted in ten geographical areas of the USA. A report of part of this study was made by Marrett *et al.* (1983). Participation was 73% for the cases and 82% for the controls. The RRs for ever *versus* never coffee drinking were 1.6 (95% CI, 1.2-2.2) for men, 1.2 (0.8-1.7) for women and 1.4 (1.1-1.8) for men and women combined, after simultaneous allowance for sex (when appropriate), age, race, geographical area and tobacco consumption. When various levels of coffee consumption were considered, the RR was significantly above unity (1.5; 1.1-1.9) only for men drinking over 63 cups of coffee per week, but no dose-response relationship was evident for either men or women. Similarly, there was no association with duration of coffee drinking. No interaction was observed with geographical area, race, occupation, artificial sweetener use or history of urinary infections. The authors noted that adjustment for smoking reduced the RR for ever/never coffee drinking from 1.8 to 1.4, and that residual confounding by tobacco (or possibly other correlates of coffee drinking) may explain the persistent but inconsistent relation between bladder cancer and coffee. Men who drank only decaffeinated coffee (ground or instant) had an estimated RR of 1.2 (0.8-1.9) compared to men who never drank coffee. The corresponding estimate for women was 1.5 (0.9-2.6). Kantor *et al.* (1988), examining the same data set by three separate histological types (squamous-cell, adeno- and transitional-cell carcinomas), found a significant trend in risk for adenocarcinomas in men and women combined, although the number was extremely low (32 cases) and none of the point estimates was significant. [The Working Group noted that the lack of significance may be the result of less precise adjustment for smoking than in the study by Hartge *et al.* (1983).]

In a population-based study carried out using the Connecticut (USA) Tumor Registry during 1978-79, Marrett *et al.* (1983) investigated the relationship between coffee consumption and bladder cancer. Data were available on 412 cases aged 21-84 (80% of those identified) and 493 controls (81% of those selected). After adjustment for age and smoking, the RR for one cup per week or more was 1.3 for males and 1.1 for females; for more than seven cups per week the RR was 1.5 for males and [1.0] for females. In males, there was some evidence of a dose-response relationship: for over 21 cups per week, the RR was 2.0. No trend in risk with dose was evident in females, nor with duration in people of either sex. The authors noted that among male and female nonsmokers combined, the RR for more than seven cups per week was 1.9 (95% CI, 1.0-3.6). There was no significant effect of the consumption of decaffeinated coffee. [The Working Group noted that there may be some overlap between this study and that of Hartge *et al.* (1983).]

In a case-control study in Aarhus, Denmark, Mommsen *et al.* (1983a,b) collected information from cases admitted to hospital and (through mailed questionnaires) from population controls (response rate of first selected controls, 85%). The overall report, based on 165 male and 47 female cases, found no association with coffee drinking, but an elevated risk was observed (RR, 2.6) among women, although the estimate was not significant and only one case and five controls were not coffee drinkers. Dose-response relationships were not analysed. [The Working Group noted the small number of cases and the limited information provided.]

In a study in Greece, Rebelakos et al. (1985) compared 300 cases of histologically confirmed bladder cancer (250 male, 50 female) admitted to the major cancer hospital in Athens with an equal number of age- and sex-matched orthopaedic controls. The refusal rate was only approximately 1%. The RR, adjusted for smoking, was not elevated in drinkers of one cup per day compared with non-coffee users; however, a significant RR of 1.7 was found when drinkers of two or more cups were compared with those drinking fewer than two cups per day. For male and female cases combined, the point estimates for five levels of coffee consumption were 1 (referent), 1.2, 1.7, 2.7 and 0.7, and the trend in risk was significant ($p = 0.02$).

Gonzáles et al. (1985) reported a hospital-based case-control study in Spain based on 58 cases; two age-matched controls were available for each case — one with non-urinary tract cancer (excluding lung cancer) and one with non-neoplastic conditions. They found a RR of [0.6] (not significant) for 'habitual coffee consumers'. [The Working Group noted the small number of cases, the limited information provided and that no allowance was made for potential confounders.]

Jensen et al. (1986) conducted a population-based case-control study in 1979-81 in Copenhagen, Denmark, of 371 (280 male, 91 female) bladder cancer cases (including papillomas) and 771 controls. The participation rate, as given in a previous paper (Jensen et al., 1983), was 94% among the cases and 75% among the controls. The RR for coffee users *versus* non-users, adjusted for age, sex, smoking (never/ever, plus a measure of pack years) was [approximately 1.4] in men and women combined, and the trend in risk with dose was not significant. The RRs were 1 (referent), 1.4, 1.2, 1.4 and 1.8 for subsequent levels of coffee use. The point estimates tended to be above unity for female coffee drinkers, but they were not dose-related.

Claude et al. (1986) conducted a case-control study of lower urinary tract cancer (90% were bladder tumours) in the Federal Republic of Germany. A total of 431 cases (340 male, 91 female) were matched for age and sex with 431 controls, who were primarily patients in hospitals for urological diseases (79%) and in homes for the elderly (21%). Only about 2% of cases refused to participate. The results were presented for each sex separately after allowance for smoking (never/ever and lifetime consumption in packs). In people of each sex, the RRs were above unity for coffee drinkers; the point estimates for more than four cups per day were 2.3 in males and 2.2 in females, and the trend in risk was significant for males. The RRs associated with coffee drinking were similar in smokers and nonsmokers. In this study, a positive association was found with total daily fluid intake, with a particularly high RR in males. The RR for drinking decaffeinated coffee *versus* that for non-users was 1.6 in males and 1.0 in females.

Piper *et al.* (1986) described a population-based case-control study of bladder cancer in women (aged 20-49) conducted in New York State in 1975-80. Information was available through telephone interviews on a total of 173 age-matched pairs, for a participation rate of 68% among cases and 71% among community controls. The crude RR for drinking brewed coffee was 1.6. The RR increased with dose, but the trend was not statistically significant.

In a study in Spain, based on 353 male and 53 female cases of bladder cancer compared with equal numbers of hospital controls without malignant or urological conditions (Bravo *et al.*, 1986, 1987), a positive association emerged among males for drinking 'espresso' coffee, with RRs of 1.9 for fewer than three cups and 2.6 for three or more cups per day. For women, the RR for daily use of coffee was [2.3], of borderline statistical significance. [The Working Group noted that details of the response rate were not given, and no allowance was made for any covariate, including smoking.]

Kabat *et al.* (1986) studied bladder cancer in nonsmokers among 76 male and 76 female cases and 238 male and 254 female hospital controls matched for sex, race, hospital and year of interview; the male controls consisted of 67% cancers not related to tobacco smoking and 33% non-neoplastic conditions; the female controls consisted of 59% and 41%, respectively. No association with brewed coffee was observed in either sex [overall RR adjusted for sex, 1.1; 95% CI, 0.8-1.5], and all subsequent risk estimates with dose were close to unity. Similarly, no association was evident with decaffeinated coffee use.

The RR for coffee drinking was significantly above unity (2.4; 95% CI, 1.4-4.4) in a study of 99 male cases of histologically confirmed bladder cancer and two groups each of 99 controls (one hospital, one neighbourhood) in La Plata, Argentina (Iscovich *et al.*, 1987). A positive trend in risk with dose was found, which persisted after allowance for smoking. The refusal rate was negligible (less than 3% of cases and 5% of controls). [The Working Group noted the limited size of the study and that an unstated number of re-interviews were undertaken to obtain missing information or to correct inconsistencies.]

In a population-based case-control study in Utah, USA, Slattery *et al.* (1988) obtained data on a total of 419 cases of bladder cancer and 889 controls (participation rate, 76% among cases and 82% among controls). A substantial proportion of the Utah population belongs to the Mormon church, which proscribes the use of coffee and tea, besides alcohol and tobacco. The RR for coffee consumption, adjusted for age, sex, diabetes, bladder infections and cigarette smoking was [approximately 1.2]. No consistent dose-response was evident, since the RR was 1.2 for up to 20 servings per week, 1.1 for 21-40 and 1.6 for over 40. Similarly, no association emerged in relation to drinking decaffeinated coffee (RR, 1.0).

In a study in Italy, Ciccone and Vineis (1988) studied coffee drinking among cases of bladder cancer (512 men, 55 women) from the main hospital of Turin; controls were 596 men and 202 women with urological or surgical conditions. The overall participation rate was 82% for cases (although there were only 2% refusals) and 98% for controls. With current coffee use, the overall RR, adjusted for smoking (never, ex- or current smoker) was [1.0] for men and [0.9] for women. There was no evidence of an increase in risk with increasing intake: in both men and women, the adjusted RR for four cups per day or more was 0.8. Similarly, no association was evident for either sex for past use (10 years before interview). The authors noted that the only subgroup with an elevated risk and a dose-response relationship was male nonsmokers.

Risch *et al.* (1988) analysed the association between drinking of coffee, tea and other beverages in a population-based case-control study on dietary factors and bladder cancer based on 826 cases of histologically confirmed bladder cancer and 792 controls in Canada. The participation rate was 67% for cases and 53% for controls. For total coffee consumption, the RR was 0.9 in males and 1.9 in females. Adjustment was made for history of diabetes and cigarette use in terms of cumulated pack-years. There was no association in either sex with frequency of use, and the RRs for the highest intake level (over six cups per day) were 0.9 for males and 1.1 for females. [The Working Group noted that the participation rates were lower than in other case-control studies.]

La Vecchia *et al.* (1989b) provided information on the coffee consumption of 163 patients with histologically confirmed bladder cancer (136 male, 27 female), from a network of hospitals in northern Italy, and of 181 controls with acute, nonneoplastic or urological conditions. The participation rate was over 98%. Compared with non- or moderate coffee drinkers, the RRs adjusted for age, sex, area of residence, social class and smoking were 2.0 for intermediate and 1.6 for heavy drinkers; the trend was not significant.

Renal pelvis and ureter. The etiology and pathogenesis of transitional-cell cancer of the renal pelvis and ureter are in several aspects similar to those of bladder cancer, although the frequency of cancer at these sites is much lower and, hence, the studies are based on small data sets.

One study in the USA (Schmauz & Cole, 1974), based on 43 cases of cancer of the renal pelvis and ureter and 451 population controls, showed a positive association with high levels of coffee consumption among men (RR for over seven cups per day, 14.9; 95% CI, 2.4-94.3).

Table 32. Summary of results of case–control studies of bladder cancer and coffee consumption: users *versus* nonusers[a]

Reference and location	Subjects (cases, controls)	Relative risk (95% CI)	Significance[b]	Comments
Cole (1971) USA	Men (345, 351)	1.2 (0.8–1.9)	NS	Adjusted for age and smoking (nonsmokers/ < ½pack/≥½ pack per day). Similar relation among nonsmokers non-occupationally exposed to carcinogens
	Women (100, 100)	2.6 (1.3–5.1)	Significant	
Dunham et al. (1968); Fraumeni et al. (1971) USA	Men and women (493, 527)	1.5	NS; significant in black women	Adjusted for age and cigarette smoking
Morgan & Jain (1974) Canada	Men (158, 158)	[0.7]	NS	Unadjusted; mailed questionnaire
	Women (74, 74)	[1.3]	NS	
Simon et al. (1975) USA	Women (135, 390)	2.1 (1.1–4.3)	Significant	[RR, 1.9] (NS) after adjustment for smoking in two categories
Wynder & Goldsmith (1977) USA	Men (574, 574)	[1.5]	NS	Adjusted for smoking (four levels)
	Women (158, 158)	[1.3]	NS	
Miller et al. (1978) Canada	Men (183, 366)	1.3	NS	
	Women (72, 144)	1.6 [1.0–2.9]	NS	
Mettlin & Graham (1979) USA	Men and women (569, 1025)	[1.5 (0.9–2.5)]	NS	Adjusted for smoking (two levels) from published data
Howe et al. (1980) Canada	Men (480, 480)	1.4 (0.9–2.0)	NS	Unadjusted estimates from matched analysis
	Women (152, 152)	1.0 (0.5–2.1)	NS	
Cartwright et al. (1981) UK	Men (631, 789)	1.1 (0.9–1.4)	NS	Adjusted for age, type of case (incident/prevalent) and smoking; no heterogeneity according to type of coffee (instant/ground)
	Women (210, 271)	0.8 (0.6–1.2)	NS	

Table 32 (contd)

Reference and location	Subjects (cases, controls)	Relative risk (95% CI)	Significance[b]	Comments
Morrison et al. (1982) USA, UK and Japan	Men and women (1417, 1839)	1.0 (0.8–1.2)	NS	Adjusted for age, sex, study area and smoking
Najem et al. (1982) USA	Men and women (75, 142)	1.8 (0.1–10.0)	NS	Unadjusted estimates; low power
Sullivan (1982) USA	Men and women (82, 169)	Not given	Significant difference in average mean intake of ground coffee in white men, decaffeinated ground in white women	No relation with duration; unadjusted covariates
Hartge et al. (1983) USA	Men and women (2982, 5782)	1.4 (1.1–1.8)	Significant	Adjusted for sex, age, race, geographical area and tobacco history
Marrett et al. (1983)[c] USA	Men Women (412, 493)	1.3 [1.1–1.6] 1.1 [0.8–1.4]	Significant NS	Adjusted for age and smoking
Mommsen et al. (1983a,b) Denmark	Men (165, 165) Women (47, 94)	No association 2.6 (0.4–18.8)	NS	Details not given for men; only one female case and five controls non-coffee drinkers
Rebelakos et al. (1985) Greece	Men and women (300, 300)	1.7 (1.2–2.3)	Significant	≥2 versus <2 cups per day; adjusted for age, sex and smoking
Gonzáles et al. (1985) Spain	Men and women (58, 116)	[0.6]	NS	'Habitual consumers'
Jensen et al. (1986) Denmark	Men and women (371, 771)	[~1.4]	NS	Including papillomas; adjusted for age, sex, smoking (never/current; lifetime pack years), tea and soft drinks
Claude et al. (1986) Federal Republic of Germany	Men (340, 340) Women (91, 91)	1.8 1.1	NS NS	Adjusted for smoking (never/ever; lifetime pack years). Significant trend in men

Table 32 (contd)

Reference and location	Subjects (cases, controls)	Relative risk (95% CI)	Significance[b]	Comments
Piper et al. (1986) USA	Women (173, 173)	1.6 (0.8–3.3)	NS	Aged 20–49; unadjusted
Bravo et al. (1986) Spain	Men (353, 353) Women (53, 53)	1.9 (1.4–2.6) [2.3 (1.1–5.1)]	Significant Significant	Matched for age and area of residence; unadjusted
Kabat et al. (1986) USA	Men (76, 238) Women (76, 254)	[1.1 (0.8–1.5)]	NS	Nonsmokers only; adjusted for sex
Iscovich et al. (1987) Argentina	Men (99, 198)	2.4 (1.4–4.4)	Significant	Adjusted for smoking
Slattery et al. (1988) USA	Men and women (419, 889)	[~1.2]	NS	Adjusted for age, sex, diabetes, bladder infections and smoking
Ciccone & Vineis (1988) Italy	Men Women (567, 798)	[1.0] [0.9]	NS	Adjusted for smoking (never, ex-, current)
Risch et al. (1988) Canada	Men Women (826, 792)	0.9 (0.6–1.3) 1.9 (1.0–3.4)	NS Significant	Adjusted for smoking (cumulated pack years) and history of diabetes
La Vecchia et al. (1989b) Italy	Men and women (163, 181)	[1.8]	Significant	Adjusted for age, sex, area of residence, social class, smoking

[a] In square brackets, calculated by the Working Group
[b] NS, not significant
[c] Some overlap with the study of Hartge et al. (1983)

Table 33. Summary of results of case–control studies of bladder cancer and coffee consumption: dose–response relationships

Reference and location	Sex	Relative risk for level of coffee consumption[a]							Significance (trend; p)
		I Lowest	II	III	IV	V	VI	VII Highest	
Cole (1971)	Men	1	1.3	1.2	1.3	–	–	–	Not given
USA	Women	1	1.6	3.8	2.2	–	–	–	
Fraumeni et al. (1971)	Men, white	1	1.4	2.0	1.7	–	–	–	Not given
	Men, black	1	2.1	2.9	2.1	–	–	–	
USA	Women, white	1	0.7	0.5	0.3	–	–	–	
	Women, black	1	10.0	4.6	2.2	–	–	–	
Morgan & Jain (1974)[b] Canada	Men and women	[1	0.6	0.9	0.8	1.1]	–	–	Nonsignificant
Simon et al. (1975)[b] USA	Women	1	2.2	1.9	2.3	–	–	–	0.28
Wynder & Goldsmith (1977) USA	Men	1	1.4	1.9	2.0	–	–	–	Nonsignificant
	Women	1	1.0	1.9	1.3	–	–	–	Nonsignificant
Mettlin & Graham (1979) USA	Men and women	1	[1.2	1.1	1.8	1.3]	–	–	Nonsignificant
Howe et al. (1980)[b] Canada	Men	1	[1.6	1.3	1.5]	–	–	–	Nonsignificant
	Women	1	[0.7	1.7	1.3]	–	–	–	Nonsignificant
Morrison et al. (1982)									
USA	Men	1	0.8	0.7	0.9	0.8	0.8	1.5	Nonsignificant
	Women	1	0.8	0.6	1.7	0.9	0.7	1.0	Nonsignificant
UK	Men	1	1.1	0.9	0.9	0.8	–	–	Nonsignificant
	Women	1	1.4	0.4	1.2	1.0	–	–	Nonsignificant
Japan	Men	1	1.0	1.2	1.3	1.9	–	–	Nonsignificant
	Women	1	0.7	–	0.7	–	–	–	Nonsignificant
Hartge et al. (1983)	Men	1	0.9	1.0	1.1	1.0	1.2	1.5	Nonsignificant
USA	Women	1	0.9	0.8	0.9	0.7	0.9	0.8	Nonsignificant
Marrett et al. (1983)[c]	Men	1	1.6	2.0	2.0	–	–	–	Significant
USA	Women	1	[1.3	1.2	1.0]	–	–	–	Nonsignificant

Table 33 (contd)

Reference and location	Sex	Relative risk for level of coffee consumption[a]							Significance (trend; p)
		I Lowest	II	III	IV	V	VI	VII Highest	
Rebelakos et al. (1985) Greece	Men and women	1	1.2	1.7	2.7	0.7	–	–	0.02
Jensen et al. (1986) Denmark	Men and women	1	1.4	1.2	1.4	1.8	–	–	0.12
Claude et al. (1986) Federal Republic of Germany	Men	1	1.4	1.4	2.3	–	–	–	< 0.05
	Women	1	1.3	1.9	2.2	–	–	–	Nonsignificant
Piper et al. (1986)[d] USA	Women	1	0.9	1.9	2.1	–	–	–	Nonsignificant
Bravo et al. (1986, 1987)[b] Spain	Men	1	1.9	2.6	–	–	–	–	< 0.01
Kabat et al. (1986)[b] USA	Men	1	0.9	1.4	1.4	0.5	–	–	Nonsignificant
	Women	1	1.5	0.8	0.7	2.4	–	–	Nonsignificant
Iscovich et al. (1987) Argentina	Men and women	1	1.1	4.5	12.0	–	–	–	< 0.01
Slattery et al. (1988) USA	Men and women	1	1.2	1.1	1.6	–	–	–	Nonsignificant
Ciccone & Vineis (1988) Italy	Men	1	0.8	1.0	1.2	0.8	–	–	Nonsignificant
	Women	1	1.4	1.0	0.7	0.8	–	–	Nonsignificant
Risch et al. (1988) Canada	Men	1	1.0	1.2	0.9	–	–	–	Nonsignificant
	Women	1	1.0	1.9	1.1	–	–	–	Nonsignificant
La Vecchia et al. (1989b) Italy	Men and women	1	2.0	1.6	–	–	–	–	Nonsignificant

[a] The levels relate to different quantities in each study; therefore, they offer information for analyses within each study but not for comparisons between studies. 1, lowest (referent) level; 7, highest level
[b] Crude risks
[c] Some overlap with the study of Hartge et al. (1983)
[d] Adjusted risks, but not stated whether smoking included

A matched hospital-based study of 33 cases of cancer of the renal pelvis and 33 controls in the UK (Amstrong *et al.*, 1976) found no positive association with coffee [RR, 0.2; $p < 0.01$]. Indeed, there was a significant excess of cases who had never consumed coffee regularly.

A population-based case-control study of 74 cases and 697 controls in the USA (McLaughlin *et al.*, 1983) showed no consistent association between cancer of the renal pelvis and coffee drinking in people of either sex after adjustment for smoking (RR, 1.6 for men, 0.5 for women).

The largest study on cancer at this site (187 case-control pairs) was conducted in Los Angeles County, USA, using telephone interviews for cases and neighbourhood controls (Ross *et al.*, 1989). Heavy coffee drinkers had an apparently elevated risk for cancer of the renal pelvis and ureter (RR for seven cups or more per day, adjusted for cigarette smoking, 1.8), but the trend in risk with dose was not significant.

Kidney. The causes of renal-cell cancer (adenocarcinoma of the kidney) are less well defined but are certainly, at least in part, different from those of cancer of the urinary tract.

In a case-control study conducted in several areas of the USA between 1965 and 1973 on 202 patients with adenocarcinoma of the kidney and 394 hospital controls, Wynder *et al.* (1974) found no significant difference in daily coffee consumption within each smoking category: [RR, 0.6, 0.9 and 1.1 for 1-2, 3-4 and ≥ 5 cups per day].

Armstrong *et al.* (1976) conducted a case-control study of 106 cases of adenocarcinoma of the renal parenchyma and 106 controls in Oxford, UK, and found neither an association with coffee use [RR, 1.1] nor a dose-response relationship.

McLaughlin *et al.* (1984) conducted a population-based case-control study on 495 cases of renal-cell carcinoma and 697 controls from the Minneapolis-St Paul seven-county metropolitan area (USA). The RR for ever having drunk coffee was 1.0 (95% CI, 0.6-1.8) in men and 1.4 (0.7-2.9) in women. In neither was a dose-response relationship observed.

Goodman *et al.* (1986) conducted a hospital-based case-control study of renal-cell carcinoma among 189 men and 78 women from various areas of the USA. For coffee drinking, the RRs (for the two sexes combined) were 0.7 for one to two cups per day and 0.8 for three or more compared with non-coffee drinkers. The RR for ever having drunk decaffeinated coffee was 1.9 (95% CI, 1.0-3.6), but people drinking one to two cups per day had a RR of 2.0 while those drinking three cups or more had a RR of 1.3.

In a study of 166 incident cases of renal-cell carcinoma and an equal number of age-, sex- and race-matched neighbourhood controls, Yu *et al.* (1986) found an association in women for daily coffee consumption (RR, 2.3; $p = 0.06$) in the absence of a direct dose-response relationship. No significant association was observed in men.

A study from Australia (McCredie *et al.*, 1988) based on 360 cases of cancer of the renal parenchyma and 985 population controls found no association with coffee consumption, but no precise information is given in the text.

(ii) *Pancreas*

Twenty-one case-control studies have reported on the relationship between coffee consumption and pancreatic cancer; these data are summarized in Table 34 on p. 140.

As part of a study of cancer at 13 sites, Lin and Kessler (1981) reported on 109 histologically confirmed cases (67 male, 42 female) of pancreatic cancer (94 adenocarcinomas and 15 islet-cell tumours) identified in 1972-75 in more than 115 hospitals in the USA. Equal numbers of hospital controls were matched for age, sex, race, hospital and year of admission. Most of the cases and controls were interviewed while in hospital by a person who was unaware of the diagnosis of the patient. Overall 86% of eligible subjects were interviewed. It was reported in a letter that an association was found with drinking decaffeinated coffee but not with total coffee consumption: 91% of the cases drank coffee compared to 93% of controls, but 41% of cases drank decaffeinated coffee compared to only 25% of controls ($p < 0.01$) (Kessler, 1981).

MacMahon *et al.* (1981a,b; the latter study was reported in a letter) reported on 367 histologically confirmed cases (216 male, 151 female) of pancreatic cancer (excluding islet-cell tumours) out of 578 patients under 80 years of age identified in 11 hospitals in Boston and Rhode Island, USA. There were 643 hospital controls, out of 1118 eligible patients, who had been at hospital at the same time as the cases; 254 had diseases other than cancer at sites other than the gastrointestinal tract, 157 had cancers other than in the gastrointestinal tract, 117 had diseases of the gastrointestinal tract other than cancer, and 115 had gastrointestinal cancer. Each case and control pair was interviewed personally by the same physician. The main reasons for failure to participate were death (20 cases, 9 controls), early discharge (35, 131), illness (78, 179), language difficulties (14, 26) and refusal (26, 73). An increased risk was found for both men and women. The RR of coffee drinkers *versus* non-coffee drinkers was 2.6 for men and 2.3 for women. No dose-response was observed in men, but a significant trend with consumption was found in women, rising to a risk of 3.1 for women who drank five or more cups per day. These risks persisted after adjustment for cigarette smoking.

Several generally smaller studies (Elinder *et al.*, 1981; Jick & Dinan, 1981; Goldstein, 1982; Severson *et al.*, 1982) reported essentially negative results. The study of Jick and Dinan (1981), published as a letter, which gave few details, was based on 83 cases and 161 hospital controls aged < 80 years in several countries matched 2:1 for age, sex, hospital and year of admission and used a standard personal hospital interview. Elinder *et al.* (1981) conducted two studies: In one, they used information from certificates of deaths in 1961-74 in two small Swedish parishes; the study was based on 21 male cases and 51 deceased male controls obtained from a random sample of deaths in the same parish and matched for age. Next-of-kin, usually wives, were interviewed. The second study was based on 41 twin pairs, born 1886-1925, both of whom were alive in 1961 and one of whom developed pancreatic cancer. Information was obtained from postal questionnaires. The study of Goldstein (1982) was based on 91 histologically verified cases of pancreatic cancer diagnosed in 1973-80 in San Diego, CA, USA; controls were patients with cancer of the prostate (45) and breast (48). Routine hospital interview data were used. Severson *et al.* (1982) based their study on 22 cases aged 40-79 from a registry that was part of the SEER (Surveillance, Epidemiology and End Results) Program in Seattle, WA, USA, 1977-80, and on a random population sample of controls. Next-of-kin were interviewed for most of the cases (20), whereas personal interviews were obtained for controls. The last two studies were also published as letters, which contained few details.

A large study of 275 histologically verified cases (153 men, 122 women) aged 20-80 interviewed in 1977-81 and of 7994 hospital controls also gave negative results, with risk ratios very near to unity after adjustment for smoking (Wynder *et al.*, 1983). This was part of a large study of tobacco-related cancers in six US cities; controls were patients with non-tobacco-related diseases: 42% had other cancers, 10% had benign neoplasms and 7% had trauma. Personal interviews were carried out within six months of diagnosis. During the last year of interviewing, 45% of potential cases and 35% of potential controls completed interviews. The main reasons for not interviewing cases were death, early discharge, illness and personal or physician refusal. The main reason for not interviewing controls was that their initial diagnosis had been made more than six months before interview.

Kinlen and McPherson (1984) re-evaluated data from the case-control study of Stocks (partly reported by Stocks, 1957) on data collected in north-west England and north Wales in 1952-54 on 216 cases (109 men, 107 women) aged > 40 years. These were compared with 432 controls, who were patients with other cancers in the original study, matched 2:1 for age, sex and area of residence; cancers of the lung, bladder, mouth, pharynx, oesophagus, gastrointestinal tract and ovary were excluded, and controls were thus patients with breast cancer (38%), prostatic cancer (19%), leukaemia or lymphoma (19%), renal cancer (7%) and other cancers

(17%). No relation with coffee consumption was found either before or after adjustment for smoking.

Subsequent studies by Gold *et al.* (1985), Mack *et al.* (1986) and Norell *et al.* (1986) all provided some evidence of an association. In the study of Gold *et al.* (1985), 201 cases (94 men, 107 women) were interviewed and included in a matched analysis out of a total of 392 patients with pancreatic cancer from 16 hospitals in Baltimore, MD, USA, in 1977-80. Seventy-two patients refused to be interviewed, physician consent was not obtained for 36, and 10 patients could not be traced or had died and no relative could be found. Of the 201, 25% had a personal interview; for 35% the spouse was interviewed and for 40%, another relative. Two control groups were used: a matched hospital series (for age, race, sex, hospital, date of admission) in which patients with other cancers were excluded (30% had heart or other circulatory disease and 13% had digestive disease) and a population-based group that was chosen by random-digit dialling, matched by age, race, sex and telephone exchange and interviewed by telephone. Participation was about 50% of 'eligible' individuals in both control series; a total of 20 706 telephone numbers and 37 033 calls were made to find eligible controls. A nonsignificant relationship was found among women only, but this was less apparent when smoking was adjusted for.

Mack *et al.* (1986) conducted a study of 490 histologically confirmed cases (282 male, 208 female) of adenocarcinoma of the exocrine pancreas in patients aged < 65 years, comprising all those registered in Los Angeles county, and an equal number of neighbourhood controls matched for age, sex, race and neighbourhood in Los Angeles, CA, USA. Home interviews were conducted; for cases, about 25% of the interviews were with the case, 53% with the spouse and 19% with a first-degree relative. Cases were selected from 736 eligible cases; losses were due to failure to locate the case (77), physician refusal (43), patient refusal (86), language problems (10) and failure to find a matched control (17). Final medical review eliminated another 13 cases. Results for coffee drinking showed a significant relationship, which persisted after adjustment for smoking.

Norell *et al.* (1986) conducted a study in Stockholm and Uppsala, Sweden, in 1982-84, based on 99 cases (55 male, 44 female) aged 40-79 out of 120 that were eligible, 138 population controls (a sample from the same parish matched for age and sex) out of 162 that were eligible and 163 hospital controls who were a random sample of patients with inguinal hernia, of whom 179 were eligible. Of the cases, 61% were verified by resection or autopsy, 33% by radiology and biopsy, and 6% by clinical examination and radiology. Cases and hospital controls were given a questionnaire at the time of diagnosis, whereas population controls were sent a postal questionnaire followed by a telephone call when necessary. The results were positive when hospital controls were used and disappeared when population controls were the basis of comparison. Results adjusted for smoking were not presented.

Wynder *et al.* (1986) undertook a study of 238 patients (127 men, 111 women) and 696 controls in 18 hospitals in six US cities, 1981-84, in which both coffee and decaffeinated coffee were examined. Controls were selected from among patients with non-tobacco-related diseases matched for age, sex, race, hospital and year of interview; 62% had other cancers. A hospital interview was used. Neither exposure was related to pancreatic cancer either before or after adjustment for smoking.

A study (reported in a letter to the Editor of *The New England Journal of Medicine*) of 172 patients (85 men, 87 women) aged < 80 years with histologically verified pancreatic cancer and 267 controls was conducted in 1981-84 in Boston and Rhode Island, MA, USA, on the basis of hospital interviews (Hsieh *et al.*, 1986). Controls had the same physician, and the main diagnoses were cancer of the breast, colon, stomach or uterus, benign tumours, hernia, colitis, enteritis and bowel obstruction. An elevated risk, of borderline significance, was found only in patients who had drunk more than five cups of coffee per day, the RR being 2.4 in men and 2.2 in women. Similar results were found for coffee and for decaffeinated coffee.

A study was carried out in northern Italy of 150 histologically verified cases aged < 75 (99 men, 51 women) and 605 hospital controls with acute conditions except cancer, digestive-tract disorders or conditions related to coffee, alcohol or tobacco consumption (33% trauma, 12% other orthopaedic, 42% general surgery) (La Vecchia *et al.*, 1987). More than 98% of eligible patients (cases and controls) agreed to participate and were given a hospital interview. Some evidence of risk was seen, but there was no dose-response relationship and the highest risk was found among people who drank one to two cups per day. Only 16 cases did not drink coffee. No relationship with decaffeinated coffee was found.

Studies by Raymond *et al.* (1987), based on 88 cases (43 male, 45 female), 67% of which were verified histologically, and 336 population controls, and by Falk *et al.* (1988), based on 363 cases (203 male, 160 female) out of 427 incident cases and 1234 hospital controls, gave negative results. In the first study, personal interviews were obtained from cases identified through the Geneva, Switzerland, registry in 1976-81 and from controls who were contacted by letter. The study by Falk *et al.* (1988) was carried out in Louisiana, USA; 82% of cases were confirmed histologically and the remainder by X-ray, ultrasound or clinical examination. Controls were matched for hospital, age, sex and race and excluded patients with cancer, diabetes, circulatory disorders and digestive or respiratory diseases. Direct interviews were carried out with 50% of cases, and 50% were with next of kin.

A small study by Gorham *et al.* (1988) of 30 cases (out of 51 eligible) and 47 controls (out of 58 eligible) was based only on death certificates in Imperial County, CA, USA, in 1978-84. Controls were matched for age, sex, race and year of death;

cancer patients were excluded, and 47% had died from heart disease, 17% from cerebrovascular disease, 4% from pneumonia and 4% from chronic obstructive pulmonary disease. The estimated RR for three or more cups of coffee a day was [2.7] compared to less than three cups, which dropped to [1.9] and was nonsignificant after adjustment for smoking. [The Working Group noted that only 30 of 51 deaths from pancreatic cancer were included; hospital records were not examined.]

Clavel *et al.* (1989) conducted a hospital interview study in Paris, France, with 161 cases (98 male, 63 female), 63% of which were histologically verified (28% by surgery and 9% by clinical examination) in 1982-85. There were 268 hospital controls: 129 had other cancers, excluding biliary, liver, stomach, oesophagus, respiratory and bladder cancers, and 139 had non-neoplastic disease. All were matched to cases for age, sex and hospital interviewer. None of the cases and about 5% of controls refused to participate. After adjustment for education, alcohol and smoking, a nonsignificant trend was found for males, giving a RR of 2.1 for four or more cups/day. In females, a significant trend was observed, and the observed risk for more than four cups per day was 9.6. Unusually high risks were seen in women and in persons who had never drunk alcohol.

A study of 216 cases (123 male, 93 female) and 279 controls was carried out in the UK for 1983-86 (Cuzick & Babiker, 1989), based on personal interview. Of the cases, 30% were verified histologically, 23% by surgery and 47% by clinical examination or imaging. The controls included 212 hospital controls without other cancers or other chronic medical conditions: 27% had fractures, 23%, hernia, 15%, varicose veins and haemorrhoids and 11%, genitourinary diseases; the remaining 67 were population controls. The study gave essentially negative results, although a slightly elevated risk was seen in cases whose current consumption was more than five cups per day (RR, 1.4). This trend disappeared when consumption approximately 10 years previously was examined.

A case-control study in the USA involved 212 cases (140 of which were confirmed pathologically) identified from death certificates, out of 262 that were eligible, and 250 population-based controls contacted by random telephone dialling and matched to cases by age within five years (Olsen *et al.*, 1989). Family members (usually widow or spouse) were interviewed on the case's use of cigarettes, alcohol, coffee and other dietary factors two years prior to death of the patient or prior to interview. Coffee was not a risk factor (odds ratio for seven cups or more per day, 0.6; 95% CI, 0.3-1.3).

Table 34. Summary of results of case-control studies of coffee drinking and pancreatic cancer

Reference and location	Subjects (cases, controls)	Coffee consumption (cups/day)	Relative risk (95% CI)	Comments
Lin & Kessler (1981); Kessler (1981) USA	Men and women (109, 109)			91% cases vs 93% controls drank coffee 41% cases vs 25% controls drank decaffeinated coffee ($p < 0.01$)
MacMahon et al. (1981a,b) USA	Men (216, 307)	0 1–2 3–4 ≥ 5	1.0 2.6 2.3 2.6	χ^2 trend = 1.5
	Women (151, 336)	0 1–2 3–4 ≥ 5	1.0 1.6 3.3 3.1	χ^2 trend = 13.7
	Men and women	0 1–2 ≥ 3	1.0 1.8 2.7	Adjusted for smoking; χ^2 trend = 10.6
Jick & Dinan (1981) Several countries	Men and women (83, 166)	0 1–5 ≥ 6	1.0 0.7 0.5	

Elinder et al. (1981) Sweden	Men (21, 51)
	  Cases
	
	  Controls
		
		5.3 ± 2.1
		(SD)
		6.1 ± 2.4
				95% CI for difference: −2.9–0.2

	Men and women (twins; 41, 41)	3.8 3.6		95% CI for difference −0.33–0.77
Goldstein (1982) USA	Men and women (91, 93)	0 1–2 3–4 ≥ 5	1.0 1.8 1.0 1.6	Crude odds ratio; χ^2 for trend nonsignificant
Severson et al. (1982) USA	Men and women (22, 485)	Current	1.0 (0.2–4.5)	Adjusted for age, sex, smoking
Wynder et al. (1983) USA	Men (153, 5469)	0 1–2 3–4 ≥ 5	1.0 [1.1] 1.0 1.4	

Table 34 (contd)

Reference and location	Subjects (cases, controls)	Coffee consumption (cups/day)	Relative risk (95% CI)	Comments
Wynder et al. (1983) (contd)	Women (122, 2525)	0 1–2 3–4 ≥5	1.0 [1.0] 1.0 1.2	
	Men	0 1–2 3–4 ≥5	1.0 [1.0] 1.0 1.0	Adjusted for smoking
	Women	0 1–2 3–4 ≥5	1.0 0.9 0.9 1.0	Adjusted for smoking
Kinlen & McPherson (1984) UK	Men (109, 218)	Never Weekly Daily	1.0 0.9 0.9	
	Women (107, 214)	Never Weekly Daily	1.0 1.3 0.9	Adjusted for tea and smoking
Gold et al. (1985) USA	Men (94, 96/96)	0 1–2 3–4 ≥5	1.0 1.6/1.5 1.5/1.0 1.0/1.3	Adjusted for age; hospital random-digit dialling controls; χ^2 for trend, [0.02/0.4]
	Women (103, 103/104)	0 1–2 3–4 ≥5	1.0 0.8/1.2 2.0/1.6 2.1/2.9	χ^2 for trend, [3.8/2.7]
Mack et al. (1986) USA	Men and women (490, 490)	0 1–4 ≥5	1.0 1.6 2.0	Crude odds ratio
	Men and women	0 1–4 ≥5	1.0 [1.4] [1.6]	Adjusted for smoking
Norell et al. (1986) Sweden	Men and women (99, 163/138)	0–1 2–4 ≥5	1.0 1.7/1.6 (0.7–3.9/0.8–3.2) 1.9/1.0 (0.8–4.9/0.4–2.6)	Hospital/population controls; 90% CI

Table 34 (contd)

Reference and location	Subjects (cases, controls)	Coffee consumption (cups/day)	Relative risk (95% CI)	Comments
Wynder et al. (1986) USA	Men (127, 371)	0 1–2 ≥3	1.0 [1.1] [1.5]	
	Women (111, 325)	0 1–2 ≥3	1.0 [0.7] [1.0]	
	Men	0 1–2 ≥3	1.0 0.8 0.7	Decaffeinated
	Women	0 1–2 ≥3	1.0 1.6 0.9	
Hsieh et al. (1986) USA	Men (85, 129)	0 1–2 3–4 ≥5	1.0 1.1 1.0 2.4	Consumption ~10 years previously; χ^2 for trend, [2.8]
	Women (87, 138)	0 1–2 3–4 ≥5	1.0 1.3 1.0 2.2	χ^2 for trend, [1.3]
	Men and women (170, 265)	0 <20.000 20–39 000 40–59 000 ≥60 000	1.0 1.0 1.3 1.8 1.4	Total consumption of coffee; χ^2 for trend, [3.3]
	Men and women (170, 265)	0 <20.000 20–39 000 40–59 000 ≥60 000	1.0 1.0 1.0 1.5 1.6	Total consumption of decaffeinated coffee; χ^2 for trend, [2.1]
	Men and women (170, 266)	0 <20.000 20–39 000 40–59 000 ≥60 000	1.0 1.4 1.2 2.0 1.5	Total consumption of both types of coffee; χ^2 for trend, [2.4]
La Vecchia et al. (1987) Italy	Men and women (150, 605)	0 1–2 3–4 ≥5	1.0 1.8 1.5 1.4	

Table 34 (contd)

Reference and location	Subjects (cases, controls)	Coffee consumption (cups/day)	Relative risk (95% CI)	Comments
La Vecchia et al. (1987) (contd)	Men and women	0 1-2 3-4 ≥5	1.0 1.7 1.4 1.1	Adjusted for smoking, alcohol, occupation
	Men and women	0 3-4	1.0 0.8	Decaffeinated coffee
	Men and women	0 3-4	1.0 0.9	Decaffeinated coffee; adjusted for smoking, alcohol, occupation
Raymond et al. (1987) Switzerland	Men and women (88, 336)	0 < 1.4 l/week ≥1.4 l/week	1.0 0.9 (0.5-1.8) 1.3 (0.7-2.3)	90% CI
	Men and women	0 Any	1.0 1.4 (0.8-2.4)	Instant coffee; 90% CI
Falk et al. (1988) USA	Men (203, 890)	0 1-2 3-4 5-7 ≥8	1.0 0.7 0.5 0.7 1.4	Adjusted for smoking, alcohol, fruit consumption, income
	Women (160, 344)	0 1-2 3-4 5-7 ≥8	1.0 0.7 0.7 1.0 0.9	Adjusted as above
Gorham et al. (1988) USA	Men and women (30, 47)	0 1-2 3-4 ≥5	1.0 [0.5] [1.2] [2.3]	
Clavel et al. (1989) France	Men (98, 161)	0 1 2-3 ≥4	1.0 1.1 1.5 2.1	χ^2 for trend, [1.2]
	Women (63, 107)	0 1 2-3 ≥4	1.0 3.9 6.7 9.6	χ^2 for trend, [6.4]

Table 34 (contd)

Reference and location	Subjects (cases, controls)	Coffee consumption (cups/day)	Relative risk (95% CI)	Comments
Cuzick & Babiker (1989) UK	Men and women (216, 279)	0 1-2 3-4 ≥5	1.0 0.9 0.6 1.4	Adjusted for smoking; χ^2 for trend, 0.23
	Men and women	0 1-2 3-4 ≥5	1.0 0.9 0.6 1.4	Coffee consumption ~10 years previously; χ^2 for trend, 0.43
Olsen et al. (1989) USA	Men and women (212, 220)	<1 1-3 4-6 ≥7	1.0 0.5 0.7 0.6	Odds ratio, adjusted for smoking, diet

(iii) *Breast cancer*

Case-control studies of breast cancer and coffee, instant coffee and decaffeinated coffee are summarized in Table 35 (p. 147).

Lawson *et al.* (1981) analysed data obtained from the Boston Collaborative Drug Surveillance Program and from a collaborative study conducted in the USA, Scotland and New Zealand. Cases were 241 women discharged with a diagnosis of breast cancer. Three controls were matched to each case for age, smoking habit, study and country. Coffee and tea drinking were grouped as 'hot beverage consumption'. Compared to those who did not drink coffee or tea, RRs for those who drank one to three, four to six and seven or more cups per day were 1.3, 1.5 and 1.1 (90% CI, 0.6-1.8 for the last category), respectively.

Lubin *et al.* (1981) reported the results of a study conducted in northern Alberta, Canada, during 1976-77. Interview was completed for 577 cases and 826 population controls. The response rate was 95% for cases and 72% for controls. Information on consumption of tea or coffee was obtained along with demographic, reproductive and medical histories and data on several food items. Tea and coffee consumption was analysed together: the age-adjusted RR when comparing more than five cups per day to five or fewer was 1.2 (95% CI, 0.9-1.5).

Mansel *et al.* (1982) in an abstract reported the results from an analysis of a computer data base of 20 000 hospital in-patients with a diagnosis of breast disease. These patients were compared with a matched non-breast disease group. As compared with non-coffee drinkers, coffee drinkers had an increased risk for breast cancer (RR, 1.3; 95% CI, 0.99-1.6). [It was not clear who was included in the control group, what variables were matched on, whether matched analyses were carried out, and thus, what confounders had been controlled. Although information was collected on several doses levels, information on any dose-effect relation was not available.]

Lubin et al. (1984, 1985) conducted a hospital-based case-control study in Israel. Cases were histologically confirmed breast cancer cases in the greater Tel Aviv metropolitan area diagnosed between 1975 and 1979. Two control series, surgical and neighbourhood, were used; each was matched individually to a case by age ($\pm$ five years), country of origin and length of residence in Israel. Neighbourhood controls were drawn from the national voting list and lived in the same voting district as the cases. Information was sought on the frequency of consumption of 250 food and beverage items as well as on selected hormonal, medical and demographic characteristics. Response rates among the eligible subjects were 96% for cases and surgical controls and 72% for neighbourhood controls. A total of 818 cases, 743 surgical controls and 813 neighbourhood controls were included in the analysis. Breast cancer cases were found to consume less coffee than both control series.

Rosenberg et al. (1984, 1985) analysed data obtained in a case-control programme for the surveillance of drug effects. Cases were 2651 in-patients in hospitals located in eastern USA who were interviewed between 1975 and 1982. There were two control groups: one consisted of 1501 women admitted for acute nonmalignant conditions (trauma or infections); the other comprised 385 women with malignancies (malignant melanoma, lymphoma and leukaemia). With either control group, RRs were close to 1.0 and there was no trend of increasing risk with increasing daily intake of coffee. Coffee drinking was not associated with breast cancer risk among subgroups of women stratified by age and reproductive history, history of fibrocystic breast disease, family history of breast cancer, or body mass index. Among a subset of subjects who did not drink caffeine-containing coffee, age-adjusted RRs were close to 1.0.

In a study in France, described by Lê et al. (1984) and reported in a letter by Lê (1985), 500 cases and 945 surgical controls with nonmalignant disease were studied. The risk for breast cancer was found to be inversely associated with reported current daily coffee consumption. Results were similar for women with and without a history of benign breast disease.

La Vecchia et al. (1986) conducted a hospital-based case-control study of breast cancer in Italy, beginning in 1980. There were 616 pairs of cases and controls. Adjusted RRs for coffee drinking were 1.0 for none, 1.6 (95% CI, 1.1-2.4) for less than two, 1.4 (1.0-2.0) for two to three and 1.1 (0.7-1.7) for four or more cups per day. There was no tendency for the risk of breast cancer to increase with increasing quantity or duration of coffee drinking.

Katsouyanni *et al.* (1986) conducted a hospital-based case-control study in Greece over a 12-month period in 1983-84. The study included 120 cases from two teaching hospitals in the Greater Athens area and 120 controls admitted for accidents and orthopaedic disorders in a third teaching hospital. Subjects were asked to indicate average frequency of consumption of 120 food or beverage items in the period preceding the onset of disease, along with information on demographic, socioeconomic, reproductive and medical variables. A test for a linear trend was not significant for coffee consumption.

Schairer *et al.* (1987) conducted a case-control study on participants in the Breast Cancer Detection Demonstration Project in the USA, a five-year screening programme begun in 1973. Cases were diagnosed from June 1977 to November 1980. Control subjects were women who had not been recommended for, and had not undergone, surgical evaluation during screening participation and were similar to breast cancer cases with regard to screening centre, age, ethnic origin, time of entry into the screening programme and length of participation in the programme. The number of daily servings of brewed, instant or decaffeinated coffee was not associated with increased risk for breast cancer.

Pozner *et al.* (1986) examined caffeine and coffee intake in women with breast cancer to determine whether it influences cell differentiation in tumours. Dietary history was obtained by interview with 106 women who had undergone mastectomy and axillary dissection for breast cancer at the Mount Sinai Medical Center in New York, USA. Information on tumour differentiation was missing for five women, leaving 101 with complete data. Tumours categorized as well or moderately differentiated were grouped (70 subjects) and compared to poorly differentiated tumours (31 subjects). Women with moderately to well differentiated tumours had had a higher intake of coffee (2.65 ± 2.23 cups per day) than women with poorly differentiated tumours (1.71 ± 1.43); the same trend was seen for caffeine and for all coffee, decaffeinated coffee, cola and tea. Stepwise logistic regression, with tumour differentiation as the dependent variable and coffee, both caffeinated and decaffeinated, tea, cola, cocoa, caffeine (mg/day), caffeine (mg per kg body weight per day), vitamin A, age and Quetelet's index as candidate independent variables, indicated that high coffee consumption is associated with moderately and well differentiated tumours; after accounting for differences in coffee intake, no other variable in the model emerged as significant. When logistic regression was performed including smoking, oral-contraceptive use, parity, number of children, age at first pregnancy, age at menarche, total calories, protein, total fat and other nutrients, however, no variable appeared to be significantly associated with degree of tumour differentiation. [The Working Group noted that this study is difficult to group with other studies of etiology. Also, factors that historically have been linked to breast cancer did not appear to influence tumour differentiation in this study.]

Mabuchi *et al.* (1985a) studied risk factors for male breast cancer as part of a larger case-control investigation of various rare cancers conducted over 1972-75 in a large number of hospitals in five US metropolitan areas. Cases were identified through continuous monitoring of documents in the hospital pathology and medical records departments. Controls were hospital patients free of cancer and matched to the cases for age (± three years), sex, race and marital status. Of the 64 eligible male breast cancer patients identified, 52 were interviewed, along with an equal number of controls. Matched analysis showed no difference in coffee or decaffeinated coffee consumption.

Table 35. **Summary of results of case–control studies of breast cancer and coffee consumption**

Reference and location	Subjects (cases, controls)	Coffee consumption (cups/day)	Relative risk (95% confidence interval)	Comments
Lawson *et al.* (1981) USA, Scotland, New Zealand	Women (241, 723)	0 1–3 4–6 ≥7	1.0 1.3 1.5 1.1 (0.6–1.8)	Coffee and tea; 90% CI
Lubin *et al.* (1981) Canada	Women (577, 826)	≤5 >5	1.0 1.2 (0.9–1.5)	Coffee and tea
Lubin *et al.* (1984, 1985) Israel	Women (738, 738) surgical controls	0 1 2–3 ≥4	1.0 0.7 (0.4–1.1) 0.7 (0.4–1.0) 0.7 (0.4–1.1)	Matched by age, country of origin, length of residence in Israel. Cases in the two comparisons involved the same series of subjects.
	(807, 807) neighbourhood controls	0 1 2–3 ≥4	1.0 0.5 (0.3–0.9) 0.5 (0.2–0.9) 0.6 (0.2–0.9)	
Rosenberg *et al.* (1984, 1985) USA	Women (2651, 1501) controls with non-malignant conditions	0 1–2 3–4 ≥5	1.0 1.2 (1.0–1.5) 1.2 (1.0–1.6) 1.2 (0.9–1.6)	Extensive adjustment made for known or suspected breast cancer risk factors
	(2651, 385) controls with cancers at other sites	0 1–2 3–4 ≥5	1.0 1.0 (0.7–1.4) 0.9 (0.7–1.3) 1.1 (0.7–1.6)	

Table 35 (contd)

Reference and location	Subjects (cases, controls)	Coffee consumption (cups/day)	Relative risk (95% confidence interval)	Comments
Rosenberg et al. (1984, 1985) (contd)	(916, 584) controls with non-malignant conditions	0 1-2 3-4 ≥5	1.0 1.2 (0.9-1.5) 1.4 (0.9-1.8) 0.6 (0.3-1.1)	Decaffeinated coffee; adjusted for age
	(916, 138) controls with cancers at other sites	0 1-2 3-4 ≥5	1.0 1.1 (0.7-1.7) 1.1 (0.6-2.0) 1.0 (0.4-2.8)	Decaffeinated coffee; adjusted for age
Lê (1985) France	Women (500, 945)	Never 1-2 ≥3	1.0 0.8 0.6	Test for trend, $p = 0.003$; adjusted for known risk factors
La Vecchia et al. (1986) Italy	Women (616, 616)	0 <2 2-3 ≥4	1.0 1.6 (1.1-2.4) 1.4 (1.0-2.0) 1.1 (0.7-1.7)	Adjusted for known risk factors
Katsouyanni et al. (1986) Greece	Women (120, 120)	Frequency of use Tertile 1 2 3		Adjusted for age, interviewer, and length of schooling; nonsignificant inverse trend
Schairer et al. (1987) USA	Women (1510, 1882)	0 <1 2 3 4 ≥5	1.0 1.0 (0.8-1.3) 1.0 (0.7-1.2) 0.9 (0.7-1.2) 0.9 (0.7-1.3) 1.0 (0.8-1.3)	Crude, unmatched analysis; adjustment for other risk factors and types of caffeine-containing beverage did not change the results.
		0 <1 2 3 4 ≥5	1.0 0.9 (0.8-1.1) 0.9 (0.7-1.2) 0.9 (0.6-1.3) 0.9 (0.5-1.7) 0.7 (0.3-1.3)	Instant coffee

Table 35 (contd)

Reference and location	Subjects (cases, controls)	Coffee consumption (cups/day)	Relative risk (95% confidence interval)	Comments
Schairer et al. (1987) (contd)		0 <1 2 3 4 ≥5	1.0 1.0 (0.9–1.2) 1.0 (0.8–1.4) 0.7 (0.4–1.1) 0.9 (0.5–1.7) 1.1 (0.6–2.2)	Decaffeinated coffee
Mabuchi et al. (1985a) USA	Men (52, 52)	<1 ≥1	(81% versus 83%, NS)	Matched on age, sex, race, marital status
		<1 ≥1	(38% versus 31%, NS)	Decaffeinated coffee

(iv) *Ovary*

Case-control studies of ovarian cancer and coffee or decaffeinated coffee are summarized in Table 36 (p. 153).

Trichopoulos et al. (1981) reported data from a relatively small case-control study in Athens, Greece, showing a suggestive positive association between coffee consumption and risk of ovarian cancer of common epithelial types. The association was significant (two-tailed $p \sim 0.03$) when dose trends (cups of coffee per day, lifetime consumption of cups of coffee) were taken into account. [The Working Group noted that this study is not considered separately, since the relevant data are part of a larger subsequent study (Trichopoulos et al., 1984; Tzonou et al., 1984).]

Subsequently, Hartge et al. (1982) reported in a letter to the Editor of *The International Journal of Cancer* data on coffee and ovarian cancer collected as part of a case-control study of ovarian cancer (McGowan et al., 1979). Cases were 158 women with pathologically confirmed primary ovarian cancer of the epithelial type treated in participating hospitals in the Washington DC area. Controls were 187 women frequency-matched to cases for age, race and hospital, treated at the same hospitals for conditions other than gynaecological, psychiatric or malignant diseases or pregnancy. Ten women had been excluded from the control series because they were hospitalized for conditions that might necessitate alterations in the diet. Women who regularly drank any amount of coffee had a nonsignificant increased risk for ovarian cancer compared to non-coffee drinkers (adjusted RR, 1.3; 95% CI, 0.8–2.2), but there was no statistically significant dose-response. [The

Working Group noted that there was no apparent confounding by the controlled variables in this study. The crude estimate of RR for drinkers of any amount of coffee was [1.3], i.e., identical to the reported adjusted figure.]

In a multicentre, hospital-based case-control study, Miller *et al.* (1984, 1987) collected data on 290 women, 20-69 years old, with epithelial ovarian cancer diagnosed within six months of the index hospital admission. Two control groups were used: women with benign conditions hospitalized more or less acutely (580) and women with malignancies (476) presumed to be unrelated to coffee (thus excluding women with pancreatic or bladder cancer) and to other factors that are considered to be predictive of ovarian cancer (thus excluding women with endometrial cancer). Women with benign conditions were *a priori* considered to be heavier consumers of coffee than the other control group (Miller *et al.*, 1984). There was no evidence of a positive association between ovarian cancer and drinking decaffeinated coffee. With respect to brewed coffee, there was evidence of a positive association with overall consumption when comparison was made with noncancer controls, but there was no such evidence when ovarian cancer cases were compared with the 'other cancers' control group. In no instance was there a clear indication of a dose-dependent trend. [The Working Group noted that, since the results with respect to the two control groups are contrary to what was predicted, it is legitimate to combine the two control groups, the results of which are given in Table 36. The crude estimate of RR for drinkers of any amount of coffee was [1.2]; from the crude and adjusted data, there seems to be no evidence of confounding.]

Byers *et al.* (1983) conducted a case-control study of dietary and nondietary factors in ovarian cancer. Cases were 274 white women, 30-79 years old, admitted to the Roswell Park Memorial Institute, Buffalo, NY, USA, between 1957-65 for ovarian cancer. Nineteen additional cases with ovarian tumours of nonepithelial origin and 36 additional cases with ovarian cancer diagnosed more than two years prior to the admission date were excluded. Controls were 1034 women, 30-79 years old [probably white only] admitted during the same period to the Institute for conditions that were found to be nonmalignant. An additional 499 women with diagnoses related to the reproductive system and 408 with conditions of the gastrointestinal system (401) or diabetes (seven) were excluded. There was no statistically significant association with any consumption category or dose trend with respect to coffee consumption. [The Working Group calculated that the age-adjusted RR for drinkers of any amount of coffee, with adjustment to age distribution of the control group by the direct method, was [1.2] (nonsignificant).]

In the Greek case-control study (Tzonou *et al.*, 1984), coffee consumption was compared between 150 women with epithelial ovarian cancer admitted to any of ten large hospitals in Athens between 1980 and 1981, and 250 control women hospitalized during the same period for fractures or orthopaedic disorders in the

Athens Hospital for Orthopaedic Disorders. In the final results, after adjustment for age, parity, menopausal status, age at menopause, use of exogenous oestrogens, tobacco smoking and consumption of alcoholic beverages, the χ^2 for trend in coffee consumption was 1.15 ($p \sim 0.27$); at no level of coffee consumption did the RR differ significantly from the value of 1.0. [The Working Group noted that the crude estimate of RR for drinkers of any amount of coffee was 1.2; comparison of crude and adjusted RR estimates indicates that there was little confounding, and that which existed was slightly 'negative'.]

Cramer et al. (1984) conducted a case-control study in the Boston, MA (USA), area between 1978 and 1981. Cases were 215 white women with newly diagnosed epithelial ovarian cancer admitted to 12 participating hospitals, whereas controls were 215 white women randomly selected from lists of Massachusetts residents, matched for age and precinct of residence. There was no evidence of an association between ovarian cancer and any of the combinations of coffee drinking, alcohol drinking or tobacco smoking. The crude RR was 1.2 for coffee drinkers. In the combinations that included coffee drinking, the RRs of coffee users *versus* nonusers of either coffee, alcohol or tobacco were between 1.2 and 1.8. [The Working Group noted that there was no evidence of overt confounding with respect to the results for coffee.]

La Vecchia et al. (1984) conducted a case-control study of ovarian cancer in Milan between 1979 and 1983. Cases were 247 women, 19-74 years of age, with epithelial ovarian cancer admitted to the university hospital and the National Cancer Institute of Milan. Controls were 494 women below the age of 75 years admitted to the university or general hospitals of the Milan area, suffering from diseases judged to be unrelated to coffee consumption or to any of the established or suspected risk factors of ovarian cancer. In the logistic regression analyses, there were statistically significant linear trends with daily consumption of coffee ($p = 0.003$) and with years of regular coffee consumption ($p = 0.02$). [The Working Group noted that comparison of crude [1.4] and adjusted RR indicates that there is some degree of confounding that incorrectly reduces the association between coffee consumption and risk of ovarian cancer ('negative' confounding).]

In a case-control study in the San Francisco Bay area, CA, USA, between 1983 and 1985, Whittemore et al. (1988) compared the exposure histories of 188 women with primary epithelial ovarian cancer admitted to one of seven participating hospitals with the exposure histories of women in two control groups. The first control group consisted of women hospitalized in one of the hospitals to which cases were admitted, whereas the second group was selected from the general population using random-digit dialling. When both control groups were combined, there was a statistically significant positive association between coffee drinking and the risk for ovarian cancer. [The Working Group noted that there may be an error, in that the risk relative to the two control groups combined is higher (2.0) than that relative to either control group (1.9 for hospital controls and 1.5 for population controls).] RRs were elevated in 23 of the 24 categories of coffee drinking by quantity (cups per day), duration (years) or by product when hospital and population controls were considered separately; they were significantly elevated ($p < 0.05$) in 11 out of 12 such categories when hospital and population controls were combined. However, no clear trend was seen with daily quantity of coffee consumed.

Overall, in all seven case-control studies of coffee use and risk for ovarian cancer, users of any amount of coffee had an increased risk, although the elevation was significant in only two. In most of the studies, the increase was small or minimal: the overall crude RR estimates were between 1.1 and 1.3 in five studies, 1.4 in a recent study and 1.9 in the last one. Use of crude estimates is legitimate, since confounding of the association between coffee drinking and ovarian cancer in these sets was either absent or negative. In only one study was there a statistically significant dose-response relationship. A Mantel-Haenszel meta-analysis by the Working Group of the crude data from these seven studies (an acceptable, although slightly conservative procedure, for the reasons indicated above) gave a significant ($p < 0.01$) pooled estimated RR of [1.3 (95% CI, 1.1-1.5)] for coffee users *versus* nonusers.

(v) *Cancers of the digestive tract*

Case-control studies of cancers of the digestive tract and coffee consumption are summarized in Tables 37-39 (pp. 158, 162, 164).

Large bowel: Higginson (1966) studied 340 cases of colorectal cancer (196 male, 144 female) from seven hospitals in the Kansas City area, USA, from 1959 to the early 1960s. Three controls per case were selected from the same hospitals. Cases had histologically confirmed diagnoses, and controls excluded patients with gastrointestinal disease or with recent dietary abnormalities. Cases and controls were matched for age, sex and race. The socioeconomic status of cases and controls were similar. No significant association was found between coffee consumption and colorectal cancer: the RR for subjects who drank one or more cups of coffee a day was [0.8 (95% CI, 0.7-1.0)]. [The Working Group noted that no adjustment was made for confounding variables other than age, sex and race.]

Haenszel *et al.* (1973) studied 179 Japanese patients (101 male, 78 female) with colorectal cancer and 357 age- and sex-matched controls from the three largest general hospital in Honolulu, Hawaii, between 1966 and 1970. All but one of the cases had been confirmed histologically. Controls did not include patients with gastric or duodenal ulcers, gastrointestinal cancer or other diseases of the large bowel; their most frequent diagnoses were circulatory diseases, external causes and genito-urinary diseases. Patients were interviewed on dietary history, habits and

Table 36. Case–control studies of ovarian cancer (common epithelial tumours) and brewed coffee intake

Reference and location	Subjects (cases, controls)	Coffee consumption (cups/day)	Relative risk (95% CI)			Comments
			Noncancer controls	Cancer controls	All controls	
Hartge et al. (1982) USA	158, 187	0 <2 2–3 ≥4	1.0 1.0 (0.5–2.2) 1.8 (0.9–3.6) 1.4 (0.6–3.0)			Adjusted for age, gravity and smoking
Byers et al. (1983) USA	274, 1034	0 <3 ≥3	1.0 [1.3] [1.0]			No significant association with any consumption category or trend
Miller et al. (1984, 1987) Several cities in the USA and Canada	287, 569/470	0 1 2 3 4 ≥5	1.0 1.6 (0.9–2.7) 1.5 (0.9–2.6) 1.6 (0.9–2.7) 1.7 (0.9–3.3) 1.1 (0.6–2.0)	1.0 1.0 (0.5–1.7) 0.9 (0.6–1.6) 0.9 (0.6–1.6) 1.6 (0.8–3.1) 1.0 (0.5–1.8)	1.0 [1.3] [1.2] [1.3] [1.7] [1.1]	Multivariate analysis
	289, 572/473	0 1–2 3–4 ≥5	1.0 1.4 (0.9–2.2) 0.8 (0.4–1.6) 0.7 (0.2–2.1)	1.0 1.0 (0.6–1.4) 0.9 (0.5–1.6) 0.7 (0.2–3.3)	1.0 [1.2] [0.9] [0.7]	Decaffeinated coffee
Trichopoulos et al. (1981, 1984); Tzonou et al. (1984) Greece	149, 250	0 0.5–1 1.5–2 2.5–3 ≥3.5	1.0 0.9 1.6 0.9 1.5			
Cramer et al. (1984) USA	215, 215	0 Any	1.0 1.1			Adjusted for smoking

Table 36 (contd)

Reference and location	Subjects (cases, controls)	Coffee consumption	Relative risk (95% CI)			Comments
La Vecchia et al. (1984) Italy	247, 494	0 ≤1 2-3 ≥4	1.0 1.5 (0.9-2.5) 1.9 (1.2-3.0) 2.2 (1.2-3.9)			Multivariate analysis
			Hospital controls	Population controls	All controls	
Whittemore et al. (1988) USA	188, 280/259					Adjusted for smoking
		0 1 2-3 ≥4	1.0 2.2 2.1 2.0	1.0 1.9 1.6 1.6	1.0 2.4 (1.2-5.1) 2.3 (1.1-4.7) 2.1 (1.0-4.4)	
		0 1-14 years 15-24 years 25-39 years ≥40 years	1.0 1.6 1.8 2.4 3.5	1.0 0.7 1.7 1.7 2.5	1.0 1.5 (0.6-3.6) 2.2 (1.0-4.8) 2.3 (1.1-4.9) 3.4 (1.5-8.0)	

socioeconomic status. Coffee drinking was associated with a RR of 0.7, which was not statistically significant.

A significant negative association between coffee consumption and colon cancer was reported from case-control studies in Norway and the USA (Bjelke, 1973).

Graham *et al.* (1978) carried out a case-control study of white male patients with histologically confirmed cancer of the colon (256 patients) or rectum (330 patients) and 1222 controls seen at the Roswell Park Memorial Institute in Buffalo, NY, USA, during 1959-65. Controls were non-cancer, non-gastrointestinal patients who were selected so as to have a similar distribution as the cases, but no individual matching was carried out. Patients attending the hospital where the study was carried out were similar to the population of the neighouring areas in terms of socioeconomic and marital status, religion and smoking habits. The interview included demographic, socioeconomic and dietary variables. Frequent drinking of coffee was associated with a 'significant but small excess risk' for cancer of the colon but not of the rectum, as was 'drinking coffee very hot'. [The Working Group noted that no figures were given, that, other than for age, there was no adjustment for possible confounding variables and that no RRs or CIs are given.]

Dales *et al.* (1979) carried out a study of black patients with colorectal cancer and matched controls from hospitals and clinics in the San Francisco Bay area, CA, USA. Cases were identified from a cancer registry covering the period September 1973 to August 1976, but 60% could not be interviewed, mostly due to death or severe illness, leaving 99 cases. Similarly, only 50% (280) of the controls who were identified were successfully interviewed. The questionnaire was answered at the patients' homes and included demographic and socioeconomic data, as well as information on dietary habits three years prior to the interview. No association between coffee drinking and colorectal cancer was found. [The Working Group noted that the low rates of participation make this study difficult to interpret and that RRs associated with coffee consumption are not given.]

Watanabe *et al.* (1984) studied 65 cases of cancer of the rectum (39 male, 26 female) and 138 cases of colon cancer (71 male, 67 female) in Kyoto, Japan. For each case, one control was selected; the sex and age distribution of cases and controls were similar. Data were collected on a number of dietary items including coffee and tea consumption. No significant association was found between coffee drinking and cancer of the rectum or of the colon, although both risks were reduced by 20-30% among coffee drinkers.

Tajima and Tominaga (1985) compared the characteristics of 42 incident cases of colon cancer (27 male, 15 female) and 51 cases of rectal cancer (25 male, 26 female) with those of 186 controls admitted to a specialized hospital in Nagoya, Japan, between 1981 and 1983. The diagnoses of the cases were confirmed histologically. There was no significant association between coffee drinking and either colon or rectal cancer (RRs for daily drinkers, 1.1 and 1.0, respectively). [The Working Group noted that almost half of the controls had gastrointestinal conditions.]

Macquart-Moulin *et al.* (1986) reported a case-control study from Marseille, France, based on 399 histologically confirmed cases of colorectal cancer and the same number of controls which was conducted between 1979 and 1984. After adjustment for age, sex, calories and weight, the risk in increasing quartiles of coffee consumption was 1.0, 0.6, 0.7 and 0.6. The test for trend was not significant.

Tuyns (1986) and Tuyns *et al.* (1988) presented the results of a study which covered approximately one-half of the cases of colorectal cancer in two Belgian provinces, Oost-Vlaanderen and Liège, in 1978-82. A total of 453 cases of colon cancer, 365 of rectal cancer and 2851 population controls were included. The response rate for controls was approximately 70%. The analyses were adjusted for age, sex and residence. 'Heavy consumers' of coffee and/or tea had crude RRs of 0.7 (95% CI, 0.6-0.9) for colon cancer and 0.8 for rectal cancer (0.6-0.9), relative to 'light consumers' (Tuyns, 1986). Separate results are not given for coffee and tea drinking, but the latter was reported to be rare.

In Yugoslavia, Jarebinski *et al.* (1989) compared 98 patients (56 male, 42 female) with histologically confirmed rectal cancer admitted to one of five hospitals in Belgrade in 1984-86 to two control groups: Hospital controls were patients admitted due to non-cancer conditions — mainly fractures and other injuries, cardiovascular diseases and hernias; a second control group consisted of neighbours of the cases. Controls were matched to cases by age, sex, place of residence and interviewer. The RRs associated with any coffee consumption were 1.7 when compared with hospital controls and 0.8 when compared with neighbourhood controls. The corresponding RRs for consumption of three or more cups per day were 1.1 and 0.8, and for having consumed coffee for 30 or more years, 1.2 and 1.2. None of these differences approached statistical significance. [The Working Group noted that no data are given on the proportions of potential cases or controls who could not be contacted.]

La Vecchia *et al.* (1988, 1989c) studied 455 histologically confirmed cases of colon cancer (221 male, 234 female), 295 cases of rectal cancer (170 male, 125 female) and 1944 hospital controls recruited from a network of teaching and general hospitals in greater Milan, Italy, between 1985 and 1988. Controls did not include patients with malignant tumours, digestive diseases or any condition related to use of coffee, alcohol or tobacco or which may have resulted in long-term dietary modification. RRs were calculated through logistic regression after adjustment for sex, age, social class, education, marital status, smoking and alcohol consumption. Compared to subjects consuming no to one cup per day, those consuming two cups per day had a RR of 0.9 for colon cancer, and those consuming three or more cups had a RR of 0.6 (p for trend, < 0.01). The corresponding figures for rectal cancer were 1.0 and 0.7 (p for trend, < 0.05). The RRs were also examined after stratification for sex, age, marital status, education, social class, smoking and alcohol consumption. The overall pattern of protection afforded by coffee against colon cancer was evident in all strata but appeared to be restricted to males.

In another case-control study, carried out among Singapore Chinese, Lee et al. (1989) studied 203 (121 male, 82 female) consecutive incident cases (132 cases of colon cancer, 71 of rectal cancer) admitted to a general hospital in 1985-87. All cases had histologically confirmed colorectal cancer. A total of 426 controls were selected among 489 patients who were free of any gastrointestinal disease, cancer or diabetes; approximately two controls were selected for each case, matched for age group and sex. The response rates for cases and controls were above 80%. Coffee intake of one or more cups per day was associated with a nonsignificant 30-40% reduction in the risk for cancer at each site. When both sites were pooled, the association was close to significance ($0.1 > p > 0.05$). The effect of coffee remained virtually unchanged after adjustment for other food items for which a significant result was found. However, there was no evidence of a dose-response relationship.

Data on coffee consumption was collected as part of a multicentre, multiorgan case-control study in the USA (Rosenberg et al., 1989). In 1978-82, data were obtained on coffee consumption one month before interview, whereas during 1983-86 the data on consumption were for one and three years before hospital admission. Cases were 717 patients with cancer of colon and 538 with rectal cancer, aged 30-69 years. A non-cancer control group consisted of 2128 trauma and 369 appendicitis patients, and a second, cancer control group was composed of 892 patients with malignant melanoma and 494 with lymphoma and bone cancer. Multiple logistic regression analyses, adjusting for age, sex, geographic area, year of interview, cigarette smoking, alcohol consumption, education, religion and race, were employed, using persons who consumed one cup of coffee per day as the referent category. For colon cancer, the adjusted RRs for drinking less than one, two and three to four cups of coffee per day compared to one cup per day were all close to one, but the risk associated with drinking five or more cups per day was significantly reduced (0.6; 95% CI, 0.4-0.8). This risk pattern was similar for men and women and when recent or past consumption was evaluated. For rectal cancer, the risks were close to unity for present or past consumption at all dose levels. The risk pattern was somewhat different for males and females: with the exception of a significantly elevated risk for drinking three to four cups per day (1.7; 95% CI, 1.0-2.8), men had nonsignificantly increased risks for all other dose categories; however, women had nonsignificantly reduced risks.

Benito *et al.* (1990) reported a case-control study of 286 incident cases of histologically confirmed colorectal cancer, 295 population controls and 203 hospital controls in Majorca, Spain. Coffee consumption was presented in quartiles. Risk in the lowest intake category was 1.0 and that in increasing quartiles of intake was 0.7, 0.5 and 0.8. The trend statistic was not significant.

Table 37. Summary of results of case–control studies on colorectal cancer and coffee consumption

Reference, location and site	Subjects (cases, controls)	Coffee consumption (cups/day)	Relative risk (95% CI)	Comments
Higginson (1966) USA Colon and rectum	Men and women (340, 1020)	0/irregular <1 <2 ≥3	1.0 [0.4] [0.7] [0.6]	Crude RR; nonsignificant
Haenszel *et al.* (1973) USA Colon and rectum	Men and women (179, 357)	0 Any	1.0 0.7	Crude RR; nonsignificant
Watanabe *et al.* (1984) Japan				
Rectum	Men and women (65, 65)	0 Any	1.0 0.7 (0.3–1.6)	
Colon	Men and women (138, 138)	0 Any	1.0 0.8 (0.5–1.3)	
Tajima & Tominaga (1985) Japan				
Rectum	Men and women (51, 186)	0 Sometimes Daily	1.0 1.3 1.0	Nonsignificant; adjusted for age, sex
Colon	Men and women (42, 186)	0 Sometimes Daily	1.0 1.2 1.1	Nonsignificant; adjusted for age, sex
Macquart-Moulin *et al.* (1986) France Colon and rectum	Men and women (399, 399)	Quartiles Low 2nd 3rd High	 1.0 0.6 0.7 0.6	Nonsignificant; adjusted for age, sex, calories, weight

Table 37 (contd)

Reference, location and site	Subjects (cases, controls)	Coffee consumption (cups/day)	Relative risk (95% CI)	Comments
Tuyns et al. (1988) Belgium				
Rectum	Men and women (365, 2851)	Quartiles Low 2nd 3rd High	1.0 0.9 0.9 0.7	Coffee and tea, but latter said to be uncommon; adjusted for age, sex, province; significant trend
Colon	Men and women (453, 2851)	Quartiles Low 2nd 3rd High	1.0 0.9 1.0 0.6	
Jarebinski et al. (1989) Yugoslavia Rectum	Men and women (98, 98)	0 Any <3 ≥3 <30 years ≥30 years	1.0 1.7 1.0 1.1 1.0 1.2	Nonsignificant; hospital controls Nonsignificant Nonsignificant
		0 Any <3 ≥3 cups/day <30 years ≥30 years	1.0 0.8 1.0 0.8 1.0 1.2	Nonsignificant; neighbourhood controls Nonsignificant Nonsignificant
La Vecchia et al. (1989c) Italy Rectum	Men (170, 1334)	0–1 2 ≥3	1.0 0.8 0.5	$p < 0.01$ for men; nonsignificant for women; adjusted for age, marital status, education, social class, smoking, alcohol consumption; 95% CI could not be calculated; p levels based on chi-squared test for linear trend
	Women (125, 610)	0–1 2 ≥3	1.0 1.2 0.9	

Table 37 (contd)

Reference, location and site	Subjects (cases, controls)	Coffee consumption (cups/day)	Relative risk (95% CI)	Comments
La Vecchia et al. (1989c) (contd)				
Colon	Men (221, 1334)	0–1 2 ≥3	1.0 0.8 0.6	$p < 0.05$
	Women (234, 610)	0–1 2 ≥3	1.0 0.9 0.6	$p < 0.05$
Lee et al. (1989) Singapore				
Colon	Men and women (132, 426)	Tertiles Low Intermediate High	1.0 0.7 (0.4–1.1) 0.7 (0.4–1.2)	Nonsignificant
Rectum	(71, 426)	Low Intermediate High	1.0 0.6 (0.3–1.1) 0.7 (0.4–1.4)	Nonsignificant
Colon and rectum	(203, 426)	Low Intermediate High	1.0 0.7 (0.4–1.0) 0.7 (0.5–1.1)	$0.1 > p > 0.05$; logistic analysis
Colon and rectum		Low Intermediate High	1.0 0.7 (0.4–1.0) 0.7 (0.5–1.2)	Nonsignificant; combined analysis; adjusted for cruciferous vegetables, total vegetables, meat/vegetable ratio, cholecystectomy history
Rosenberg et al. (1989) USA				Adjusted for age, sex, cigarette smoking, alcohol consumption, several other potential confounding factors
Colon	Men and women (717, 3883)	<1 1 2 3–4 ≥5	1.1 (0.8–1.4) 1.0 1.0 (0.8–1.3) 0.9 (0.7–1.2) 0.6 (0.4–0.8)	

Table 37 (contd)

Reference, location and site	Subjects (cases, controls)	Coffee consumption (cups/day)	Relative risk (95% CI)	Comments
Rosenberg et al. (1989) (contd)				
Rectum	(538, 3883)	<1	1.2 (0.9–1.6)	
		1	1.0	
		2	1.1 (0.8–1.5)	
		3–4	1.1 (0.8–1.5)	
		≥5	1.2 (0.8–1.8)	
Benito et al. (1990) Spain	Men and women (286, 498)	0	1.0	Nonsignificant; adjusted for age, sex, weight
Colon and rectum		1–30/month	0.7	
		31–60/month	0.5	
		≥60/month	0.8	

Stomach: In the study of Higginson (1966), described on p. 152, 93 cases of histologically confirmed stomach cancer and 279 age-, sex- and race-matched controls were studied. No significant association was found between coffee drinking and stomach cancer.

Graham et al. (1967) compared 276 cases (188 male, 88 female) of gastric cancer and 2221 controls (800 male, 1421 female) with non-neoplastic, non-digestive conditions seen at the Roswell Park Memorial Institute in Buffalo, NY, USA, between 1957 and 1965. Interviews on dietary habits prior to the onset of symptoms were carried out at admission. Separate analyses were made for each sex and for four age groups. The authors infer that the frequency of drinking coffee was not significantly associated with the risk for gastric cancer, but no figures were given.

Tajima and Tominaga (1985), in the study described above (p. 155), reported on 93 cases of histologically confirmed stomach cancer and 186 controls admitted to a specialized hospital in Nagoya, Japan. There was no significant association between coffee drinking and cancer of the stomach. [The Working Group noted that almost half of the controls had gastrointestinal conditions.]

Trichopoulos et al. (1985) studied 110 consecutive incident cases (57 male, 53 female) of histologically confirmed adenocarcinoma of the stomach admitted to two hospitals in Piraeus, Greece, between 1981 and 1984. Controls were 100 patients admitted to a nearby hospital due to accidents, fractures and orthopaedic disorders. Age, sex and years of schooling were controlled for in the statistical analysis. The association between the consumption of coffee and tea and the risk for stomach cancer was not statistically significant.

La Vecchia et al. (1989c) studied 397 histologically confirmed cases of stomach cancer (243 male, 154 female) and 1944 hospital controls from greater Milan, Italy. No association between coffee drinking and stomach cancer was found after adjustment for sex and age. The lack of association remained when the data were also adjusted for social class, education, marital status, smoking and alcohol consumption.

Table 38. Summary of results of case–control studies on stomach cancer and coffee consumption

Reference, location and site	Subjects (cases, controls)	Coffee consumption (cups/day)	Relative risk (95% CI)	Comments
Higginson (1966) USA	Men and women (93, 279)	0/irregular <1 <2 ≥3	1.0 [0.7] [1.3] [1.3]	Crude RR; nonsignificant
Graham et al. (1967) USA	Men and women (276, 2221)			No association
Tajima & Tominaga (1985) Japan	Men and women (93, 186)	0 Not daily Daily	1.0 0.8 1.0	Nonsignificant; adjusted for age, sex
Trichopoulos et al. (1985) Greece	Men and women (110, 100)	1 (low) 2 3 4 5 (high)	1.0 [1.7] [1.8] [2.7] [3.2]	Nonsignificant after adjustment for age, sex, years of schooling; p values based on chi-squared test for linear trend; coffee and tea
La Vecchia et al. (1989c) Italy	Men and women (397, 1944)	0–1 2 ≥3	1.0 0.9 1.3	Nonsignificant; adjusted for age, marital status, education, social class, smoking, alcohol consumption; 95% CI could not be calculated; p values based on chi-squared test for linear trend

Upper digestive tract: Martinez (1969) studied 400 cases of cancer of the oesophagus (179 cases; 120 male, 59 female), mouth (153 cases; 115 male, 38 female) and pharynx (68 cases; 55 male, 13 female), comprising all histologically confirmed cases reported to the Puerto Rico cancer registry in 1966. For each case, three age- and sex-matched controls were selected: one non-cancer patient from the same hospital and two community controls. The results were presented for cancer of the mouth, pharynx and oesophagus taken together. For men, there was a significant association between drinking hot coffee and cancer at these three sites; there was a similar, but nonsignificant trend for women. There was no association between drinking coffee with milk and the occurrence of cancer.

de Jong *et al.* (1974) carried out a hospital-based case-control study of oesophageal cancer among Singapore Chinese in 1970-72. For each case, four age- and sex-matched control patients were selected: two non-cancer patients from the same ward and two orthopaedic controls from a general hospital. Neither in the unadjusted analysis nor after adjustment for dialect group was there an association between coffee drinking and oesophageal cancer. Reported drinking of 'burning hot' coffee, however, was associated with a five- to six-fold higher crude risk of cancer. [The Working Group noted that the control groups included a large number of patients with digestive disorders.]

Yen *et al.* (1987) studied 67 patients with cancer of the extrahepatic bile ducts (40 men, 27 women) who had originally been recruited as controls in a case-control study of pancreatic cancer carried out in 11 large hospitals in Massachusetts and Rhode Island, USA, in 1975-79. The cases were obtained from a group of 104 patients with histologically confirmed cancer of the extrahepatic bile ducts, 37 of whom could not be interviewed. A control group was selected comprising 275 patients with other cancers not known to be related to tobacco or alcohol consumption — mainly of the breast (65 patients) and colon (60 patients). The analysis was stratified by age and sex. No association was found betweeen cancer occurrence and coffee drinking. [The Working Group noted that the study was not designed to study extrahepatic bile duct cancer, and a large proportion of the potential cases could not be interviewed.]

Victora *et al.* (1987), in a study described in detail in the monograph on mate, compared 171 cases of oesophageal cancer in southern Brazil with 342 hospital controls matched for age and sex. They found no effect of coffee drinking. [The Working Group noted that data are not given.]

In the study of La Vecchia *et al.* (1989c), described on p. 156, the association between coffee drinking and oesophageal cancer was examined by comparing 209 histologically confirmed cases (162 male, 47 female) with 1944 controls. The data were initially adjusted for age and sex, and later also for a number of confounding variables. Neither analysis showed any association. These authors also studied 50 cases of cancer of the mouth and pharynx (43 male, seven female) and 151 cases of liver cancer (115 male, 36 female). No association was found between coffee drinking and cancer of the mouth or pharynx, either in the analysis adjusted for sex and age or after adjustment for a number of confounding variables. In the first type of analysis, the RR for liver cancer for those drinking two cups per day was 0.7, and that for people drinking more than three cups per day, 0.6. This trend was less marked and no longer significant after adjustment for other confounding variables, when the corresponding RRs were 0.8 and 0.8.

Franco *et al.* (1989) carried out a case-control study of cancer of the mouth in three Brazilian cities. A total of 232 incident cases (201 male, 31 female) of histologically confirmed cancer of the tongue, gum, floor of the mouth and other parts of the oral cavity were recruited in three head-and-neck surgery services. Two hospital controls matched for age, sex, hospital and time of admission were selected for each case. Patients with cancer or with mental disorders were not included as controls. The crude analysis showed a clear trend of increasing risk with greater frequency of coffee drinking ($p = 0.01$). After adjustment for tobacco and alcohol consumption, however, this association was no longer significant. There was no indication that the temperature at which coffee was drunk affected the risk. [The Working Group noted that approximately one-third of the controls had digestive conditions.]

Table 39. Summary of results of case–control studies on other digestive cancers and coffee consumption

Reference, location and site	Subjects (cases, controls)	Coffee consumption (cups/day)	Relative risk (95% CI)	Comments
Martinez (1969) Puerto Rico Oesophagus, mouth and pharynx	Men (290, 870)	0 Cold or warm Hot	1.0 [1.3] [2.7]	Black coffee; $p < 0.01$
		0 Cold or warm Hot	1.0 [0.8] [1.2]	With milk; non-significant
	Women (110, 330)	0 Cold or warm Hot	1.0 [1.6] [3.4]	Black coffee; non-significant
		0 Cold or warm Hot	1.0 [1.0] [1.6]	With milk; nonsignificant
de Jong *et al.* (1974) Singapore Oesophagus	Men (95, 465)	Not daily Daily Burning hot	1.0 0.9 5.1 crude RR 4.2 adjusted RR	Nonsignificant $p < 0.01$ for both
	Women (36, 200)	Not daily Daily Burning hot	1.0 1.4 6.6 crude RR 4.1 adjusted RR	Nonsignificant $p < 0.01$ for both; RR crude and adjusted for dialect group

Table 39 (contd)

Reference, location and site	Subjects (cases, controls)	Coffee consumption (cups/day)	Relative risk (95% CI)	Comments
Yen et al. (1987) USA Extrahepatic bile ducts	Men and women (67, 275)	0 Any 1–2 3–4 ≥5	1.0 0.8 (0.3–2.0) 0.8 (0.3–2.0) 1.0 (0.4–2.8) 0.6 (0.2–1.9)	Adjusted for age, sex
Victora et al. (1987) Brazil Oesophagus	Men and women (171, 342)			No association
La Vecchia et al. (1989c) Oesophagus	Men and women (209, 1944)	0–1 2 ≥3	1.0 0.9 1.0	Nonsignificant; adjusted for age, sex, marital status, education, social class, smoking, alcohol consumption; 95% CI could not be calculated; p values based on chi-squared test for linear trend
Mouth and pharynx	Men and women (50, 1944)	0–1 2 ≥3	1.0 0.9 0.8	
Liver	(151, 1944)	0–1 2 ≥3	1.0 0.8 0.8	
Franco et al. (1989) Brazil Oral cavity	Men and women (232, 464)	0–1 2–5 ≥6	1.0 1.3 (0.8–1.9) 1.9 (1.2–3.2)	$p = 0.01$; crude matched analysis; p value based on test for linear trend
		0–1 2–5 ≥6	1.0 1.1 (0.7–1.8) 1.5 (0.9–2.6)	Nonsignificant; adjusted for tobacco, alcohol consumption

(vi) *Cancers at other sites*

These studies are summarized in Table 40 (p. 166).

Henderson et al. (1976) studied 156 (105 male, 51 female) patients with *nasopharyngeal* squamous-cell *carcinoma* from three cancer registries and 267 controls in California, USA. From the main registry included in the study, 41% of the cases could not be interviewed. Controls were selected from inpatient and outpatient facilities and were matched to the cases for age, sex, race and socioeconomic status. No association was found between coffee drinking and nasopharyngeal carcinoma. [The Working Group noted that the description of the selection of cases and controls is confusing, as several different sources were used, and that a high proportion of cases could not be interviewed.]

Mabuchi et al. (1985b) studied 149 patients with histologically confirmed *carcinoma of the vulva* from five metropolitan areas in the USA between 1972 and 1975. Cases were identified from more than 115 hospitals. One non-cancer patient was matched to each case according to age, race, marital status and hospital. Drinking one or more cups of coffee daily was associated with a doubling of the RR for cancer of the vulva, but this was not significant. The risk was significantly higher, however, among women drinking three or more cups per day. There was no dose-response relationship.

Mettlin (1989) reported a case-control study of 569 cases of histologically diagnosed *lung cancer* and the same number of controls who had no diagnosis or history of malignant or benign neoplasms, selected from patients seen at Roswell Park Memorial Institute in Buffalo, NY, USA. After adjustment for sex, smoking history, beta-carotene intake and education level relative to the risk in people who had never drunk coffee (1.0), the risk in increasing categories of coffee consumption was 1.0 (0.7-1.5) for less than one cup per day, 1.0 (0.7-1.4) for two to three cups per day and 1.3 (0.9-1.8) for four or more cups per day. The study also presented data regarding intake of decaffeinated coffee, and for the same categories of consumption the RRs were 1.0, 0.7 (0.5-0.9), 0.5 (0.3-0.7) and 0.8 (0.5-1.3).

In a case-control study of 208 cases of *non-Hodgkin's lymphoma* and 401 hospital controls in northeastern Italy, Franceschi et al. (1989) found a direct trend in risk, of borderline statistical significance, for coffee drinking in a multivariate analysis (RR for the upper tertile, 1.6). Only total methylxanthine-containing beverage consumption was correlated in multivariate analysis, which seemed to flatten out the relationship moderately.

Table 40. Summary of results of case–control studies on other cancers and coffee consumption

Reference, location and site	Subjects (cases, controls)	Coffee consumption (cups/day)	Relative risk	Comments
Henderson et al. (1976) USA Nasopharynx	Men and women (156, 267)	0 Any	1.0 1.1	Nonsignificant; adjusted for sex, race, socioeconomic status, place of residence
Paffenbarger et al. (1978) USA				Case–control analysis of cohort study described on p. 118
Hodgkin's disease	Men (45, 180)	0 Any	1.0 2.5	Nonsignificant; matched analysis

Table 40 (contd)

Reference, location and site	Subjects (cases, controls)	Coffee consumption (cups/day)	Relative risk (95% CI)	Comments
Paffenbarger et al. (1978) (contd)				
Non-Hodgkin's lymphoma	Men (89, 356)	0 Any	1.0 1.6	Nonsignificant
Malignant melanoma	Men (45, 180)	0 Any	1.0 1.3	Nonsignificant
Lymphatic leukaemia	Men (27, 108)	0 Any	1.0 2.7	Nonsignificant
Myeloid leukaemia	Men (41, 164)	0 Any	1.0 3.2	$p = 0.02$
Other/unspecified leukaemias	Men (30, 120)	0 Any	1.0 0.8	Nonsignificant
Mabuchi et al. (1985b) USA Vulva	Women (149, 149)	< 1 1-2 3-4 ≥5	1.0 1.5 3.0 2.4	Unmatched analysis Nonsignificant $p < 0.05$ $p < 0.05$
Franceschi et al. (1989) Italy Non-Hodgkin's lymphoma	Men and women (208, 401)	Low Intermediate High	1.0 1.2 1.6	Borderline significance

4. Summary of Data Reported and Evaluation

4.1 Exposure data

Coffee is a beverage that has been consumed in many parts of the world for centuries. The two main types of cultivated coffee are arabica and robusta. Green coffee is one of the major commodities of world trade and is exported mainly from tropical countries. Ground roasted coffee is brewed in many different ways, including decoction/boiling, infusion, filtration and percolation. Instant (soluble) coffee and decaffeinated coffee are more recent developments. Instant coffee is the dried pure water extract of ground roasted coffee and is used directly to prepare the beverage. Caffeine, the major pharmacologically active purine present in coffee, can be effectively and selectively removed from green coffee beans to give, ultimately, decaffeinated coffee.

Worldwide consumption of roasted coffee was estimated to be 4.3 million tonnes per year in 1983-87. Per-caput consumption in Nordic countries is two or three times higher than that in Canada, the USA and other countries of Europe. These regions have higher consumption levels than in the rest of the world.

Over 700 volatile compounds in many structural categories have been identified in roasted coffee, as well as numerous nonvolatile components (e.g., polysaccharides, melanoidins, protein-like products, chlorogenic acids). Arabica and robusta green coffees contain average caffeine levels of 1.2% and 2.2%, respectively, on a dry weight basis. Depending on the brewing method and species of coffee used, caffeine levels in the beverage are generally in the range of 70-150 mg per cup. Many volatile aldehydes and ketones have been characterized in coffee, including glyoxal and methylglyoxal. Occasional contamination of green coffees with mycotoxins has been reported.

4.2 Experimental carcinogenicity data

Coffee was tested for carcinogenicity in one study in mice and in two studies in rats by oral administration. The mice received instant coffee in the diet for their lifetime, including the gestation period; no increase in tumour incidence was reported. Rats were given brewed coffee as the drinking fluid in one study; a slight increase in the number of tumour-bearing animals was seen only among males in the lowest dose group. In another study, rats were given different samples of instant coffee, decaffeinated coffee or decaffeinated coffee supplemented with caffeine; no increase in tumour incidence was observed.

These three studies are suggestive of an absence of relationship between coffee and cancer in experimental animals, but the incomplete reporting of the study in mice precludes a definitive evaluation at present.

In a number of studies, various known carcinogens were administered by different routes either simultaneously or sequentially with coffee in water as the drinking fluid or in the diet. Several of these studies, however, suffered from various limitations and were not considered for the evaluation.

In one of the adequate studies, coffee reduced the number of pancreatic tumours per animal in azaserine-treated rats maintained on a high-fat diet; the result may have been due in part to impaired growth. No significant effect of coffee was found on the number of pancreatic tumours per animal induced in hamsters by *N*-nitrosobis(2-oxypropyl)amine. In separate experiments, rats on two different diets were treated intravenously or orally with a single dose of 7,12-dimethylbenz[*a*]anthracene in combination with coffee. No difference in the number of rats with mammary tumours was found as compared to animals receiving 7,12-dimethylbenz[*a*]anthracene only; a significant decrease in the number of mammary tumours per animal was observed after administration of coffee only in rats treated intravenously and not in those treated orally with 7,12-dimethylbenz[a]anthracene.

4.3 Human carcinogenicity data

(a) Descriptive studies

The risk for cancer associated with coffee consumption has been investigated in several descriptive geographical and temporal studies. There was no consistent association between coffee intake, usually estimated indirectly from trade data, and cancer risk, although significant results were occasionally reported in a number of studies. Pancreatic cancer was correlated with coffee consumption in all of the studies in which the relationship was examined. None of the ecological studies showed an association with risk for bladder cancer.

(b) Analytical studies

(i) All sites

A cohort study in which a case-control analysis was used showed a nonsignificant reduction in risk for mortality from cancer at all sites with increased coffee consumption. A second cohort study with longer follow-up reported a nonsignificant increase in mortality after adjustment for age, smoking and other confounders.

(ii) Bladder and urinary tract cancer

Two cohort studies reported findings on bladder cancer incidence. In one, there was a nonsignificant increase in risk; the second showed neither an increase nor a decrease.

Of the 26 case-control studies considered that provided information on the possible relationship between coffee drinking and the occurrence of urinary tract cancers, predominantly of the bladder, in very different populations, 22 were used to make the evaluation. In 16 studies, a weak positive association was seen with consumption of coffee as compared to nonconsumption; in seven of these the association was significant, with a dose-response relationship in three. No association was seen in the six remaining studies. The association persisted, but was less clear, when reported nonsmokers were considered in seven of the 16 studies, suggesting that confounding by tobacco smoking is unlikely to be the sole explanation for this finding. The association was also found in men and women separately, suggesting that occupational factors could not fully explain the finding.

Of the four available case-control studies, three indicated a slightly increased risk for transitional-cell cancers of the renal pelvis and ureter, but none of the results was significant. Six case–control studies and one cohort study do not provide evidence of a consistent association between adenocarcinoma of the kidney and coffee drinking.

Although drinking of decaffeinated coffee was addressed in six case–control studies, it was not possible to distinguish the effects from those of coffee containing caffeine.

Taken as a whole, these data are consistent with a weak positive relationship between coffee consumption and the occurrence of bladder cancer, but the possibility that this is due to bias or confounding cannot be excluded.

(iii) *Breast cancer*

None of the seven case–control studies has suggested the existence of an association between breast cancer risk and the consumption of coffee. All of the studies gave relative risk estimates that were near unity. One study presented results on instant coffee separately and also found no association; three studies showed no association with decaffeinated coffee consumption. Confounding due to recognized risk factors for breast cancer was controlled in most studies. There is no reason to believe that measurement error or confounding was responsible for the finding.

(iv) *Cancer of the large bowel*

Cohort studies that addressed the issue of coffee drinking and risk for cancer of the colon or rectum were not particularly informative but have generally been interpreted as showing no association.

Of the 12 informative case–control studies, 11 indicated inverse ('protective') associations between coffee consumption and risk for colorectal cancer, which reached significance in five. A significant dose–response relationship was seen in one study. At present, it is not possible to exclude bias and confounding as the source of the apparent inverse association, but the collective evidence is also compatible with a 'protective' effect.

(v) *Pancreatic cancer*

Six cohort studies provide data on the relationship between coffee consumption and pancreatic cancer. None reported a significant association with increased consumption; any nonsignificant increase was reduced following adjustment for smoking.

Twenty-one case–control studies have reported on the relationship between coffee consumption and pancreatic cancer. An early report showed a positive relationship, with a significant dose–response, in women but not in men, which persisted after removing those controls with digestive disorders. Another study reported a significant relationship with decaffeinated coffee but not with consumption of all kinds of coffee. Nineteen subsequent reports have been less positive overall. In ten of these studies, a positive association was seen; in three of these, the findings were significant, with a dose–response relationship in two studies. No association was seen in seven studies, and a weakly negative association was found in another. A nonsignificant increase in risk for the highest exposure group has been a more consistent finding, but this has generally become weaker after adjustment for smoking and may be the result of residual confounding. Potential biases associated with the comparability of case and control groups also complicate interpretation, and methodological problems were noted in some studies.

Taken as a whole, the data are suggestive of a weak relationship between high levels of coffee consumption and the occurrence of pancreatic cancer, but the possibility that this is due to bias or confounding is tenable.

The results with regard to decaffeinated coffee are less comprehensive but have generally been negative.

(vi) *Ovarian cancer*

In two case–control studies of coffee drinking and risk for ovarian cancer, a significant increase in risk was found, whereas in five others small, nonsignificant increases were noted. An overall analysis of the data indicates a marginal, significant increase in relative risk, but bias from unidentified sources or even chance cannot be ruled out.

The few available studies do not suggest that drinking decaffeinated coffee increases the risk for ovarian cancer.

(vii) *Gastric cancer*

The relationship between coffee drinking and gastric cancer was studied in five case–control investigations, none of which showed an association.

(viii) *Cancers of the upper digestive tract*

Six case–control studies assessed the association between coffee drinking and cancers of the oesophagus, mouth and pharynx. After adjustment for confounding variables, the frequency of coffee drinking was not associated with risk for cancer in any of these studies. Overall, no association was found between coffee drinking and cancers of the upper digestive tract, except when populations who drink coffee at very high temperatures were studied.

(ix) *Cancers at other sites*

In one case-control study, no association with the occurrence of liver cancer was found among coffee drinkers after adjustment for smoking and alcohol consumption.

Two cohort studies and one case-control study showed no association with lung cancer.

A cohort study reported associations between coffee drinking and Hodgkin's disease and lymphatic and myeloid leukaemia; no association was reported with the occurrence of non-Hodgkin's lymphoma, malignant melanoma, or other and unspecified leukaemias. One case-control study showed an increased incidence of carcinoma of the vulva among coffee drinkers. A single cohort study showed an association with cervical cancer.

4.4 Other relevant data

(a) *Toxic effects*

The available evidence cannot be used to establish a significant, independent relationship between coffee consumption and morbidity or mortality from coronary heart disease. The question remains open, however, especially in view of the finding that some methods of coffee preparation are associated with an elevation in plasma levels of cholesterol and low-density lipoproteins.

(b) *Effects on reproduction and prenatal toxicity*

The teratogenic potential of coffee and caffeine-containing beverages was investigated in two cohort and four case-control studies. Two studies (one cohort and one case-control) found significant positive associations between the consumption of caffeine-containing drinks and the risk for malformations. The remaining four studies (one cohort and three case-control), which included the three most informative reports, failed to find an association. Taken together, these studies do not provide evidence of a teratogenic effect of coffee intake.

Eight studies, from Costa Rica, the Federal Republic of Germany, the UK and the USA, reported an association between decreased birth weight and intake of coffee and caffeine-containing beverages, which was statistically significant in the crude analyses. After correction for confounding variables, including smoking, four of the studies reported positive associations which were significant. Of two other studies, one reported an increased risk among heavy consumers which, however, was not significant, and the other reported a positive association of only borderline significance. The two remaining studies did not show an association after adjustment for confounding. Reporting of coffee consumption was usually most complete for the first and second trimesters, while the greatest impact on birth weight may be from consumption during the last trimester. Overall, the data provide an indication that maternal coffee drinking reduces the birth weight of offspring.

Of the three studies with adequate design and interpretation, only one showed a clear dose–response relationship.

Information concerning prematurity was insufficient for conclusions to be drawn about an effect of coffee consumption. One study provided evidence of a relationship between late spontaneous abortions and moderate to heavy coffee consumption.

No effect on reproduction was observed in rats given percolated or drip (filtered) coffee as the drinking fluid. Developmental delays were observed in the offspring of coffee-treated rats, including decreased fetal and neonatal body weights and delayed ossification. No teratogenic effect was observed.

No teratogenic effect or effect on reproduction was observed in rats given instant coffee as the drinking fluid or as crystals in the diet. In the offspring of treated rats, delayed development was observed, including decreased fetal and neonatal body weight and delayed ossification shortly before birth.

No teratogenic effect or effect on reproduction was observed in rats given decaffeinated coffee (either brewed or instant) as the drinking fluid, although a decrease in body weight of offspring was observed.

The reproductive effects seen in these studies occurred only at levels of coffee much higher than those to which humans are exposed.

(c) *Genetic and related effects*

Otherwise healthy splenectomized coffee drinkers, some of whom occasionally drank tea, had an increased frequency of micronuclei in both reticulocytes and mature erythrocytes.

The urine of coffee drinkers was not mutagenic to bacteria but induced chromosomal aberrations in cultured mammalian cells.

Brewed coffee induced chromosomal aberrations and sister chromatid exchange in cultured human lymphocytes. Sister chromatid exchange was also induced in cultured mammalian cells. In insects, negative results were obtained for aneuploidy, chromosomal aberrations, dominant lethal effects and sex-linked recessive lethal mutation; brewed coffee gave weakly positive results in assays for somatic cell mutation and mitotic recombination. In bacteria, it was mutagenic, particularly to strains with enhanced sensitivity to oxidative mutagens, and induced DNA damage.

Instant coffee did not induce sister chromatid exchange or micronuclei in the bone-marrow cells of rodents treated *in vivo*. It induced chromosomal aberrations in cultured human lymphocytes and induced mutations and sister chromatid exchange in cultured mammalian cells. In insects, negative results were obtained for aneuploidy, chromosomal aberrations, dominant lethal effects and sex-linked recessive lethal mutations; instant coffee gave weakly positive results in assays for somatic cell mutation and mitotic recombination. In bacteria, instant coffee was mutagenic, particularly to strains sensitive to oxidative mutagens, and induced DNA damage; it was not mutagenic in host-mediated bacterial mutagenicity assays.

Decaffeinated coffee induced chromosomal aberrations in cultured human lymphocytes and sister chromatid exchange in cultured mammalian cells. It gave negative results in assays for somatic cell mutation and mitotic recombination assays in insects. In bacteria, decaffeinated coffee was mutagenic, particularly in strains with enhanced sensitivity to oxidative mutagens, and induced DNA damage.

Coffee reduced the genotoxic activity of several model mutagens both *in vivo* and *in vitro*.

4.5 Evaluation[1]

There is *limited evidence* in humans that coffee drinking is carcinogenic in the urinary bladder.

There is *evidence suggesting lack of carcinogenicity* of coffee drinking in the human female breast and in the large bowel.

There is *inadequate evidence* in humans that coffee drinking is carcinogenic in the pancreas, ovary and other body sites.

There is *inadequate evidence* in experimental animals for the carcinogenicity of coffee.

Overall evaluation[2,3]

Coffee is *possibly carcinogenic to the human urinary bladder (Group 2B)*.

---

[1]For description of the italicized terms, see Preamble, pp. 27-31.

[2]There is some evidence of an inverse relationship between coffee drinking and cancer of the large bowel; coffee drinking could not be classified as to its carcinogenicity to other organs.

[3]M.J. Arnaud dissociated himself from the overall evaluation.

5. References

Abraham, S.K. (1989) Inhibition of in vivo genotoxicity by coffee. *Food chem. Toxicol.*, 27, 787-792

Aeschbacher, H.U. (1990) Mutagenic and antimutagenic compounds in beverages. In: Hayatsu, H., ed., *Mutagens in Food-Detection and Prevention*, Boca Raton, FL, CRC Press (in press)

Aeschbacher, H.U. & Chappuis, C. (1981) Nonmutagenicity of urine from coffee drinkers compared with that from cigarette smokers. *Mutat. Res.*, 89, 161-177

Aeschbacher, H.U. & Würzner, H.P. (1980) An evaluation of instant and regular coffee in the Ames mutagenicity test. *Toxicol. Lett.*, 5, 139-145

Aeschbacher, H.U., Chappuis, C. & Würzner, H.P. (1980) Mutagenicity testing of coffee: a study of problems encountered with the Ames Salmonella test system. *Food Cosmet. Toxicol.*, 18, 605-513

Aeschbacher, H.U., Meier, H., Ruch, E., Wolleb, U. & Würzner, H.P. (1984a) Risk evaluation of coffee based on in vitro and in vivo mutagenicity testing. In: MacMahon, B. & Sugimura, T., eds, *Coffee and Health* (Banbury Report 17), Cold Spring Harbor, NY, CSH Press, pp. 89-98

Aeschbacher, H.U., Meier, H., Ruch, E. & Würzner, H.P. (1984b) Investigation of coffee in sister chromatid exchange and micronucleus tests *in vivo*. *Food chem. Toxicol.*, 22, 803-807

Aeschbacher, H.U., Ruch, E., Meier, H., Würzner, H.P. & Munoz-Box, R. (1985) Instant and brewed coffees in the in vitro human lymphocyte mutagenicity test. *Food chem. Toxicol.*, 23, 747-752

Aeschbacher, H.U., Wolleb, U., Löliger, J., Spadone, J.C. & Liardon, R. (1989) Contribution of coffee aroma constituents to the mutagenicity of coffee. *Food chem. Toxicol.*, 27, 227-232

Albertini, S., Friederich, U., Schlatter, C. & Würgler, F.E. (1985) The influence of roasting procedure on the formation of mutagenic compounds in coffee. *Food chem. Toxicol.*, 23, 593-597

Angelucci, E., Yokomizo, Y., de Moraes, R.M., de Campos, R.B., Miya, E.E. & Figueiredo, I.B. (1973) Chemical and sensory evaluation of the main Brazilian instant coffee. In: *6e Colloque Scientifique International sur le Café, Bogotá, 1973*, Paris, Association Scientifique International du Café, pp. 178-182

Anon. (1987) Coffee (Marketing Report No. 4). *Retail Bus.*, 356, 57-67

Anon. (1988) Coffee in Italy (Special Report No. 1). *Marketing Europe*, 311, 44-55

Anon. (1989) Indicators of market size for 117 countries. Part I, Section II. *Business int.*, 3 July

Ariza, R.R., Dorado, G., Barbancho, M. & Pueyo, C. (1988) Study of the causes of direct-acting mutagenicity in coffee and tea using the Ara test in *Salmonella typhimurium*. *Mutat. Res.*, 201, 89-96

Armstrong, B. & Doll, R. (1975) Environmental factors and cancer incidence and mortality in different countries, with special reference to dietary practices. *Int. J. Cancer*, *15*, 617–631

Armstrong, B., Garrod, A. & Doll, R. (1976) A retrospective study of renal cancer with special reference to coffee and animal protein consumption. *Br. J. Cancer*, *33*, 127–136

Arnandova, R. & Kaculov, A. (1978) Coffee and pregnancy (Russ.). *Akush. Ginekol. (Sofia)*, *17*, 57–61

Aro, A., Kostiainen, E., Huttunen, J.K., Seppälä, E. & Vapaatalo, H. (1985) Effects of coffee and tea on lipoproteins and prostanoids. *Atherosclerosis*, *57*, 123–128

Aro, A., Tuomilehto, J., Kostiainen, E., Uusitalo, U. & Pietinen, P. (1987) Boiled coffee increases serum low density lipoprotein concentration. *Metabolism*, *36*, 1027–1030

Aro, A., Pietinen, P., Uusitalo, M. & Tuomilehto, J. (1989) Coffee and tea consumption, dietary fat intake and serum cholesterol concentration of Finnish men and women. *J. int. Med.*, *226*, 127–132

Bak, A.A.A. & Grobbee, D.E. (1989) The effect on serum cholesterol levels of coffee brewed by filtering or boiling. *New Engl. J. Med.*, *321*, 1432–1437

Barone, J.J. & Roberts, H.R. (1984) Human consumption of caffeine. In: Dews, P.B., ed., *Caffeine. Perspectives from Recent Research*, Berlin, Springer, pp. 59–73

Benarde, M.A. & Weiss, W. (1982) Coffee consumption and pancreatic cancer: temporal and spatial correlation. *Br. med. J.*, *284*, 400–402

Benito, E., Obrador, A., Stiggelbout, A., Bosch, F.X., Mulet, M., Muñoz, N. & Kaldor, J. (1990) A population-based case-control study of colorectal cancer in Majorca. I. Dietary factors. *Int. J. Cancer*, *45*, 69–76

van den Berg, B.J. (1977) Epidemiologic observations of prematurity: effects of tobacco, coffee and alcohol. In: Reed, D.M. & Stanley, F.J., eds, *The Epidemiology of Prematurity*, Baltimore, MD, Urban & Schwarzenberg, pp. 157–176

Berkowitz, G.S., Holford, T.R. & Berkowitz, R.L. (1982) Effects of cigarette smoking, alcohol, coffee and tea consumption on preterm delivery. *Early Hum. Dev.*, *7*, 239–250

Berry, N.E. & Walters, R.H. (1943) *Process of Decaffeinating Coffee*, US Patent 2,309,092 (General Foods Corp., New York)

Binstock, M., Krakow, D., Stamler, J., Reiff, J., Persky, V., Liu, K. & Moss, D. (1983) Coffee and pancreatic cancer: an analysis of international mortality data. *Am. J. Epidemiol.*, *118*, 630–640

Bjelke, E. (1973) *Epidemiologic Studies of Cancer of the Stomach, Colon and Rectum; With Special Emphasis on the Role of Diet*, Thesis, University of Minnesota

Blanc, M. (1977) Carboxylic acids of coffee (Fr.) In: *8e Colloque Scientifique sur le Café, Abidjan, 1977*, Paris, Association Scientifique Internationale du Café, pp. 73–77

Borlée, I., Lechat, M.F., Bouckaert, A. & Misson, C. (1978) Coffee, risk factor during pregnancy? (Fr.) *Louvain méd.*, *97*, 279–284

Boston Collaborative Drug Surveillance Program (1972) Coffee drinking and acute myocardial infarction. *Lancet*, *ii*, 1278–1281

Bravo, P., del Rey, J., Sánchez, J. & Conde, M. (1986) Coffee and analgesics as risk factors for bladder cancer (Sp.). *Arch. esp. Urol.*, *39*, 337–341

Bravo, P., del Rey-Calero, J. & Conde, M. (1987) Risk factors of bladder cancer in Spain. *Neoplasma*, *34*, 633–637

Brooke, O.G., Anderson, H.R., Bland, J.M., Peacock, J.L. & Stewart, C.M. (1989) Effects on birth weight of smoking, alcohol, caffeine, socioeconomic factors, and psychosocial stress. *Br. med. J.*, *298*, 795–801

Bross, I.D.J. & Tidings, J. (1973) Another look at coffee drinking and cancer of the urinary bladder. *Prev. Med.*, *2*, 445–451

Bunker, M.L. & McWilliams, M. (1979) Caffeine content of common beverages. *J. Am. diet. Assoc.*, *74*, 28–32

Burg, A.W. (1975) Effects of caffeine on the human system. *Tea Coffee Trade J.*, *147*, 40

Butcher, R.E., Vorhees, C.V. & Wootten, V. (1984) Behavioral and physical development of rats chronically exposed to caffeinated fluids. *Fundam. appl. Toxicol.*, *4*, 1–13

Byers, T., Marshall, J., Graham, S., Mettlin, C. & Swanson, M. (1983) A case–control study of dietary and nondietary factors in ovarian cancer. *J. natl Cancer Inst.*, *71*, 681–686

Caan, B.J. & Goldhaber, M.K. (1989) Caffeinated beverages and low birthweight: a case–control study. *Am. J. public Health*, *79*, 1299–1300

Callahan, M.M., Rohovsky, M.W., Robertson, R.S. & Yesair, D.W. (1979) The effect of coffee consumption on plasma lipids, lipoproteins, and the development of aortic atherosclerosis in rhesus monkeys fed an atherogenic diet. *Am. J. clin. Nutr.*, *32*, 834–845

Cartwright, R.A., Adib, R., Glashan, R. & Gray, B.K. (1981) The epidemiology of bladder cancer in West Yorkshire. A preliminary report on non-occupational aetiologies. *Carcinogenesis*, *2*, 343–347

Chen, A.T.L., Reidy, J.A., Annest, J.L., Welty, T.K. & Zhou, H.-G. (1989) Increased chromosome fragility as a consequence of blood folate levels, smoking status, and coffee consumption. *Environ. mol. Mutagenesis*, *13*, 319–324

Christianson, R.E., Oechsli, F.W. & van den Berg, B.J. (1989) Caffeinated beverages and decreased fertility (Letter to the Editor). *Lancet*, *i*, 378

Ciccone, G. & Vineis, P. (1988) Coffee drinking and bladder cancer. *Cancer Lett.*, *41*, 45–52

Clarke, R.J. (1985) Water and mineral contents. In: Clarke, R.J. & Macrae, R., eds, *Coffee*, Vol. 1, *Chemistry*, London, Elsevier Applied Science, pp. 42–82

Clarke, R.J. (1986) The flavour of coffee. In: Morton, I.D. & MacLeod, A.J., eds, *Food Flavours*, Part B, *The Flavour of Beverages*, Amsterdam, Elsevier, pp. 1–47

Clarke, R.J. (1987) Coffee technology. In: Herschdoefer, S.H., ed., *Quality Control in the Food Industry*, 2nd ed., Vol. 4, London, Academic Press, pp. 161–191

Clarke, R.J. & Macrae, R., eds (1985) *Coffee*, Vol. 1, *Chemistry*, London, Elsevier Applied Science

Clarke, R.J. & Macrae, R., eds (1987a) *Coffee*, Vol. 5, *Related Beverages*, London, Elsevier Applied Science

Clarke, R.J. & Macrae, R., eds (1987b) *Coffee*, Vol. 2, *Technology*, London, Elsevier Applied Science

Clarke, R.J. & Macrae, R., eds (1988a) *Coffee*, Vol. 4, *Agronomy*, London, Elsevier Applied Science

Clarke, R.J. & Macrae, R., eds (1988b) *Coffee*, Vol. 3, *Physiology*, London, Elsevier Applied Science

Claude, J., Kunze, E., Frentzel-Beyme, R., Paczkowski, K., Schneider, J. & Schubert, H. (1986) Life-style and occupational risk factors in cancer of the lower urinary tract. *Am. J. Epidemiol.*, *124*, 578–589

Clavel, F., Benhamou, E., Auquier, A., Tarayre, M. & Flamant, R. (1989) Coffee, alcohol, smoking and cancer of the pancreas: a case–control study. *Int. J. Cancer*, *43*, 17–21

Clifford, M.N. (1985) Chlorogenic acids. In: Clarke, R.J. & Macrae, R., eds, *Coffee*. Vol. 1, *Chemistry*, London, Elsevier Applied Science, pp. 153–202

Clinton, W.P. (1985) The chemistry of coffee. In: *11e Colloque Scientifique International sur le Café, Lomé, 1985*, Paris, Association Scientifique Internationale du Café, pp. 87–92

Cole, P. (1971) Coffee-drinking and cancer of the lower urinary tract. *Lancet*, *ii*, 1335–1337

Commission of the European Communities (1977) Council Directive of 27 June 1977 on the approximation of the laws of the Member States relating to coffee extracts and chicory extracts. *Off. J. Eur. Commun.*, *L172*, 20–24

Commission of the European Communities (1985) Council Directive of 19 December 1985 amending Directive 77/436/EEC on the approximation of the laws of the Member States relating to coffee extracts and chicory extracts. *Off. J. Eur. Commun.*, *L372*, 22–24

Cramer, D.W., Welch, W.R., Hutchison, G.B., Willett, W. & Scully, R.E. (1984) Dietary animal fat in relation to ovarian cancer risk. *Obstet. Gynaecol.*, *63*, 833–838

Cuckle, H.S. & Kinlen, L.J. (1981) Coffee and cancer of the pancreas. *Br. J. Cancer*, *44*, 760–761

Curb, J.D., Reed, D.M., Kautz, J.A. & Yano, K. (1986) Coffee, caffeine, and serum cholesterol in Japanese men in Hawaii. *Am. J. Epidemiol.*, *123*, 648–655

Cuzick, J. & Babiker, A.G. (1989) Pancreatic cancer, alcohol, diabetes mellitus and gall-bladder disease. *Int. J. Cancer*, *43*, 415–421

Dales, L.G., Friedman, G.D., Ury, H.K., Grossman, S. & Williams, S.R. (1979) A case–control study of relationships of diet and other traits to colorectal cancer in American blacks. *Am. J. Epidemiol.*, *109*, 132–144

Dart, S.K. & Nursten, H.E. (1985) Volatile components. In: Clarke, R.J. & Macrae, R., eds, *Coffee*, Vol. 1, *Chemistry*, London, Elsevier Applied Sciences, pp. 223–265

Davis, B.R., Curb, J.D., Borhani, N.O., Prineas, R.J. & Molteni, A. (1988) Coffee consumption and serum cholesterol in the hypertension detection and follow-up program. *Am. J. Epidemiol.*, *128*, 124–136

Dawber, T.R., Kannel, W.B. & Gordon, T. (1974) Coffee and cardiovascular disease. Observations from the Framingham study. *New Engl. J. Med.*, *291*, 871–874

Debry, G. (1989) *Le Café* [Coffee], Nancy, Centre de Nutrition humaine

Decarli, A. & La Vecchia, C. (1986) Environmental factors and cancer mortality in Italy: correlational exercise. *Oncology*, *43*, 116–126

Donahue, R.P., Orchard, T.J., Stein, E.A. & Kuller, L.H. (1987) Lack of an association between coffee consumption and lipoprotein lipids and apolipoproteins in young adults: the Beaver County study. *Prev. Med.*, *16*, 796–802

Dorado, G., Barbancho, M. & Pueyo, C. (1987) Coffee is highly mutagenic in the L-arabinose resistance test in *Salmonella typhimurium*. *Environ. Mutagenesis*, 9, 251–260

Douwe-Egberts Ltd (1989) *Coffee*, Utrecht

Dunham, L.J., Rabson, A.S., Stewart, H.L., Frank, A.S. & Young, J.L. (1968) Rates, interview, and pathology study of cancer of the urinary bladder in New Orleans, Louisiana. *J. natl Cancer Inst.*, 41, 683–709

Dunn, B.P. & Curtis, J.R. (1985) Clastogenic agents in the urine of coffee drinkers and cigarette smokers. *Mutat. Res.*, 147, 179–188

Elinder, C.-G., Millqvist, K., Floderus-Myrhed, B. & Pershagen, G. (1981) Swedish studies do not support the hypothesis concerning a relationship between coffee and pancreatic cancer (Sw.). *Läkartidningen*, 78, 3676–3677

Enstrom, J.E. (1975) Cancer mortality among Mormons. *Cancer*, 36, 825–841

Enstrom, J.E. (1978) Cancer and total mortality among active Mormons. *Cancer*, 42, 1943–1951

Enstrom, J.E. (1980) Cancer mortality among Mormons in California during 1968–75. *J. natl Cancer Inst.*, 65, 1073–1082

Ernster, V.L. (1984) Epidemiologic studies of caffeine and human health. In: Spiller, G.A., ed., *The Methylxanthine Beverages and Foods: Chemistry, Consumption, and Health Effects*, New York, Alan R. Liss, pp. 377–400

Falk, R.T., Pickle, L.W., Fontham, E.T., Correa, P. & Fraumeni, J.F., Jr (1988) Life-style risk factors for pancreatic cancer in Louisiana: a case–control study. *Am. J. Epidemiol.*, 128, 324–336

Fischer, A. & Kummer, P. (1979) *Verfahren zum Entcoffeinieren von Rohkaffee* [Process for Decaffeination of Raw Coffee], European Patent 0,008,398 A1 (Coffex AG)

Flament, I. (1987) From assamar to kahweofuran, a century and a half of research into coffee aroma (Fr.). In: *12e Colloque Scientifique International sur le Café, Montreux, 1987*, Paris, Association Scientifique Internationale du Café, pp. 146–150

Folstar, P. (1985) Lipids. In: Clarke, R.J. & Macrae, R., eds, *Coffee*, Vol. 1, *Chemistry*, London, Elsevier Applied Sciences, pp. 203–222

Førde, O.H., Knutsen, S.F., Arnesen, E. & Thelle, D.S. (1985) The Tromsø heart study: coffee consumption and serum lipid concentrations in men with hypercholesterolaemia: a randomised intervention study. *Br. med. J.*, 290, 893–895

Franceschi, S., Serraino, D., Carbone, A., Talamini, R. & La Vecchia, C. (1989) Dietary factors and non-Hodgkin's lymphoma: a case–control study in the northeastern part of Italy. *Nutr. Cancer*, 12, 333–341

Franco, E.L., Kowalski, L.P., Oliveira, B.V., Curado, M.P., Pereira, R.N., Silva, M.E., Fava, A.S. & Torloni, H. (1989) Risk factors for oral cancer in Brazil: a case–control study. *Int. J. Cancer*, 43, 992–1000

Fraumeni, J.F., Jr, Scotto, J. & Dunham, L.J. (1971) Coffee-drinking and bladder cancer (Letter to the Editor). *Lancet*, ii, 1204

Friederich, U., Hann, D., Albertini, S., Schlatter, C. & Würgler, F.E. (1985) Mutagenicity studies on coffee. The influence of different factors on the mutagenic activity in the *Salmonella*/mammalian microsome assay. *Mutat. Res.*, 156, 39–52

Fujii, M., Mori, H., Nishikawa, A. & Takahashi, M. (1980) Effect of coffee on carcinogenicity of N-2-fluorenylacetamide. *Acta schol. med. Univ. Gifu*, 28, 295-298

Fujita, Y., Wakabayashi, K., Nagao, M. & Sugimura, T. (1985a) Implication of hydrogen peroxide in the mutagenicity of coffee. *Mutat. Res.*, 144, 227-230

Fujita, Y., Wakabayashi, K., Nagao, M. & Sugimura, T. (1985b) Characteristics of major mutagenicity of instant coffee. *Mutat. Res.*, 142, 145-148

Furuhashi, N., Sato, S., Suzuki, M., Hiruta, M., Tanaka, M. & Takahashi, T. (1985) Effects of caffeine ingestion during pregnancy. *Gynecol. obstet. Invest.*, 19, 187-191

Gilbert, R.M. (1984) Caffeine consumption. In: Spiller, G.A., ed., *The Methylxanthine Beverages and Foods: Chemistry, Consumption and Health Effects*, New York, Alan R. Liss, pp. 185-213

Gilbert, R.M., Marshman, J.A., Schwieder, M. & Berg, R. (1976) Caffeine content of beverages as consumed. *Can. med. Assoc. J.*, 114, 205-208

Gold, E.B., Gordis, L., Diener, M.D., Seltser, R., Boitnott, J.K., Bynum, T.E. & Hutcheon, D.F. (1985) Diet and other risk factors for cancer of the pancreas. *Cancer*, 55, 460-467

Goldman, P. (1984) Coffee and health: what's brewing? *New Engl. J. Med.*, 310, 783-785

Goldstein, H.R. (1982) No association found between coffee and cancer of the pancreas (Letter to the Editor). *New Engl. J. Med.*, 306, 997

Gonzáles, C.A., Lopez-Abente, G., Errezola, M., Castejón, J., Estrada, A., Garcia-Milá, M., Gili, P., Huguet, M., Serrat, M., Soler, F. & Rodriguez, C. (1985) Occupation, tobacco use, coffee and bladder cancer in the county of Mataro (Spain). *Cancer*, 55, 2031-2034

Goodman, M.T., Morgenstern, H. & Wynder, E.L. (1986) A case-control study of factors affecting the development of renal cell cancer. *Am. J. Epidemiol.*, 124, 926-941

Gorham, E.D., Garland, C.F., Garland, F.C., Benenson, A.S. & Cottrell, L. (1988) Coffee and pancreatic cancer in a rural California county. *West. J. Med.*, 148, 48-53

Graf, U. & Würgler, F.E. (1986) Investigation of coffee in *Drosophila* genotoxicity tests. *Food chem. Toxicol.*, 24, 835-842

Graham, S., Lilienfeld, A.M. & Tidings, J.E. (1967) Dietary and purgation factors in the epidemiology of gastric cancer. *Cancer*, 20, 2224-2234

Graham, S., Dayal, H., Swanson, M., Mittelman, A. & Wilkinson, G. (1978) Diet in the epidemiology of cancer of the colon and rectum. *J. natl Cancer Inst.*, 61, 709-714

Green, D. & Blanc, M. (1981) *Process for the Removal of Caffeine from Green Coffee and Process for the Recovery of Caffeine*, European Patent 0,040,712 B2 (Société des Produits Nestlé)

Groisser, D.S., Rosso, P. & Winick, M. (1982) Coffee consumption during pregnancy: subsequent behavioral abnormalities of the offspring. *J. Nutr.*, 112, 829-832

Haenszel, W., Berg, J.W., Segi, M., Kurihara, M. & Locke, F.B. (1973) Large-bowel cancer in Hawaiian Japanese. *J. natl Cancer Inst.*, 51, 1765-1779

Hartge, P., Lesher, L.P., McGowan, L. & Hoover, R. (1982) Coffee and ovarian cancer (Letter to the Editor). *Int. J. Cancer*, 30, 531-532

Hartge, P., Hoover, R., West, D.W. & Lyon, J.L. (1983) Coffee drinking and risk of bladder cancer. *J. natl Cancer Inst.*, 70, 1021-1026

Hattox, R.S. (1988) *Coffee and Coffeehouses. The Origins of a Social Beverage in the Medieval Near East*, Seattle, WA, University of Washington Press

Hayashi, T. & Shibamoto, T. (1985) Analysis of methyl glyoxal in foods and beverages. *J. agric. Food Chem.*, 33, 1090-1093

Hayashi, T., Reece, C.A. & Shibamato, T. (1986) Gas chromatographic determination of formaldehyde in coffee *via* thiazolidine derivative. *J. Assoc. off. anal. Chem.*, 69, 101-105

Heller, J. (1987) What do we know about the risks of caffeine consumption in pregnancy? *Br. J. Addict.*, 82, 885-889

Henderson, B.E., Louie, E., Jing, J.S., Buell, P. & Gardner, M.B. (1976) Risk factors associated with nasopharyngeal carcinoma. *New Engl. J. Med.*, 295, 1101-1106

Hennekens, C.H., Drolette, M.E., Jesse, M.J., Davies, J.E. & Hutchison, G.B. (1976) Coffee drinking and death due to coronary heart disease. *New Engl. J. Med.*, 294, 633-636

Heuch, I., Kvåle, G., Jacobsen, B.K. & Bjelke, E. (1983) Use of alcohol, tobacco and coffee, and risk of pancreatic cancer. *Br. J. Cancer*, 48, 637-643

Heyden, S., Heyden, F., Heiss, G. & Hames, C.G. (1979) Smoking and coffee consumption in three groups: cancer deaths, cardiovascular deaths and living controls. A prospective study in Evans County, Georgia. *J. chron. Dis.*, 32, 673-677

Hiatt, R.A., Klatsky, A.L. & Armstrong, M.A. (1988) Pancreatic cancer, blood glucose and beverage consumption. *Int. J. Cancer*, 41, 794-797

Higginson, J. (1966) Etiological factors in gastrointestinal cancer in man. *J. natl Cancer Inst.*, 37, 527-545

Hofman, A., van Laar, A., Klein, F. & Valkenburg, H.A. (1983) Coffee and cholesterol (Letter to the Editor). *New Engl. J. Med.*, 309, 1248-1249

Hogue, C.J. (1981) Coffee in pregnancy (Letter to the Editor). *Lancet*, i, 554

Howe, G.R., Burch, J.D., Miller, A.B., Cook, G.M., Estève, J., Morrison, B., Gordon, P., Chambers, L.W., Fodor, G. & Winsor, G.M. (1980) Tobacco use, occupation, coffee, various nutrients, and bladder cancer. *J. natl Cancer Inst.*, 64, 701-713

Hsieh, C.-C., MacMahon, B., Yen, S., Trichopoulos, D., Warren, K. & Nardi, G. (1986) Coffee and pancreatic cancer (Chapter 2) (Letter to the Editor). *New Engl. J. Med.*, 315, 587-589

Hudler, K. (1988) Coffee market snapshot - West Germany. *Aroma Q. Rev.*, Winter, 24, 26

IARC (1976a) *IARC Monographs on the Evaluation of Carcinogenic Risk of Chemicals to Man*, Vol. 10, *Some Naturally Occurring Substances*, Lyon, pp. 51-72

IARC (1976b) *IARC Monographs on the Evaluation of Carcinogenic Risk of Chemicals to Man*, Vol. 10, *Some Naturally Occurring Substances*, Lyon, pp. 245-251

IARC (1979) *IARC Monographs on the Evaluation of the Carcinogenic Risk of Chemicals to Humans*, Vol. 20, *Some Halogenated Hydrocarbons*, Lyon, pp. 545-572

IARC (1982) *IARC Monographs on the Evaluation of the Carcinogenic Risk of Chemicals to Humans*, Vol. 29, *Some Industrial Chemicals and Dyestuffs*, Lyon, pp. 345-389

IARC (1983) *IARC Monographs on the Evaluation of the Carcinogenic Risk of Chemicals to Humans*, Vol. 31, *Some Food Additives, Feed Additives and Naturally Occurring Substances*, Lyon, pp. 191-206

IARC (1986a) *IARC Monographs on the Evaluation of the Carcinogenic Risk of Chemicals to Humans*, Vol. 41, *Some Halogenated Hydrocarbons and Pesticide Exposures*, Lyon, pp. 43–85

IARC (1986b) *IARC Monographs on the Evaluation of the Carcinogenic Risk of Chemicals to Humans*, Vol. 40, *Some Naturally Occurring and Synthetic Food Components, Furocoumarins and Ultraviolet Radiation*, Lyon, pp. 275–281

IARC (1987) *IARC Monographs on the Evaluation of Carcinogenic Risks to Humans*, Suppl. 7, *Overall Evaluations of Carcinogenicity: An Updating of* IARC Monographs *Volumes 1–42*, Lyon, pp. 194–195, 364–366, 83–87, 271–272, 211–216

International Coffee Organization (1982) *International Coffee Agreement 1983*, London

International Coffee Organization (1988a) *Federal Republic of Germany. Summary of National Coffee Drinking Study 1987* (PC-558/88), London

International Coffee Organization (1988b) *Japan; Proposal by the All Japan Coffee Association for the Continuation of Generic Promotion Activities in Coffee Year 1988-89* (PC-538/88), London

International Coffee Organization (1989a) *Supply – Stocks, Production and Availability of Coffee in Exporting Member Countries, Crop Years and Coffee Years 1968 to 1988* (WP Agreement No. 11/88 (E) Rev. 2), London

International Coffee Organization (1989b) *Prospectus of Coffee Education and Training Activity*, London

International Coffee Organization (1989c) *ICO Basic Information. Objectives, Structure, History and Operation*, London

International Coffee Organization (1989d) *Supply – Production of Arabica and Robusta Coffees* (WP Agreement No. 16/88 (E) Rev. 1), London

International Coffee Organization (1989e) *Exports – Exports by Exporting Members to Members and Non-members, May 1989 and the Eight Months October–May 1988/89* (EB 3149/89 (E)), London

International Coffee Organization (1989f) *Demands – Imports, Re-exports, Net Imports, Inventories, Disappearance and Household Purchases, Quarter October–December 1988 and the Twelve Months January–December 1988* (EB 3150/89 (E)), London

International Coffee Organization (1989g) *Non-member Countries – Imports and Consumption of Coffee* (WP Agreement No. 48/89 (E)), London

International Coffee Organization (1989h) *USA. Coffee Drinking Study, Winter 1989* (PC-585/89), London

International Coffee Organization (1990) *Importing Members. Imports, Re-exports, Net Imports and Disappearance, Coffee Year 1988/89* (WP Board No. 723/90 (E)), London

Iscovich, J., Castelletto, R., Estève, J., Muñoz, N., Colanzi, R., Coronel, A., Deamezola, I., Tassi, V. & Arslan, A. (1987) Tobacco smoking, occupational exposure and bladder cancer in Argentina. *Int. J. Cancer*, 40, 734–740

Jacobsen, B.K., Bjelke, E., Kvåle, G. & Heuch, I. (1986) Coffee drinking, mortality and cancer incidence: results from a Norwegian prospective study. *J. natl Cancer Inst.*, 76, 823–831

Jacobson, M.F., Goldman, A.S. & Syme, R.H. (1981) Coffee and birth defects (Letter to the Editor). *Lancet, i*, 1415-1416

James, J.E. & Paull, I. (1985) Caffeine and human reproduction. *Rev. environ. Health, 5*, 151-167

Jarebinski, M., Adanja, B. & Vlajinac, H. (1989) Case-control study of relationship of some biosocial correlates to rectal cancer patients in Belgrade, Yugoslavia. *Neoplasma, 36*, 369-374

Jensen, O.M., Knudsen, J.B., Sørensen, B.L. & Clemmesen, J. (1983) Artificial sweeteners and absence of bladder cancer risk in Copenhagen. *Int. J. Cancer, 32*, 577-582

Jensen, O.M., Wahrendorf, J., Knudsen, J.B. & Sørensen, B.L. (1986) The Copenhagen case-control study of bladder cancer. II. Effect of coffee and other beverages. *Int. J. Cancer, 37*, 651-657

Jick, H. & Dinan, B.J. (1981) Coffee and pancreatic cancer (Letter to the Editor). *Lancet, ii*, 92

Jick, H., Miettinen, O.S., Neff, R.K., Shapiro, S., Heinonen, O.P. & Slone, D. (1973) Coffee and myocardial infarction. *New Engl. J. Med., 289*, 63-67

Joesoef, R., Beral, V., Rolfs, R.T., Aral, S.O. & Cramer, D.W. (1990) Are caffeinated beverages risk factors for delayed conception? *Lancet, i*, 136-137

de Jong, U.W., Breslow, N., Hong, J.G.E., Sridharan, M. & Shanmugaratnam, K. (1974) Aetiological factors in oesophageal cancer in Singapore Chinese. *Int. J. Cancer, 13*, 291-303

Kabat, G.C., Dieck, G.S. & Wynder, E.L. (1986) Bladder cancer in nonsmokers. *Cancer, 57*, 362-367

Kam, J.K.-H. (1980) Mutagenic activity of caffeinated and decaffeinated coffee. *Cancer Detect. Prev., 3*, 507-511

Kantor, A.F., Hartge, P., Hoover, R.N. & Fraumeni, J.F., Jr (1988) Epidemiological characteristics of squamous cell carcinoma and adenocarcinoma of the bladder. *Cancer Res., 48*, 3853-3855

Kark, J.D., Friedlander, Y., Kaufmann, N.A. & Stein, Y. (1985) Coffee, tea, and plasma cholesterol: the Jerusalem Lipid Research Clinic prevalence study. *Br. med. J., 291*, 699-704

Kasai, H., Kumeno, K., Yamaizumi, Z., Nishimura, S., Nagao, M., Fujita, Y., Sugimura, T., Nukaya, H. & Kosuge, T. (1982) Mutagenicity of methylglyoxal in coffee. *Gann, 73*, 681-683

Katsouyanni, K., Trichopoulos, D., Boyle, P., Xirouchaki, E., Trichopoulou, A., Lisseos, B., Vasilaros, S. & MacMahon, B. (1986) Diet and breast cancer: a case-control study in Greece. *Int. J. Cancer, 38*, 815-820

Katz, S.N. (1980) Decaffeination of coffee. In: *9e Colloque Scientifique International sur le Café, London, 16-20 June 1980*, Paris, Association Scientifique Internationale du Café, pp. 295-302

Katz, S.N. (1987) Decaffeination. In: Clarke, R.J. & Macrae, R., eds, *Coffee*, Vol. 2, *Technology*, London, Elsevier Applied Science, pp. 59-71

Katz, S.N. & Proscia, G.E. (1981) *Carbon–caffeine Separation*, US Patent 4,298,736 (General Foods Corp.)

Kazi, T. (1985) Determination of caffeine and other purine alkaloids in coffee and tea products by high performance liquid chromatography. In: *11e Colloque Scientifique International sur le Café, Lomé, 1985*, Paris, Association Scientifique Internationale du Café, pp. 227-244

Kessler, I.I. (1981) Coffee and cancer of the pancreas (Letter to the Editor). *New Engl. J. Med.*, 304, 1605

Kikugawa, K., Kato, T. & Takahashi, S. (1989) Possible presence of 2-amino-3,4-dimethylimidazo[4,5-f]quinoline and other heterocyclic amine-like mutagens in roasted coffee beans. *J. agric. Food Chem.*, 37, 881-886

Kinlen, L.J. & McPherson, K. (1984) Pancreas cancer and coffee and tea consumption: a case–control study. *Br. J. Cancer*, 49, 93-96

Kinlen, L.J., Goldblatt, P., Fox, J. & Yudkin, J. (1984) Coffee and pancreas cancer: controversy in part explained? *Lancet*, i, 282-283

Klatsky, A.L., Friedman, G.D. & Siegelaub, A.B. (1973) Coffee drinking prior to acute myocardial infarction. Results from the Kaiser-Permanente epidemiologic study of myocardial infarction. *J. Am. med. Assoc.*, 226, 540-543

Klatsky, A.L., Petitti, D.B., Armstrong, M.A. & Friedman, G.D. (1985) Coffee, tea and cholesterol. *Am. J. Cardiol.*, 55, 577-578

Kosugi, A., Nagao, M., Suwa, Y., Wakabayashi, K. & Sugimura, T. (1983) Roasting coffee beans produces compounds that induce prophage λ in *E. coli* and are mutagenic in *E. coli* and *S. typhimurium*. *Mutat. Res.*, 116, 179-184

Kovar, M.G., Fulwood, R. & Feinleib, M. (1983) Coffee and cholesterol (Letter to the Editor). *New Engl. J. Med.*, 309, 1249

Kraft General Foods (1989) *Coffee Consumption*, White Plains, NY

Kršnjavi, H. & Mimica, M. (1987) Coffee and alcohol consumption, and smoking habit in pregnancy (Slav.). *Arh. hig. rada Toksikol.*, 38, 141-147

de Kruijf, N., Schouten, T. & van der Stegen, G.H.D. (1987) Rapid determination of benzo[a]pyrene in roasted coffee and coffee brew by high-performance liquid chromatography with fluorescence detection. *J. agric. Food Chem.*, 35, 545-549

Kung, J.T., McNaught, R.P. & Yeransian, J.A. (1967) Determining volatile acids in coffee beverages by NMR and gas chromatography. *J. Food Sci.*, 32, 455-458

Kurppa, K., Holmberg, P.C., Kuosma, E. & Saxén, L. (1983) Coffee consumption during pregnancy and selected congenital malformations: a nationwide case–control study. *Am. J. public Health*, 73, 1397-1399

Kuzma, J.W. & Sokol, R.J. (1982) Maternal drinking behavior and decreased intrauterine growth. *Alcohol. clin. exp. Res.*, 6, 396-402

LaCroix, A.Z., Mead, L.A., Liang, K.-Y., Thomas, C.B. & Pearson, T.A. (1986) Coffee consumption and the incidence of coronary heart disease. *New Engl. J. Med.*, 315, 977-982

La Vecchia, C., Franceschi, S., Decarli, A., Gentile, A., Liati, P., Regallo, M. & Tognoni, G. (1984) Coffee drinking and the risk of epithelial ovarian cancer. *Int. J. Cancer*, *33*, 559–562

La Vecchia, C., Talamini, R., Decarli, A., Franceschi, S., Parazzini, F. & Tognoni, G. (1986) Coffee consumption and the risk of breast cancer. *Surgery*, *100*, 477–481

La Vecchia, C., Liati, P., Decarli, A., Negri, E. & Franceschi, S. (1987) Coffee consumption and risk of pancreatic cancer. *Int. J. Cancer*, *40*, 309–313

La Vecchia, C., Negri, E., Decarli, A., D'Avanzo, B., Gallotti, L., Gentile, A. & Franceschi, S. (1988) A case–control study of diet and colo-rectal cancer in northern Italy. *Int. J. Cancer*, *41*, 492–498

La Vecchia, C., Gentile, A., Negri, E., Parazzini, F. & Franceschi, S. (1989a) Coffee consumption and myocardial infarction in women. *Am. J. Epidemiol.*, *130*, 481–485

La Vecchia, C., Negri, E., Decarli, A., D'Avanzo, B., Liberati, C. & Franceschi, S. (1989b) Dietary factors in the risk of bladder cancer. *Nutr. Cancer*, *12*, 93–101

La Vecchia, C., Ferraroni, M., Negri, E., D'Avanzo, B., Decarli, A., Levi, F. & Franceschi, S. (1989c) Coffee consumption and digestive tract cancers. *Cancer Res.*, *49*, 1049–1051

Lawson, D.H., Jick, H. & Rothman, K.J. (1981) Coffee and tea consumption and breast disease. *Surgery*, *90*, 801–803

Lê, M.G. (1985) Coffee consumption, benign breast disease, and breast cancer (Letter to the Editor). *Am. J. Epidemiol.*, *122*, 721

Lê, M.G., Hill, C., Kramar, A. & Flamant, R. (1984) Alcoholic beverage consumption and breast cancer in a French case–control study. *Am. J. Epidemiol.*, *120*, 350–357

Lecos, C. (1984) The latest caffeine scorecard. *FDA Consumer*, March, 14–16

Lee, H.P., Gourley, L., Duffy, S.W., Estève, J., Lee, J. & Day, N.E. (1989) Colorectal cancer and diet in an Asian population – a case–control study among Singapore Chinese. *Int. J. Cancer*, *43*, 1007–1016

LeGrady, D., Dyer, A.R., Shekelle, R.B., Stamler, J., Liu, K., Paul, O., Lepper, M. & MacMillan Shryock, A. (1987) Coffee consumption and mortality in the Chicago Western Electric Company study. *Am. J. Epidemiol.*, *126*, 803–812

Leviton, A. (1984) Epidemiologic studies of birth defects. In: Dews, P.B., ed., *Caffeine: Perspectives from Recent Research*, Berlin, Springer, pp. 188–200

Leviton, A. (1988) Caffeine consumption and the risk of reproductive hazards. *J. reprod. Med.*, *33*, 175–178

Lin, R.S. & Kessler, I.I. (1981) A multifactorial model for pancreatic cancer in man. Epidemiologic evidence. *J. Am. med. Assoc.*, *245*, 147–152

Linn, S., Schoenbaum, S.C., Monson, R.R., Rosner, B., Stubblefield, P.G. & Ryan, K.J. (1982) No association between coffee consumption and adverse outcomes of pregnancy. *New Engl. J. Med.*, *306*, 141–145

Little, J.A., Shanoff, H.M., Csima, A. & Yano, R. (1966) Coffee and serum-lipids in coronary heart-disease. *Lancet*, *i*, 732–734

Lubin, J.H., Burns, P.E., Blot, W.J., Ziegler, R.G., Lees, A.W. & Fraumeni, J.F., Jr (1981) Dietary factors and breast cancer risk. *Int. J. Cancer*, *28*, 685–689

Lubin, F., Ron, E., Wax, Y., Funaro, M., Shitrit, A., Black, M. & Modan, B. (1984) Coffee and methylxanthine in benign and malignant breast diseases. In: MacMahon, B. & Sugimura, T., eds, *Coffee and Health* (Banbury Report 17), Cold Spring Harbor, NY, CSH Press, pp. 177-187

Lubin, F., Ron, E., Wax, Y. & Modan, B. (1985) Coffee and methylxanthines and breast cancer: a case-control study. *J. natl Cancer Inst.*, 74, 569-573

Lyon, J.L., Klauber, M.R., Gardner, J.W. & Smart, C.R. (1976) Cancer incidence in Mormons and non-Mormons in Utah, 1966-1970. *New Engl. J. Med.*, 294, 129-132

Lyon, J.L., Gardner, J.W. & West, D.W. (1980) Cancer incidence in Mormons and non-Mormons in Utah during 1967-75. *J. natl Cancer Inst.*, 65, 1055-1061

Maarse, H. & Visscher, C.A. (1986) *Volatile Compounds in Foods. Qualitative Data. Roast Coffee* (Supplement 3), Zeist, Central Institute for Nutrition and Food Research, TNO

Mabuchi, K., Bross, D.S. & Kessler, I.I. (1985a) Risk factors for male breast cancer. *J. natl Cancer Inst.*, 74, 371-375

Mabuchi, K., Bross, D.S. & Kessler, I.I. (1985b) Epidemiology of cancer of the vulva. A case-control study. *Cancer*, 55, 1843-1848

Mack, T.M., Yu, M.C., Hanisch, R. & Henderson, B.E. (1986) Pancreas cancer and smoking, beverage consumption, and past medical history. *J. natl Cancer Inst.*, 76, 49-60

MacMahon, B., Yen, S., Trichopoulos, D., Warren, K. & Nardi, G. (1981a) Coffee and cancer of the pancreas. *New Engl. J. Med.*, 304, 630-633

MacMahon, B., Yen, S., Trichopoulos, D., Warren, K. & Nardi, G. (1981b) Coffee and cancer of the pancreas (Letter to the Editor). *New Engl. J. Med.*, 304, 1605-1606

Macquart-Moulin, G., Riboli, E., Cornee, J., Charnay, B., Berthezène, P. & Day, N. (1986) Case-control study on colorectal cancer and diet in Marseilles. *Int. J. Cancer*, 38, 183-191

Macrae, R. (1985) Nitrogenous compounds. In: Clarke, R.J. & Macrae, R., eds, *Coffee*, Vol. 1, *Chemistry*, London, Elsevier Applied Science, pp. 115-152

Maier, H.G. (1981) *Kaffee*, Berlin, Paul Parey, pp. 33-35, 63

Maier, H.G. (1987a) The acids of coffee. In: *12e Colloque Scientifique International sur le Café, Montreux, 1987*, Paris, Association Scientifique Internationale du Café, pp. 229-237

Maier, H.G. (1987b) Introduction. In: Clarke, R.J. & Macrae, R., eds, *Coffee*, Vol. 5, *Related Beverages*, London, Elsevier Applied Science, pp. 1-18

Malizia, P.D. & Trumbetas, J.F. (1984) *Decaffeination of a Coffee Extract*, US Patent 4,446,162 (General Foods Corp.)

Mann, J.I. & Thorogood, M. (1975) Coffee-drinking and myocardial infarction (Letter to the Editor). *Lancet*, ii, 1215

Mansel, R.E., Webster, D.J.T., Burr, M. & St Leger, S. (1982) Is there a relationship between coffee consumption and breast disease? (Abstract No. 69). *Surg. Res. Soc.*, 69, 295-296

Marrett, L.D., Walter, S.D. & Meigs, J.W. (1983) Coffee drinking and bladder cancer in Connecticut. *Am. J. Epidemiol.*, 117, 113-127

Martin, H. (1982) Selective extraction of caffeine from green coffee beans and the application of similar processes on other natural products. In: *10e Colloque Scientifique International sur le Café, Salvador (Bahia), 1982*, Paris, Association Scientifique Internationale du Café, pp. 21-28

Martin, T.R. & Bracken, M.B. (1987) The association between low birth weight and caffeine consumption during pregnancy. *Am. J. Epidemiol.*, 126, 813-821

Martinez, I. (1969) Factors associated with cancer of the esophagus, mouth, and pharynx in Puerto Rico. *J. natl Cancer Inst.*, 42, 1069-1094

Mathias, S., Garland, C., Barrett-Connor, E. & Wingard, D.L. (1985) Coffee, plasma cholesterol, and lipoproteins. A population study in an adult community. *Am. J. Epidemiol.*, 121, 896-905

Mätzel, U. & Maier, H.G. (1983) Diterpenes in coffee. II. Glycosides of atractyligenin (Ger.). *Z. Lebensmittel. Untersuch. Forsch.*, 176, 281-284

Mau, G. & Netter, P. (1974) Coffee and alcohol consumption. Risk factors during pregnancy? (Ger). *Geburtsh. Frauenheilk.*, 34, 1018-1022

McCredie, M., Ford, J.M. & Stewart, J.H. (1988) Risk factors for cancer of the renal parenchyma. *Int. J. Cancer*, 42, 13-16

McGowan, L., Parent, L., Lednar, W. & Norris, H.J. (1979) The woman at risk for developing ovarian cancer. *Gynecol. Oncol.*, 7, 325-344

McLaughlin, J.K., Blot, W.J., Mandel, J.S., Schuman, L.M., Mehl, E.S. & Fraumeni, J.F., Jr (1983) Etiology of cancer of the renal pelvis. *J. natl Cancer Inst.*, 71, 287-291

McLaughlin, J.K., Mandel, J.S., Blot, W.J., Schuman, L.M., Mehl, E.S. & Fraumeni, J.F., Jr (1984) A population-based case-control study of renal cell carcinoma. *J. natl Cancer Inst.*, 72, 275-284

Mettlin, C. (1989) Milk drinking, other beverage habits, and lung cancer risk. *Int. J. Cancer*, 43, 608-612

Mettlin, C. & Graham, S. (1979) Dietary risk factors in human bladder cancer. *Am. J. Epidemiol.*, 110, 255-263

Meyer, J.F., Jr (1906) *Improvement Relating to the Preparation or Treatment of Coffee*, British Patent 6375, London, His Majesty's Stationery Office

Meyer, J.F., Jr, Roselius, L. & Wimmer, K. (1908) *Removing Caffeine from Coffee*, US Patent 897,763 [*Chem. Abstr.*, 1909, 3, p. 344]

Miller, A.B. (1977) The etiology of bladder cancer from the epidemiological viewpoint. *Cancer Res.*, 37, 2939-2942

Miller, C.T., Neutel, C.I., Nair, R.C., Marrett, L.D., Last, J.M. & Collins, W.E. (1978) Relative importance of risk factors in bladder carcinogenesis. *J. chron. Dis.*, 31, 51-56

Miller, D.R., Rosenberg, L., Helmrich, S.P., Kaufman, D.W. & Shapiro, S. (1984) Ovarian cancer and coffee drinking. In: MacMahon, B. & Sugimura, T., eds, *Coffee and Health* (Banbury Report 17), Cold Spring Harbor, NY, CSH Press, pp. 157-165

Miller, D.R., Rosenberg, L., Kaufman, D.W., Helmrich, S.P., Schottenfeld, D., Lewis, J., Stolley, P.D., Rosenshein, N. & Shapiro, S. (1987) Epithelial ovarian cancer and coffee drinking. *Int. J. Epidemiol.*, 16, 13-17

Miller, E.G., Formby, W.A., Rivera-Hidalgo, F. & Wright, J.M. (1988) Inhibition of hamster buccal pouch carcinogenesis by green coffee beans. *Oral Surg. oral Med. oral Pathol.*, *65*, 745–749

Mills, P.K., Beeson, W.L., Abbey, D.E., Fraser, G.E. & Phillips, R.L. (1988) Dietary habits and past medical history as related to fatal pancreas cancer risk among Adventists. *Cancer*, *61*, 2578–2585

Mitchell, H.W. (1988) Cultivation and harvesting of the arabica coffee tree. In: Clarke, R.J. & Macrae, R., eds, *Coffee*, Vol. 4, *Agronomy*, London, Elsevier Applied Science, pp. 43–90

Mommsen, S., Aagaard, J. & Sell, A. (1983a) An epidemiological study of bladder cancer in a predominantly rural district. *Scand. J. Urol. Nephrol.*, *17*, 307–312

Mommsen, S., Aagaard, J. & Sell, A. (1983b) A case-control study of female bladder cancer. *Eur. J. Cancer clin. Oncol.*, *19*, 725–729

Morgan, R.W. & Jain, M.G. (1974) Bladder cancer: smoking, beverages and artificial sweeteners. *Can. med. Assoc. J.*, *111*, 1067–1070

Mori, H. & Hirono, I. (1977) Effect of coffee on carcinogenicity of cycasin. *Br. J. Cancer*, *35*, 369–371

Morrison, A.S. (1978) Geographic and time trends of coffee imports and bladder cancer. *Eur. J. Cancer*, *14*, 51–54

Morrison, R.L., Jr & Phillips, J.H. (1983) *Accelerated Decaffeinated Process*, European Patent 0,114,426 A1 (Procter & Gamble Co.)

Morrison, A.S., Buring, J.E., Verhoek, W.G., Aoki, K., Leck, I., Ohno, Y. & Obata, K. (1982) Coffee drinking and cancer of the lower urinary tract. *J. natl Cancer Inst.*, *68*, 91–94

Müller-Henniges, H.-G. & Rothfos, B. (1989) *European Coffee Report 1988*, Amsterdam, European Coffee Federation

Muñoz, L., Keen, C.L., Lönnerdal, B. & Dewey, K.G. (1986) Coffee intake during pregnancy and lactation in rats: maternal and pup hematological parameters and liver iron, zinc and copper concentration. *J. Nutr.*, *116*, 1326–1333

Muñoz, L., Lönnerdal, B., Keen, C.L. & Dewey, K.G. (1988) Coffee consumption as a factor in iron deficiency anemia among pregnant women and their infants in Costa Rica. *Am. J. clin. Nutr.*, *48*, 645–651

Murphy, S.J. & Benjamin, C.P. (1981) The effects of coffee on mouse development. *Microbios. Lett.*, *17*, 91–100

Nagao, M., Takahashi, Y., Yamanaka, H. & Sugimura, T. (1979) Mutagens in coffee and tea. *Mutat. Res.*, *68*, 101–106

Nagao, M., Suwa, Y., Yoshizumi, H. & Sugimura, T. (1984) Mutagens in coffee. In: MacMahon, B. & Sugimura, T., eds, *Coffee and Health* (Banbury Report 17), Cold Spring Harbor, NY, CSH Press, pp. 69–77

Nagao, M., Fujita, Y. & Sugimura, T. (1986a) Methylglyoxal in beverages and foods: its mutagenicity and carcinogenicity. In: Singer, B. & Bartsch, H., eds, *The Role of Cyclic Nucleic Acid Adducts in Carcinogenesis and Mutagenesis* (IARC Scientific Publications No. 70), Lyon, IARC, pp. 283–291

Nagao, M., Fujita, Y., Wakabayashi, K., Nukaya, H., Kosuge, T. & Sugimura, T. (1986b) Mutagens in coffee and other beverages. *Environ. Health Perspect.*, *67*, 89–91

Naismith, D.J., Akinyanju, P.A. & Yudkin, J. (1969) Influence of caffeine-containing beverages on the growth, food utilization and plasma lipids of the rat. *J. Nutr.*, *97*, 375–381

Najem, G.R., Louria, D.B., Seebode, J.J., Thind, I.S., Prusakowski, J.M., Ambrose, R.B. & Fernicola, A.R. (1982) Life time occupation, smoking, caffeine, saccharine, hair dyes and bladder carcinogenesis. *Int. J. Epidemiol.*, *11*, 212–217

Nakasato, F., Nakayasu, M., Fujita, Y., Nagao, M., Terada, M. & Sugimura, T. (1984) Mutagenicity of instant coffee on cultured Chinese hamster lung cells. *Mutat. Res.*, *141*, 109–112

Nestlé (1989) *Coffee Consumption*, Vevey

Nichols, A.B., Ravenscroft, C., Lamphiear, D.E. & Ostrander, L.D., Jr (1976) Independence of serum lipid levels and dietary habits: the Tecumseh study. *J. Am. med. Assoc.*, *236*, 1948–1953

Nishikawa, A., Tanaka, T. & Mori, H. (1986) An inhibitory effect of coffee on nitrosamine-hepatocarcinogenesis with aminopyrine and sodium nitrite in rats. *J. Nutr. Growth Cancer*, *3*, 161–166

Nolen, G.A. (1981) The effect of brewed and instant coffee on reproduction and teratogenesis in the rat. *Toxicol. appl. Pharmacol.*, *58*, 171–183

Nolen, G.A. (1982) A reproduction/teratology study of brewed and instant decaffeinated coffees. *J. Toxicol. environ. Health*, *10*, 769–783

Nomura, A., Stemmermann, G.N. & Heilbrun, L.K. (1981) Coffee and pancreatic cancer (Letter to the Editor). *Lancet*, *ii*, 415

Nomura, A., Heilbrun, L.K. & Stemmermann, G.N. (1984) Coffee and pancreatic cancer (Letter to the Editor). *Lancet*, *i*, 917

Nomura, A., Heilbrun, L.K. & Stemmermann, G.N. (1986) Prospective study of coffee consumption and the risk of cancer. *J. natl Cancer Inst.*, *76*, 587–590

Norell, S.E., Ahlbom, A., Erwald, R., Jacobson, G., Lindberg-Navier, I., Olin, R., Törnberg, B. & Wiechel, K.-L. (1986) Diet and pancreatic cancer: a case–control study. *Am. J. Epidemiol.*, *124*, 894–902

Obana, H., Nakamura, S.-I. & Tanaka, R.-I. (1986) Suppressive effects of coffee on the SOS responses induced by UV and chemical mutagens. *Mutat. Res.*, *175*, 47–50

Ohno, Y., Aoki, K., Obata, K. & Morrison, A.S. (1985) Case–control study of urinary bladder cancer in metropolitan Nagoya. *Natl Cancer Inst. Monogr.*, *69*, 229–234

Olsen, G.W., Mandel, J.S., Gibson, R.W., Wattenberg, L.W. & Schuman, L.M. (1989) A case–control study of pancreatic cancer and cigarettes, alcohol, coffee and diet. *Am. J. publ. Health*, *79*, 1016–1019

Paffenbarger, R.S., Jr., Wing, A.L. & Hyde, R.T. (1978) Characteristics in youth predictive of adult-onset malignant lymphomas, melanomas and leukemias: brief communication. *J. natl Cancer Inst.*, *60*, 89–92

Pagliaro, F.A., Franklin, J.G. & Gasser, R.J. (1984) *Decaffeination Process*, US Patent 4,465,669 (Société d'Assistance Technique pour Produits Nestlé)

Palm, P.E., Arnold, E.P., Rachwall, P.C., Leyczek, J.C., Teague, K.W. & Kensler, C.J. (1978) Evaluation of the teratogenic potential of fresh-brewed coffee and caffeine in the rat. *Toxicol. appl. Pharmacol.*, *44*, 1-16

Palm, P.E., Arnold, E.P., Nick, M.S., Valentine, J.R. & Doerfler, T.E. (1984) Two-year toxicity/carcinogenicity study of fresh-brewed coffee in rats initially exposed *in utero*. *Toxicol. appl. Pharmacol.*, *74*, 364-382

Pannelli, F., La Rosa, F., Saltalamacchia, G., Vitali, R., Petrinelli, A.M. & Mastrandrea, V. (1989) Tobacco smoking, coffee, cocoa and tea consumption in relation to mortality from urinary bladder cancer in Italy. *Eur. J. Epidemiol.*, *5*, 392-397

Paoletti, R., Corsini, A., Tremoli, E., Fumagalli, R. & Catapano, A.L. (1989) Effects of coffee on plasma lipids, lipoproteins and apolipoproteins. *Pharmacol. Res.*, *21*, 27-38

Patel, J.M. & Wolfson, A.B. (1972) *Semi-continuous Countercurrent Decaffeination Process*, US Patent 3,671,263 (Procter & Gamble Co.)

Petracco, M. (1990) Physico-chemical and structural characterisation of 'espresso' coffee brew. In: *13e Colloque Scientifique International sur le Café, Paipa, Colombia, 1990*, Paris, Association Scientifique Internationale du Café (in press)

Phelps, H.M. & Phelps, C.E. (1988) Caffeine ingestion and breast cancer. A negative correlation. *Cancer*, *61*, 1051-1054

Phillips, R.L. & Snowdon, D.A. (1983) Association of meat and coffee use with cancers of the large bowel, breast and prostate among Seventh-day Adventists: preliminary results. *Cancer Res.*, *43* (Suppl.), 2403s-2408s

Phillips, R.L. & Snowdon, D.A. (1985) Dietary relationships with fatal colorectal cancer among Seventh-day Adventists. *J. natl Cancer Inst.*, *74*, 307-317

Phillips, N.R., Havel, R.J. & Kane, J.P. (1981) Levels and interrelationships of serum and lipoprotein cholesterol and triglycerides. Association with adiposity and the consumption of ethanol, tobacco, and beverages containing caffeine. *Arteriosclerosis*, *1*, 13-24

Pictet, G. (1987) Home and catering brewing of coffee. In: Clarke, R.J. & Macrae, R., eds, *Coffee*, Vol. 2, *Technology*, London, Elsevier Applied Science, pp. 221-256

Pieters, J.J.L. (1985) Nutritional teratogens: a survey of the epidemiological literature. *Progr. clin. biol. Res.*, *163B*, 419-429

Pietinen, P., Geboers, J. & Kesteloot, H. (1988) Coffee consumption and serum cholesterol: an epidemiological study in Belgium. *Int. J. Epidemiol.*, *17*, 98-104

Pietinen, P., Aro, A., Tuomilehto, J., Uusitalo, U. & Korhonen, H. (1990) Consumption of boiled coffee is correlated with serum cholesterol in Finland. *Int. J. Epidemiol.*, *19*, 586-590

Piper, J.M., Matanoski, G.M. & Tonascia, J. (1986) Bladder cancer in young women. *Am. J. Epidemiol.*, *123*, 1033-1042

Pozner, J., Papatestas, A.E., Fagerstrom, R., Schwartz, I., Saevitz, J., Feinberg, M. & Aufses, A.H., Jr (1986) Association of tumor differentiation with caffeine and coffee intake in women with breast cancer. *Surgery*, *100*, 482-488

Raymond, L., Infante, F., Tuyns, A.J., Voirol, M. & Lowenfels, A.B. (1987) Diet and cancer of the pancreas (Fr.). *Gastroenterol. clin. biol.*, *11*, 488-492

Rebelakos, A., Trichopoulos, D., Tzonou, A., Zavitsanos, X., Velonakis, E. & Trichopoulou, A. (1985) Tobacco smoking, coffee drinking and occupation as risk factors for bladder cancer in Greece. *J. natl Cancer Inst.*, 75, 455–461

Reidy, J.A., Annest, J.L., Chen, A.T.L. & Welty, T.K. (1988) Increased sister chromatid exchange associated with smoking and coffee consumption. *Environ. mol. Mutagenesis*, 12, 311–318

Risch, H.A., Burch, J.D., Miller, A.B., Hill, G.B., Steele, R. & Howe, G.R. (1988) Dietary factors and the incidence of cancer of the urinary bladder. *Am. J. Epidemiol.*, 127, 1179–1191

Roberts, H.R. & Barone, J.J. (1983) Caffeine. History and use. *Food Technol.*, September, 32–39

Roebuck, B.D., MacMillan, D.L., Baumgartner, K.J. & Ruggiero, M.L. (1985) Evaluation of the carcinogenic potential of coffee for the rat pancreas (Abstract No. 59). *Toxicologist*, 5, 15

Rosenberg, L., Slone, D., Shapiro, S., Kaufman, D.W., Stolley, P.D. & Miettinen, O.S. (1980) Coffee drinking and myocardial infarction in young women. *Am. J. Epidemiol.*, 111, 675–681

Rosenberg, L., Mitchell, A.A., Shapiro, S. & Slone, D. (1982) Selected birth defects in relation to caffeine–containing beverages. *J. Am. med. Assoc.*, 247, 1429–1432

Rosenberg, L., Miller, D.R., Helmrich, S.P., Kaufman, D.W. & Shapiro, S. (1984) Breast cancer and coffee drinking. In: MacMahon, B. & Sugimura, T., eds, *Coffee and Health* (Banbury Report 17), Cold Spring Harbor, NY, CSH Press, pp. 189–195

Rosenberg, L., Miller, D.R., Helmrich, S.P., Kaufman, D.W., Schottenfeld, D., Stolley, P.D. & Shapiro, S. (1985) Breast cancer and the consumption of coffee. *Am. J. Epidemiol.*, 122, 391–399

Rosenberg, L., Werler, M.M., Kaufman, D.W. & Shapiro, S. (1987) Coffee drinking and myocardial infarction in young women: an update. *Am. J. Epidemiol.*, 126, 147–149

Rosenberg, L., Palmer, J.R., Kelly, J.P., Kaufman, D.W. & Shapiro, S. (1988) Coffee drinking and nonfatal myocardial infarction in men under 55 years of age. *Am. J. Epidemiol.*, 128, 570–578

Rosenberg, L., Werler, M.M., Palmer, J.R., Kaufman, D.W., Warshauer, M.E., Stolley, P.D. & Shapiro, S. (1989) The risks of cancers of the colon and rectum in relation to coffee consumption. *Am. J. Epidemiol.*, 130, 895–903

Ross, R.K., Paganini-Hill, A., Landolph, J., Gerkins, V. & Henderson, B.E. (1989) Analgesics, cigarette smoking, and other risk factors for cancer of the renal pelvis and ureter. *Cancer Res.*, 49, 1045–1048

Rothfos, B. (1986) *Coffee Consumption*, Hamburg, Gordian-Max Rieck

Ruschenburg, U. (1985) Benzo[a]pyrene content of coffee and some other foodstuffs (Ger.). In: *11e Colloque Scientifique International sur le Café, Lomé, 1985*, Paris, Association Scientifique Internationale du Café, pp. 205–212

Schairer, C., Brinton, L.A. & Hoover, R.N. (1987) Methylxanthines and breast cancer. *Int. J. Cancer*, 40, 469–473

Schmauz, R. & Cole, P. (1974) Epidemiology of cancer of the renal pelvis and ureter. *J. natl Cancer Inst.*, 52, 1431–1434

Schneider, K.T.M. (1987) Caffeine and pregnancy (Ger). *Gynäkologe*, 20, 123–128

Schormüller, J., Brandenburg, W. & Langner, H. (1961) Organic acids in coffee replacement compounds as well as in dry extract powder of coffee and replacement compounds and of coffee (Ger.). *Z. Lebensmittel. Untersuch. Forsch.*, 119, 226–235

Scott, N.R., Chakraborty, J. & Marks, V. (1989) Caffeine consumption in the United Kingdom: a retrospective survey. *Food Sci. Nutr.*, 42F, 183–191

Sen, N.P. & Seaman, S.W. (1981) Volatile N-nitrosamines in dried foods. *J. Assoc. off. anal. Chem.*, 64, 1238–1242

Sen, N.P., Seaman, S.W. & Weber, D. (1990) Mass spectrometric confirmation of the presence of N-nitrosopyrrolidine in instant coffee. *J. Assoc. off. anal. Chem.* (in press)

Severson, R.K., Davis, S. & Polissar, L. (1982) Smoking, coffee and cancer of the pancreas (Letter to the Editor). *Br. med. J.*, 285, 214

Shane, B.S., Troxclair, A.M., McMillin, D.J. & Henry, C.B. (1988) Comparative mutagenicity of nine brands of coffee to *Salmonella typhimurium* TA100, TA102 and TA104. *Environ. mol. Mutagenesis*, 11, 195–206

Shennan, D.H. (1973) Renal carcinoma and coffee consumption in 16 countries. *Br. J. Cancer*, 28, 473–474

Shimizu, M. & Yano, E. (1987) Mutagenicity of instant coffee and its interaction with dimethylnitrosamine in the micronucleus test. *Mutat. Res.*, 189, 307–311

Shirlow, M.J. & Mathers, C.D. (1984) Caffeine consumption and serum cholesterol levels. *Int. J. Epidemiol.*, 13, 422–427

Silwar, R. (1982) *Gaschromatographisch–massenspeckrometrische untersuchungen schwefelhaltiger Verbindungen in Röstkaffee und Cystein/Methionin – Modellsystemen* [Gas Chromatographic–Mass Spectrometric Investigation of Sulfur Containing Compounds in Roasted Coffee and Cysteine/methionine – Model Systems], Thesis, University of Berlin

Silwar, R., Kamperschröer, H. & Tressl, R. (1986a) Gas chromatographic–mass spectrometric analyses of roasted coffee aroma. Quantitative determination of steam-volatile aroma constituents (Ger.). *Mikrobiol. Technol. Lebensmittel*, 10, 176–187

Silwar, R., Bendig, J., Walter, G. & Dommers, D. (1986b) Capillary gas chromatographic study of volatile sulfur compounds of coffee aroma by FID/FPD-detection (Ger). *Lebensmittel. Gerichtl. Chem.*, 40, 84–88

Simon, D., Yen, S. & Cole, P. (1975) Coffee drinking and cancer of the lower urinary tract. *J. natl Cancer Inst.*, 54, 587–591

Simpson, P.R. (1988) Caffeine sources in the diet and caffeine intakes. *Food Technol. Austr.*, January, *Suppl.*, ii–iv

Singer, G.M. & Lijinsky, W. (1976) Naturally occurring nitrosatable compounds. I. Secondary amines in foodstuffs. *J. agric. Food Chem.*, 24, 550–553

Slattery, M.L., West, D.W. & Robison, L.M. (1988) Fluid intake and bladder cancer in Utah. *Int. J. Cancer*, 42, 17–22

Smith, D.F., MacGregor, J.T., Hiatt, R.A., Hooper, N.K., Wehr, C.M., Peters, B., Goldman, L.R., Yuan, L.A., Smith, P.A. & Becker, C.E. (1990) Micronucleated erythrocytes as an index of cytogenetic damage in humans: demographic and dietary factors associated with micronucleated erythrocytes in splenectomized subjects. *Cancer Res.*, *50*, 5049-5054

Snoeck, J. (1988) Cultivation and harvesting of the robusta coffee tree. In: Clarke, R.J. & Macrae, R., eds, *Coffee*, Vol. 4, *Agronomy*, London, Elsevier Applied Science, pp. 91-128

Snowdon, D.A. & Phillips, R.L. (1984) Coffee consumption and risk of fatal cancers. *Am. J. publ. Health*, *74*, 820-823

Spiller, M.A. (1984a) The chemical components of coffee. In: Spiller, G.A., ed., *The Methylxanthine Beverages and Foods: Chemistry, Consumption, and Health Effects*, New York, Alan R. Liss, pp. 91-147

Spiller, M.A. (1984b) Coffee plant and processing. In: Spiller, G.A., ed., *The Methylxanthine Beverages and Foods: Chemistry, Consumption and Health Effects*, New York, Alan R. Liss, pp. 75-89

Spiller, G.A., ed. (1984c) *The Methylxanthine Beverages and Foods: Chemistry, Consumption and Health Effects*, New York, Alan R. Liss

Srisuphan, W. & Bracken, M.B. (1986) Caffeine consumption during pregnancy and association with late spontaneous abortion. *Am. J. Obstet. Gynecol.*, *154*, 14-20

Stalder, R., Luginbühl, H., Bexter, A. & Würzner, H.-P. (1984) Preliminary findings of a carcinogen bioassay of coffee in mice. In: MacMahon, B. & Sugimura, T., eds, *Coffee and Health* (Banbury Report 17), Cold Spring Harbor, New York, CSH Press, pp. 79-88

Stavric, B., Klassen, R., Watkinson, B., Karpinski, K., Stapley, R. & Fried, P. (1988) Variability in caffeine consumption from coffee and tea: possible significance for epidemiological studies. *Food chem. Toxicol.*, *26*, 111-118

van der Stegen, G.H.D. (1979) The effect of dewaxing of green coffee on the coffee brew. In: Birch, G.G. & Green, L.F., eds, *Food Chemistry*, Vol. 4, London, Applied Science, pp. 23-29

van der Stegen, G.H.D. & van Duijn, J. (1987) Analysis of normal organic acids in coffee. In: *12e Colloque Scientifique International sur le Café, Montreux, 1987*, Paris, Association Scientifique Internationale du Café, pp. 238-246

Stensvold, I., Tverdal, A. & Foss, O.P. (1989) The effect of coffee on blood lipids and blood pressure. Results from a Norwegian cross-sectional study, men and women, 40-42 years. *J. clin. Epidemiol.*, *42*, 877-884

Stich, H.F., Rosin, M.P. & Bryson, L. (1982) Inhibition of mutagenicity of a model nitrosation reaction by naturally occurring phenolics, coffee and tea. *Mutat. Res.*, *95*, 119-128

Stocks, P. (1957) Statistical survey of cancer in North Wales and Liverpool region. *Br. Empire Cancer Cgn., 35th Ann. Rep.*, Part II, 496-501

Stocks, P. (1970) Cancer mortality in relation to national consumption of cigarettes, solid fuel, tea and coffee. *Br. J. Cancer*, *24*, 215-225

Stone, M.C. (1987) Coffee and coronary heart disease. *J. R. Coll. gen. Pract.*, *37*, 146-147 van Straten, S., Maarse, H., de Beauvaser, J.C. & Visscher, C.A., eds (1983) *Volatile Compounds in Food*, Vol. 2, *Quantitative Data* (Sections 72.1–72.11), Zeist, Central Institute for Nutrition and Food Research, TNO

Strobel, R.G.K. (1988a) Polycyclic aromatic hydrocarbon contaminants in coffee. In: Clarke, R.J. & Macrae, R., eds, *Coffee*, Vol. 3, *Physiology*, London, Elsevier Applied Science, pp. 321–364

Strobel, R.G.K. (1988b) Allergens and mould toxin contaminants. In: Clarke, R.J. & Macrae, R., eds, *Coffee*, Vol. 3, *Physiology*, London, Elsevier Applied Science, pp. 215–320

Strubelt, O., Siegers, C.-P., Breining, H. & Steffen, J. (1973) Experimental studies on chronic toxicity of coffee and caffeine (Ger.). *Z. Ernährungsw.*, *12*, 252–260

Sugimura, T. (1982) Mutagens in cooked food. In: Fleck, R.A. & Hollaender, A., eds, *Genetic Toxicology*, New York, Plenum Press, pp. 243–269

Sugimura, T. & Sato, S. (1983) Mutagens–carcinogens in foods. *Cancer Res.*, *43* (*Suppl.*), 2415s–2421s

Sugimura, T., Nagao, M., Suwa, Y. & Takayama, S. (1984) Mutagens in coffee – background and present knowledge of mutagens/carcinogens produced by pyrolysis. In: MacMahon, B. & Sugimura, T., eds, *Coffee and Health* (Banbury Report 17), Cold Spring Harbor, NY, CSH Press, pp. 59–67

Sullivan, J.W. (1982) Epidemiologic survey of bladder cancer in greater New Orleans. *J. Urol.*, *128*, 281–283

Suwa, Y., Nagao, M., Kosugi, A. & Sugimura, T. (1982) Sulfite suppresses the mutagenic property of coffee. *Mutat. Res.*, *102*, 383–391

Swain, A.R., Dutton, S.P. & Truswell, A.S. (1985) Salicylates in foods. *J. Am. Diet. Assoc.*, *85*, 950–960

Tajima, K. & Tominaga, S. (1985) Dietary habits and gastro–intestinal cancers: a comparative case–control study of stomach and large intestinal cancers in Nagoya, Japan. *Jpn. J. Cancer Res. (Gann)*, *76*, 705–716

Takahashi, E. (1964) Coffee consumption and mortality for prostate cancer. *Tohoku J. exp. Med.*, *82*, 218–223

Takahashi, S., Kato, T. & Kikugawa, K. (1989) Formation and content of 2-amino-3,4-dimethylimidazo[4,5-f]quinoline in roasted coffee beans (Abstract No. 57). *Mutat. Res.*, *216*, 380

Thelle, D.S., Arnesen, E. & Førde, O.H. (1983) The Tromsø heart study. Does coffee raise serum cholesterol? *New Engl. J. Med.*, *308*, 1454–1457

Thelle, D.S., Heyden, S. & Fodor, J.G. (1987) Coffee and cholesterol in epidemiological and experimental studies. *Atherosclerosis*, *67*, 97–103

Tikkanen, J. & Heinonen, O.P. (1988) Cardiovascular malformations and organic solvent exposure during pregnancy in Finland. *Am. J. ind. Med.*, *14*, 1–8

Tohnai, I., Oka, T. & Ohno, Y. (1984) A case-control study on cleft lip and/or palate: maternal dietary practices in early pregnancy (Abstract). *Teratology*, *30*, 23A

Tressl, R. (1977) Di- and triphenols in arabica, robusta and arabusta coffees (Ger.). In: *8e Colloque Scientifique International sur le Café, Abidjan, 1977*, Paris, Association Scientifique Internationale du Café, pp. 117-120

Tressl, R. (1980) Formation of aromatic compounds through the Maillard reaction (Ger.). In: *9e Colloque Scientifique International sur le Café, London, 1980*, Paris, Association Scientifique Internationale du Café, pp. 55-76

Tressl, R. & Silwar, R (1981) Investigation of sulfur-containing components in roasted coffee. *J. agric. Food Chem.*, 29, 1078-1082

Tressl, R., Bahri, D., Köppler, H. & Jensen, A. (1978a) Diphenols and caramel compounds in roasted coffees of different varieties. II. (Ger). *Z. Lebensmittel Untersuch. Forsch.*, 167, 111-114

Tressl, R., Grünewald, K.G., Köppler, H. & Silwar, R. (1978b) Volatile phenols in roasted coffee of different varieties. I. (Ger). *Z. Lebensmittel Untersuch. Forsch.*, 167, 108-110

Tressl, R., Grünewald, K.G. & Silwar, R. (1981) Gas chromatographic-mass spectrometric investigation of N-alkyl- and N-furfurylpyrroles in roasted coffee (Ger.). *Chem. Mikrobiol. Technol. Lebensmittel*, 7, 28-32

Trichopoulos, D., Papapostolou, M. & Polychronopoulou, A. (1981) Coffee and ovarian cancer. *Int. J. Cancer*, 28, 691-693

Trichopoulos, D., Tzonou, A., Polychronopoulou, A. & Day, N.E. (1984) A case-control investigation of a possible association between coffee consumption and ovarian cancer in Greece. In: MacMahon, B. & Sugimura, T., eds, *Coffee and Health* (Banbury Report 17), Cold Spring Harbor, NY, CSH Press, pp. 149-155

Trichopoulos, D., Ouranos, G., Day, N.E., Tzonou, A., Manousos, O., Papadimitriou, C. & Trichopoulou, A. (1985) Diet and cancer of the stomach: a case-control study in Greece. *Int. J. Cancer*, 36, 291-297

Trugo, L.C. (1984) *HPLC in Coffee Analysis*, PhD Thesis, University of Reading

Trugo, L.C. (1985) Carbohydrates. In: Clarke, R.J. & Macrae, R., eds, *Coffee*, Vol. 1, *Chemistry*, London, Elsevier Applied Science, pp. 83-114

Trugo, L.C. & Macrae, R. (1984a) A study of the effect of roasting on the chlorogenic acid composition of coffee using HPLC. *Food Chem.*, 15, 219-227

Trugo, L.C. & Macrae, R. (1984b) Chlorogenic acid composition of instant coffees. *Analyst*, 109, 263-266

Trugo, L.C., Macrae, R. & Dick, J. (1983) Determination of purine alkaloids and trigonelline in instant coffee and other beverages using high performance liquid chromatography. *J. Sci. Food Agric.*, 34, 300-306

Tucker, J.D., Taylor, R.T., Christensen, M.L., Strout, C.L. & Hanna, M.L. (1989) Cytogenetic response to coffee in Chinese hamster ovary AUXB1 cells and human peripheral lymphocytes. *Mutagenesis*, 4, 343-348

Tuomilehto, J., Tanskanen, A., Pietinen, P., Aro, A., Salonen, J.T., Happonen, P., Nissinen, A. & Puska, P. (1987) Coffee consumption is correlated with serum cholesterol in middle-aged Finnish men and women. *J. Epidemiol. Community Health*, 41, 237-242

Tuyns, A.J. (1986) A case-control study on colorectal cancer in Belgium. Preliminary results. *Soz. Präventivmed.*, 31, 81-82

Tuyns, A.J., Kaaks, R. & Haelterman, M. (1988) Colorectal cancer and the consumption of foods: a case–control study in Belgium. *Nutr. Cancer*, *11*, 189–204

Tzonou, A., Day, N.E., Trichopoulos, D., Walker, A., Saliaraki, M., Papapostolou, M. & Polychronopoulou, A. (1984) The epidemiology of ovarian cancer in Greece: a case–control study. *Eur. J. Cancer clin. Oncol.*, *20*, 1045–1052

Vandenbroucke, J.P., Kok, F.J., Van't Bosch, G., van den Dungen, P.J.C., van der Heide-Wessel, C. & van der Heide, R.M. (1986) Coffee drinking and mortality in a 25-year follow-up. *Am. J. Epidemiol.*, *123*, 359–361

Viani, R. (1986) Coffee. In: *Ullmann's Encyclopedia of Industrial Chemistry*, Vol. A7, Weinheim, VCH Verlagsgesellschaft, pp. 315–339

Viani, R. (1988) Physiologically active substances in coffee. In: Clarke, R.J. & Macrae, R., eds, *Coffee*, Vol. 3, *Physiology*, London, Elsevier Applied Science, pp. 1–31

Viani, R. (1989) *Coffee*, Vevey, Nestec

Victora, C.G., Muñoz, N., Day, N.E., Barcelos, L.B., Peccin, D.A. & Braga, N.M. (1987) Hot beverages and oesophageal cancer in southern Brazil: a case–control study. *Int. J. Cancer*, *39*, 710–716

Vitzthum, O.G. (1976) Chemistry and processing of coffee. In: Eichler, O., ed., *Coffee and Caffeine* (Ger.), Berlin, Springer, pp. 3–64

Watanabe, Y., Tada, M., Kawamoto, K., Uozumi, G., Kajiwara, Y., Hayashi, K., Yamaguchi, K., Murakami, K., Misaki, F., Akasaka, Y. & Kawai, K. (1984) A case–control study of cancer of the rectum and the colon (Jpn.). *Nippon Shokakibyo Gakkai Zasshi*, *81*, 185–193

Watkinson, B. & Fried, P.A. (1985) Maternal caffeine use before, during and after pregnancy and effects upon offspring. *Neurobehav. Toxicol. Teratol.*, *7*, 9–17

Wattenberg, L.W. & Lam, L.K.T. (1984) Protective effects of coffee constituents on carcinogenesis in experimental animals. In: MacMahon, B. & Sugimura, T., eds, *Coffee and Health* (Banbury Report 17), Cold Spring Harbor, New York, CSH Press, pp. 137–145

Wellman, F.L. (1961) *Coffee. Botany, Cultivation and Utilization*, London, Leonard Hill

Welsch, C.W. & DeHoog, J.V. (1988) Influence of caffeine consumption on 7,12-dimethylbenz[*a*]anthracene-induced mammary gland tumorigenesis in female rats fed a chemically defined diet containing standard and high levels of unsaturated fat. *Cancer Res.*, *48*, 2074–2077

Welsch, C.W., DeHoog, J.V. & O'Connor, D.H. (1988) Influence of caffeine and/or coffee consumption on the initiation and promotion phases of 7,12-dimethylbenz[*a*]-anthracene-induced rat mammary gland tumorigenesis. *Cancer Res.*, *48*, 2068–2073

Whittemore, A.S., Paffenbarger, R.S., Jr, Anderson, K. & Halpern, J. (1983) Early precursors of pancreatic cancer in college men. *J. chron. Dis.*, *36*, 251–256

Whittemore, A.S., Wu, M.L., Paffenbarger, R.S., Jr, Sarles, D.L., Kampert, J.B., Grosser, S., Jung, D.L., Ballon, S. & Hendrickson, M. (1988) Personal and environmental characteristics related to epithelial ovarian cancer. *Am. J. Epidemiol.*, *128*, 1228–1240

Wilcox, A., Weinberg, C. & Baird, D. (1988) Caffeinated beverages and decreased fertility. *Lancet*, *ii*, 1453–1456

Wilhelmsen, L., Tibblin, G., Elmfeldt, D., Wedel, H. & Werkö, L. (1977) Coffee consumption and coronary heart disease in middle-aged Swedish men. *Acta med. scand.*, *201*, 547–552

Woodman, J.S. (1985) Carboxylic acids. In: Clarke, R.J. & Macrae, R., eds, *Coffee*, Vol. 1, *Chemistry*, London, Elsevier Applied Science, pp. 266–289

Woutersen, R.A., van Garderen-Hoetmer, A., Bax, J. & Scherer, E. (1989) Modulation of dietary fat-promoted pancreatic carcinogenesis in rats and hamsters by chronic coffee ingestion. *Carcinogenesis*, *10*, 311–316

Wrigley, G. (1988) *Coffee*, Harlow, Longman Scientific & Technical

Wu, A.H., Paganini-Hill, A., Ross, R.K. & Henderson, B.E. (1987) Alcohol, physical activity and other risk factors for colorectal cancer: a prospective study. *Br. J. Cancer*, *55*, 687–694

Würzner, H.-P., Lindström, E., Vuataz, L. & Luginbühl, H. (1977a) A 2-year feeding study of instant coffee in rats. I. Body weight, food consumption, haematological parameters and plasma chemistry. *Food Cosmet. Toxicol.*, *15*, 7–16

Würzner, H.-P., Lindström, E., Vuataz, L. & Luginbühl, H. (1977b) A 2-year feeding study of instant coffees in rats. II. Incidence and types of neoplasms. *Food Cosmet. Toxicol.*, *15*, 289–296

Wynder, E.L. & Goldsmith, R. (1977) The epidemiology of bladder cancer. A second look. *Cancer*, *40*, 1246–1268

Wynder, E.L., Mabuchi, K. & Whitmore, W.F., Jr (1974) Epidemiology of adenocarcinoma of the kidney. *J. natl Cancer Inst.*, *53*, 1619–1634

Wynder, E.L., Hall, N.E.L. & Polansky, M. (1983) Epidemiology of coffee and pancreatic cancer. *Cancer Res.*, *43*, 3900–3906

Wynder, E.L., Dieck, G.S. & Hall, N.E.L. (1986) Case-control study of decaffeinated coffee consumption and pancreatic cancer. *Cancer Res.*, *46*, 5360–5363

Yen, S., Hsieh, C.-C. & MacMahon, B. (1987) Extrahepatic bile duct cancer and smoking, beverage consumption, past medical history, and oral-contraceptive use. *Cancer*, *59*, 2112–2116

Yu, M.C., Mack, T.M., Hanisch, R., Cicioni, C. & Henderson, B.E. (1986) Cigarette smoking, obesity, diuretic use, and coffee consumption as risk factors for renal cell carcinoma. *J. natl Cancer Inst.*, *77*, 351–356

Zeitlin, B.R. (1972) Coffee and bladder cancer (Letter to the Editor). *Lancet*, *i*, 1066

Zock, P.L., Katan, M.B., Merkus, M.P., van Dusseldorp, M. & Harryvan, J.L. (1990) Effect of lipid-rich fraction from boiled coffee on serum cholesterol. *Lancet*, *335*, 1235–1237

Zosel, K. (1981) *Process for the Decaffeination of Coffee*. US Patent 4,260,639 (Studiengesellschaft Kohle MbH)

Appendix 1
Chemical formulae of selected components of coffee

1. **Nonvolatile compounds**

    (a) *Caffeine and other purines*

    $R_1 = R_2 = R_3 = CH_3$: Caffeine, 1,3,7-trimethylxanthine
    $R_1 = H, R_2 = R_3 = CH_3$: Theobromine, 3,7-dimethylxanthine
    $R_1 = R_2 = CH_3, R_3 = H$: Theophylline, 1,3-dimethylxanthine
    $R_1 = R_3 = CH_3, R_2 = H$: Paraxanthine, 1,7-dimethylxanthine

    $R_1 = R_2 = R_3 = R_4 = CH_3$: Theacrine, 1,3,7,9-tetramethyluric acid

    $R_1 = R_4 = CH_3, R_3 = H$: Liberine, O(2), 1,9-trimethyluric acid

(b) Chlorogenic acid and related substances

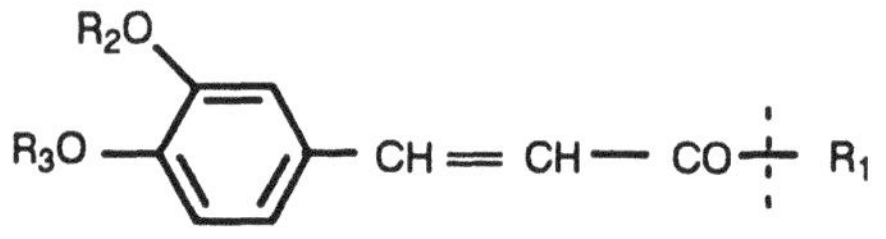

A ($R_2 = R_3 = $ H): Caffeoyl

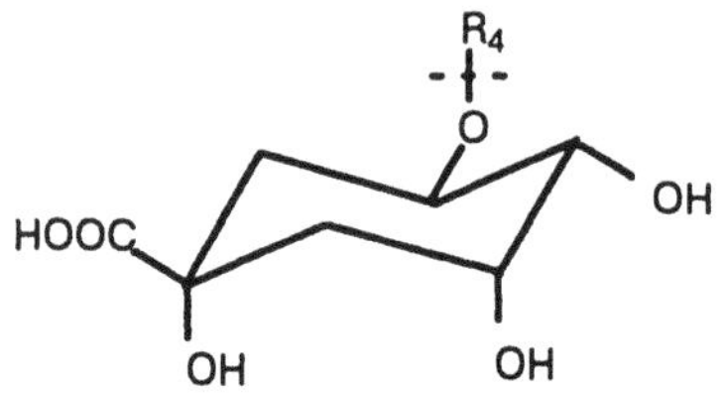

B: Quinyl

$R_1 = $ B, $R_2 = R_3 = $ H, $R_4 = $ A: Chlorogenic acid
$R_1 = $ OH, $R_2 = R_3 = $ H: Caffeic acid
$R_1 = $ OH, $R_2 = $ H, $R_3 = CH_3$: Ferulic acid
$R_1 = $ OH, $R_2 = CH_3$, $R_3 = $ H: Isoferulic acid
$R_4 = $ H: Quinic acid

A chlorogenic acid (taken as 5-caffeoylquinic acid) and component acids

(c) Glycosides

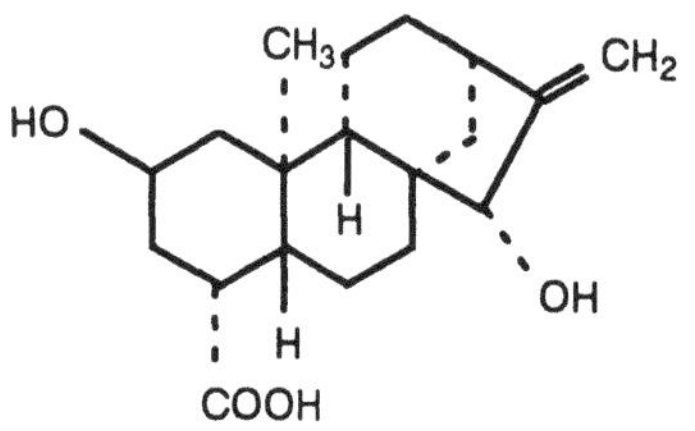

Atractyligenin

(d) Lipids

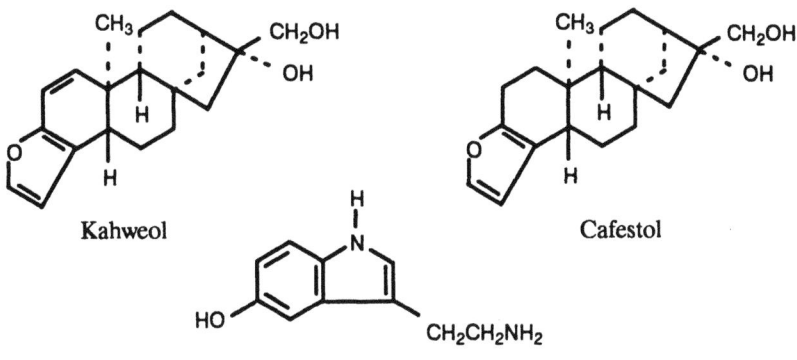

Kahweol

Cafestol

5-Hydroxytryptamine

(e) Trigonelline and nicotinic acid

Trigonelline

Nicotinic acid

(f) Acids

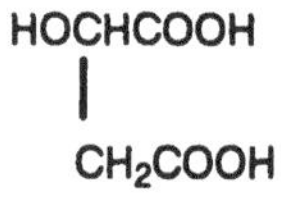

Malic acid
HOCHCOOH
|
CH$_2$COOH

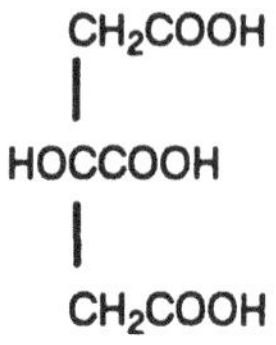

Citric acid
CH$_2$COOH
|
HOCCOOH
|
CH$_2$COOH

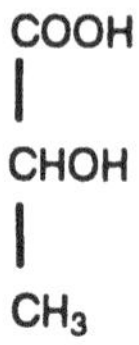

Lactic acid
COOH
|
CHOH
|
CH$_3$

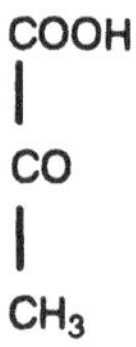

Pyruvic acid
COOH
|
CO
|
CH$_3$

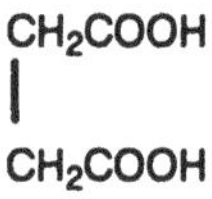

Succinic acid
CH$_2$COOH
|
CH$_2$COOH

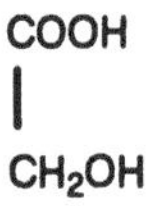

Glycolic acid
COOH
|
CH$_2$OH

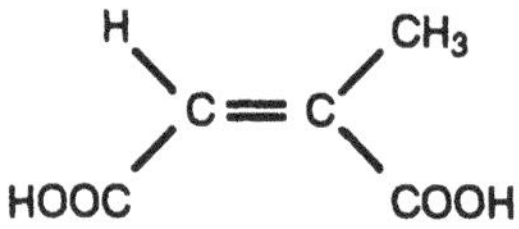

Citraconic acid
(H)(HOOC)C=C(CH$_3$)(COOH)

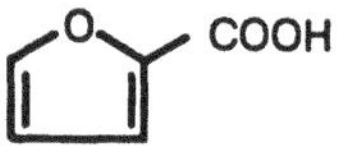

2-Furoic acid
(furan ring)—COOH

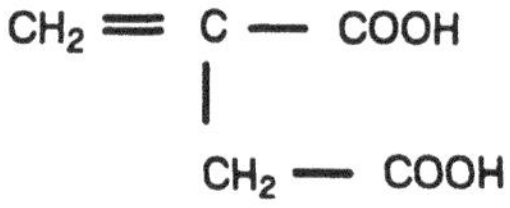

Itaconic acid
CH$_2$=C—COOH
|
CH$_2$—COOH

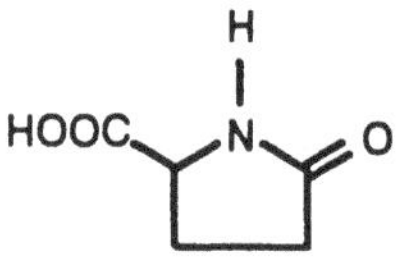

Pyrrolidone carboxylic acid
(pyrrolidone ring with HOOC and N-H, C=O)

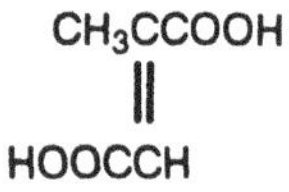

Mesaconic acid
CH$_3$CCOOH
‖
HOOCCH

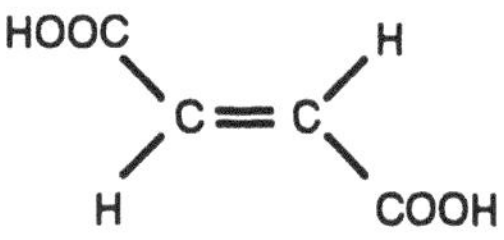

Fumaric acid
(HOOC)(H)C=C(H)(COOH)

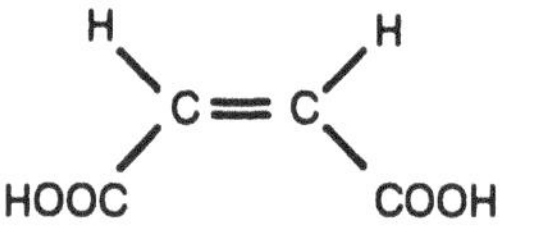

Maleic acid
(H)(HOOC)C=C(H)(COOH)

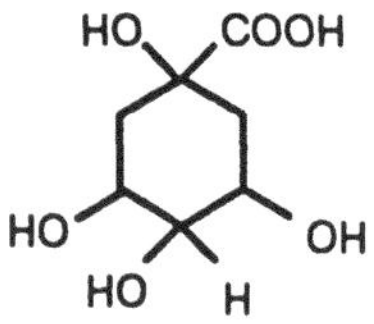

Quinic acid
(cyclohexane ring with HO, COOH, OH, HO, HO, H substituents)

2. Volatile compounds

(a) Carbonyl compounds

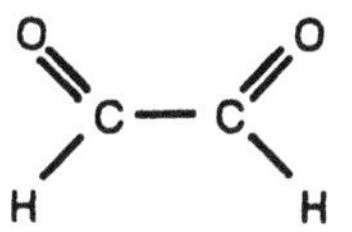

Glyoxal

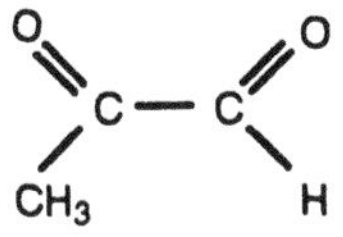

Methylglyoxal

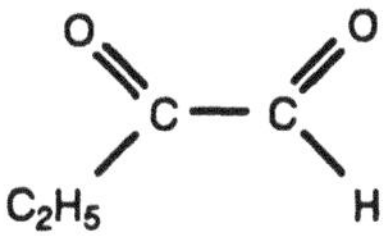

Ethylglyoxal

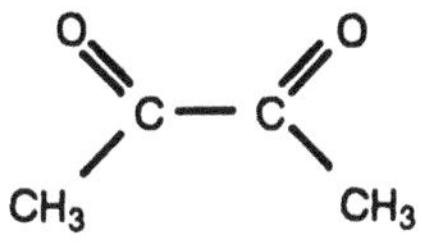

Diacetyl

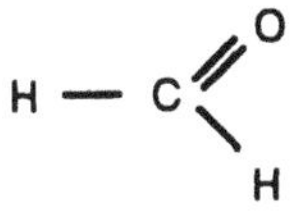

Formaldehyde

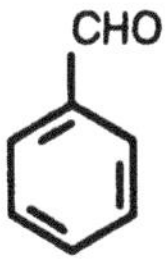

Benzaldehyde

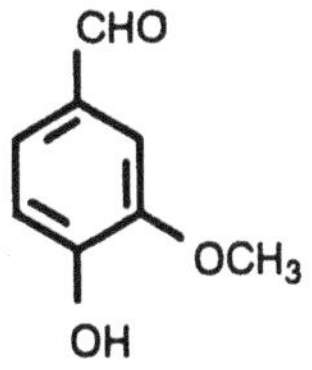

Vanillin

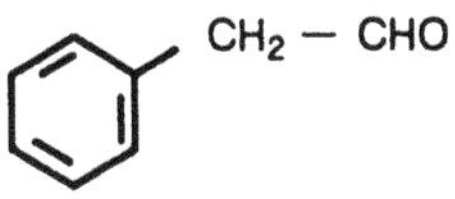

2-Phenylacetaldehyde

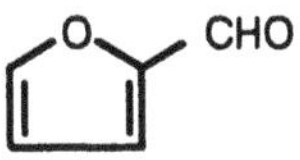

Furfural

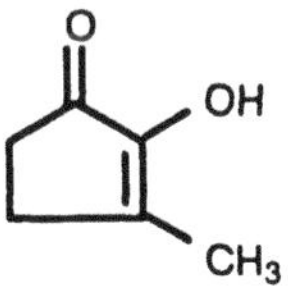

Cyclotene

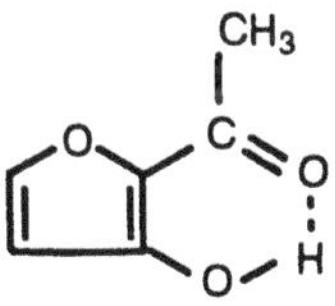

Isomaltol

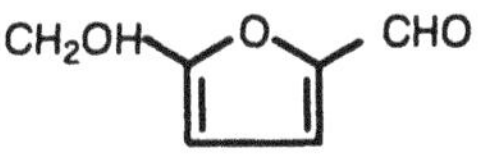

5-(Hydroxymethyl)-2-furfural

(b) *Alcohols*

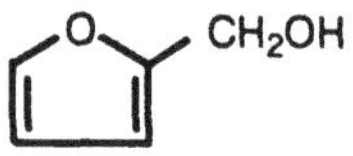

Furfuryl alcohol

(c) *Acids*

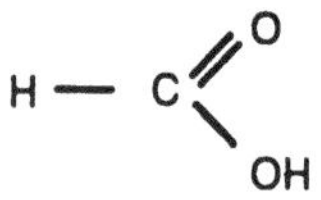

Formic acid

(d) *Esters, ethers and lactones*

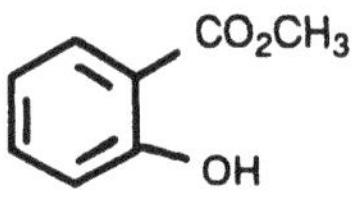

Methyl salicylate

(e) *Nitrogen compounds*

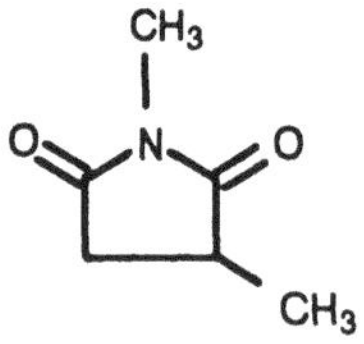

N-α-Dimethylsuccinimide

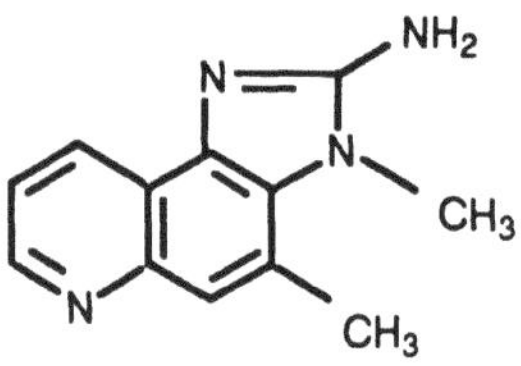

MeIQ

(f) Furan-based compounds

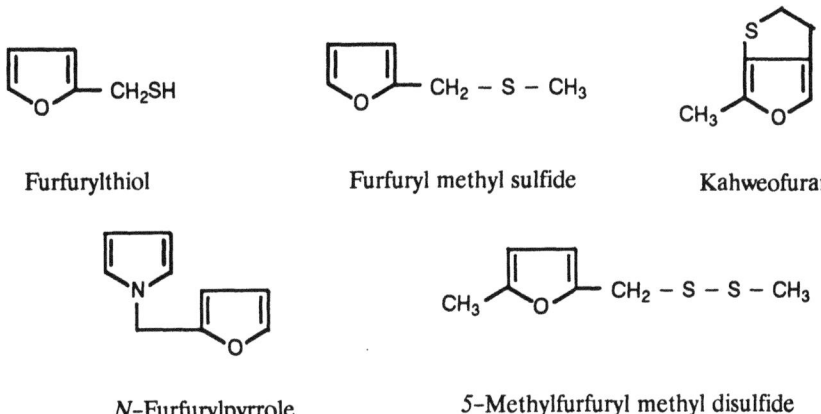

Furfurylthiol

Furfuryl methyl sulfide

Kahweofuran

N-Furfurylpyrrole

5-Methylfurfuryl methyl disulfide

(g) Phenols

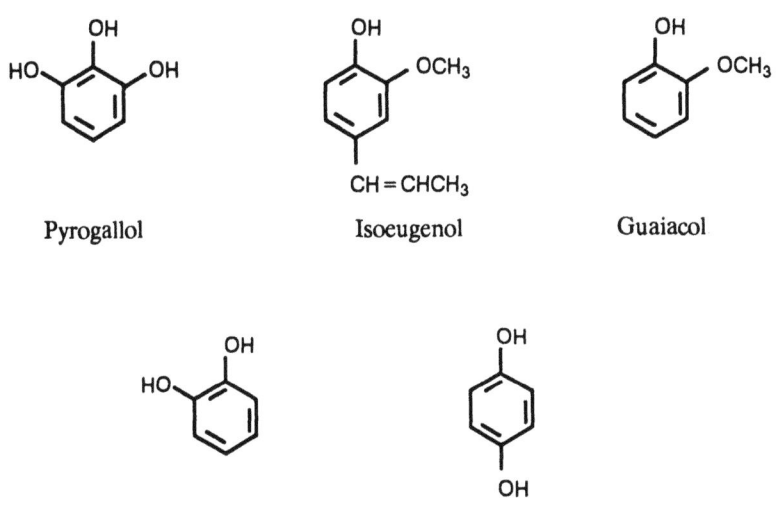

Pyrogallol

Isoeugenol

Guaiacol

Pyrocatechol

Hydroquinone

(h) Pyrones

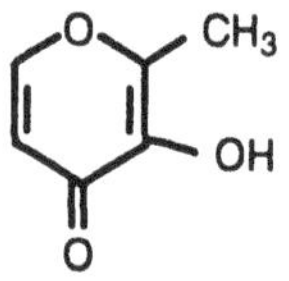

Maltol

(i) Contaminants

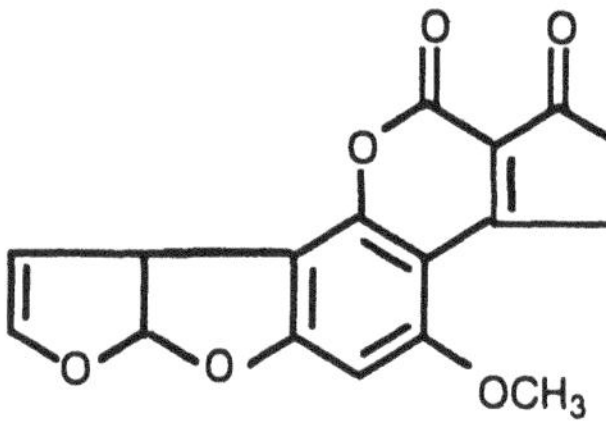

Aflatoxin B$_1$

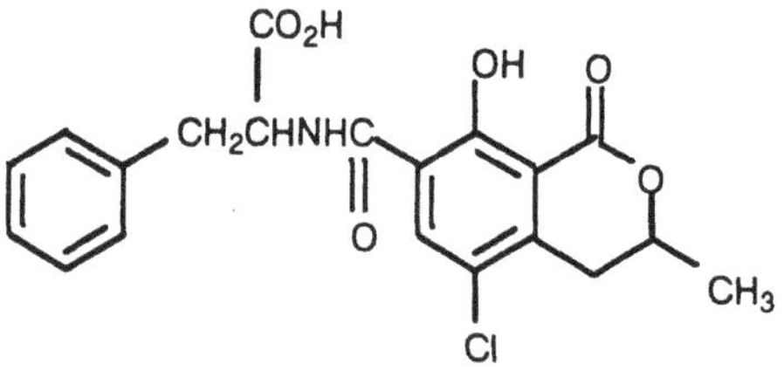

Ochratoxin A

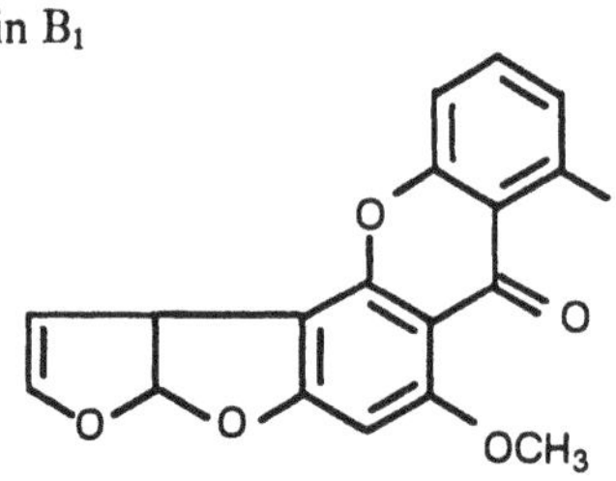

Sterigmatocystin

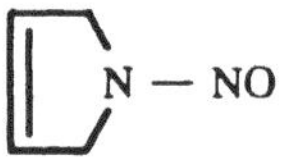

N-Nitrosopyrrolidine

TEA

1. Production and Use

1.1 Introduction

The origin of tea is lost in ancient history, although legend dates it at about 2700 BC (Woodward, 1980). The first generally accepted reference to tea is found in a Chinese dictionary from 350 AD which stated that the beverage was used as a medicine for various ills (Schapira *et al.*, 1975). Tea achieved popularity in the west only during the late seventeenth and eighteenth centuries, although it was brought to Europe in 1559 (Wickremasinghe, 1978). The first public sale of tea in England was held in 1657. The beverage's popularity grew, and its trade became an economic mainstay. Today, tea is arguably the most popular beverage in the world (Graham, 1984).

Black and green tea are the two main types, defined by their respective manufacturing techniques. Green tea is consumed mostly in Japan, China, North Africa and the Middle East; the remainder of the world uses black tea. Oolong tea, found in some regions of China, is an intermediate variant between black and green tea (Graham, 1983). Black and green teas lightly flavoured with other botanicals are sometimes seen; these include jasmine tea, scented with jasmine blossoms, and Earl Grey tea, flavoured with bergamot, a type of citrus fruit (Graham, 1984).

1.2 Production processes

A general description of tea manufacture and terms used is provided by Eden (1976) and, more briefly, by Graham (1984) and by Millin (1987).

(a) Botany and culture

Tea was first cultivated in China and then in Japan. With the opening of ocean routes to the east by European traders during the fifteenth, sixteenth and seventeenth centuries, commercial cultivation gradually expanded to Indonesia and then to the Indian subcontinent, including Sri Lanka. Tea is now grown commercially in tropical and subtropical regions of Asia, Africa and South America. Major exporting countries include Argentina, China, India, Kenya and Sri Lanka (Forrest, 1985).

All varieties and cultivars of tea belong to a single species, *Camellia sinensis* (L.) O. Kuntze (Cloughley, 1983), formerly called *Thea sinensis* (Graham, 1984). The plant is a tender evergreen that can grow to heights of 12-14 m (Forrest, 1985). The bushes are usually kept about 1 m tall by pruning and periodic harvesting of new growth, called flush. Flush is used for the manufacture of finished tea (Graham, 1984).

Throughout many of the world's tea growing regions, harvesting is done by hand as it has been for centuries. Mechanical harvesting is practised to some extent; however, uniformity and, therefore, quality are considered to be superior with the precise selection of leaf that is achievable only by hand selection (Graham, 1984; Forrest, 1985).

(b) Manufacture

Following harvest, fresh tea flush is subjected to a series of treatment steps that result in the manufacture of either black, Oolong or green tea. Black tea results from promoting enzymic oxidation of fresh leaves; the process was originally called 'fermentation' but does not involve microbial action; for the production of green tea 'fermentation' is prevented. The third type, Oolong, is produced by short fermentation (Graham, 1984).

(i) *Black tea*

Withering: After transport to the tea factory, freshly harvested leaves are spread in layers on trays and belts for up to 18 h in order to reduce the initial moisture content to approximately 60% of the leaf weight (Graham, 1983). Warm or ambient air may be circulated through the beds of tea leaves depending on local climatic conditions. A uniform moisture distribution is dependent on the uniformity of the flush and is important in maintaining the quality of the finished tea. Chemical changes, including an increase in caffeine content, begin during this step (Cloughley, 1983).

Rolling: The leaves are crushed and macerated, partially destroying cell structure, to allow enzymic oxidation of the flavanols in the presence of oxygen from the atmosphere. Orthodox rolling involves use of traditional devices that impart a characteristic curl to the leaf. Other types of maceration equipment are now becoming popular, for example, crush, tear, curl (CTC) is gradually replacing orthodox processing in some growing regions (Graham, 1983).

'Fermentation': During 'fermentation', tea undergoes significant compositional changes leading to the characteristic colour and flavour of black tea

(Sanderson, 1972). 'Fermentation' actually begins during rolling when endogenous enzymes are freed to comingle with other leaf components, primarily flavanols. This enzymatically catalysed aerobic oxidation and subsequent reactions constitute the 'fermentation' process. After rolling, the tea is spread in layers to optimize temperature, moisture and air circulation. The time for which the macerated leaf is allowed to ferment varies according to temperature and other local conditions but ranges from 45 min to 3 h. During this step, the tea begins to develop its characteristic aroma and copper-coloured appearance. Duration is judged subjectively and the reaction is stopped by the next step in manufacture (Graham, 1983). Some caffeine is lost during 'fermentation' (Cloughley, 1983).

Firing: Passing the tea on trays through hot air driers halts the enzymic fermentation step. Moisture content is reduced to 3% in about 20 min. During firing, nonenzymic chemical changes, resulting in further flavour and aroma development, continue. The tea takes on the black colour characteristic of black tea (Graham, 1983). Small amounts of caffeine are lost through sublimation (Cloughley, 1983).

Grading: The last step is to sort the black tea into appropriate grades. The dried leaves are passed through a series of screens with varying mesh sizes to yield tea corresponding to particular grades such as Orange Pekoe, Pekoe, broken Orange Pekoe, fannings and dust. Traditionally, bulk tea has been shipped in aluminium foil-lined plywood chests (Millin, 1987) holding 45-60 kg, depending on the tea's density (Graham, 1983). More recently, tea 'sacks', which are also foil-lined, have begun to replace the chests.

Specification: The International Organization for Standardization (ISO) (1981) has established a standard for black tea (ISO 3720-1981), which includes the following specifications:

"*Definition*: Tea derived solely and exclusively, and produced by acceptable processes, notably 'fermentation' and drying, from the leaves, buds and tender stems of varieties of the species *Camellia sinensis* (Linnaeus) O. Kuntze known to be suitable for making tea for consumption as a beverage.

"*General requirements*: The tea shall be clean and reasonably free from extraneous matter.

"*Chemical requirements*: (1) The tea shall comply with the requirements specified in Table 1, in which all the figures given are calculated on the basis of the material oven-dried to constant mass at $103 \pm 2°C$.

"Table 1. Chemical requirements for black tea

Characteristic	Requirement	Test method
Water extract, % (w/w) minimum	32	ISO 1574
Total ash, % (w/w)		
maximum	8	ISO 1575
minimum	4	
Water-soluble ash, as percentage of total ash, minimum	45	ISO 1576
Alkalinity of water-soluble ash (as KOH), % (w/w)		
minimum	1.0[a]	ISO 1578
maximum	3.0	
Acid-insoluble ash, % (w/w) maximum	1.0	ISO 1577
Crude fibre, % (w/w) maximum	16.5	Annex

[a] When the alkalinity of water-soluble ash is expressed in terms of milliequivalents per 100 g of ground sample, the limits are: minimum, 17.8; maximum, 53.6.

"(2) No limit is specified for the 'moisture' content of the tea. If desired, the actual loss in mass at 103°C of the sample under test may be determined and the result recorded in the test report. The determination shall be carried out by the method described in ISO 1573."

(ii) *Green tea*

Green tea is made from the same species as black tea, although the varieties used are suited to the specific climatic conditions prevailing in the growing region and local taste preferences. Green tea is not allowed to ferment. Harvesting is similar to that for black tea, but the fresh leaves are quickly subjected to heat in order to inactivate enzymes, thus preventing any oxidative fermentation from occurring. This is accomplished by either steaming the fresh leaves (Japanese type) or roasting in pans with dry heat (Chinese type) (Yamanishi, 1986). Prior to final drying, the leaves are pressed and rolled, which develops their characteristic shape and sizes. After drying, the leaf fragments are sorted into various grades. International standards have not been finalized for green tea (Graham, 1984).

(iii) *Oolong tea*

Oolong teas are only partially oxidized and retain a considerable amount of the original polyphenolic material. Manufacture is usually a cottage industry; the teas are prepared by a series of withering, gentle rolling and drying steps, which vary greatly from facility to facility. Sun drying is often utilized as the first step. The appearance of the leaf is considered an important aspect of quality, and a significant amount of hand labour is often utilized. The colour of Oolong tea is intermediate between that of green and black tea (Graham, 1984).

(iv) *Instant tea*

Instant tea is used almost entirely to prepare iced tea. It is manufactured by a fairly exhaustive extraction of black tea with hot water. After separation of leaf matter from the extract, the latter is usually stripped of volatile substances (aroma) and concentrated. Drying of such a concentrate without further processing would result in a product incompletely soluble in cold water, so the extract is precooled to precipitate cold water-insoluble fractions, known as 'cream'. These may be processed to improve solubility and then added to the main extract. The preserved aroma fraction is added back to the total extract concentrate before spray or freeze drying (Graham, 1984).

In the USA approximately 15% of tea is used in the instant form. Production in 1981 was about 6000 tonnes; Kenya, India and Sri Lanka together manufactured about 1000 tonnes, much of which was exported to the USA (Graham, 1984).

(v) *Decaffeinated tea*

The most prevalent process for decaffeinating tea is extraction using supercritical carbon dioxide as the solvent. Conditions of temperature and pressure are chosen to favour the selective extraction of caffeine. Carbon dioxide is removed by allowing it to vapourize (Graham, 1984).

1.3 Preparation of tea beverage

(a) *Traditional*

Tea beverage is prepared by steeping tea leaves in water at 90-100°C in teapots or cups. Additional hot water may be added to residual leaf in teapots to produce more but often weaker beverage. In Japan, different varieties of green tea are steeped in water at the temperature considered appropriate for the tea used.

(b) *Tea bags*

Tea is confined in porous bags chosen to retain solids but allow free diffusion of water and beverage without imparting taste to the tea. In the USA, tea bags now account for well over 95% of home use. Their use is increasing throughout the world.

(c) *Brick tea*

In China, Outer Mongolia and the USSR, tea is sometimes compressed into bricks, pieces of which are used to prepare the infusion (Graham, 1984).

(d) Iced tea

This beverage may be prepared by cooling traditionally brewed tea, but it is sometimes prepared by the prolonged (8-24 h) steeping of tea at room temperature or in chilled water. Cold water-soluble instant teas, which may be sweetened and flavoured, are also used. Instant tea products are usually used at levels of 0.6-1.0 g of tea solids per 100 ml water. Iced tea beverage is also available in canned form.

(e) Tea-gruel

Tea leaves packed in a cotton pouch are boiled in water in an iron pan for several minutes. Washed or unwashed rice is then added and the mixture is reboiled. The product is usually eaten burning hot (Anon., 1974).

1.4 Production, trade and consumption

(a) Production

World production of manufactured tea in 1988 was nearly 2.5 million tonnes (Table 2). Four of the top five producing areas are in Asia. Green tea comprises about 21% of the total (International Tea Committee, 1989).

Table 2. World tea production in 1983-88 (in thousand tonnes)[a]

Continent or country	1983	1984	1985	1986	1987	1988
Asia (including Oceania)	1630.3	1748.0	1820.3	1817.0	1921.6	2026.5
Africa	224.9	236.1	271.8	260.3	263.9	282.3
USSR	145.6	151.1	152.1	146.6	120.0	120.0
South America	53.1	57.6	44.6	55.9	50.0	50.0
Total	2054.0	2192.8	2288.8	2279.8	2355.5	2478.8

[a]From International Tea Committee (1989)

Eight countries account for 86% of world production (Table 3); six of these eight account for 95% of green tea production. Virtually all tea produced in Japan and about 60% of that produced in China is green tea. India is the largest tea producer, nearly all of which is black tea.

Table 3. Tea production by country in 1988 (in thousand tonnes)[a]

Country	All tea	Green tea
India	701.1	8.0
China	545.4	338.5
Sri Lanka	228.2	1.2
Kenya	164.0	-
Turkey	153.2	-
Indonesia	135.6	30.0
USSR	120.0	24.0
Japan	89.8	89.8
Other	341.6	28.1

[a]From International Tea Committee (1989)

(b) Exports

About 40% of total tea production is exported, and five countries account for over 80% of these exports (Table 4). Of the eight most important producing countries, China is the only significant exporter of green tea. In Japan, Turkey and the USSR, nearly all the production is consumed within the country.

Table 4. Tea exports by country in 1988 (in thousand tonnes)[a]

Country	All tea	Green tea
India	221.5	2.0
Sri Lanka	219.7	1.3
China	198.3	78.6
Kenya	138.2	-
Indonesia	92.7	0.1
Other	183.1	12.5

[a]From International Tea Committee (1989)

(c) Imports

Total tea imports (adjusted for re-export) in 1988 were approximately 1030 thousand tonnes. The 15 leading importing countries in 1988 accounted for 80% of all imports. Imports over the last six years from these countries are shown in Table 5.

Table 5. Tea imports for consumption by country in 1983-88 (in thousand tonnes)[a]

Country	1983	1984	1985	1986	1987	1988
UK	155.2	184.2	155.4	171.1	142.6	162.7
USSR	55.8	70.0	95.8	109.9	134.8	140.0
Pakistan	86.7	85.7	89.1	84.8	90.1	85.5
USA	77.1	88.2	79.1	89.5	77.3	90.1
Egypt	65.5	75.0	76.2	72.9	64.9	76.4
Iran	27.4	29.1	32.6	25.5	28.4	40.3
Iraq	37.8	45.5	34.6	44.7	41.8	57.7
Poland	25.9	25.5	34.7	29.9	32.1	33.6
Japan	12.0	15.6	22.9	26.3	26.3	27.3
Morocco	16.6	22.6	22.3	20.4	23.4	30.0
Saudi Arabia	18.0	20.5	20.6	17.6	19.0	19.0
Australia	21.8	20.6	20.7	20.6	18.2	19.4
Germany, Federal Republic of	14.1	17.1	15.5	15.5	15.2	13.6
Canada	17.5	18.4	15.7	17.5	14.2	14.1
Sudan	12.9	10.7	14.0	11.1	13.0	13.0

[a] From International Tea Committee (1989)

(d) *Consumption*

Consumption data based on import, export and production statistics provide a sound estimate for economic purposes; however, determination of actual human consumption or ingestion must take into account the methods of beverage preparation and varying levels of extraction of tea leaves into finished beverages. In addition to the nature of the manufactured leaf, brewing variables, such as leaf to water ratio, temperature and time, all affect the amount of solid extracted.

The estimates of the International Tea Committee of actual consumption take into account imports, exports and, when possible, locally grown tea. Tables 6 and 7 show total and per-caput consumption, respectively.

Table 6. Total average tea consumption by country (in thousand tonnes)[a]

Country	Consumption		Country or region	Consumption	
	1984-86	1985-87		1984-86	1985-87
India	415.10	430.00	Ireland	10.77	10.95
China	~ 350.00 (1988)		Netherlands	9.34	9.51
USSR	236.35	NA	Hong Kong	9.22	9.14
UK	166.97	160.03	France	9.21	9.45
Turkey	130.81	139.42	New Zealand	5.76	5.61
Japan	113.49	120.28	Algeria	5.18	4.90
Pakistan	86.56	88.02	Kuwait	4.37	4.16
USA	85.61	81.97	Jordan	3.92	4.07
Egypt	74.70	73.03	Tanzania, United	4.39	4.80
Iran	50.20	NA	Republic of		
Iraq	43.20	41.40	Italy	3.43	3.55
Poland	30.06	32.25	Sweden	2.98	2.99
Sri Lanka	22.70	23.00	German Democratic	2.72	2.60
Morocco	21.75	22.03	Republic		
South Africa	20.96	20.23	Denmark	2.36	2.30
Australia	20.64	19.87	Czechoslovakia	2.25	2.20
Saudi Arabia	19.54	19.05	Switzerland	1.89	1.80
Canada	17.22	15.79	Belgium/Luxembourg	1.36	1.34
Kenya	16.36	17.35	Austria	1.23	1.15
Germany, Federal	16.03	15.40	Qatar	1.16	0.99
Republic of			Norway	0.87	0.93
Syria	14.72	13.83	Finland	0.85	0.94
Tunisia	13.10	13.56	Bahrain	0.64	0.62
Sudan	11.89	12.68	Thailand	0.55	0.54
Afghanistan	11.33	NA	Greece	0.30	NA
Chile	11.01	11.43	Portugal	0.22	NA
			Spain	0.71	NA

[a]From International Tea Committee (1989)
NA, not available

Table 7. Average tea consumption *per caput*[a]

Country or region	Amount (kg)		Country or region	Amount (kg)	
	1984-86	1985-87		1984-86	1985-87
Qatar	3.74	3.21	Afghanistan	0.63	NA
Ireland	3.03	3.09	South Africa	0.56	0.53
United Kingdom	2.94	2.81	Sudan	0.55	0.56
Iraq	2.72	2.51	India	0.55	0.55
Turkey	2.65	2.72	Denmark	0.46	0.45
Kuwait	2.55	2.23	Sweden	0.36	0.35
Tunisia	1.81	1.82	USA	0.36	0.34
New Zealand	1.77	1.71	China	~ 0.35 (1988)	
Hong Kong	1.69	1.63	Switzerland	0.29	0.27
Saudi Arabia	1.69	1.40	Germany, Federal Republic of	0.26	0.25
Egypt	1.54	1.44			
Bahrain	1.52	1.45	Algeria	0.24	0.22
Sri Lanka	1.43	1.41	Norway	0.21	0.22
Syria	1.43	1.26	Tanzania, United Republic of	0.20	0.21
Australia	1.31	1.22			
Jordan	1.12	1.12	Finland	0.17	0.19
Iran	1.05	NA	France	0.17	0.17
Morocco	0.99	0.97	German Democratic Republic	0.16	0.16
Japan	0.94	0.99			
Chile	0.91	0.93	Austria	0.16	0.15
Pakistan	0.90	0.86	Czechoslovakia	0.14	0.14
USSR	0.85	NA	Belgium/Luxembourg	0.13	0.13
Poland	0.81	0.86	Italy	0.06	0.06
Kenya	0.80	0.76	Portugal	0.02	NA
Canada	0.68	0.62	Spain	0.02	NA
Netherlands	0.65	0.65	Thailand	0.01	0.01

[a] From International Tea Committee (1989)
NA, not available

2. Chemical Composition

2.1 Compounds present in black tea and its beverage

The precise composition of black tea is markedly influenced by the nature of the green shoots used and by procedures in their subsequent processing which take place in the producing countries. Differences in chemical composition are reflected in the various flavour grades and origins offered on the market, which are from mixed seedling populations with characteristics intermediate between two extreme genotypes, *Camellia sinensis* var. assamica (larger leaves) and *C. sinensis* var. sinensis (small leaves) (Millin, 1987).

The flavour aspects of black and green tea have been described (Millin, 1987), and a review of tea volatiles is available (Bokuchava & Skobeleva, 1986). A listing of the volatile compounds identified in black, Oolong and green tea has been provided by Maarse and Visscher (1986); 404 volatile compounds are listed for black tea, 48 in Oolong tea and 230 in green tea. Groups and subgroups of volatile compounds in black tea leaves are shown in Tables 8 and 9. Table 10 gives a broad tabulation of the components of fresh leaf (Millin, 1987); the structures of some of the components are given in Figure 1. Table 11 gives the composition of black tea beverage.

Table 8. Classification of volatile compounds in black tea leaf[a]

Group/subgroup	Numbers of compounds			
	Total	Aliphatic	Benzenoid	Alicyclic
Hydrocarbons	22			
Saturated		1	11	0
Unsaturated		4	1	5
Alcohols	39			
Saturated		12	3	0
Unsaturated		19	0	5
Aldehydes	54			
Saturated		11	4	0
Unsaturated		30	4	3
Hydroxy-		0	1	0
Methoxy-		0	1	0

Table 8 (contd)

Group/subgroup	Numbers of compounds			
	Total	Aliphatic	Benzenoid	Alicyclic
Ketones	48			
Mono-				
Saturated		10	9	1
Unsaturated		11	0	12
Hydroxy-		1	0	1
Di-				
Saturated		2	0	0
Unsaturated		0	0	1
Hydroxy-		0	0	0
Acids	72			
Saturated		38	2	0
Unsaturated		28	0	0
Hydroxy-		2	1	0
Oxo-		1	0	0
Esters	52			
Saturated		16	12	2
Unsaturated		19	1	2
Acetal	1	1	0	-
Nitrogen-containing	19			
Nitriles		4	1	0
Amides		2	0	0
Amines				
Primary		5	2	0
Secondary		0	3	0
Aza-, Diaza-		2	0	0
Sulfur-containing	5			
Thiols		3	0	0
Thioether		1	0	0
Other		1	0	0
Phenols	11			
Monohydroxy-		-	8	-
Alkoxy- (ethers)		-	3	-
Totals	323	224	67	32

[a] From Maarse & Visscher (1986)
0, none found
-, not applicable

Table 9. Classification of heterocyclic (oxygen-, nitrogen- and sulfur-containing) volatile compounds in dry black tea[a]

Group/subgroup	Epoxides	Furans	Pyrans	Lactones	Pyrroles	Benzo-pyrrole (indole)	Pyrazines	Pyridines	Benzo-pyridines (quinolines)	Thiophene	Thiazoles	Benzo-xazoles	Total
Simple	–	1	–	–	–	1	–	1	–	1	–	1	
Hydrogenated	–	3	2	1	–	–	–	–	–	–	–	–	
Alkyl-	6	4	–	13	–	–	11	11	7	–	5	–	
Alkoxy-	–	1	–	–	–	–	–	1	–	–	–	–	
Aldehydes	–	2	–	–	–	–	–	–	–	–	–	–	
Alcohols	–	1	–	–	–	–	–	–	–	–	–	–	
Acyl-	–	–	–	–	3	–	–	1	–	–	–	–	
Aryl-	–	–	–	–	–	–	–	2	–	–	2	–	
Totals	6	12	2	14	3	1	11	16	7	1	7	1	81

[a] From Maarse & Visscher (1986)
–, not reported

Table 10. Composition of fresh tea leaf, var. assamica[a]

Substance	% dry weight
Flavanols	25
Epi-gallocatechin gallate	9-13
Epi-catechin gallate	3-6
Epi-gallocatechin	3-6
Epi-catechin	1-3
Others	1-2
Flavonols and flavonol glycosides	3-4
Flavanediols	2-3
Polyphenolic acids and depsides	5
Other polyphenols	3
Caffeine	3-4
Theobromine	0.2
Theophylline	0.04
Amino acids	4
Organic acids	0.5
Monosaccharides	4
Polysaccharides	13-14
Protein	15
Cellulose	7
Lignin	6
Lipids	3
Chlorophyll and other pigments	0.5
Ash	5
Volatiles	0.01-0.02

[a] Adapted from Sanderson (1972), Graham (1984) and Millin (1987)

Black tea beverage differs in composition from fresh leaf in that most of the flavanols and some of the other phenolic materials are converted to the oxidized forms known as theaflavins and thearubigins. The total flavanol level is reduced to 10%, and theaflavins may be present at a level of 1-3% and thearubigins at a level of 10-40% (Graham, 1984; Ullah *et al.*, 1984). Changes in pigmentation and aroma also take place. All other components are virtually unchanged (Millin, 1987).

Fig. 1. Structures of some important tea components (From Millin, 1987)

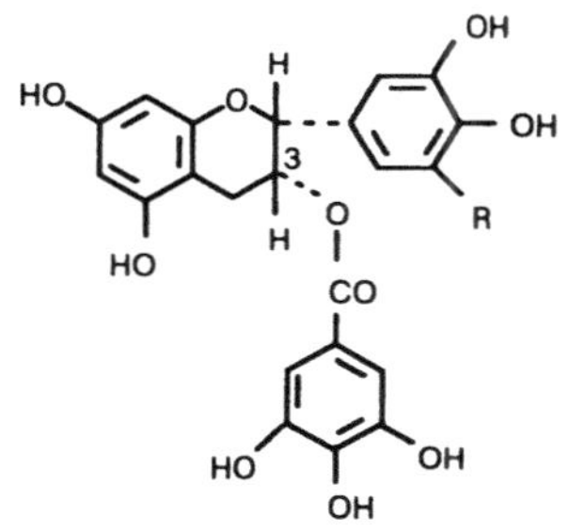

Flavanols

(−) epi-gallocatechin gallate, R = OH
(−) epi-catechin gallate, R = H
(−) epi-gallocatechin, R = OH
(without galloyl ester group, position 3)
(−) epi-catechin, R = H
(without galloyl ester group, position 3)

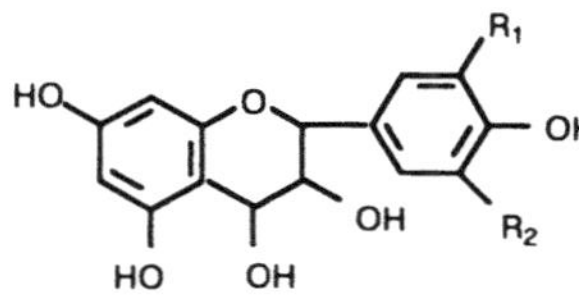

Flavan - 3,4 - diols

(leucoanthocyanins)
R_1, R_2 = H or OH

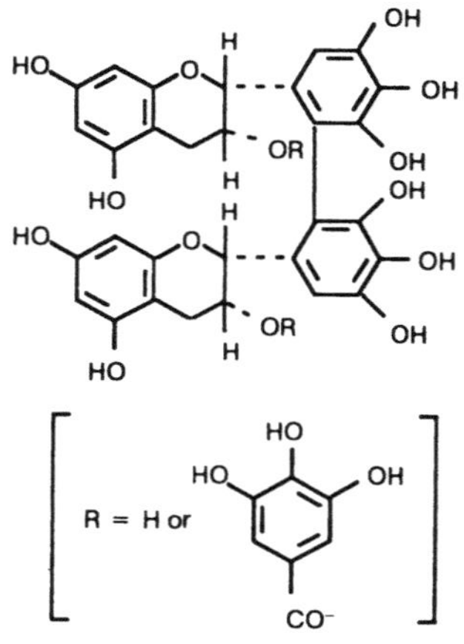

Bisflavanols

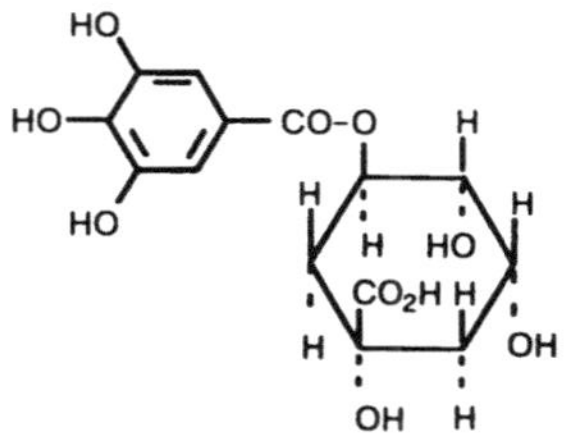

Theogallin

(3-galloylquinic acid)

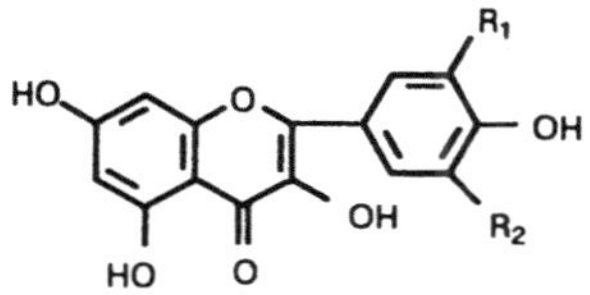

Flavonols

Kaempferol, $R_1 = R_2 = H$
Quercetin, $R_1 = OH$, $R_2 = H$
Myricetin, $R_1 = R_2 = OH$

$$HO_2C-\underset{NH_2}{CH}-CH_2-CH_2-\underset{NHC_2H_5}{CO}$$

Theanine

(γ-N-ethylglutamine)

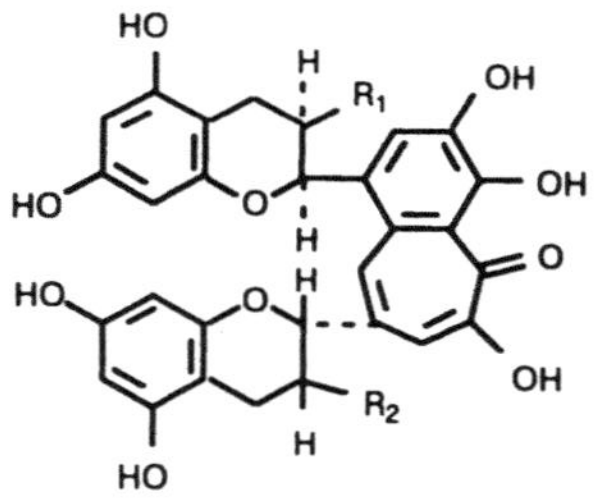

Theaflavins

Theaflavin ($R_1 = R_2 = OH$)
Theaflavin monogallates (R_1 = galloyl, R_2 = OH) or R_1 = OH, R_2 = galloyl)
Theaflavin digallate ($R_1 = R_2$ = galloyl)

Table 11. Composition of a black tea beverage[a]

Substance	% dry weight
Epi-gallocatechin gallate	4.6
Epi-gallocatechin	1.1
Epi-catechin gallate	3.9
Epi-catechin	1.2
Flavonol glycosides	trace
Bisflavanols	trace
Theaflavins	2.6
Theaflavic acid	trace
Thearubigins	35.9
Caffeine	7.6
Theobromine	0.7
Theophylline	0.3
Gallic acid	1.2
Chlorogenic acid	0.2
Oxalic acid	1.5
Malonic acid	0.02
Succinic acid	0.1
Malic acid	0.3
Aconitic acid	0.01
Citric acid	0.8
Lipids	4.8
Monosaccharides	6.9
Pectin	0.2
Polysaccharides	4.2
Peptides	6.0
Theanine	3.6
Other amino acids	3.0
Potassium	4.8
Other minerals	4.7
Volatiles	0.01

[a] Adapted from Graham (1984)

The quantitative data given below generally refer to the content in dry black tea. In order to provide representative values for the content in hot beverage prepared by steeping loose tea (or in tea bags), it is convenient and realistic to assume usage of 13.5 g black tea per litre of hot water, providing six 150-ml cups of consumable brew (or 6.67 cups in all). Thus, 200 cups are available from 450 g black tea, giving 2.25 g black tea per cup. Spiller (1984) assumed an average of 2.27 g per teabag in a cup for US usage.

At a yield of 23-28% w/w soluble solids in black tea from, say, a 3-5 min brew or first withdrawal, 2.25 g per cup would provide 0.3% w/w soluble solids per cup.

(a) Nonvolatile compounds

Considerable information is given by Yamanishi (1986) on the changes in composition of both nonvolatile and volatile components during storage under both normal and accelerated conditions.

(i) *Caffeine and other purines*

Because brewing techniques vary widely according to cultural customs around the world (Woodward, 1980), estimation of caffeine intake from tea is subject to considerable variation (Stavric *et al.*, 1988). There is little published information on extraction efficiency under household conditions, but examination of the caffeine contents of brewed tea (Bunker & McWilliams, 1979) allowed the Working Group to calculate an extraction efficiency of total solids in the range of 20-30%.

Caffeine has been reported to be present in dry black tea at 3-4% (Millin, 1987), depending upon the type of leaf used (e.g., there is more in fresh shoots). More detailed information is available from Cloughley (1983). In five samples of commercial blended black tea available in the UK, Kazi (1985) found caffeine contents ranging from 2.7-3.2% by a high-performance liquid chromatography procedure.

Table 12 provides estimates of probable caffeine contents per cup of brewed tea, together with directly obtained data. Bunker and McWilliams (1979) provided data on the caffeine content of black tea brews after various brewing times (Table 13). Caffeine tends to form complexes with oxidized polyphenols in black tea (especially theaflavins and thearubigins); when the latter possess gallate ester groupings, such complexes are poorly soluble in cold water.

Kazi (1985) found theobromine at 0.09-0.28% and theophylline at 0.02-0.06% in dry black tea, which were calculated by the Working Group to correspond to 2.6-8.4 mg and 0.5-1.8 mg per cup.

(ii) *Flavanols and their gallic acid esters*

Four flavanols and their gallic acid esters occur in large amounts among the polyphenols present in tea shoots (34% on a dry basis), i.e., epi-gallocatechin and epi-catechin and their corresponding gallates. Normally, only 5-10% of these flavanols survive the processing of black tea, e.g., 1-3% in dry black tea and 3-8% in its total soluble solids (Millin, 1987). Minimal amounts of other flavanols have been reported (Millin, 1987; Hashimoto *et al.*, 1989). Flavandiols, which are originally present in small quantities, disappear totally on processing (Millin, 1987).

Table 12. Caffeine content of black tea brews

Reference	Type of brew	Caffeine content (mg/cup)	
		Average	Range
Kazi (1985)	-		[57-67][a]
Barone & Roberts (1984)	Bag	42	-
	Leaf tea	41	30-48
	Bag	-	28-44
	Instant tea	28	24-31
	NS	27	8-91
US Food and Drug Administration (1984)	NS (US brands)	40	20-90
	NS (imported brands)	60	25-110

[a] Estimates based upon average caffeine content in dry black tea of 3.0% (Kazi, 1985) and range given for 85-100% extraction efficiencies on addition of 150 ml boiling water; 2.25 g tea per cup

NS, not specified; -, not reported

Table 13. Mean caffeine content by brand and brewing time of black and Oolong teas[a]

Type of tea	Weight of tea leaf (g)	Caffeine content (mg/140 ml; mean ± SD) with brewing time of:		
		1 min	3 min	5 min
Bagged				
Black				
Brand A	NS	33±0.4	46±7.0	50±5.0
Brand B	NS	29±0.2	44±6.0	48±4.8
Brand C	NS	21±1.0	35±1.8	39±2.4
Oolong	NS	13±2.9	30±1.7	40±1.6
Leaf				
Black, Brand A	3	31±1.1	38±1.9	40±6.7
Black, Brand E	1.7	19±2.7	25±1.7	28±3.3
Oolong	2	17±0.3	20±0.6	24±0.2

[a] From Bunker & McWilliams (1979)

NS, not stated; bag used as purchased, one bag per cup of beverage

(iii) *Flavonols and their glycosides*

Three flavonols are present: kaempferol (see IARC, 1983a), quercetin (see IARC, 1983b) and myricetin, predominantly as their 3-glycosides. A portion survives the processing stages unchanged and is present in the final product (Millin, 1987).

(iv) *Phenolic acids and depsides*

A depside is an ester formed by the condensation of two naturally occurring hydroxy acids. Gallic acid is the most important phenolic acid, while theogallin (3-galloylquinic acid) is the major depside, up to 4% occurring in dry black tea, and is substantially water soluble. The depsides are often referred to as hydrolysable tannins and are the gallo-equivalent of chlorogenic acid in coffee. They are virtually unchanged by processing (Millin, 1987).

(v) *Theaflavins and their gallates*

These are of major significance in determining the quality and flavour of tea. They are formed in black tea by oxidation of quinones derived from the epicatechins. They are present to the extent of 1-2% in dry black tea and are substantially water extractable (Millin, 1987).

(vi) *Bisflavanols*

Bisflavanols result from the condensation of *ortho*-quinones, derived from the gallocatechins. They are present at low levels (2-4%) in black tea and are largely water extractable (Millin, 1987).

(vii) *Thearubigins*

Thearubigin is a collective name for the largely unidentified, highly coloured flavanol oxidation products. They are highly heterogeneous in molecular weight and molecular structure and comprise a significant proportion of non-dialysable material. They are often structurally linked to small quantities of peptides or proteins. Their quantity in dry black tea has been given as 10-20% (Ullah *et al.*, 1984), and they are substantially water extractable.

(viii) *Amino acids and peptides*

These compounds are present to a significant extent in black tea (5% on a dry basis); among the amino acids, theanine (γ-N-ethylglutamine) is a major component (Millin, 1987).

(ix) *Other organic acids*

These comprise only a small proportion of black tea (0.5%) and are water extractable (see Table 10).

(x) *Trace elements*

Minerals including fluoride and potassium are present in black and green teas. The tea plant is known to accumulate aluminium and manganese (Graham, 1984).

(xi) *Other nonvolatile compounds*

The remaining compounds consist of partially soluble proteins, polysaccharides, lignins and sugars (monosaccharides).

(b) *Volatile substances*

van Straten *et al.* (1983) compiled quantitative data on 56 volatile substances in black tea; 404 such compounds were listed by Maarse and Visscher (1986). Volatile essences (obtained by steam distillation) were reported to account for only 0.02% by weight of black tea, i.e., 200 mg/kg (Sanderson, 1972). It is notable that different groups of workers emphasize different groups of substances as being important to the flavour of tea.

(i) *Carbonyls*

van Straten *et al.* (1983) listed quantatitive data for nine aliphatic and two aromatic aldehydes. The quantities reported are generally very small, except that for *trans*-2-hexenal (1.6-25 mg/kg) derived from lipids in the mature leaf; this compound is generally recognized as being undesirable with regard to flavour.

van Straten *et al.* (1983) listed only one ketone and one diketone, both aliphatic, present in very small quantities (0.004-0.2 mg/kg). β-Ionone, a mixed alicyclic-aliphatic ketone, is regarded as important for flavour and has been quantified by Skobeleva *et al.* (1979) at 1.3-4.4 mg/kg (0.13-0.44 mg %) in a range of black teas. 2,3-Butanedione (diacetyl) is reported to be present (Wickremasinghe & Swain, 1965) at 0.01-0.2 mg/kg [corresponding to 0.02-0.45 µg per cup (2.25 g/cup black tea)]. Small quantities (0.05 mg/l) of methylglyoxal were reported in black tea by Nagao *et al.* (1986); 2.4 mg/kg (0.7 µg per serving) were reported in instant tea (Hayashi & Shibamoto, 1985).

(ii) *Alcohols*

Quantitative data are reported by van Straten *et al.* (1983) for 15 aliphatic alcohols, including citronellol and geraniol. Higher quantities of linalool and its oxides, citronellol and geraniol are present in more 'flavourful' teas (e.g., from India) than in lower grades (e.g., from Georgia) (Skobeleva *et al.*, 1979). The listing by von Straten *et al.* (1983) included three other alcohols: benzyl alcohol, 2-phenylethanol and α-terpineol. Of the simpler aliphatic alcohols, 1-butanol is reported to be present in the largest quantity (12-89 mg/kg); of the others, linalool is reported at 1-29 mg/kg.

(iii) *Volatile acids*

Maarse and Visscher (1986) listed 72 volatile acids in black tea. van Straten *et al.* (1983) gave quantitative data for only three of these: formic, acetic and butanoic acids were reported at levels of 0.4, 5.3 and 1.0 mg/kg, respectively, in one sample.

(iv) *Esters*

Quantitative data on five aliphatic and three aromatic esters were listed by van Straten *et al.* (1983). The largest reported amount is for hexyl benzoate, at 4-22 mg/kg; methyl salicylate is present at 4.8-4.9 mg/kg.

(v) *Nitrogen compounds*

Two amines have been reported to be present in substantial quantities: ethylamine at 288 mg/kg and propylamine at 20-29 mg/kg (van Straten *et al.*, 1983). Although a number of N, N/S and N/O-heterocyclic compounds have been reported (see Table 9), none has been quantified. Yamanishi (1986) reported the occurrence of benzyl cyanide and indole in black tea.

(vi) *Furans*

Two complex furans were listed by van Straten *et al.* (1983): one, *cis*-5-(2-hydroxyisopropyl)-2-methyl-2-vinyltetrahydrofuran, was reported to occur at 4-20 mg/kg.

(vii) *Sulfur compounds*

Methylthiomethane was reported to be present in black tea at 0.05-0.1 mg/kg (van Straten *et al.*, 1983)

(viii) *Phenols*

Eleven phenols were listed as present (Maarse & Visscher, 1986); only phenol was quantified and found at 7-15 mg/kg (Skobeleva *et al.*, 1979).

(ix) *Epoxides*

cis- and *trans*-Linalool oxides were reported to be present in small amounts (Saijo & Kuwabara, 1967). Yamanishi (1986) additionally identified pyranoid and furanoid forms of these two substances. In conjunction with linalool itself, they are regarded as being important for flavour.

(x) *Hydrocarbons*

Twenty-two hydrocarbons have been reported in black tea (Maarse & Visscher, 1986). Ruschenburg (1985) reported quantities of polycyclic aromatic hydrocarbons ranging from 0.5 to 3.12 µg/kg in 11 samples of black tea. Four other samples of black teas had levels ranging from 13.3 to 18.7 µg/kg; 51.5-64.6 µg/kg were found in five samples of smoked tea. In a 5-min black tea brew, the quantities were less than 0.01 µg/l.

(xi) *Hydrogen peroxide*

The hydrogen peroxide content of tea brews was found to increase with the length of incubation and the concentration of tea: for example, a solution of 1 mg/ml tea contained 11.8 nmol/ml [0.4 µg/ml] hydrogen peroxide 1 min after it was prepared; a solution of 0.5 mg/ml tea contained 270.4 nmol/ml [9.2 µg/ml] hydrogen peroxide after standing at 30°C for about 24 h (Ariza *et al.*, 1988).

(xii) *Summarized data*

Table 14 gives estimates of the contents per cup of the groups of volatile compounds considered above. The approximate calculated total is 570 mg/kg (0.06%) in black tea, which is higher than the figure obtained for essence weight (0.02%). [The Working Group suggested that the determined quantity of amines had been overestimated.]

Table 14. Estimated content of various groups of volatile compounds in brewed black tea

Group	Number identified[a]	Number quantified[b]	Total average amount (mg/cup)[c]
Carbonyls	102	13	0.115 (mainly *trans*-2-hexanol and hexanal)
Alcohols	39	18	0.31 (mainly 1-butanol, linalool, 2-phenyl ethanol)
Acids	72	3	0.013 (mainly acetic acid)
Ester	52	8	0.074 (mainly hexyl benzoate)
Amines	12	2	0.68 (substantially ethylamine)
Sulfur compounds	13	1	0.0002
Phenols	11	1	0.015-0.034
Furans	12	3	0.05
Epoxides/lactones	20	2	0.014
Hydrocarbons	22	3	0.0001
Others	49	-	-
Total	404	54	1.3 (578 mg/kg)

[a] From Maarse & Visscher (1986)
[b] From van Straten *et al.* (1983)
[c] Calculated by the Working Group assuming 100% extraction from 2.25 g of dry black tea

Table 15 provides quantitative data on the most abundant aroma compounds in a high-quality black Darjeeling tea (Schreier & Mick, 1984).

Table 15. Principal aroma components in a dry Darjeeling tea[a]

Component	Quantity (mg/kg)
Linalool oxides	23
Linalool	18
Geraniol and benzyl alcohol	7.5
Methyl salicylate	5.5
cis-3-Hexen-1-ol	4.2
2-Phenylethanol	3.3
trans-2-Hexenal	2.5
Hexanal	1.7
1-Penten-3-ol	1.6
trans-2-penten-1-ol	1.3
Phenylacetaldehyde	1.3
trans,trans-2,4-Heptadienal	1.2
trans-2-Hexen-1-ol	1.2

[a]From Schreier & Mick (1984)

(d) Additives and contaminants

Allowable levels of pesticide residues are given by the US Department of Agriculture (1989). Most teas in international trade comply with these regulations.

Some black tea has traditionally been flavoured with various natural agents; the most famous is the 'Earl Grey' blend, prepared by the addition of oil of bergamot (main constituent, linalool) (Millin, 1987). Another popular additive is jasmine flowers, added at the time of drying to both black and green tea. Lapsang Souchong teas are smoked during processing (Graham, 1984).

2.2 Compounds present in green tea and its beverage

The flavour of the green tea beverage is considered to depend upon a suitable balance between the largely unoxidized polyphenols and amino acids, especially theanine (Graham, 1984). The volatile fraction is derived from the original volatiles present in the fresh leaf and pyrolysis products produced during firing. Like black tea, the most important desirable flavour characteristics are associated with higher-boiling terpenid and aromatic substances (Millin, 1987). A total of 230 volatile compounds has been identified in green tea (Maarse & Visscher, 1986).

The quantitative data presented below refer to the content in dry green tea, assuming that the quantity of green tea used per cup is similar to that for black tea, i.e., 2.25-3.0 g.

(a) Nonvolatile compounds

(i) Caffeine

The caffeine content of green tea is similar to that of black tea (Table 16).

Table 16. Mean caffeine content by brand and brewing time of green tea[a]

Type of tea	Weight of tea leaf (g)	Caffeine content (mg/140 ml; mean ± SD) with brewing time of:		
		1 min	3 min	5 min
Bagged				
Brand A	NS	19±1.0	33±2.7	36±2.7
Brand B	NS	9±0.2	20±0.2	26±0.2
Leaf				
Brand A	2.7	28±1.5	33±5.8	35±1.6
Brand C	1.2	15±0.1	-	20±1.8
Pan-fired	1.7	14±0.9	20±2.7	21±3.5

[a]From Bunker & McWilliams (1979)
NS, not stated; bag used as purchased, one bag per cup of beverage

(ii) Flavanols, flavonols and their glycosides

As no 'fermentation' is involved, there is very little polyphenol oxidation; polyphenols amount to 38% of the total soluble solids of dry extract (Graham, 1984).

(iii) Phenolic acids and their depsides

Depsides are present in the green tea shoots and are largely unchanged by processing (Millin, 1987).

(iv) Theaflavins and thearubigins

Green tea has little or none of these transformation products.

(v) Ascorbic acid

Ascorbic acid (vitamin C) is present in green tea at an average level of 2.0-2.5 g/kg (Yamanishi, 1986).

(vi) Amino acids and peptides

Theanine (γ-N-ethylglutamine) is the most important constituent of green tea, constituting some 4.70% of the dry weight of extract. Other free amino acids are present, in particular glutamic acid (0.50%), aspartic acid (0.50%) and arginine (0.74%); others are present to a total of 0.74% (Graham, 1984).

(b) *Volatile compounds*

van Straten *et al.* (1983) listed data on 113 volatile compounds in green tea. The total volatile compound content is reported to be one-third to one-quarter of that in black tea, and quantitative data are available for a large number of compounds.

(i) *Carbonyls*

van Straten *et al.* (1983) reported quantitative data for three aliphatic aldehydes, one aromatic aldehyde, β-cyclocitral and safranal. Only *trans*-2-hexenal was reported to be present in a significant quantity, i.e., 10 mg/kg. These authors also reported quantitative data for 13 complex ketones and diketones, all present in very small quantity, except β-ionone at 0.4-6.4 mg/kg. Traces of methylglyoxal have been reported in green tea (Nagao *et al.*, 1986).

(ii) *Alcohols*

van Straten *et al.* (1983) gave quantitative data for 26 alcohols, including geraniol, nerol and linalool. The concentration of geraniol ranged from 0.2 to 13.8 mg/kg, and that of linalool from 0.4 to 50 mg/kg.

(iii) *Acids*

van Straten *et al.* (1983) reported that six aliphatic acids up to decanoic occurred at low levels.

(iv) *Esters*

van Straten *et al.* (1983) reported data for 11 mainly aliphatic esters, including methyl jasmonate (0.2 mg/kg).

(v) *Nitrogen compounds*

van Straten *et al.* (1983) reported ethylamine at 210-457 mg/kg and diphenylamine at 1.5 mg/kg. They also reported data on four pyrroles, two indoles and three pyrazines, presumably arising from the 'firing' stage, but in small quantities, except for indole at 1.2-9.7 mg/kg.

(vi) *Furans*

The same furans as in black tea are reported to be present in very small quantities.

(vii) *Others*

van Straten *et al.* (1983) reported figures for five lactones, benzylcyanide, three phenols, 1,2,4-trichlorobenzene and three epoxides. They also reported figures for 20 hydrocarbons, of which δ-cadinene occurred in the largest amount (23.5 mg/kg).

(viii) *Summarized data*

Belitz and Grosch (1986) listed the percentages of volatile compounds, ranging from linalool (19.9%) and δ-cadinene (9.4%) down to heptanol (0.1%). Table 17 gives estimates of the contents per cup of the groups of volatile compounds considered above.

Table 17. Estimated content of various groups of volatile compounds in brewed green tea

Group	Number identified[a]	Number quantified[b]	Total average amount (mg/cup)[c]
Carbonyls	55	19	0.11
Alcohols	34	15	1.1
Acids	15	6	0.007
Esters	20	11	0.0018
Amines	3	2	0.9 (mainly ethylamine)
Pyroles and indoles	10	6	0.03
Pyrazines	23	3	0.0018
Phenols	14	3	0.0039
Furans	8	7	0.048
Lactones	5	5	0.006
Epoxides	6	3	0.018
Hydrocarbons	30	20	0.15
Others	7	28	0.009
Total	230	128	2.4

[a]From Maarse & Visscher (1986)
[b]From van Straten *et al.* (1983)
[c]Calculated by the Working Group assuming 100% extraction from 3 g green tea

Kosuge *et al.* (1981) determined the aroma composition in high-quality pan-fired green Japanese teas. One example is shown in Table 18.

Table 18. Volatile compounds in a Japanese pan-fired green tea[a]

Compound	%
Geraniol	17.9
Linalool oxides	16.1
Linalool	9.5
Nerolidol	8.8
cis-Jasmone	7.5
2,6,6-Trimethyl-2-hydroxycyclohexane-1-one	7.0

Table 18 (contd)

Compound	%
β-Tonone	5.5
Benzyl alcohol	4.7
cis-3-Hexenyl hexanoate	3.5
5,6-Epoxy-β-ionone	2.7
1-Penten-3-ol	2.7
α-Terpineol	2.2
cis-3-Hexen-1-ol	2.0
Acetylpyrrole	1.8
2-Phenylethanol	1.3
cis-2-Penten-1-ol	1.1
Pentanol	0.7
2,5-Dimethylpyrazine	0.6

a From Kosuge *et al.* (1981)

3. Biological Data Relevant to the Evaluation of Carcinogenic Risk to Humans

3.1 Carcinogenicity studies in animals

(a) *Subcutaneous administration*

Rat: Groups of 15 male and 15 female NIH Black rats, one to two months of age, received weekly subcutaneous injections of 12 mg of the total aqueous extract or 8 mg of the tannin fraction of Assam tea leaf alternately into each flank for 69-70 weeks (extract) or 45-77 weeks (fraction). A group of 15 male and 15 female controls received injections of saline. Whereas a high number of local tumours (malignant fibrous histiocytomas) developed in the rats receiving the tannin fraction (10/15 males and 11/15 females), a nonsignificant number of local tumours developed in rats treated with the aqueous extract (1/15 males and 1/15 females). No local tumour developed in the controls (Kapadia *et al.*, 1976).

(b) *Administration with known carcinogens*

(i) *Polycyclic aromatic hydrocarbons*

Mouse: A group of 15 young Swiss mice [sex unspecified] received a single skin application in the neck region of a 1% solution of benzo[*a*]pyrene in acetone, followed by applications of black tea solution (1 g tea brewed for 5 min in 155 ml boiling water) on alternate days for 55 paintings. A control group of 15 mice received benzo[a]pyrene alone. [The duration of the study was not stated]. In the group treated with benzo[a]pyrene and tea, 6/15 mice developed epithelial-cell carcinomas in the neck region. Other mice in this group developed various preneoplastic lesions of the squamous epithelium. No skin lesion was observed in the group treated with benzo[a]pyrene alone (Kaiser, 1967). [The Working Group noted the absence of an appropriate control group and the inadequate reporting of histological findings.]

Two groups of 25 male and 25 female Charles River CD-1 random-bred albino mice, six weeks old, were treated with a single application of 50 μl of a 1% solution of benzo[a]pyrene (0.53-0.6 mg benzo[a]pyrene) in acetone on the shaved interscapular area. One group received no further treatment and served as controls. The other group received 80 applications three times per week of an infusion of black Chinese (Keemun) tea containing 1% tannin. Mice were observed for 567-580 days, at which time all survivors were killed. Survival was similar in both groups. The incidence of hepatomas was 10% in the group receiving benzo[a]pyrene alone and 6% in the group also given tea. Skin tumour occurrence in the interscapular area was similar in both groups: the incidences of benign and malignant (carcinomas) tumours in the group given benzo[a]pyrene were 15/50 and 2/50, respectively; those in animals also given tea were 15/50 and 3/50, respectively. In the group treated with benzo[a]pyrene plus tea, skin tumours occurred significantly earlier than in those given benzo[a]pyrene alone (Bogovksi *et al.*, 1977).

Eight groups of 20 female Sencar mice, six weeks old, were pretreated with plant phenols (tannic acid or quercetin; 3000 nmol), green tea polyphenols (24 mg/mouse) or acetone for seven days, after which they received a single topical application of 200 nmol ($\pm$)-7β,8α-dihydroxy-9α,10α-epoxy-7,8,9,10-tetrahydro-benzo[a]pyrene as the initiating agent or acetone. Beginning seven days after initiation, animals received applications of 3.24 nmol 12-*O*-tetradecanoylphorbol 13-acetate three times per week until termination of the experiment at 18 weeks. The formation of skin tumours [probably papillomas] > 1 mm in diameter and persisting for two weeks or more was recorded weekly and included in the cumulative total. Tannic acid and green tea phenols afforded significant protection ($p < 0.01$) against the induction of skin tumours; quercetin gave only moderate protection (Khan *et al.*, 1988).

Four groups of 20 female BALB/c mice, six weeks of age, were painted on shaved dorsal skin as follows: Group 1 received 0.2 ml acetone daily for seven days then 0.2 ml acetone twice weekly for 16 weeks; Group 2 received acetone daily for seven days and then 3-methylcholanthrene twice weekly for 16 weeks; Group 3 received 1.2 mg green tea polyphenols in acetone daily for seven days and then

3-methylcholanthrene in acetone 1 h following the green tea polyphenols twice weekly for 16 weeks; Group 4 received green tea polyphenols daily for seven days and then green tea polyphenols 1 h following acetone twice weekly for 16 weeks, at which time the experiment was terminated. The number of skin tumours > 1 mm in diameter and persisting for two weeks or more was 11.6 ± 0.5 in mice receiving 3-methylcholanthrene (Group 2) as compared with 5.8 ± 0.9 in those pretreated with green tea polyphenols followed by 3-methylcholanthrene (Group 3). In a parallel experiment, protection by green tea polyphenols was obtained in female Sencar mice pretreated by topical application or in the drinking-water against initiation by 7,12-dimethylbenz[a]anthracene or promotion by 12-O-tetradecanoyl phorbol 13-acetate; i.e., there was a longer latent period and 28.8 ± 1.7 or 29.1 ± 3.7 versus 51.3 ± 3.6 tumours per animals. Green tea polyphenols did not initiate skin tumours. Furthermore, when administered topically or orally, they significantly inhibited polycyclic aromatic hydrocarbon-DNA adduct formation in epidermis after topical administration of ^{3}H-7,12-dimethylbenz[a]anthracene or ^{3}H-benzo[a]-pyrene (Wang et al., 1989a).

(ii) *N-Nitroso compounds*

Mouse: Thirty-one male C57Bl/6 mice, eight weeks of age, received 100 mg/l *N*-ethyl-*N'*-nitro-*N*-nitrosoguanidine in the drinking-water for four weeks; 15 animals subsequently received 0.005% epi-gallocatechin gallate (the main polyphenolic constituent of green tea infusion) in the drinking-water for 11 weeks; 16 animals received tap-water only for 11 weeks. All mice were sacrificed in the 16th week after the start of treatment with the nitrosamide. The incidences of duodenal tumours were 3/15 (20%) in the group receiving epi-gallocatechin gallate and 10/16 (63%; $p < 0.001$) in the group treated with the nitrosamide alone. Similar results were obtained when the experiment was repeated (Fujita et al., 1989).

3.2 Other relevant data

(a) *Experimental systems*

(i) *Absorption, distribution, metabolism and excretion*

No data were available to the Working Group.

(ii) *Toxic effects*

Green and black teas have been reported to decrease significantly the activity of transketolase in whole blood of rats. The activity of liver transketolase was decreased by green tea only. Neither type of tea had any effect on the activity of intestinal transketolase. The activity of lactate dehydrogenase was not affected by the teas, while both green and black teas decreased the activity of lactate dehydrogenase in whole blood. Neither tea had an effect on intestinal alkaline phosphatase, but thiamine diphosphatase activity was decreased by both teas (Ali *et al.*, 1989).

(iii) *Effects on reproduction and prenatal toxicity*

No data were available to the Working Group.

(iv) *Genetic and related effects*

The genetic and related effects of tea have been reviewed (Sugimura, 1982; Sugimura & Sato, 1983; Nagao *et al.*, 1986).

Tea has been studied in experimental genetic and related systems following preparation by various methods (Nagao *et al.*, 1979; Uyeta *et al.*, 1981), including adding water at various temperatures to tea leaves, followed by decanting or filtering the solution. Variations included the use of different types of tea, water:leaf ratios and steeping times. The tea beverage was evaporated and the residue redissolved in a solvent (e.g., dimethylsulfoxide) for testing. The doses are expressed either as the original weight of tea leaves from which the extract was obtained or as the original volume of the tea beverage (infusion). Tea preparations were hydrolysed by various methods (e.g., acid, enzymes or bacteria), the hydrolysates extracted with organic solvents, the solvents evaporated and the residue redissolved in a solvent (e.g., dimethylsulfoxide) suitable for genetic assays.

Several studies addressed the nature of the components of green and black tea that are mutagenic to bacteria. Mutagenic activity suppressed by catalase may be attributed in part to hydrogen peroxide (Ariza *et al.*, 1988) and dicarbonyls present in tea (Nagao *et al.*, 1986). In addition, tea has been shown to contain precursors (flavonoid glycosides) of mutagenic flavonols (e.g., kaempferol, quercetin and myricetin) which are released when the tea is treated to produce hydrolysates. In these studies, treatment of dried teas with acid, glycosidase enzymes (e.g., hesperidinase) or bacteria (e.g., human intestinal bacteria) increased their mutagenic activity in *Salmonella typhimurium* TA98 and TA100, especially when an exogenous metabolic activation system was added (Nagao *et al.*, 1979; Uyeta *et al.*, 1981).

The results described in this section are listed at the end, in Table 19, with the evaluation of the Working Group, as positive, negative or inconclusive, as defined in the footnotes. The results are tabulated separately for the presence and absence of an exogenous metabolic system. The lowest effective dose (LED), in the case of positive results, or the highest ineffective dose (HID), in the case of negative results, are shown, together with the appropriate reference. The studies are summarized briefly below.

Black tea: Black teas were mutagenic to *S. typhimurium*. Oolong, Lapsang Souchong and jasmine teas inhibited DNA synthesis in cultured lymphocytes (Yang *et al.*, 1979).

Green tea: Green teas were mutagenic to *S. typhimurium*. An antioxidant fraction of green tea did not affect gap-junctional intercellular communication in cultured mouse hepatocytes and human keratinocytes.

Japanese green tea was found to contain a considerable amount of epi-gallocatechin gallate; this tannin effectively reduced the spontaneous mutation rate in NIG 1125 *Bacillus subtilis* carrying a mutation in DNA-polymerase III, but failed to lower the frequency of chemically or ultra-violet radiation-induced reverse mutations in *S. typhimurium* or *Escherichia coli* (Kada *et al.*, 1985).

Unspecified teas: Tea (Horniman's brand, puchased in Córdoba, Spain [unspecified as black or green, but probably black]) was mutagenic to *S. typhimurium* TA104 in the histidine reversion assay and to *S. typhimurium* BA13 in the arabinose-resistance forward mutation assay.

Tea in combination with other agents: Both green and black teas decreased the mutagenic activity of *N*-methyl-*N'*-nitro-*N*-nitrosoguanidine in *E. coli* and *S. typhimurium* TA100, both *in vitro* and in an in-vivo/in-vitro assay in which the gastric contents of rats were sampled and tested 1 h after oral administration of the nitrosamide either alone or with tea extracts (Jain *et al.*, 1989a).

Green tea and black tea decreased the mutagenic activity of nitrosation products of methylurea and salted fish in *S. typhimurium* TA1535 (Stich *et al.*, 1982a,b) and decreased the mutagenic activity of benzo[*a*]pyrene in *S. typhimurium* TA100 (Joner & Dommarsnes, 1983). Both Oolong and green teas similarly decreased the mutagenicity induced by benzo[*a*]pyrene in *S. typhimurium*; and the frequency of chromosomal aberrations induced by benzo[*a*]pyrene in Chinese hamster lung (CHL) cells was decreased by the addition of Oolong tea (Kojima *et al.*, 1989). Oolong tea also decreased the mutagenicity induced in *S. typhimurium* by gasoline vehicle exhaust, cooked salmon, 1,6-dinitropyrene, 3-amino-1-methyl-5*H*-pyrido[4,3-*b*]indole (Trp-P-2) and 2-amino-3-methylimidazo[4,5-*f*]quinoline (IQ) (Kojima *et al.*, 1989).

The frequency of chromosomal aberrations in rat bone marrow following intraperitoneal injection of aflatoxin B_1 was reduced by hot-water extracts of green tea but not of black tea. This effect was observed when the teas were administered 24 h before the aflatoxin, and was attributed to green tea tannins (Ito *et al.*, 1989).

An antioxidant fraction from green tea containing catechins prevented the inhibition of gap-junctional intercellular communication induced by paraquat, glucose oxidase and phenobarbital in mouse hepatocytes, and by 12-*O*-tetradecanoylphorbol 13-acetate in human keratinocytes (Ruch *et al.*, 1989).

Green tea and polyphenols from green tea inhibited the mutagenicity of benzo[a]pyrene, aflatoxin B_1, 2-aminofluorene and coal-tar pitch in *S. typhimurium* TA100 and/or TA98. The polyphenols from green tea also inhibited aflatoxin B_1-induced mutations, decreased sister chromatid exchange and chromosomal aberrations in V79 cells and inhibited benzo[a]pyrene-induced mutations in V79 cells (Wang *et al.*, 1989b).

In one study, green tea and black tea reduced the induction of anchorage-independent growth of mouse epidermal JB6 cells by 12-*O*-tetradecanoylphorbol 13-acetate (Jain *et al.*, 1989b).

(b) *Humans*

(i) *Absorption, distribution, metabolism and excretion*

No data were available to the Working Group.

(ii) *Toxic effects*

In a number of studies in which coffee drinking was associated with increased serum cholesterol levels, participants who consumed tea showed either no association or a negative correlation with serum cholesterol levels (Arab *et al.*, 1983; Haffner *et al.*, 1985; Klatsky *et al.*, 1985; Curb *et al.*, 1986; Green & Jucha, 1986; Little *et al.*, 1986; Tuomilehto *et al.*, 1987).

Several studies, including the Boston Collaborative Drug Surveillance Program (1972), that showed a correlation between coffee consumption and the risk of coronary heart disease (see p. 104) showed no difference between patients and controls for tea drinking (Jick *et al.*, 1973; Rosenberg *et al.*, 1980).

Cases of asthma due to sensitivity to tea dust have been reported in workers who process tea in the tea industry (Lewis & Morgan, 1989).

A positive association between the consumption of tea and other caffeine-containing beverages and the premenstrual syndrome was suggested (Rossignol, 1985; Rossignol *et al.*, 1989). [The Working Group noted the limitation of the methodology and the small number of subjects.]

(iii) *Effects on reproduction and prenatal toxicity*

No association was found between tea consumption during pregnancy and the occurrence of malformations in offspring (Rosenberg *et al.*, 1982) (for a description of the study, see the monograph on coffee, p. 105).

In a study by Berkowitz *et al.* (1982), described on p. 109, tea drinking was compared among women who had had preterm infants and women who had had full-term infants. Drinking four or more cups daily was more frequent among cases than controls (odds ratios, 1.5-2.0 in the three trimesters), but these differences were

Table 19. Genetic and related effects of black, green and unspecified teas

Test system	Results without exogenous metabolic activation	Results with exogenous metabolic activation	Dose[a] LED/HID	Reference
Black tea				
SA0, Salmonella typhimurium TA100, reverse mutation	+	–	7500.0000[b]	Nagao et al. (1979)
SA0, Salmonella typhimurium TA100, reverse mutation	–	+	0.0000 (hydrolysate)	Nagao et al. (1979)
SA0, Salmonella typhimurium TA100, reverse mutation	+	+	0.0000 (hydrolysate)	Uyeta et al. (1981)
SA9, Salmonella typhimurium TA98, reverse mutation	–	–	0.0000 (hydrolysate)	Nagao et al. (1979)
SA9, Salmonella typhimurium TA98, reverse mutation	+	+	0.0000 (hydrolysate)	Uyeta et al. (1981)
SA9, Salmonella typhimurium TA98, reverse mutation	–	+	0.0000 (hydrolysate)	Nagao et al. (1979)
Green tea				
SA0, Salmonella typhimurium TA100, reverse mutation	+	–	8000.0000[b]	Nagao et al. (1979)
SA0, Salmonella typhimurium TA100, reverse mutation	–	+	0.0000 (hydrolysate)	Nagao et al. (1979)
SA0, Salmonella typhimurium TA100, reverse mutation	+	+	0.0000 (hydrolysate)	Uyeta et al. (1981)
SA9, Salmonella typhimurium TA98, reverse mutation	–	–	0.0000 (hydrolysate)	Nagao et al. (1979)
SA9, Salmonella typhimurium TA98, reverse mutation	+	+	0.0000 (hydrolysate)	Uyeta et al. (1981)
SA9, Salmonella typhimurium TA98, reverse mutation	–	+	0.0000 (hydrolysate)	Nagao et al. (1979)
ICR, Cell communication, mouse hepatocytes in vitro	–	0	50.0000[c]	Ruch et al. (1989)
ICH, Cell communication, human keratinocytes in vitro	–	0	50.0000[c]	Ruch et al. (1989)
Tea unspecified				
SAF, Salmonella typhimurium BA13, forward mutation ara[R]	+	0	220.0000	Alejandre-Duran et al. (1987)
SA2, Salmonella typhimurium TA102, reverse mutation	–	0	880.0000	Alejandre-Duran et al. (1987)
SA4, Salmonella typhimurium TA104, reverse mutation	+	0	880.0000	Alejandre-Duran et al. (1987)
SA5, Salmonella typhimurium BA13, reverse mutation	–	0	880.0000	Alejandre-Duran et al. (1987)

[a] Expressed as dry weight of extract
[b] Weight of material from which extract was prepared
[c] Green tea antioxidant fraction

not significant. The odds ratio was 1.6 (95% confidence interval (CI), 0.7-3.7) after adjustment for smoking and alcohol and coffee consumption.

Brooke *et al.* (1989), in a study described on p. 110, found an association between tea consumption and low birth weight in their crude data. The birthweight ratios, adjusted to 40 weeks' gestation, were 1.050, 1.043, 1.034 and 1.012 in babies born to mothers drinking 0, 1-14, 15-43 and more than 43 cups of tea per week. While the difference among the groups and the linear trend were statistically significant, no significance remained when the data were additionally adjusted for smoking.

In the papers of Watkinson and Fried (1985) and Martin and Bracken (1987) tea drinkers were included but data were not given separately. The studies of Furuhashi *et al.* (1985) and Caan and Goldhaber (1989) showed no association between tea drinking and low birth weight. (These studies are discussed on pp. 109, 110, 106 and 111.)

In a study described on p. 111, late spontaneous abortions were studied by Srisuphan and Bracken (1986) in relation to caffeine intake from various beverages including tea. Tea was apparently not associated with spontaneous abortions (crude relative risk (RR), 1.1).

(iii) *Genetic and related effects*

No data were available to the Working Group.

3.3 Case reports and epidemiological studies of cancer in humans

In comparison with coffee, less attention has been paid to the possible relationship between tea and cancer. No study has been specifically designed to study this issue, but data on tea have been published in several studies in which coffee and other possible risk factors for cancer were considered.

(*a*) *Descriptive epidemiology*

In the study of Phelps and Phelps (1988), described on p. 114, no association was found with breast cancer; no distinction was made between tea and coffee.

An ecological study examining the association between annual tea consumption, estimated from trade data, and age-adjusted cancer mortality rates for 1964-65 from 20 different countries (Stocks, 1970) noted that mean death rates from cancers at the following sites were significantly associated with tea consumption: intestine ($p < 0.01$), breast (women; $p < 0.01$), larynx (women; $0.01 < p < 0.05$), lung and bronchus (women; $0.01 < p < 0.05$). There was no association with oesophageal cancer.

A comprehensive examination of the correlation between cancer incidence (27 cancers in 23 countries) and mortality (14 cancers in 32 countries) and a variety of dietary and other environmental variables (Armstrong & Doll, 1975) showed weak positive correlations between tea consumption and cancers of the colon and rectum, although the adjusted correlation coefficients for tea were not noted. Lung cancer incidence in women was significantly associated with tea consumption ($p < 0.01$).

(i) *Pancreatic cancer*

In an early Japanese paper (Ishii *et al.*, 1973), information on diet, smoking and occupation was collected from a case series of 311 male patients with pancreatic cancer. A comparison group of the same age [but unspecified sex] was identified from a separate prospective study. In a ridit analysis, patients had a nonsignificantly higher prevalence of drinking hot tea.

(ii) *Oesophageal cancer*

A number of the studies investigating the association between oesophageal cancer and tea consumption have focused on the Caspian littoral of Iran, where oesophageal cancer rates are the highest in the world (Hormozdiari *et al.*, 1975; Joint Iran-IARC Study Group, 1977; Mahboubi & Aramesh, 1980; Ghadirian, 1987). Within this region, incidence rates for oesophageal cancer vary by 30 fold in women and by six fold in men (Hormozdiari *et al.*, 1975). A household survey showed that in the villages in the areas with the highest cancer rates there was higher tea consumption than in the lowest incidence villages, although the intermediate incidence region reported the highest tea consumption overall. These data were confirmed in a subsequent report (Joint Iran-IARC Study Group, 1977).

The effect of differences in the temperature at which the tea was consumed was reported (Ghadirian, 1987), and this was related to incidence rates in high- and low-risk regions of the littoral. In the low-risk region, tea was consumed at an average temperature of 50.1°C compared with an average temperature of 61.3°C ($p < 0.0001$) in the high incidence area.

In an ecological study by Segi (1975) in Japan, a geographical correlation was found between rates for cancer of the oesophagus and consumption of tea-gruel.

(*b*) *Cohort studies*

These studies are summarized in Table 20.

(i) *All sites*

In the study of Heilbrun *et al.* (1986), 7833 Hawaiian Japanese men were interviewed about their consumption of black tea in 1965-68, and incident cases of cancer were identified. The RRs for rectal cancer, adjusted for age at examination and alcohol consumption, showed a significant dose-response relationship (p for trend = 0.0007) when the tea consumption category 'almost never' was used as the standard. The excess risk for rectal cancer was confined to men aged 58 years or over at examination. The authors also reported that none of the examined variables that were associated with tea intake (height, weight, pack-years of smoking and physical activity level) was associated with rectal cancer risk. Prostate cancer risk, adjusted for age at examination, showed a significant negative association with tea consumption, although there was no clear dose-response relationship. There was a nonsignificant, steady inverse association between the risk for liver cancer and tea consumption.

Kinlen *et al.* (1988) examined the relationship between tea consumption and rectal and other cancers in a mortality study of 14 453 men in London, UK, aged 45-60, who were administered a questionnaire about diet and smoking in 1967; 97% were traced to the end of 1986 (14 085 men). Only deaths that occurred after the first 18 months of follow-up were included in analyses. Expected numbers of deaths were calculated using age-specific mortality rates for men in England and Wales for the appropriate time periods. Rectal cancer showed no trend with tea consumption, while colon cancer showed a negative trend with increasing consumption; the risk associated with tea consumption was similar among older and younger men. The authors reported positive trends between increasing tea consumption and the risk for stomach, lung and kidney cancers. The association with stomach and lung cancer persisted after limited adjustment for social class and smoking. [The Working Group noted that there were inconsistencies in the paper in reporting the number of rectal cancer deaths.]

(ii) *Pancreatic cancer*

In the study by Hiatt *et al.* (1988; described on p. 117), cancer patients had drunk 0.32 cup of tea per day, while the controls from within the cohort had drunk 0.62 cup per day (p = 0.10). These figures were adjusted for age and smoking.

The nested case-control study of Whittemore *et al.* (1983; described on p. 116) found a RR of 0.6 for drinking ≥2 cups per day. The authors stated that adjustment for smoking at college did not alter the findings. The reduction remained after adjustment for coffee drinking.

Table 20. Summary of results of cohort studies on cancer and tea consumption

Reference, location, site	Subjects	Tea consumption	RR (95% CI)	Comments
Heilbrun et al. (1986) Hawaii	7833 Japanese men			
Rectum	76 cases	Almost never Twice/week 2–4×/week Almost daily >Once daily	1.0 1.3 2.0 2.1 significant 4.2 significant	p for trend = 0.0007; adjusted for age at examination and alcohol consumption
Pancreas	30 cases	Almost never Twice/week 2–4×/week Almost daily } >Once daily } 0.9	1.0 0.6 1.4	p for trend = 0.87; adjusted for age at examination and pack-years of smoking
Prostate	149 cases	Almost never Twice/week 2–4×/week Almost daily } >Once daily } 0.6	1.0 0.8 0.4	p for trend = 0.02; adjusted for age at examination
Bladder	57 cases	Almost never Twice/week 2–4×/week Almost daily } >Once daily } 0.8	1.0 1.4 1.0	p for trend = 0.68; adjusted for age at examination and pack-years of smoking
Liver	25 cases	Almost never Twice/week 2–4×/week } Almost daily } 0.6 >Once daily }	1.0 0.8	p for trend = 0.134; adjusted for age at examination and alcohol consumption
Rectum	37 cases <58 years old at examination	Almost never Twice/week 2–4×/week Almost daily >Once daily	1.0 1.4 1.4 1.1 1.4	p for trend = 0.67; adjusted for age at examination and alcohol consumption
Rectum	39 cases ≥58 years old at examination	Almost never Twice/week 2–4×/week Almost daily >Once daily	1.0 1.0 2.9 3.5 significant 8.7 significant	p for trend < 0.0001; adjusted for age at examination and alcohol consumption

Table 20 (contd)

Reference, location, site	Subjects	Tea consumption	RR (95% CI)	Comments
Kinlen *et al.* (1988) London, UK	14 085 men		Observed:expected ratios	Expected no. of deaths calculated using national age-specific data
Rectum	62 cases	0-3 cups/day 4-6 cups/day 7-9 cups/day ≥10 cups/day	0.5 0.9 0.8 0.5	*p* for trend = 0.94
Pancreas	70 cases	0-3 cups/day 4-6 cups/day 7-9 cups/day ≥10 cups/day	0.6 0.8 1.1 0.9	*p* for trend = 0.28
Prostate	88 cases	0-3 cups/day 4-6 cups/day 7-9 cups/day ≥10 cups/day	0.6 0.8 1.0 0.8	*p* for trend = 0.30
Bladder	71 cases	0-3 cups/day 4-6 cups/day 7-9 cups/day ≥10 cups/day	1.0 0.7 1.2 1.4	*p* for trend < 0.13
Stomach	172 cases	0-3 cups/day 4-6 cups/day 7-9 cups/day ≥10 cups/day	0.6 0.8 1.2 1.4	*p* for trend < 0.0005
Colon	79 cases	0-3 cups/day 4-6 cups/day 7-9 cups/day ≥10 cups/day	1.0 0.8 0.5 0.7	*p* for trend = 0.066
Lung	718 cases	0-3 cups/day 4-6 cups/day 7-9 cups/day ≥10 cups/day	0.6 0.8 1.1 1.4	*p* for trend = 0.0001
Kidney	26 cases	0-3 cups/day 4-6 cups/day 7-9 cups/day ≥10 cups/day	0.4 0.7 1.2 1.8	*p* for trend = 0.04

Table 20 (contd)

Reference, location, site	Subjects	Tea consumption	RR (95% CI)	Comments
Whittemore et al. (1983) USA	50 000 men			
Pancreas	126 cases	Nondrinkers	1.00	Adjusted for age,
		Drinkers	0.5 (0.3-0.9)	college and class year
		< 2 cups/day	1.0	Adjusted for age,
		≥2 cups/day	0.6 (0.3-1.1)	college and class year

(c) *Case-control studies*

(i) *Bladder and urinary tract*

These studies are summarized in Table 21, at the end of this section.

Bladder: In a Canadian case-control study of patients with histologically confirmed bladder cancer (Morgan & Jain, 1974; described on p. 122), there was no association with tea intake (overall RR for drinkers *versus* non-drinkers adjusted for sex, 0.7).

In the US study of Simon *et al.* (1975; described on p. 122), no relation between tea drinking and cancer of the lower urinary tract (renal pelvis, ureter, bladder and urethra) was revealed.

In the study by Miller *et al.* (1978; described on p. 123) of cases of bladder cancer in Ottawa, Canada, the RR for drinking tea (users *versus* nonusers) was close to unity for people of each sex. No quantitative data were provided on doses.

In the Canadian study of Howe *et al.* (1980; described on p. 123), the RRs for tea drinkers *versus* nondrinkers were 1.0 for men and 0.5 for women.

In the largest case-control study on bladder cancer carried out in the USA (Hartge *et al.*, 1983; described on p. 124), the relation between tea consumption and bladder cancer risk was examined among subjects who drank no more than seven cups of coffee per week. No evidence of an association was found for people of either sex, and the trends in risk with dose were nonsignificant.

In a case-control study conducted in 1976-78 in metropolitan Nagoya, Japan (Ohno *et al.*, 1985; described on p. 124), no relation was evident with consumption of black tea.

In the study by Jensen *et al.* (1986); described on p. 126) on bladder cancer in Denmark, a significant, direct relationship with dose of tea emerged among men, but not among women. The overall trend in risk associated with tea drinking in the two sexes combined, adjusted for age, sex, smoking, coffee and soft drinks, was significant. The authors noted that the association with tea might be related to the unexpected finding of a positive association between total beverage consumption and bladder cancer risk in this study.

In a case-control study of bladder cancer in the Federal Republic of Germany (Claude *et al.*, 1986; described on p. 126), the estimated RRs for drinking black tea were above unity in men and women, but the trends in risk with dose were not significant. In this study, a positive association was found with total daily fluid intake, with a particularly high RR in men. [The Working Group noted the possible influence of the use of urological controls on these estimates.]

In the study by Iscovich *et al.* (1987; described on p. 127) in La Plata, Argentina, the RR for tea drinking was above unity. However, only four cases drank three or more cups per day, and the trend in risk with dose was not significant.

In a population-based case-control study from Utah, USA (Slattery *et al.*, 1988; described on p. 127), data for tea consumption were presented separately for people who had never smoked and those who had ever smoked. The authors stated that the risk increased in nonsmokers with number of cups of tea per week. [The Working Group noted that, when the data were examined globally, however, there was no appreciable association with tea. The RRs, as calculated by the Working Group, were 1.0 for one to three cups per week and 1.2 for more than three cups per week.]

In the study by Risch *et al.* (1988; described on p. 128), on bladder cancer in Canada, no association was found with various measures of tea consumption: the RR for 100 cup-years, derived from a multiple logistic model, was 1.0 for men and women.

In a study from northern Italy (La Vecchia *et al.*, 1989; described on p. 128), univariate analysis suggested a reduced bladder cancer risk among tea drinkers (RR, 0.5; [95%, 0.3-0.8]), but the risk rose to 0.8 (nonsignificant) after multivariate analysis.

Renal pelvis and ureter: The etiology and pathogenesis of transitional-cell cancer of the renal pelvis and ureter are in several aspects similar to those of bladder cancer, although the frequency of cancers at these sites is much lower and, hence, the studies are based on small data sets.

A matched hospital-based study of 33 cases of cancer of the renal pelvis and 33 controls in the UK (Amstrong *et al.*, 1976) found no association with tea drinking, although no risk estimate was reported.

Table 21. Summary of results of case–control studies of bladder cancer and tea consumption

Reference, location	Subjects (cases, controls)	Tea consumption	Relative risk (95% CI)	Comments
Morgan & Jain (1974) Canada	Men and women (232, 232)	0 <1 cup/day 1–<3 cups/day 3–<5 cups/day ≥5 cups/day	1 [0.5] [0.6] [1.1] [1.0]	Nonsignificant; adjusted for sex only
Simon et al. (1975) USA	Men and women (132, 384)	Nonuser <1 cup/day 1–2 cups/day ≥3 cups/day	1 1.0 1.3 0.8	Nonsignificant; unadjusted
Miller et al. (1978) Canada	Men (183, 366) Women (72, 144)	Users versus nonusers	1.1 0.9	Nonsignificant; unadjusted Nonsignificant
Howe et al. (1980) Canada	Discordant pairs[a] Men (80/79) Women (12/26)	Users versus nonusers	1.0 (0.7–1.4) 0.5 (0.2–1.0)	Nonsignificant; unadjusted estimates from matched analysis Nonsignificant
Hartge et al. (1983) USA	Men (455, 1106)	Nonuser <7 cups/week 7–14 cups/week >14 cups/week	1 1.1 1.1 1.0	Nonsignificant; adjusted for age, race, geographical area, tobacco and coffee
	Women (204, 452)	Nonuser <7 cups/week 7–14 cups/week >14 cups/week	1 1.1 1.7 1.2	Nonsignificant
Ohno et al. (1985) Japan	Men (227, 443) Women (65, 146)	Users versus nonusers	1.0 (0.7–1.3) 0.6 (0.3–1.0)	Nonsignificant; adjusted for age and smoking Nonsignificant
Jensen et al. (1986) Denmark	Men and women (371, 771)	0 <0.5 l/day 0.5–0.99 l/day ≥1 l/day	1 0.8 2.0 1.5	$p = 0.03$; adjusted for age, sex, smoking (never/current and lifetime pack-years), coffee and soft drinks

Table 20 (contd)

Reference, location	Subjects (cases, controls)	Tea consumption	Relative risk (95% CI)	Comments
Claude et al. (1986) Federal Republic of Germany	Men (340, 340)	0 1–2 cups/day 3–4 cups/day >4 cups/day	1 1.0 1.5 1.9	Nonsignificant; adjusted for smoking (never/ever and lifetime packs)
	Women (91, 91)	0 1–2 cups/day 3–4 cups/day >4 cups/day	1 1.9 1.3 1.9	Nonsignificant
Iscovich et al. (1987) Argentina	Men and women (99, 99)	0 1 cup/day 2 cups/day ≥3 cups/day	1 1.5 1.2 1.4	Nonsignificant; adjusted for smoking
Slattery et al. (1988) USA	Men and women (413, 886)	0 1–3 cups/week ≥4 cups/week	1 [1.0] [1.2]	Nonsignificant; adjusted for smoking (never/ever) from published data; calculated by the Working Group
Risch et al. (1988) Canada	Men and women (826, 792)	Per 100 cup-years	1.0 (0.9–1.1) 1.0 (0.8–1.2)	Adjusted for smoking (cumulated pack-years) and history of diabetes
La Vecchia et al. (1989) Italy	Men and women (163, 181)	Users versus nonusers	0.8 [0.4–1.3]	Adjusted for age, area of residence, social class and selected indicator foods

^aPatient ever used, control never used/patient never used, control ever used

A population-based case-control study of 74 cases (50 men and 24 women) of cancer of the renal pelvis and 697 controls from the USA (McLaughlin et al., 1983) showed a positive trend with tea drinking in women only. The RRs, adjusted for smoking, were 2.6 for two cups per day, based on three cases, and 18.8 for three cups or more, based on nine cases. [The Working Group noted that the same control group was used in this study and in that on renal-cell cancer described below.]

Kidney: Among the studies in which tea was considered in the epidemiology of renal-cell cancers, four (Armstrong et al., 1976; Goodman et al., 1986, ≥2 cups/day; RR, 1.4 (0.9–2.2); Yu et al., 1986, RR for daily consumption, 0.6; McCredie et al., 1988) found no association, and one (McLaughlin et al., 1984) found an association with drinking ≥3 cups/day in women only (RR, 3.4; 95% CI, 1.4–8.9), although the trend in risk was largely inconsistent.

(ii) *Pancreas* (see Table 22)

In the study of Kinlen and McPherson (1984), described on p. 136, a positive trend for tea consumption was found, which was not significant.

In several other case-control studies (MacMahon *et al.*, 1981; Mack *et al.*, 1986; La Vecchia *et al.*, 1987; Raymond *et al.*, 1987; Cuzik & Babiker, 1989; described on pp. 135, 137, 138, 139), no association was found between tea consumption and pancreatic cancer.

Table 22. Summary case–control studies of tea consumption and pancreatic cancer

Reference, location	Subjects (cases, controls)	Tea consumption (cups/day)	RR	Comments
MacMahon *et al.* (1981) USA	Men (216, 306)	0	1.0	$\chi^2 = 1.4$
		1–2	0.7	
		≥ 3	0.8	
	Women (150, 336)	0	1.0	$\chi^2 = 1.9$
		1–2	0.7	
		≥ 3	0.6	
Kinlen & McPherson (1984) UK	Men and women (216, 432)	0–2	1.0	
		3–4	2.2	Significant
		5–9	2.3	Significant
		≥ 10	2.5	
	Men and women	0–2	1.0	Adjusted for smoking and coffee
		3–4	2.3	Significant
		5–9	2.3	Significant
		≥ 10	2.6	
Mack *et al.* (1986) USA	Men and women (490, 490)	0	1.0	Crude odds ratio
		1–4	0.7	
		≥ 5	0.7	
La Vecchia *et al.* (1987) Italy	Men and women (150, 605)	0	1.0	
		1	0.9	
		≥ 2	1.3	
	Men and women	0	1.0	Adjusted for smoking and occupation
		1	0.8	
		≥ 2	1.1	

Table 22 (contd)

Reference, location	Subjects (cases, controls)	Tea consumption (cups/day)	RR	Comments
Raymond et al. (1987) Switzerland	Men and women (88, 336)	0 <910 ml/week >910 ml/week	1.0 2.2 (1.1–4.3) 1.0 (0.5–2.0)	90% CI
Cuzik & Babiker (1989) UK	Men and women (216, 279)	0–2 3–4 5–6 ≥7	1.0 0.8 0.9 0.9	Adjusted for smoking; $\chi^2 = 0.01$
	Men and women	0–2 3–4 5–6 ≥7	1.0 1.2 1.1 1.5	Consumption ~10 years previously; adjusted for smoking; $\chi^2 = 1.0$

(iii) *Breast*

Case-control studies of breast cancer and tea consumption are summarized in Table 23.

A study by Lawson et al. (1981), in which coffee and tea drinking were grouped, is described on p. 144.

In the hospital-based case-control study in Israel of Lubin et al. (1984, 1985; described on p. 144), no association between tea consumption and breast cancer risk was found.

In the study of Rosenberg et al. (1984, 1985; described on p. 145), using data from a case-control study in eastern USA, the consumption of tea was similar among all cases and controls and among those cases and controls who did not drink caffeine-containing coffee.

In the study by La Vecchia et al. (1986; described on p. 145), the RRs for drinkers of one and two or more cups per day were 1.3 and 1.0.

In the study by Schairer et al. (1987; described on p. 146), results were given on consumption of non-herbal tea: RRs were 0.9, 0.8, 1.3, 1.0 and 0.6 for increasing levels of consumption.

In the study of Mabuchi et al. (1985a; see p. 147), on risk factors for male breast cancer in a large number of hospitals in five US metropolitan areas, 42% of cases and 54% of controls drank one cup or more of tea per day; the difference was not significant.

Table 23. Summary of results of case–control studies of breast cancer and tea consumption

Reference, location	Subjects (cases, controls)	Tea consumption (cups/day)	Relative risk (95% confidence interval)	Comments
Lubin et al. (1984, 1985) Israel	Women (731, 731) surgical controls	0 1 2–3 ≥4	1.0 1.0 (0.6–1.4) 0.9 (0.5–1.2) 0.9 (0.4–1.8)	Matched for age, country of origin, length of residence in Israel
	(804, 804) neighbourhood controls	0 1 2–3 ≥4	1.0 0.8 (0.6–1.4) 0.8 (0.5–1.2) 0.8 (0.4–1.8)	
Rosenberg et al. (1985) USA	Women (2651, 1501) noncancer controls	0 1–2 3–4 ≥5	1.0 1.0 (0.8–1.1) 0.8 (0.6–1.0) 0.6 (0.5–0.9)	Adjusted for age within five years
	(2651, 385) cancer controls	0 1–2 3–4 ≥5	1.0 0.9 (0.7–1.2) 1.1 (0.7–1.6) 0.8 (0.5–1.4)	
La Vecchia et al. (1986) Italy	Women (616, 616)	0 1 ≥2	1.0 1.3 1.0	
Schairer et al. (1987) USA	Women (1510, 1882)	0 ≤1 2 3 4 ≥5	1.0 0.9 (0.8–1.1) 0.8 (0.6–1.1) 1.3 (0.8–2.1) 1.0 (0.5–2.3) 0.6 (0.2–1.9)	
Mabuchi et al. (1985a) USA	Men (52, 52)	<1 ≥1		42% versus 54%; nonsignificant; matched on age, race, marital status

(iv) *Ovary* (see Table 24)

In the study by Byers *et al.* (1983; described on p. 150), there was no significant association with any consumption category or dose trend of tea among ovarian cancer patients in Buffalo, NY, USA .

In the North American multicentre study of Miller *et al.* (1984, 1987; described on p. 150), no association was found between tea consumption and ovarian cancer.

Table 24. Summary of case–control studies of ovarian cancer (common epithelial tumours) and tea intake

Reference, location	Subjects (cases, controls)	Tea consumption (cups/day)	Relative risk (95% confidence interval)	Comment
Byers et al. (1983) USA	274, 1034	0 <3 ≥3	1.0 1.1 0.8	No significant association with any consumption category or trend
Miller et al. (1984, 1987) Several cities in the USA and Canada	290 cases 480 noncancer controls	0 1-2 3-4 ≥5	1.0 0.8 (0.6–1.2) 0.8 (0.5–1.4) 0.5 (0.2–1.0)	
	376 cancer controls	0 1-2 3-4 ≥5	1.0 0.7 (0.5–1.0) 1.1 (0.6–2.1) 0.7 (0.3–1.6)	
	856 combined controls	0 1-2 3-4 ≥5	1.0 [0.8] [1.0] [0.6]	

(v) *Cancers of the digestive tract*

Large bowel: Case-control studies on colorectal cancer and tea consumption are summarized in Table 25.

In the study of Higginson (1966; described on p. 152), no significant association was found between tea consumption and colorectal cancer in patients in Kansas City, USA.

In the study by Watanabe et al. (1984; described on p. 155), drinking black tea was negatively associated with the risk for rectal cancer in cases in Kyoto, Japan. There was a possible dose-response relationship (the RR for non-daily drinkers was 0.5 and for daily drinkers, 0.4). The positive association between rectal cancer and drinking green tea was not significant, nor were the associations between colon cancer and the consumption of black or green tea.

In the study of Tajima and Tominaga (1985; described on p. 155) in Nagoya, Japan, there was no significant association between black or green tea drinking and cancers of the colon or rectum.

In the large case-control study in Milan, Italy, conducted by La Vecchia et al. (1988; described on p. 156), subjects with a higher intake of tea had RRs of 1.4 for colon cancer [$p = 0.06$] and 1.5 for rectal cancer ($p < 0.05$).

Table 25. Summary of results of case–control studies on colorectal cancer and tea consumption

Reference, location, site	Subjects (cases, controls)	Tea consumption	Relative risk (95% CI)	Comments
Higginson (1966) USA Colon and rectum	Men and women (340, 1020)	Never/irregular <1 cup/day <2 cups/day ≥3 cups/day	1.0 [1.0] [1.1] [0.5]	Nonsignificant

Watanabe et al. (1984) Japan Rectum	Men and women (65, 65)	Green tea
		  Nondrinkers
		  Drinkers
		Black tea
		  Nondrinkers
		  Drinkers
		Frequency
		  Never
		  Daily
		  Sometimes
			
			1.0
			3.0 (0.4–25.8)
			
			1.0
			0.5 (0.2–1.0)
			
			1.0
			0.4 (0.1–1.6)
			0.5 (0.2–1.1)
				Crude RR

Colon	Men and women (138, 138)	Green tea
		  Nondrinkers
		  Drinkers
		Black tea
		  Nondrinkers
		  Drinkers
			
			1.0
			1.3 (0.3–5.9)
			
			1.0
			1.1 (0.7–1.7)	

Tajima & Tominaga (1985) Japan Rectum	Men and women (51, 186)	Green tea
		  0–3 times/day
		  ≥4 times/day
		Black tea
		  Nondrinkers
		  Drinkers
			
			1.0
			0.9
			
			1.0
			0.9
				Adjusted for age and sex; nonsignificant
				
				Nonsignificant

Colon	Men and women (42, 186)	Green tea
		  0–3 times/day
		  ≥4 times/day
		Black tea
		  Nondrinkers
		  Drinkers
			
			1.0
			1.0
			
			1.0
			1.7
				
				Nonsignificant
				
				Nonsignificant

La Vecchia et al. (1988) Italy Rectum	Men and women (236, 778)	Low tertile Intermediate/ high tertiles	1.0 1.5	$p < 0.05$; adjusted for age, marital status, education, social class, smoking and alcohol consumption

Table 25 (contd)

Reference, location, site	Subjects (cases, controls)	Tea consumption	Relative risk (95% CI)	Comments
Colon	Men and women (339, 778)	Low tertile Intermediate/ high tertiles	1.0 1.4	 Nonsignificant

Stomach: Case-control studies on stomach cancer and tea consumption are summarized in Table 26.

In the studies of Higginson (1966; see p. 152), in the Kansas City area, USA, of Graham *et al.* (1967; see p. 161) in Buffalo, NY, USA, of Tajima and Tominaga (1985; see p. 155) in Nagoya, Japan, and of Trichopoulos *et al.* (1985; see p. 161) in Piraeus, Greece, there was no significant association between drinking tea and cancer of the stomach.

Kono *et al.* (1988) studied 139 incident cases of gastric cancer in Kyushu, Japan. Two control groups were used: 2574 controls were subjects screened for gastrointestinal conditions but found to be healthy, and 278 (two per case) were population controls from ten neighbouring municipalities, matched to the cases by sex and year of birth. Individuals consuming ten or more cups of green tea per day tended to have a lower risk for gastric cancer. There was no difference, however, between individuals drinking none to four cups and five to nine cups per day.

Table 26. Summary of results of case–control studies on gastric cancer and tea consumption

Reference, location	Subjects (cases, controls)	Tea consumption	Relative risk (95% CI)	Comments
Higginson (1966) USA	Men and women (93, 279)	Never/irregular <1 cup/day <2 cups/day ≥3 cups/day	1.0 [0.9] [1.3] [1.3]	Nonsignificant
Graham *et al.* (1967) USA	Men and women (276, 2221)			No association
Tajima & Tominaga (1985) Japan	Men and women (93, 186)	Green tea 0–4 times/day ≥5 times/day Black tea Nondrinkers Drinkers	 1.0 0.6 1.0 0.8	Nonsignificant; adjusted for age and sex Nonsignificant

Table 26 (contd)

Reference, location	Subjects (cases, controls)	Tea consumption	Relative risk (95% CI)	Comments
Trichopoulos et al. (1985) Greece	Men and women (110, 100)	1 (low) 2 3 4 5 (high)	1.0 [1.7] [1.8] [2.7] [3.2]	Nonsignificant; adjusted for age, sex, years of schooling; p value based on chi-squared test for linear trend; coffee and tea intakes added
Kono et al. (1988) Japan	Men and women (139, 2574)	0-9 cups/day ≥10 cups/day	1.0 0.5 (0.3-1.1)	$p = 0.10$; hospital controls; adjusted for age, sex, smoking, consumption of oranges and other fruit
	Men and women (139, 278)	0-9 cups/day ≥10 cups/day	1.0 0.3 (0.1-0.7)	$p = 0.007$; population controls

Oesophagus: Case-control studies on oesophageal cancer and tea consumption are summarized in Table 27.

Kaufman et al. (1965) studied 82 cases of oesophageal cancer and 73 controls in Kazakhstan, USSR, and later added 51 cases from another area (effective numbers, 127 cases and 72 controls). Drinking very hot tea was associated with a three-fold higher risk of cancer.

In the same region, Bashirov et al. (1968) carried out a comparison of 301 cases of oesophageal cancer (142 men and 159 women) and 301 healthy population controls. Cases and controls had smoked for similar durations and used nass to the same extent. Oesophageal cancer was more common among those who reported drinking six or more cups of hot black tea at a single sitting than among those who did not.

In the study of de Jong et al. (1974; described on p. 163) among Singapore Chinese, there was no association between tea drinking and oesophageal cancer; however, drinking of 'burning hot' tea was associated with a three- to four-fold higher risk.

In northern Iran, Cook-Mozaffari et al. (1979) studied 344 patients with oesophageal cancer registered at the Caspian cancer registry between January 1975 and 1976. These comprised 54% of the patients registered during that period. Two population controls were chosen per case, matched for village of residence, age, sex and language group. A second group of 181 patients with other cancers (of whom approximately 50% had stomach cancer) were also matched to two neighbourhood controls. Drinking hot tea was associated with a doubling in the risk of oesophageal cancer in males and females ($p < 0.01$). Hot-tea drinking was also associated with a three-fold higher risk of the other cancers studied among men, but with no excess among women.

In the study of Victora et al. (1987; see p. 280) in southern Brazil, cases and controls did not differ significantly in the frequency of tea intake, although no data were given.

Table 27. Summary of results of case–control studies on oesophageal cancer and tea consumption

Reference, location	Subjects (cases, controls)	Tea consumption	Relative risk	Comments
Kaufman et al. (1965) USSR	Men and women (127, 72)	Drinking of very hot tea No Yes	 1.0 [3.2]	[$p < 0.001$]
Bashirov et al. (1968) USSR	Men (142, 142)	Glasses of hot tea at a time <7 ≥7	 1.0 [2.6]	[$p < 0.01$]
	Women (159, 159)	Glasses of hot tea at a time <7 ≥7	 1.0 [3.0]	Nonsignificant
de Jong et al. (1974) Singapore	Men (95, 465)	Not daily Daily Burning hot	1.0 0.8 3.7	Nonsignificant; adjusted for dialect group $p < 0.01$
	Women (36, 200)	Not daily Daily Burning hot	1.0 0.8 3.5	 Nonsignificant $p < 0.05$
Cook-Mozaffari et al. (1979) Iran	Men (217, 434)	Drinking hot tea No Yes	 1.0 1.7	$p < 0.01$
	Women (127, 254)	No Yes	1.0 2.2	$p < 0.01$
Victora et al. (1987) Brazil	Men and women (171, 342)			No association

Other digestive tract (Table 28): In the study of Yen et al. (1987; described on p. 163) in eastern USA, subjects who consumed tea had half the risk for cancer of the extrahepatic bile ducts than people who had never drunk tea. This difference was marginally significant, but there was no suggestion of a dose-response relationship.

In the study of Franco et al. (1989; described on p. 164), in Brazil, no association was found between the frequency of tea drinking and oral cancer.

Table 28. Summary of results of case–control studies on other digestive tract cancers

Reference, location, site	Subjects (cases, controls)	Tea consumption	Relative risk (95% CI)	Comments
Yen et al. (1987) USA Extrahepatic bile duct	Men and women (67, 275)	0 Ever Occasionally 1–2 cups/day 3–4 cups/day ≥5 cups/day	1.0 0.5 (0.3–1.0) 0.4 (0.2–0.9) 0.6 (0.3–1.3) 0.5 (0.2–1.4) 0.8 (0.2–3.3)	Adjusted for age and sex
Franco et al. (1989) Brazil Oral cavity	Men and women (232, 464)	< 1 cup/month 1–30 cups/month > 30 cups/month	1.0 0.9 (0.6–1.3) 1.0 (0.6–1.7)	Nonsignificant; crude matched analysis; p level based on test for linear trend
		< 1 cup/month 1–30 cups/month > 30 cups/month	1.0 0.9 (0.6–1.3) 1.3 (0.7–2.3)	Nonsignificant; adjusted for tobacco and alcohol consumption

(vi) *Nasopharynx*

Case-control studies of nasopharyngeal cancers (NPC) and tea consumption are summarized in Table 29.

Lin et al. (1973) studied 343 patients with NPC and 1017 controls in Taiwan. No association was found between tea drinking and NPC, but no data were given.

In the study of Henderson et al. (1976; described on p. 165), tea drinking was associated with a significantly decreased risk for NPC ($p = 0.02$). Cases with other pharyngeal cancers, however, were not more likely to drink tea (RR, 1.4; $p = 0.3$).

Shanmugaratnam et al. (1978) investigated the association between tea drinking and NPC in Singapore. The case series consisted of 379 Chinese patients (266 men, 113 women) with histologically confirmed NPC in Singapore between 1966 and 1968. Two control groups were recruited: the first were 595 Chinese patients from the ear, nose and throat department at the same hospital, and the second were 1044 Chinese patients in the medical, surgical and orthopaedic wards of another hospital. No difference was found regarding the frequency of consumption of Chinese tea between cases and ear, nose and throat controls; the comparison with other hospital controls showed no consistent association.

Table 29. Summary of results of case–control studies on nasopharyngeal cancers and tea consumption

Reference, location	Subjects (cases, controls)	Tea consumption	Relative risk (95% CI)	Comments
Henderson et al. (1976) USA	Men and women (156, 267)	0 Drinkers	1.0 0.5 [0.3–1.0]	$p = 0.02$; adjusted for age, sex, race, socio-economic status and place of residence
Shanmugaratnam et al. (1978) Singapore	Men and women (379, 595)	< once/month < once/day Daily	0.9 0.9 1.2	Nonsignificant; ear, nose and throat controls; adjusted for sex, age and interviewer
	Men and women (379, 1044)	< once/month < once/day Daily	1.1 0.7 1.3	$p < 0.05$; other hospital controls

(vii) *Other sites*

Case-control studies of cancers at other sites and tea consumption are summarized in Table 30.

In the study of Mabuchi et al. (1985b; described on p. 166) of carcinoma of the vulva in five US metropolitan areas, no association was found between the consumption of tea and cancer of the vulva.

Bunin et al (1987) studied tea drinking during pregnancy and Wilms' tumour in the offspring. Cases were white children under 15 years of age identified through the registries of the three main childhood cancer hospitals in Philadelphia, PA, during 1970-83. About 30% of eligible cases could not be interviewed. Tea consumption during pregnancy was associated with a doubling of the risk for Wilms' tumour in the offspring ($p < 0.05$).

[The Working Group noted that, unless otherwise specified, the studies did not distinguish different types of tea (green, black or herbal). Furthermore, the effect of the consumption of other hot beverages was not considered in most of the studies. Consequently, non-drinkers of tea could represent drinkers of other hot beverages, including coffee.]

Table 30. Summary of results of case–control studies on other cancers and tea consumption

Reference, location, site	Subjects (cases, controls)	Tea consumption	Relative risk (95% CI)	Comments
Mabuchi et al. (1985b) USA Vulva	Women (149, 149)	< 1 cup/day 1–2 cups/day 3–4 cups/day ≥5 cups/day	1.0 0.8 1.1 1.1	Nonsignificant; unmatched analysis
Bunin et al. (1987) USA Wilms' tumour	Boys and girls (88, 88)	Tea intake of mother during pregnancy 0 Drinkers	 1.0 2.2 (1.0–4.7)	Matched analysis $p < 0.05$

4. Summary of Data Reported and Evaluation

4.1 Exposure data

Tea is an aqueous infusion prepared from the dried leaves of *Camellia sinensis*, which has been consumed since ancient times in Asia and since the late seventeenth century in most other parts of the world. Tea is the most widely consumed beverage in the world. About 80% of world production of tea is in Asian countries. Depending on manufacturing techniques, teas can be divided into two main types: black tea, which has undergone an enzymic oxidation called 'fermentation' during processing, and green tea, which has not. Black tea represents about 80% of world production.

Annual tea consumption varies from country to country, ranging from a high level of about 3 kg *per caput* to negligible values in many countries. World consumption is approximately 0.5 kg *per caput*. Green tea is the primary form consumed in China, Japan and some Middle Eastern countries. Instant tea and decaffeinated tea consumption is small, but the latter is becoming more significant in the USA.

Over 400 volatile compounds comprising many structural categories have been identified in black teas and over 200 in green teas; these contribute to the flavour and aroma of the beverage. In addition to the expected components of leaf matter (e.g., flavonols, flavanols and phenolic acids), other nonvolatile components are present; bisflavanols, theaflavins and thearubigins are found in black tea. Average caffeine levels in both black and green teas are 3-4% on a dry weight basis, resulting in about 30-50 mg caffeine per cup. Some black and green teas have traditionally been flavoured with natural agents such as oil of bergamot and jasmine flowers.

4.2 Experimental carcinogenicity data

Tea was tested for carcinogenicity in one study in rats by repeated subcutaneous injection of a total aqueous extract of tea leaves. A nonsignificant increase in the incidence of local tumours was observed.

In a number of studies, various known carcinogens were administered by different routes either simultaneously or sequentially with tea or its constituents by various routes. In one study in mice, skin application of black tea infusion containing 1% tannin after a single application of benzo[a]pyrene did not affect the incidence of skin tumours.

Administration of polyphenolic extracts of green tea in combination with known carcinogens resulted in decreased incidences of skin tumours in mice treated with benzo[a]pyrene diol epoxide, 3-methylcholanthrene or 7,12-dimethylbenz[a]anthracene and of duodenal tumours in mice treated with N-ethyl-N'-nitro-N-nitrosoguanidine, within a limited period of observation.

4.3 Human carcinogenicity data

Correlation studies on cancer risk associated with tea consumption have provided inconsistent reports of increased risks for cancers of the breast, intestine, larynx, lung and colon. Ecological studies of villages in the Caspian littoral have shown a broad correspondence between the occurrence of oesophageal cancer and tea consumption. An additional report found a relationship with the temperature at which the tea was drunk. A geographical study showed that in areas of Japan with high reported consumption of tea-gruel there were higher mortality rates from oesophageal cancer.

(a) Bladder and urinary tract cancer

In two cohort studies in which bladder cancer risk was examined, no association was reported.

The overall evidence from 12 case-control studies indicates no consistent association between measures of tea consumption and risk for bladder cancer. Although the data are limited, a similar pattern of trend was apparent for transitional-cell cancers of the renal pelvis and ureter.

One cohort study found a positive dose-response relationship for cancer of the kidney, but there was inadequate adjustment for confounding. Case-control studies on adenocarcinoma of the kidney are scarce and do not provide evidence of an association with tea drinking.

(b) Pancreatic cancer

The effect of tea consumption was examined in four cohort studies: three reported no association, and one documented a small protective effect.

Six case-control studies were designed to evaluate the relationship between tea consumption and pancreatic cancer: one showed a positive association.

(c) Breast cancer

None of five studies in which results on tea consumption were presented showed an association with breast cancer.

(d) Ovarian cancer

In two case-control studies, there was no association between tea consumption and ovarian cancer.

(e) Cancer of the large bowel

One cohort study found a strong positive dose-response relationship for cancer of the rectum, but another indicated no relationship with rectal cancer and a nonsignificant 'protective' effect for colon cancer.

The association between tea consumption and cancer of the colon and rectum was investigated in four case-control studies. Two showed no association. One study found a decreased risk for cancer of the rectum but not for cancer of the colon among drinkers of black tea relative to nondrinkers; another found an increased risk in the high consumption group. Taken together, these studies do not suggest the existence of an association.

(f) Gastric cancer

One cohort study found an increased risk for gastric cancer, which remained after inadequate adjustment for social class.

The role of tea drinking as a risk factor for cancer of the stomach was considered in five case-control studies. Four of these found no association. A negative association was observed in one study, but no dose-response relationship was seen.

(g) Cancer of the oesophagus

Five case-control studies were carried out, in Iran, the USSR, Brazil and Singapore, to investigate the effect of tea drinking on the frequency of cancer of the oesophagus. One study in Brazil did not show an association between tea drinking and oesophageal cancer, but the subjects were not asked about the temperature at which they drank tea. The other four studies, three of which were conducted in the Caspian area, stressed the role of the temperature of tea. All four studies showed that ingestion of very hot tea was associated with a two- to three-fold increase in the risk for oesophageal cancer. Only one of these studies investigated the effect of frequency of tea ingestion irrespective of temperature; no association was found. Taken together, these studies suggest that the temperature may be more important than the composition of the beverage, but the results are not conclusive.

One case-control study on oral cancer and one on cancer of the extrahepatic bile ducts reported no clear association with tea drinking.

(h) Nasopharyngeal cancer

Three case-control studies showed no evidence of an association between tea drinking and nasopharyngeal cancer.

(i) Cancers at other sites

One cohort study found no association with liver cancer. Another showed a significant positive dose-response relationship for lung cancer after adjusting for age and smoking; these findings could, however, be attributed to residual confounding by smoking.

One case-control study showed no association between tea drinking and cancer of the vulva. Another indicated a possible effect of maternal tea drinking during pregnancy on the frequency of Wilms' tumour in the offspring.

4.4 Other relevant data

The few informative studies concerning the effect of tea consumption during pregnancy on the frequency of adverse reproductive effects did not show an association.

In a number of studies, no association was seen between consumption of tea and the frequency of coronary heart disease.

Black tea, green tea and several unspecified teas were mutagenic to bacteria. Teas were found to reduce the activity of known mutagens both *in vivo* and *in vitro*.

4.5 Evaluation[1]

There is *inadequate evidence* for the carcinogenicity in humans of tea drinking. There is *inadequate evidence* for the carcinogenicity in experimental animals of tea.

Overall evaluation

Tea is *not classifiable as to its carcinogenicity to humans (Group 3)*.

5. References

Alejandre-Durán, E., Alonson-Moraga, A. & Pueyo, C. (1987) Implication of active oxygen species in the direct-acting mutagenicity of tea. *Mutat. Res.*, *188*, 251-257

Ali, M., Hayat, L.H.J., Al Saleh, J. & Gubler, C.J. (1989) Effect of consumption of green and black tea on the level of various enzymes in rats. *Experientia*, *45*, 112-114

Anon. (1974) 'Tea-gruel' as a possible factor of the esophagus. *Indian J. Cancer*, *11*, 232-233

Arab, L., Kohlmeier, M., Schlierf, G. & Schettler, G. (1983) Coffee and cholesterol (Letter to the Editor). *New Engl. J. Med.*, *309*, 1250

Ariza, R.R., Dorado, G., Barbancho, M. & Pueyo, C. (1988) Studies of the causes of direct-acting mutagenicity in coffee and tea using the Ara test in *Salmonella typhimurium*. *Mutat. Res.*, *201*, 89-96

Armstrong, B. & Doll, R. (1975) Environmental factors and cancer incidence and mortality in different countries, with special reference to dietary practices. *Int. J. Cancer*, *15*, 617-631

Armstrong, B., Garrod, A. & Doll, R. (1976) A retrospective study of renal cancer with special reference to coffee and animal protein consumption. *Br. J. Cancer*, *33*, 127-136

Barone, J.J. & Roberts, H.R. (1984) Human consumption of caffeine. In: Dews, P.B., ed., *Caffeine. Perspectives from Recent Research*, Berlin, Springer, pp. 59-73

Bashirov, M.S., Nugmanov, S.N., Kolycheva, N.I. (1968) Epidemiological study of oesophageal cancer in the Akhtubinsk region of the Kazakh Socialist Republic (Russ.). *Vopr. Onkol.*, *14*, 3-7

Belitz, H.D. & Grosch, W. (1986) *Food Chemistry*, Berlin, Springer, pp. 693-701

Berkowitz, G.S., Holford, T.R. & Berkowitz, R.L. (1982) Effects of cigarette smoking, alcohol, coffee and tea consumption on preterm delivery. *Early human Dev.*, *7*, 239-250

Bogovski, P., Day, N., Chvedoff, M. & Lafaverges, F. (1977) Accelerating action of tea on mouse skin carcinogenesis. *Cancer Lett.*, *3*, 9-13

---

[1]For definition of the italicized terms, see Preamble, pp. 27-31.

Bokuchava, M.A. & Skobeleva, N.I. (1986) Tea aroma. In: Morton, I.D. & MacLeod, A.J., eds, *Food Flavours*, Part B, *The Flavour of Beverages*, Amsterdam, Elsevier, pp. 49-84

Boston Collaborative Drug Surveillance Program (1972) Coffee drinking and acute myocardial infarction. *Lancet*, ii, 1278-1281

Brooke, O.G., Anderson, H.R., Bland, J.M., Peacock, J.L. & Stewart, C.M. (1989) Effects on birth weight of smoking, alcohol, caffeine, socioeconomic factors and psychosocial stress. *Br. med. J.*, 298, 795-801

Bunker, M.L. & McWilliams, M. (1979) Caffeine content of common beverages. *J. Am. diet. Assoc.*, 74, 28-32

Bunin, G.R., Kramer, S., Marrero, O. & Meadows, A.T. (1987) Gestational risk factors for Wilms' tumor: results of a case-control study. *Cancer Res.*, 47, 2972-2977

Byers, T., Marshall, J., Graham, S., Mettlin, C. & Swanson, M. (1983) A case-control study of dietary and nondietary factors in ovarian cancer. *J. natl Cancer Inst.*, 71, 681-686

Caan, B.J. & Goldhaber, M.K. (1989) Caffeinated beverages and low birthweight: a case-control study. *Am. J. public Health*, 79, 1299-1300

Claude, J., Kunze, E., Frentzel-Beyme, R., Paczkowski, K., Schneider, J. & Schubert, H. (1986) Life-style and occupational risk factors in cancer of the lower urinary tract. *Am. J. Epidemiol.*, 124, 578-589

Cloughley, J.B. (1983) Factors influencing the caffeine content of black tea. Part 2. The effect of production variables. *Food Chem.*, 10, 25-34

Cook-Mozaffari, P.J., Azordegan, F., Day, N.E., Ressicaud, A., Sabai, C. & Aramesh, B. (1979) Oesophageal cancer studies in the Caspian littoral of Iran: results of a case-control study. *Br. J. Cancer*, 39, 293-309

Curb, J.D., Reed, D.M., Kautz, J.A. & Yano, K. (1986) Coffee, caffeine, and serum cholesterol in Japanese men in Hawaii. *Am. J. Epidemiol.*, 123, 648-655

Cuzick, J. & Babiker, A.G. (1989) Pancreatic cancer, alcohol, diabetes mellitus and gall-bladder disease. *Int. J. Cancer*, 43, 415-421

Eden, T. (1976) *Tea*, 3rd ed., London, Longman

Forrest, D. (1985) *The World Tea Trade: A Survey of the Production, Distribution and Consumption of Tea*, Cambridge, Woodhead-Faulkner Ltd

Franco, E.L., Kowalski, L.P., Oliveira, B.V., Curado, M.P., Pereira, R.N., Silva, M.E., Fava, A.S. & Torloni, H. (1989) Risk factors for oral cancer in Brazil: a case-control study. *Int. J. Cancer*, 43, 992-1000

Fujita, Y., Yamane, T., Tanaka, M., Kuwata, K., Okuzumi, J., Takahashi, T., Fujiki, H. & Okuda, T. (1989) Inhibitory effect of (-)-epigallocatechin gallate on carcinogenesis with N-ethyl-N'-nitro-N-nitrosoguanidine in mouse duodenum. *Jpn. J. Cancer Res.*, 80, 503-505

Furuhashi, N., Sato, S., Suzuki, M., Hiruta, M., Tanaka, M. & Takahashi, T. (1985) Effects of caffeine ingestion during pregnancy. *Gynecol. obstet. Invest.*, 19, 187-191

Ghadirian, P. (1987) Thermal irritation and esophageal cancer in northern Iran. *Cancer*, 60, 1909-1914

Goodman, M.T., Morgenstern, H. & Wynder, E.L. (1986) A case-control study of factors affecting the development of renal cell cancer. *Am. J. Epidemiol.*, 124, 926-941

Graham, H.N. (1983) Tea. In: Mark, H.F., Othmer, D.R., Overberger, C.G., Seaborg, G.T. & Grayson, M., eds, *Kirk-Othmer Encyclopedia of Chemical Technology*, 3rd ed., Vol. 22, New York, John Wiley & Sons, pp. 628-644

Graham, H.N. (1984) Tea; the plant and its manufacture; chemistry and consumption of the beverage. In: Spiller, G.A., ed., *The Methylxanthine Beverages and Foods: Chemistry, Consumption and Health Effects*, New York, Alan R. Liss, pp. 29-74

Graham, S., Lilienfeld, A.M. & Tidings, J.E. (1967) Dietary and purgation factors in the epidemiology of gastric cancer. *Cancer*, 20, 2224-2234

Green, M. & Jucha, E. (1986) Association of serum lipids with coffee, tea, and egg consumption in free-living subjects. *J. Epidemiol. Community Health*, 40, 324-329

Haffner, S.M., Knapp, J.A., Stern, M.P., Hazuda, H.P., Rosenthal, M. & Franco, L.J. (1985) Coffee consumption, diet, and lipids. *Am. J. Epidemiol.*, 122, 1-12

Hartge, P., Hoover, R., West, D.W. & Lyon, J.L. (1983) Coffee drinking and risk of bladder cancer. *J. natl Cancer Inst.*, 70, 1021-1026

Hashimoto, F., Nonaka, G.-I. & Nishioka, I. (1989) Tannins and related compounds. LXXVII. Novel chalcan-flavan dimers, assamicains A, B and C, and a new flavan-3-ol and proanthocyanidins from the fresh leaves of *Camellia sinensis* L. var. *assamica* Kitamura. *Chem. pharm. Bull.*, 37, 77-85

Hayashi, T. & Shibamoto, T. (1985) Analysis of methyl glyoxal in foods and beverages. *J. agric. Food Chem.*, 33, 1090-1093

Heilbrun, L.K., Nomura, A. & Stemmermann, G.N. (1986) Black tea consumption and cancer risk: a prospective study. *Br. J. Cancer*, 54, 677-683

Henderson, B.E., Louie, E., Jing, J.S.-H., Buell, P. & Gardner, M.B. (1976) Risk factors associated with nasopharyngeal carcinoma. *New Engl. J. Med.*, 295, 1101-1106

Hiatt, R.A., Klatsky, A.L. & Armstrong, M.A. (1988) Pancreatic cancer, blood glucose and beverage consumption. *Int. J. Cancer*, 41, 794-797

Higginson, J. (1966) Etiological factors in gastrointestinal cancer in man. *J. natl Cancer Inst.*, 37, 527-545

Hormozdiari, H., Day, N.E., Aramesh, B. & Mahboubi, E. (1975) Dietary factors and esophageal cancer in the Caspian littoral of Iran. *Cancer Res.*, 35, 3493-3498

Howe, G.R., Burch, J.D., Miller, A.B., Cook, G.M., Estève, J., Morrison, B., Gordon, P., Chambers, L.W., Fodor, G. & Winsor, G.M. (1980) Tobacco use, occupation, coffee, various nutrients and bladder cancer. *J. natl Cancer Inst.*, 64, 701-713

IARC (1983a) *IARC Monographs on the Evaluation of the Carcinogenic Risk of Chemicals to Humans*, Vol. 31, *Some Food Additives, Feed Additives and Naturally Occurring Substances*, Lyon, pp. 171-178

IARC (1983b) *IARC Monographs on the Evaluation of the Carcinogenic Risk of Chemicals to Humans*, Vol. 31, *Some Food Additives, Feed Additives and Naturally Occurring Substances*, Lyon, pp. 213-229

International Organization for Standardization (1981) *Black Tea — Specification* (International Standard (ISO 3720)), London

International Tea Committee (1989) *Annual Bulletin of Statistics*, London

Iscovich, J., Castelletto, R., Estève, J., Munõz, N., Colanzi, R., Coronel, A., Deamezola, I., Tassi, V. & Arslan, A. (1987) Tobacco smoking, occupational exposure and bladder cancer in Argentina. *Int. J. Cancer*, *40*, 734-740

Ishii, K., Nakamura, K., Takeuchi, T. & Hirayama, T. (1973) Chronic calcifying pancreatitis and pancreatic carcinoma in Japan. *Digestion*, *9*, 429-437

Ito, Y., Ohnishi, S. & Fujie, K. (1989) Chromosome aberrations induced by aflatoxin B_1 in rat bone marrow cells *in vivo* and their suppression by green tea. *Mutat. Res.*, *222*, 253-261

Jain, A.K., Shimoi, K., Nakamura, Y., Kada, T., Hara, Y. & Tomita, I. (1989a) Crude tea extracts decrease the mutagenic activity of *N*-methyl-*N*'-nitro-*N*-nitrosoguanidine *in vitro* and in intragastric tract of rats. *Mutat. Res.*, *210*, 1-8

Jain, A.K., Shimoi, K., Nakamura, Y., Sano, M. & Tomita, I. (1989b) Effect of tea on 12-0-tetradecanoyl-phorbol-13 acetate (TPA) induced promotion of transformation in JB6 mouse epidermal cells. *Indian J. Cancer*, *26*, 92-98

Jensen, O.M., Wahrendorf, J., Knudsen, J.B. & Sørensen, B.L. (1986) The Copenhagen case-control study of bladder cancer. II. Effect of coffee and other beverages. *Int. J. Cancer*, *37*, 651-657

Jick, H., Miettinen, O.S., Neff, R.K., Shapiro, S., Heinonen, O.P. & Slone, D. (1973) Coffee and myocardial infarction. *New Engl. J. Med.*, *289*, 63-67

Joint Iran-International Agency for Research on Cancer Study Group (1977) Esophageal cancer studies in the Caspian littoral of Iran: results of population studies — a prodrome. *J. natl Cancer Inst.*, *59*, 1127-1138

Joner, P.E. & Dommarsnes, K. (1983) Effects of herbal and ordinary teas on the mutagenicity of benzo[*a*]pyrene in the Ames test. *Acta agric. scand.*, *33*, 53-56

de Jong, U.W., Breslow, N., Hong, J.G.E., Sridharan, M. & Shanmugaratnam, K. (1974) Aetiological factors in oesophageal cancer in Singapore Chinese. *Int. J. Cancer*, *13*, 291-303

Kada, T., Kaneko, K., Matsuzaki, S., Matsuzaki, T. & Hara, Y. (1985) Detection and chemical identification of natural bio-antimutagens. *Mutat. Res.*, *150*, 127-132

Kaiser, H.E. (1967) Cancer-promoting effects of phenols in tea. *Cancer*, *20*, 614-616

Kapadia, G.J., Paul, B.D., Chung, E.B., Ghosh, B. & Pradhan, S.N. (1976) Carcinogenicity of *Camellia sinensis* (tea) and some tannin-containing folk medicinal herbs administered subcutaneously in rats. *J. natl Cancer Inst.*, *57*, 207-209

Kaufman, B.D., Liberman, I.S. & Tyshetsky, V.I. (1965) Some data concerning the incidence of oesophageal cancer in the Gurjev region of the Kazakh SSR (Russ.). *Vopr. Onkol.*, *11*, 78-85

Kazi, T. (1985) Determination of caffeine and other pure alkaloids in coffee and tea products by high performance liquid chromatography. In: *11e Colloque Scientifique International sur le Café, Lomé, 1985*, Paris, Association Scientifique Internationale du Café, pp. 227-244

Khan, W.A., Wang, Z.Y., Athar, M., Bickers, D.R. & Mukhtar, H. (1988) Inhibition of the skin tumorigenicity of ($\pm$)-7β,8α-dihydroxy-9α,10α-epoxy-7,8,9,10-tetrahydrobenzo-[*a*]pyrene by tannic acid, green tea polyphenols and quercetin in Sencar mice. *Cancer Lett.*, *42*, 7-12

Kinlen, L.J. & McPherson, K. (1984) Pancreas cancer and coffee and tea consumption: a case-control study. *Br. J. Cancer, 49*, 93-96

Kinlen, L.J., Willows, A.N., Goldblatt, P. & Yudkin, J. (1988) Tea consumption and cancer. *Br. J. Cancer, 58*, 397-401

Klatsky, A.L., Petitti, D.B., Armstrong, M.A. & Friedman, G.D. (1985) Coffee, tea and cholesterol. *Am. J. Cardiol., 55*, 577-578

Kojima, H., Miwa, N., Mori, M., Osaki, M. & Konishi, H. (1989) Desmutagenic effect of Oolong tea. *J. Food Hyg. Soc. Jpn, 30*, 233-239

Kono, S., Ikeda, M., Tokudome, S. & Kuratsune, M. (1988) A case-control study of gastric cancer and diet in northern Kyushu, Japan. *Jpn. J. Cancer Res. (Gann), 79*, 1067-1074

Kosuge, M., Aisaka, H. & Yamanishi, T. (1981) Flavor constituents of chinese and Japanese pan-fired green teas (Jpn.). *Eiyot Shokuryo, 34*, 545-549

La Vecchia, C., Talamini, R., Decarli, A., Franceschi, S., Parazzini, F. & Tognoni, G. (1986) Coffee consumption and the risk of breast cancer. *Surgery, 100*, 477-481

La Vecchia, C., Liati, P., Decarli, A., Negri, E. & Francheschi, S. (1987) Coffee consumption and risk of pancreatic cancer. *Int. J. Cancer, 40*, 309-313

La Vecchia, C., Negri, E., Decarli, A., D'Avanzo, B., Gallotti, L., Gentile, A. & Franceschi, S. (1988) A case-control study of diet and colo-rectal cancer in northern Italy. *Int. J. Cancer, 41*, 492-498

La Vecchia, C., Negri, E., Decarli, A., D'Avanzo, B., Liberati, C. & Franceschi, S. (1989) Dietary factors in the risk of bladder cancer. *Nutr. Cancer, 12*, 93-101

Lawson, D.H., Jick, H. & Rothman, K.J. (1981) Coffee and tea consumption and breast disease. *Surgery, 90*, 801-803

Lewis, J. & Morgan, W.K.C. (1989) Tea asthma: response to specific and non-specific challenges. *Br. J. ind. Med., 46*, 350-351

Lin, T.M., Chen, K.P., Lin, C.C., Hsu, M.M., Tu, S.M., Chiang, T.C., Jung, P.F. & Hirayama, T. (1973) Retrospective study of nasopharyngeal carcinomas. *J. natl Cancer Inst., 51*, 1403-1408

Little, J.A., Snanoff, H.M., Csima, A. & Yano, R. (1986) Coffee and serum-lipids in coronary heart-disease. *Lancet, i*, 732-734

Lubin, F., Ron, E., Wax, Y., Funaro, M., Shitrit, A., Black, M. & Modan, B. (1984) Coffee and methylxanthine in benign and malignant breast diseases. In: MacMahon, B. & Sugimura, T., eds, *Coffee and Health* (Banbury Report 17), Cold Spring Harbor, NY, CSH Press, pp. 177-187

Lubin, F., Ron, E., Wax, Y. & Modan, B. (1985) Coffee and methylxanthines and breast cancer: a case-control study. *J. natl Cancer Inst., 74*, 569-573

Maarse, H. & Visscher, C.A. (1986) *Volatile Compounds in Food. Qualitative Data* (Supplement 3), Zeist, Central Institute for Nutrition and Food Research, TNO

Mabuchi, K., Bross, D.S. & Kessler, I.I. (1985a) Risk factors for male breast cancer. *J. natl Cancer Inst., 74*, 371-375

Mabuchi, K., Bross, D.S. & Kessler, I.I. (1985b) Epidemiology of cancer of the vulva. A case-control study. *Cancer, 55*, 1843-1848

Mack, T.M., Yu, M.C., Hanisch, R. & Henderson, B.E. (1986) Pancreas cancer and smoking, beverage consumption, and past medical history. *J. natl Cancer Inst.*, *76*, 49-60

MacMahon, B., Yen, S., Trichopoulos, D., Warren, K. & Nardi, G. (1981) Coffee and cancer of the pancreas. *New Engl. J. Med.*, *304*, 630-633

Mahboubi, E.O. & Aramesh, B. (1980) Epidemiology of esophageal cancer in Iran, with special reference to nutritional and cultural aspects. *Prev. Med.*, *9*, 613-621

Martin, T.R & Bracken, M.B. (1987) The association between low birth weight and caffeine consumption during pregnancy. *Am. J. Epidemiol.*, *126*, 813-821

McCredie, M., Ford, J.M. & Stewart, J.H. (1988) Risk factors for cancer of the renal parenchyma. *Int. J. Cancer*, *42*, 13-16

McLaughlin, J.K., Blot, W.J., Mandel, J.S., Schuman, L.M., Mehl, E.S. & Fraumeni, J.F., Jr (1983) Etiology of cancer of the renal pelvis. *J. natl Cancer Inst.*, *71*, 287-291

McLaughlin, J.K., Mandel, J.S., Blot, W.J., Schuman, L.M., Mehl, E.S. & Fraumeni, J.F. (1984) A population-based case-control study of renal cell carcinoma. *J. natl Cancer Inst.*, *72*, 275-284

Miller, C.T., Neutel, C.I., Nair, R.C., Marrett, L.D., Last, J.M. & Collins, W.E. (1978) Relative importance of risk factors in bladder carcinogenesis. *J. chron. Dis.*, *31*, 51-56

Miller, D.R., Rosenberg, L., Helmrich, S.P., Kaufman, D.W. & Shapiro, S. (1984) Ovarian cancer and coffee drinking. In: MacMahon, B. & Sugimura, T., eds, *Coffee and Health* (Banbury Report 17), Cold Spring Harbor, NY, CSH Press, pp. 157-165

Miller, D.R., Rosenberg, L., Kaufman, D.W., Helmrich, S.P., Schottenfeld, D., Lewis, J., Stolley, P.D., Rosenshein, N. & Shapiro, S. (1987) Epithelial ovarian cancer and coffee drinking. *Int. J. Epidemiol.*, *16*, 13-17

Millin, D.J. (1987) Factors affecting the quality of tea. In: Herschdoerfer, S.M., ed., *Quality Control in the Food Industry*, 2nd ed, Vol. 4, London, Academic Press, pp. 127-160

Morgan, R.W. & Jain, M.G. (1974) Bladder cancer: smoking, beverages and artificial sweeteners. *Can. med. Assoc. J.*, *111*, 1067-1070

Morrison, A.S., Buring, J.E., Verhoek, W.G., Aoki, K., Leck, I., Ohno, Y. & Obata, K. (1982) Coffee drinking and cancer of the lower urinary tract. *J. natl Cancer Inst.*, *68*, 91-94

Nagao, M., Takahashi, Y., Yamanaka, H. & Sugimura, T. (1979) Mutagens in tea and coffee. *Mutat. Res.*, *68*, 101-106

Nagao, M., Fujita, Y., Wakabayashi, K., Nukaya, H., Kosuge, T. & Sugimura, T. (1986) Mutagens in coffee and other beverages. *Environ. Health Perspect.*, *67*, 89-91

Ohno, Y., Aoki, K., Obata, K. & Morrison, A.S. (1985) Case-control study of urinary bladder cancer in metropolitan Nagoya. *Natl Cancer Inst. Monogr.*, *69*, 229-234

Phelps, H.M. & Phelps, C.E. (1988) Caffeine ingestion and breast cancer. A negative correlation. *Cancer*, *61*, 1051-1054

Raymond, L., Infante, F., Tuyns, A.J., Voirol, M. & Lowenfels, A.B. (1987) Diet and cancer of the pancreas (Fr.). *Gastroenterol. clin. Biol.*, *11*, 488-492

Risch, H.A., Burch, J.D., Miller, A.B., Hill, G.B., Steele, R. & Howe, G.R. (1988) Dietary factors and the incidence of cancer of the urinary bladder. *Am. J. Epidemiol.*, *127*, 1179-1191

Rosenberg, L., Slone, D., Shapiro, S., Kaufman, D.W., Stolley, P.D. & Miettinen, O.S. (1980) Coffee drinking and myocardial infarction in young women. *Am. J. Epidemiol.*, *111*, 675-681

Rosenberg, L., Mitchell, A.A., Shapiro, S. & Slone, D. (1982) Selected birth defects in relation to caffeine-containing beverages. *J. Am. med. Assoc.*, *247*, 1429-1432

Rosenberg, L., Miller, D.R., Helmrich, S.P., Kaufman, D.W. & Shapiro, S. (1984) Breast cancer and coffee drinking. In: MacMahon, B. & Sugimura, T., eds, *Coffee and Health* (Banbury Report 17), Cold Spring Harbor, NY, CSH Press, pp. 189-195

Rosenberg, L., Miller, D.R., Helmrich, S.P., Kaufman, D.W., Schottenfeld, D., Stolley, P.D. & Shapiro, S. (1985) Breast cancer and the consumption of coffee. *Am. J. Epidemiol.*, *122*, 391-399

Rossignol, A.M. (1985) Caffeine-containing beverages and premenstrual syndrome in young women. *Am. J. public Health*, *75*, 1335-1337

Rossignol, A.M., Zhang, J., Chen, Y. & Xiang, Z. (1989) Tea and premenstrual syndrome in the People's Republic of China. *Am. J. public Health*, *79*, 67-69

Ruch, R.J., Cheng, S.-J. & Klaunig, J.E. (1989) Prevention of cytotoxicity and inhibition of intercellular communication by antioxidant catechins isolated from Chinese green tea. *Carcinogenesis*, *10*, 1003-1008

Ruschenburg, U. (1985) Benzo[a]pyrene content of coffee and some other foodstuffs (Ger.). In: *11e Colloque Scientifique International sur le Café, Lomé, 1985*, Paris, Association Scientifique Internationale du Café, pp. 205-212

Saijo, R. & Kuwabara, Y. (1967) Volatile flavor of black tea. Part I. Formation of volatile components during black tea manufacture. *Agric. biol. Chem.*, *31*, 389-396

Sanderson, G.W. (1972) The chemistry of tea and tea manufacturing. In: Runeckles, V.C. & Tso, T.C., eds, *Recent Advances in Phytochemistry*, Vol. 5, *Structural and Functional Aspects of Phytochemistry*, New York, Academic Press, pp. 247-316

Schairer, C., Brinton, L.A. & Hoover, R.N. (1987) Methylxanthines and breast cancer. *Int. J. Cancer*, *40*, 469-473

Schapira, J., Schapira, D. & Schapira, K. (1975) *The Book of Coffee and Tea*, New York, St Martin's Press

Schreier, P. & Mick, W. (1984) Analytical differentiation of two qualities of black tea by capillary gas chromatography-mass spectrometry (Ger.). *Chem. Mikrobiol. Technol. Lebensmittel.*, *8*, 97-104

Segi, M. (1975) Tea-gruel as a possible factor for cancer of the esophagus. *Gann*, *66*, 199-202

Shanmugaratnam, K., Tye, C.Y., Goh, E.H. & Chia, K.B. (1978) Etiological factors in nasopharyngeal carcinoma: a hospital-based, retrospective, case-control, questionnaire study. In: de-Thé, G. & Ito, Y., eds, *Nasopharyngeal Carcinoma. Etiology and Control* (IARC Scientific Publications No. 20), Lyon, IARC, pp. 199-212

Simon, D., Yen, S. & Cole, P. (1975) Coffee drinking and cancer of the lower urinary tract. *J. natl Cancer Inst.*, *54*, 587-591

Skobeleva, N.I., Bezzubov, A.A., Petrova, T.A. & Bokuchava, M.A. (1979) Aroma-forming substances in black tea. *Appl. Biochem. Microbiol.*, *15*, 682-687

Slattery, M.L., West, D.W. & Robison, L.M. (1988) Fluid intake and bladder cancer in Utah. *Int. J. Cancer*, *42*, 17-22

Spiller, G.A., ed. (1984) *The Methylxanthine Beverages and Foods: Chemistry, Consumption, and Health Effects*, New York, Alan R. Liss

Srisuphan, W. & Bracken, M.B. (1986) Caffeine consumption during pregnancy and association with late spontaneous abortion. *Am. J. Obstet. Gynecol.*, *154*, 14-20

Stavric, B., Klassen, R., Watkinson, B., Karpinski, K., Stapley, R. & Fried, P. (1988) Variability in caffeine consumption from coffee and tea: possible significance for epidemiological studies. *Food chem. Toxicol.*, *26*, 111-118

Stich, H.F., Chan, P.K.L. & Rosen, M.P. (1982a) Inhibitory effects of phenolics, teas and saliva on the formation of mutagenic nitrosation products of salted fish. *Int. J. Cancer*, *30*, 719-724

Stich, H.F., Rosin, M.P. & Bryson, L. (1982b) Inhibition of mutagenicity of a model nitrosation reaction by naturally occurring phenolics, coffee and tea. *Mutat. Res.*, *95*, 119-128

Stocks, P. (1970) Cancer mortality in relation to national consumption of cigarettes, solid fuel, tea and coffee. *Br. J. Cancer*, *24*, 215-225

van Straten, S., Maarse, H., de Beauvaser, J.C. & Visscher, C.A., eds (1983) *Volatile Compounds in Food — Quantitative Data*, Vol. 2 (Sections 73.1-73.10), Zeist, Central Institute for Nutrition and Food Research, TNO

Sugimura, T. (1982) Mutagens in cooked food. In: Fleck, R.A. & Hollaender, A., eds, *Genetic Toxicology*, New York, Plenum Press, pp. 243-269

Sugimura, T. & Sato, S. (1983) Mutagens-carcinogens in foods. *Cancer Res.*, *43 (Suppl.)*, 2415s-2421s

Tajima, K. & Tominaga, S. (1985) Dietary habits and gastro-intestinal cancers: a comparative case-control study of stomach and large intestinal cancers in Nagoya, Japan. *Jpn. J. Cancer Res. (Gann)*, *76*, 705-716

Trichopoulos, D., Ouranos, G., Day, N.E., Tzonou, A., Manousos, O., Papadimitriou, C. & Trichopoulou, A. (1985) Diet and cancer of the stomach: a case-control study in Greece. *Int. J. Cancer*, *36*, 291-297

Tuomilehto, J., Tanskanen, A., Pietinen, P., Aro, A., Salonen, J.T., Happonen, P., Nissinen, A. & Puska, P. (1987) Coffee consumption is correlated with serum cholesterol in middle-aged Finnish men and women. *J. Epidemiol. Community Health*, *41*, 237-242

Ullah, M.R., Gogoi, N. & Baruah, D. (1984) The effect of withering on fermentation of tea leaf and development of liquor characters of black teas. *J. Sci. Food Agric.*, *35*, 1142-1147

US Department of Agriculture (1989) *World Tea Situation* (FTEA 3-89), Washington DC

US Food and Drug Administration (1984) The latest caffeine scorecard. *FDA Consumer*, March, 14

Uyeta, M., Taue, S. & Mazaki, M. (1981) Mutagenicity of hydrolysates of tea infusions. *Mutat. Res.*, *88*, 233-240

Victora, C.G., Muñoz, N., Day, N.E., Barcelos, L.B., Peccin, D.A. & Braga, N.M. (1987) Hot beverages and oesophageal cancer in southern Brazil: a case-control study. *Int. J. Cancer*, *39*, 710-716

Wang, Z.Y., Khan, W.A., Bickers, D.R. & Mukhtar, H. (1989a) Protection against polycyclic aromatic hydrocarbon-induced skin tumor initiation in mice by green tea polyphenols. *Carcinogenesis*, 10, 411-415

Wang, Z.Y., Cheng, S.J., Zhou, Z.C., Athar, M., Khan, W.A., Bickers, D.R. & Mukhtar, H. (1989b) Antimutagenic activity of green tea polyphenols. *Mutat. Res.*, 223, 273-285

Watanabe, Y., Tada, M., Kawamoto, K., Uozumi, G., Kajiwara, Y., Hayashi, K., Yamaguchi, K., Murakami, K., Misaki, T., Akasaka, Y. & Kawai, K. (1984) A case-control study of cancer of the rectum and the colon (Jpn.). *Nippon Shokakibyo Gakkai Zasshi*, 81, 185-193

Watkinson, B. & Fried, P.A. (1985) Maternal caffeine use before, during and after pregnancy and effects upon offspring. *Neurobehav. Toxicol. Teratol.*, 7, 9-17

Whittemore, A.S., Paffenbarger, R.S., Jr, Anderson, K. & Halpern, J. (1983) Early precursors of pancreatic cancer in college men. *J. chron. Dis.*, 36, 251-256

Wickremasinghe, R.L. (1978) Tea. In: Chichester, C.O., Mark, E.M. & Stewart, G.E., eds, *Advances in Food Research*, Vol. 24, New York, Academic Press, pp. 229-286

Wickremasinghe, R. & Swain, T. (1965) Studies on the quality and flavour of Ceylon tea. *J. Sci. Food Agric.*, 16, 57-64

Woodward, N.H. (1980) *Teas of the World*, New York, Collier, p. 184

Yamanishi, T. (1986) Chemical changes during storage of tea. In: Charalambous, G., ed., *Handbook of Food and Beverage Stability*, London, Academic Press, pp. 665-683

Yang, J.A., Huber, S.A. & Lucas, Z.J. (1979) Inhibition of DNA synthesis in cultured lymphocytes and tumor cells by extracts of betel nut, tobacco, and miang leaf, plant substances associated with cancer of the ororespiratory epithelium. *Cancer Res.*, 39, 4802-4809

Yen, S., Hsieh, C.-C. & MacMahon, B. (1987) Extrahepatic bile duct cancer and smoking, beverage consumption, past medical history, and oral-contraceptive use. *Cancer*, 59, 2112-2116

Yu, M.C., Mack, T.M., Hanisch, R., Cicioni, C. & Henderson, B.E. (1986) Cigarette smoking, obesity, diuretic use, and coffee consumption as risk factors for renal cell carcinoma. *J. natl Cancer Inst.*, 77, 351-356

MATE

1. Production and Use

1.1 Introduction

Mate is native to the area of South America between 18° and 25° S latitude and from the Atlantic Ocean to the Paraguay River. This area takes in a portion of southern Brazil and Paraguay, Uruguay and northern Argentina. The plant was used to make a beverage by the indigenous populations of the area long before the first Spanish colonists arrived early in the sixteenth century. Jesuit priests who arrived in the middle of the century gradually took over control of most of the producing areas and began cultivation of selected varieties to ensure supply. Virtually all of Argentinian and Brazilian production is now cultivated, while much of Paraguayan production is derived from wild plants (Graham, 1984).

1.2 Production processes

(a) Botany and culture

Mate ('Yerba mate', 'Jesuits' tea', 'Paraguayan tea', 'yerba') is prepared from the leaves of *Ilex paraguariensis* St. Hil, a member of the Aquifoliaceae (holly) family, which is native to Paraguay and Argentina. The tree can grow to 12-16 m in the wild but is usually cultivated as a shrub 3-6 m tall with numerous stems. The leaves are dark-green, 15-20 cm long and short-stalked with an acuminate tip and finely dentated edges. It has small white flowers, which grow in forked clusters in the axils of the leaves, and violet-black berries, each of which contains four to eight seeds (Graham, 1984; Vázquez & Moyna, 1986).

Mate is propagated by seed; the seedlings are transplanted to a shaded nursery where they remain for 9-12 months, and are finally transferred to the plantation when they reach a height of 30-80 cm. During the first year, the plant must be protected against wind and low temperatures. Plantations consist of 800-1000 trees per hectare pruned to a height of 3-6 m to facilitate harvesting. Harvesting, which can start in the fourth or fifth year, is annual and takes place from May to October;

it consists of cutting off smaller leafy branches with a knife. A good plantation yields 20-25 kg fresh leaves per tree (Graham, 1984).

(b) Processing

Information obtained from Graham (1984).

(i) *Traditional*

The trees are cleared of vines and smaller branches are cut off. These leaf-bearing branches are 'toasted' momentarily over an open fire to reduce the moisture content, but avoiding 'blackening'; this process is known as *supeco*. They are dried further by heating for 12-24 h on a platform of poles suspended over an open fire. An alternative procedure involves the use of a dome-shaped structure (*barbaqua*), over which the toasted branches are spread; hot air is conducted through a tunnel from a fire some distance away. This procedure avoids direct deposition of smoke on the leaf and requires 5-15 h.

Threshing separates leaf from bark and twigs. Further grading by sifting is carried out, and the product is packed in 30-60-kg bags and aged. Additional grading and blending is practised to provide greater uniformity.

(ii) *Modern*

The toasting step is now frequently carried out by passing the branches through a perforated rotating metal cylinder in an inclined position over an open fire for a very short time. The cylinders used are about 2-2.5 m in diameter and 4 m in length. This process is known as *sepecadora*.

The *barbaqua* step may be carried out in a specially constructed room with a frame above the floor to contain the leaves, which are dried with hot air conducted from a fire. Leaf temperatures reach 80-100°C. Some caffeine is lost at the higher temperature.

Further grinding and sifting are carried out, and many different grades of mate are made available. Ageing, which is extremely important to produce a palatable beverage, may take place over 6-18 months.

1.3 Production, trade and consumption

Production of all types of mate is concentrated in Argentina (Misiones, Corrientes; 172 000 tonnes in 1987), Brazil (Parana, Santa Catarina, Rio Grande do Sul; 80 000-120 000 tonnes per year) and Paraguay (60 000 tonnes per year) (Graham, 1984).

To prepare the mate, ground leaves are poured into a gourd to three-quarters of its internal volume, with the gourd's hole tilted about 30° from the vertical. The gourd is then held upright and warm water (60-80°C) is poured on the depressed side of the surface of the mate. The wet mate swells within 3-5 min, and a metal straw with a filtering head (known as a *bombilla*) is introduced to the bottom of the gourd. This step eliminates the possibility that the consumer will suck up powdered mate. Small volumes of hot water (90-95°C) are then poured onto the mate around the *bombilla*, and the consumer sips through the *bombilla* until the sound of air rushing in makes a typical chirping noise. This operation is repeated (and the gourd circulates around a group of drinkers if there are more than one) until the flavour diminishes. The *bombilla* is then removed and inserted into a different place in the mate ('turning the mate round'). Once the drink has lost its taste, the *cebadura* (the charge of yerba used and the operation of adding water) is finished (Vázquez & Moyna, 1986).

Mate is consumed mainly in Argentina, Bolivia, Brazil, Chile, Ecuador, Paraguay and Uruguay, usually as a hot beverage. To a much lesser extent, it is drunk in Germany as a cold beverage. It is also drunk chilled in Paraguay and southwestern Brazil, with milk or water and sugar. Burnt sugar, lemon or lime juice are sometimes added instead of milk; 20% of mate is drunk in this manner in Brazil. Consumption of mate in Argentina is increasing and was 162 329 tonnes in 1987 (equivalent to 5.14 kg *per caput*). Uruguay imports 18 000-24 000 tonnes per year, with an average annual consumption of 6-8 kg per person (Vázquez & Moyna, 1986).

Table 1 gives data on production, trade and consumption of mate in South America in 1977.

Table 1. Mate production, trade and consumption (in thousands of tonnes) in 1977[a]

Country	Production	Exports	Waste	Consumption	Consumption per caput (kg/year)
Paraguay	20	1	2	17	6.2
Uruguay	18	0	0	18	6.2
Argentina	143	4	0	139	5.4
Brazil	100	23	5	72	0.6
Chile	0	0	0	4	0.3
Total	281	28	7	250	

[a]From Gilbert (1984)

In Argentina, the commercial product must be free from extraneous matter, well preserved and must contain less than 11% moisture, 9% total ash, 1.5% ash in

10% hydrochloric acid and 15% fibre and more than 0.6% caffeine and 25% aqueous extract (Ministerio de Agricultura y Ganadería, 1971).

2. Chemical Composition

Two early accounts were given of the composition of the beverage mate, especially as consumed in several South American countries (Hauschild, 1935; Hegnauer, 1964). More recent estimates of its composition have been compiled by Graham (1984) and by Belitz and Grosch (1986), although these are brief and contain negligible reference to volatile components. Clifford and Ramirez-Martinez (1990) determined the caffeine and chlorogenic acid contents of a number of commercial packets of mate.

2.1 Nonvolatile compounds

(a) Caffeine and other purines

Graham (1984) stated that the caffeine content of the mate leaf was 0.9-2.2%, depending on the age of the leaf; whilst Belitz and Grosch (1986) stated that, while one-third of the total dry matter is solubilized with hot water, only half of the available caffeine is released, to give 19-28 mg/100 g of solution (brew). Côrtes (1953) measured 25 mg per 120-ml cup. These figures are reasonably consistent.

Dried mate leaves were analysed for methylxanthines by high-performance liquid chromatography, and caffeine was found at 0.56%, theobromine at 0.03% and theophylline at 0.02% (Vázquez & Moyna, 1986).

Stavric *et al.* (1988) analysed two samples of mate leaves (purchased in Ottawa, Canada) for extractable methylxanthines. After steeping 1 g of loose leaves for 2 min in 44 ml water, they found 7 mg (157 µg/ml) caffeine and 2 mg (45.7 µg/ml) theobromine. When the steeping time was increased to 5 min, the extractable caffeine and theobromine contents were 9 and 3 mg, respectively.

Clifford and Ramirez-Martinez (1990) recently examined five commercial samples of two types of mate leaf of South American origin, purchased in the UK and the Federal Republic of Germany, using high-performance liquid chromatography, and reported caffeine at 0.89-1.73% and theobromine at 0.45-0.88%, with very small quantities of other unidentified purine alkaloid-like components. Theophylline was not detected in these samples. Quantities were also assessed per cup, after following the instructions for use given on the packet, which were not necessarily South American practices; the amount of caffeine per cup was 12-33 mg and that of theobromine, 6-17 mg.

(b) *Chlorogenic acids*

Chlorogenic acids are a family of mono- and di-acyl quinic acids. Quinic acid is 1L-1(OH),3,4/5-tetrahydroxycyclohexane carboxylic acid. The common acylating residues are caffeic acid (3,4-dihydroxycinnamic acid), ferulic acid (3-methoxy-4-hydroxycinnamic acid) and *para*-coumaric acid (4-hydroxycinnamic acid), thus producing caffeoylquinic acids, dicaffeoylquinic acids, feruloylquinic acids, *para*-coumaroylquinic acids and caffeoylferuloylquinic acids. Two samples of mate leaf that yielded brown extracts contained 1.11-1.27% caffeoylquinic acids, 0.39-0.42% feruloylquinic acids, 0.62-1.12% dicaffeoylquinic acids and 2.88-2.89% total chlorogenic acids; levels of 4.53-4.71%, 0, 4.03-4.56% and 9.16-9.76%, respectively, were found in three samples yielding greenish extracts (Clifford & Ramirez-Martinez, 1990). The authors could not define which processes or species were responsible. They also analysed the brews and found that those made with the first two samples contained 16-41 mg caffeoylquinic acids and 1.8-9.5 mg dicaffeoylquinic acids per cup; the last three contained 107-133 mg caffeoylquinic acids and 36-44 mg per cup dicaffeoylquinic acids.

(c) *Other components*

Some other components are listed in Table 2.

Table 2. **Components of mate other than caffeine and other purines and chlorogenic acids**[a]

Component	Amount
Sucrose	3.33 (% dry wt of leaf)
Raffinose	0.44 (% dry wt of leaf)
Glucose	0.27 (% dry wt of leaf)
Fructose	0.16 (% dry wt of leaf)
Trigonelline	0.50 (% dry wt of leaf)
Choline	15 µg/g
Thiamine	1 µg/g
Riboflavin	Trace
Ascorbic acid	20 µg/g
Folic acid	16 µg/g
Total extractable ash	5.99 (% dry wt of leaf)

[a]From Graham (1984)

Some 60 species of plants occur in some samples of mate along with *I. paraguariensis* (Graham, 1984).

Aglycones of the family Aquifoliaceae that have been identified in mate are rutin (quercetin-3-*O*-rutinoside), quercetin-3-*O*-glucoside and kaempferol-3-*O*-

rutinoside. Triterpenes can also be found. The main component is ursolic acid (Ohem & Hölzl, 1988).

2.2 Volatile compounds

No data were available.

2.3 Contaminants

Ruschenburg (1985) reported the presence of relatively large quantities (24-461 µg/kg) of benzo[*a*]pyrene in eight commercial samples of mate leaf bought in the Federal Republic of Germany, but only 0.02-0.12 µg/l in the beverage (made from 15 g mate leaf and 1 l of water).

3. Biological Data Relevant to the Evaluation of Carcinogenic Risk to Humans

3.1 Carcinogenicity studies in animals

No data were available to the Working Group.

3.2 Other relevant data

(*a*) *Experimental systems*

No data were available to the Working Group.

(*b*) *Humans*

(i) *Absorption, distribution, metabolism and excretion*

No relevant data were available to the Working Group.

(ii) *Toxic effects*

A brief report on mate drinking in Uruguay suggested that some of its pharmacological effects were probably due to its caffeine content (Pronczuk *et al.*, 1987; see also the monograph on caffeine, p. 299).

An endoscopic survey was carried out in southern Brazil by Muñoz *et al.* (1987) to investigate the presence of lesions of the oesophagus presumed to be precancerous (chronic oesophagitis, atrophy and dysplasia) in relation to mate drinking. A total of 120 male unskilled workers were interviewed at their work places on mate intake, alcohol drinking and smoking habits. Of these, 36 were non-mate drinkers or drank mate less than once a week, and they were matched to 36 daily drinkers of similar age, smoking and alcohol drinking habits. Of the 72 subjects selected, 60 (83%) agreed to undergo an endoscopy of the oesophagus during which biopsy samples were taken. The samples were examined independently by two pathologists, who agreed on 57 out the 60. There was virtually no difference in the endoscopic findings in the oesophagi of drinkers and nondrinkers of mate. The presence of histopathological oesophagitis, however — which had been defined *a priori* as the most valid outcome — was 2.2 times more frequent ($p < 0.05$) among drinkers in an unmatched analysis. A matched analysis showed that this ratio was [3.3].

(iii) *Effects on reproduction and prenatal toxicity*

No data were available to the Working Group.

(iv) *Genetic and related effects*

No data were available to the Working Group.

3.3 Case reports and epidemiological studies of cancer in humans

(a) *Descriptive epidemiology and cohort studies*

No data were available to the Working Group.

(b) *Case-control studies*

The studies are summarized in Table 3, at the end of this section.

(i) *Oesophagus*

Vassallo *et al.* (1985) studied 226 incident cases (185 male, 41 female) of histopathologically confirmed squamous-cell carcinoma of the oesophagus treated at the Oncology Institute of Montevideo, Uruguay, between 1979 and 1984. A total of 469 unmatched controls (386 men, 83 women) with cancers at other sites were obtained from the same institute; these constituted mainly cancers of the skin (24%), colon or rectum (14%) and prostate (11%). Information on sociodemographic variables and on consumption of tobacco, alcohol and mate was obtained during the routine interviews to which patients were submitted prior to diagnostic evaluation. Men who drank more than one litre of mate per day were five times more likely to develop oesophageal cancer than nondrinkers of mate, after adjustment for age, tobacco and alcohol intake. For women, the corresponding age-adjusted relative risk (RR) was 34.6. For men and women together, a clear dose-response relationship was observed. The joint effects of mate and tobacco and of mate and alcohol appeared to be multiplicative. [The Working Group noted that the issue of information bias, reflecting the assumption among health professions that mate drinking is involved in the etiology of oesophageal cancer, was not adequately addressed.]

Victora *et al.* (1987) studied all cases of oesophageal cancer treated in 11 main hospitals and radiotherapy units in the two largest cities in a southern Brazilian state in 1985-86. Of 190 patients with histologically confirmed squamous-cell carcinoma, 171 (90%) were included in the study (135 male, 36 female). For each case, two sex-, age- and hospital-matched controls were selected, who did not include patients with diseases of the upper gastrointestinal tract or with conditions associated with use of tobacco or alcohol. Cases and controls were interviewed about intake of mate, other hot beverages, alcohol and a number of foodstuffs, as well as on smoking and socioeconomic status. A matched analysis was carried out. Relative to controls, cases had lower socioeconomic status, were more likely to smoke, to drink alcohol and to eat meat, and were less likely to eat fruit. In the crude matched analysis, daily mate drinkers were 1.9 times more likely to have oesophageal cancer than nondaily drinkers ($p = 0.006$). Dose-response trends with daily intake and with duration of the habit were observed. After adjustment for alcohol consumption, smoking, place of residence and meat and fruit intake, the RR associated with daily drinking of mate was reduced to 1.5 (nonsignificant; one-tailed test). Cases were no more likely than controls to report drinking mate hot or very hot. [The Working Group noted that no data were available to assess whether the range of temperatures was wide enough to permit an informative analysis.]

De Stefani *et al.* (1990) carried out a case-control study in Uruguay on 261 oesophageal cancer patients (199 male, 62 female) at the four main hospitals in Montevideo in 1985-88. Of 268 patients with histologically confirmed squamous-cell carcinoma of the oesophagus, seven (3%) could not be interviewed. For each case, two controls matched by age, sex and hospital were selected, who did not have a diagnosis of tobacco- or alcohol-related disease; the most common diagnoses among controls were hernia (15%) and diseases of the eye (14%) and gall-bladder (11%). An unconditional analysis was carried out; RRs were adjusted for age, sex, region, alcohol, duration of smoking and type of tobacco. Mate was drunk by 98% of cases and 91% of controls. There was a strong dose-response relationship between the daily amount of mate drunk and the risk of oesophageal cancer; this effect was observed in men and in women. There was also a significant association with the duration of the habit, but the dose-response curve was not as clear as for the daily amount drunk. The authors reported no consistent association between the reported temperature at which mate was drunk and the risk for cancer. [The Working Group noted that the dose-effect relationships within temperature strata (very hot, hot, warm) were evaluated, but the effect of temperature *per se* was not reported.]

(ii) *Mouth and pharynx*

In the case-control study by Franco *et al.* (1989), described in detail on p. 164, a dose-response relationship for oral cancer was observed in a crude matched analysis for daily drinkers of mate in three Brazilian cities; they had a nonsignificant two-fold increase in risk over that in nondrinkers of mate. After adjustment for smoking and alcohol, mate drinking was associated with a nonsignificant RR of 1.6, and no dose-response effect was seen.

In another case-control study from Uruguay, the association between mate drinking and cancer of the oral cavity and pharynx was investigated. A total of 108 male cases of squamous-cell carcinoma of the oral cavity (excluding lip and salivary glands) and of the pharynx admitted to a university hospital in 1985-86 were included; 286 controls from the same hospital with diagnoses other than diseases related to smoking and alcohol consumption were selected. Interviews were carried out by social workers who were unaware of the diagnosis of the patients. A dose-response association between daily intake of mate and risk for oropharyngeal cancer was observed (crude RR, 1.0, 2.8 and 7.8 for < 1 l per day, 1-1.99 l per day and > 2 l per day). This trend was still present after adjustment for confounding variables (age, smoking and alcohol intake) (De Stefani *et al.*, 1988). [The Working Group noted that no attempt was made to compare the temperature at which mate was drunk by cases and controls.]

(iii) *Larynx*

A case-control study in Montevideo, Uruguay, included 107 histologically confirmed male incident cases of squamous-cell carcinoma of the larynx diagnosed at one hospital and 290 controls selected from the same hospital between June 1985 and May 1986. A questionnaire eliciting information on tobacco, alcohol, diet and mate drinking was administered by three trained interviewers. Controls were patients who had diseases other than those associated with tobacco and alcohol consumption. A significantly increased risk was found for mate drinking *versus* no drinking of mate (RR, 3.4; 95% confidence interval, 1.8-6.6), and there was a significant dose-response relationship after adjustment for age, tobacco and alcohol (De Stefani *et al.*, 1987).

(iv) *Bladder*

A case-control study of 99 male cases of histologically confirmed bladder cancer and two groups each of 99 controls (one hospital, one neighbourhood) identified between March 1983 and December 1985 in La Plata, Argentina, included information on mate, besides coffee and tea drinking. The participation rate was 97% of cases and 96% of controls. Although a significant positive trend with dose was observed for coffee (see p. 127), no such association was found for mate (see Table 3) (Iscovich *et al.*, 1987). [The Working Group noted that no adjustment was made for coffee consumption.]

4. Summary of Data Reported and Evaluation

4.1 Exposure data

Mate, an aqueous infusion prepared from dried leaves of *Ilex paraguariensis*, is consumed mainly in Argentina, Bolivia, Brazil, Chile, Ecuador, Paraguay and Uruguay. It is usually drunk very hot following repeated addition of almost boiling water to the infusion; in Paraguay and southwestern Brazil, however, it is also drunk cold. Among numerous constituents, caffeine, theobromine and a number of chlorogenic acids have been identified in mate.

4.2 Experimental carcinogenicity data

No data were available to the Working Group.

4.3 Human carcinogenicity data

Three case-control studies in South America have investigated the association between mate drinking and oesophageal cancer. Two studies from Uruguay reported an increased risk among drinkers and dose-response relationships, even after adjustment for confounding variables, including alcohol consumption and smoking. Heavy drinkers of mate were approximately ten times more likely to develop cancer than people who did not drink mate. Another study in southern Brazil showed a nonsignificant increase in risk for oesophageal cancer among daily drinkers of mate after adjustment for confounding variables; however, intake levels were lower than in the previous studies, and no attempt was made to assess a possible dose-response relationship.

The role of mate in oral cancer was the subject of another case-control investigation in Brazil. The crude analysis showed a dose-response effect with the frequency of mate drinking, but this effect was no longer present after adjustment for smoking and alcohol consumption. After such adjustment, mate drinkers were 1.6 times more likely to have oral cancer than nondrinkers of mate — a nonsignificant difference. A case-control study from Uruguay reported a dose-response association between mate drinking and oropharyngeal cancer, which remained after adjustment for age, alcohol and smoking.

Table 3. Summary of results of case–control studies on cancer and mate consumption

Reference, location	Site	Subjects (cases, controls)	Mate consumption	Relative risk (95% CI)	Comments
Vassallo et al. (1985) Uruguay	Oesophagus	Men (185, 386)	None 0.01–0.49 l/day 0.50–0.99 l/day ≥ 1 l/day	1.0 1.1 (0.2–5.0) 3.1 (1.2–7.8) 4.8 (1.9–12.1)	$p < 0.001$; adjusted for age, tobacco and alcohol consumption
		Women (41, 83)	None 0.01–0.49 l/day 0.50–0.99 l/day ≥ 1 l/day	1.0 2.1 (0.1–31.7) 12.5 (2.0–80.1) 34.6 (4.9–246.5)	$p < 0.001$; adjusted for age
Victora et al. (1987) Brazil	Oesophagus	Men and women (171, 342)	Less than daily Daily	1.0 1.5 (0.9–2.5)	Nonsignificant; adjusted for alcohol, smoking, residence, fruit and meat intake; 90% confidence interval
De Stefani et al. (1990) Uruguay	Oesophagus	Men and women (261, 522)	None 0.01–0.49 l/day 0.50–1.49 l/day 1.50–2.49 l/day ≥ 2.50 l/day	1.0 2.5 (0.8–8.4) 3.6 (1.3–9.9) 6.1 (2.1–17.3) 12.2 (3.8–39.6)	Adjusted for age, sex, region, alcohol and smoking
Franco et al. (1989) Brazil	Mouth	Men and women (232, 464)	< 1 cup/month 1–30 cups/month > 30 cups/month	1.0 1.6 (0.8–3.3) 1.6 (0.8–3.3)	Nonsignificant; adjusted for alcohol and smoking
De Stefani et al. (1988) Uruguay	Oral cavity and pharynx	Men (108, 286)	< 1 l/day 1.0–1.99 l/day ≥ 2 l/day	1.0 2.5 (1.1–5.7) 5.2 (2.1–13.1)	$p < 0.001$; adjusted for age, smoking and alcohol

Table 3 (contd)

Reference, location	Site	Subjects (cases, controls)	Mate consumption	Relative risk (95% CI)	Comments
De Stefani et al. (1987) Uruguay	Larynx	Men (107, 290)	0.0–0.49 l/day 0.5–0.99 l/day 1.0–1.49 l/day ≥1.5 l/day	1.0 3.2 (0.9–10.3) 2.6 (0.8–8.2) 4.9 (1.7–14.3)	$p < 0.001$; adjusted for age, tobacco and alcohol
Iscovich et al. (1987) Argentina	Bladder	Men (99, 198)	None < 10 drinks/day 10–19 drinks/day ≥20 drinks per day	1.0 2.0 0.9 0.8	Trend not significant; adjusted for age and smoking

One study from Uruguay reported a three-fold increased risk for laryngeal cancer among mate drinkers, with a significant dose-response relationship after adjustment for age, tobacco and alcohol.

The results of a case-control study of bladder cancer in Argentina showed no evidence of trend in risk with increasing consumption of mate.

Overall, the case-control studies on mate drinking and cancer of the upper gastrointestinal tract suggest a strong association, whereas no such association was seen in one study of bladder cancer. These findings would be compatible with an effect of mate drinking due either to the composition of the beverage or to the temperature at which it is consumed or both, since all of these studies were conducted in populations that consume hot mate. No data were available on populations that drink cold mate. Some issues must be resolved before a conclusive result is obtained: (i) Awareness of the possibility that mate drinking may increase the risk for cancer of the upper gastrointestinal tract may have led to increased reporting of mate drinking for cancer cases as compared to controls. (ii) The results require confirmation by other groups of investigators. (iii) The possibility of residual confounding by alcohol drinking and tobacco smoking cannot be excluded entirely, although this was adjusted for in all of the studies.

4.4 Other relevant data

An endoscopic survey from southern Brazil showed that daily drinkers of hot mate had a prevalence of histologically confirmed oesophagitis which was three times higher than that of nondrinkers of mate.

4.5 Evaluation[1]

There is *limited evidence* for the carcinogenicity of hot mate drinking in humans. No data were available on the drinking of cold mate.

There are no data on the carcinogenicity of mate in experimental animals.

Overall evaluation

Mate is *not classifiable as to its carcinogenicity to humans* (Group 3).
Hot mate drinking is *probably carcinogenic to humans* (Group 2A).

---

[1]For description of the italicized terms, see Preamble, pp. 27-31.

5. References

Belitz, M.D. & Grosch, W. (1986) *Food Chemistry*, Berlin, Springer, p. 702

Clifford, M.N. & Ramirez-Martinez, J.R. (1990) Chlorogenic acids and purine alkaloid contents of mate (*Ilex paraguariensis*) leaf and beverage. *Food Chem.*, 35, 13-21

Côrtes, F.F. (1953) Doses of caffeine in infusions of coffee, tea and mate (Sp.). *Arq. Bromat*, 1, 47

De Stefani, E., Correa, P., Oreggia, F., Leiva, J., Rivero, S., Fernandez, G., Deneo-Pellegrini, H., Zavala, D. & Fontham, E. (1987) Risk factors for laryngeal cancer. *Cancer*, 60, 3087-3091

De Stefani, E., Correa, P., Oreggia, F., Deneo-Pellegrini, H., Fernandez, G., Zavala, D., Carzoglio, J., Leiva, J., Fontham, E. & Rivero, S. (1988) Black tobacco, wine and mate in oropharyngeal cancer. A case-control study from Uruguay. *Rev. Epidémiol. Santé publ.*, 36, 389-394

De Stefani, E., Muñoz, N., Estève, J., Vassallo, A., Victora, C.G. & Teuchmann, S. (1990) Mate drinking, alcohol, tobacco, diet, and esophageal cancer in Uruguay. *Cancer Res.*, 50, 426-431

Franco, E.L., Kowalski, L.P., Oliveira, B.V., Curado, M.P., Pereira, R.N., Silva, M.E., Fava, A.S. & Torloni, H. (1989) Risk factors for oral cancer in Brazil: a case-control study. *Int. J. Cancer*, 43, 992-1000

Gilbert, R.M. (1984) Caffeine consumption. In: Spiller, G.A., ed., *The Methylxanthine Beverages and Foods: Chemistry, Consumption and Health Effects*, New York, Alan R. Liss, pp. 185-213

Graham, H. (1984) Mate. In: Spiller, G.A., ed., *The Methylxanthine Beverages and Foods: Chemistry, Consumption and Health Effects*, New York, Alan R. Liss, pp. 179-183

Hauschild, W. (1935) Study of the constituents of mate (Ger.). *Mitt. Lebensmittel. Hyg.*, 26, 329-350

Hegnauer, R. (1964) *Chemotaxonomie der Pflanzen* [Chemotaxonomy of Plants], Vol. 3, Basel, Birkhauser, pp. 163-173

Iscovich, J., Castelletto, R., Estève, J., Muñoz, N., Colanzi, R., Coronel, A., Deamezola, I., Tassi, V. & Arslan, A. (1987) Tobacco smoking, occupational exposure and bladder cancer in Argentina. *Int. J. Cancer*, 40, 734-740

Ministerio de Agricultura y Ganadería (Ministry of Agriculture and Husbandry) (1971) *La Yerba Mate* [Yerba Mate], Buenos Aires

Muñoz, N., Victora, C.G., Crespi, M., Saul, C., Braga, N.M. & Correa, P. (1987) Hot mate drinking and precancerous lesions of the oesophagus: an endoscopic survey in southern Brazil. *Int. J. Cancer*, 39, 708-709

Ohem, N. & Hölzl, J. (1988) Some new investigations on *Ilex paraguariensis*: flavonoids and triterpenes (Abstract No. P1-12). *Planta med.*, 516, 576

Pronczuk, J., Laborde, A., Heuhs, L., Moyna, P., Romaniello, P. & Vazquez, A. (1987) Mate-drinking: another source of caffeine. *Vet. hum. Toxicol.*, 29 (*Suppl. 2*), 70-71

Ruschenburg, U. (1985) Benzo[a]pyrene content of coffee and some other foodstuffs (Ger.). In: *11e Colloque Scientifique International sur le Café, Lomé 1985*, Paris, Association Scientifique Internationale du Café, pp. 205-212

Stavric, B., Klassen, R., Watkinson, B., Karpinski, K., Stapley, R. & Fried, P. (1988) Variability in caffeine consumption from coffee and tea: possible significance for epidemiological studies. *Food chem. Toxicol.*, 26, 111-118

Vassallo, A., Correa, P., De Stefani, E., Cendán, M., Zavala, D., Chen, V., Carzoglio, J. & Ceneo-Pellegrini, H. (1985) Esophageal cancer in Uruguay: a case-control study. *J. natl Cancer Inst.*, 75, 1005-1009

Vázquez, A. & Moyna, P. (1986) Studies on mate drinking. *J. Ethnopharmacol.*, 18, 267-272

Victora, C.G., Muñoz, N., Day, N.E., Barcelos, L.B., Peccin, D.A. & Braga, N.M. (1987) Hot beverages and oesophageal cancer in southern Brazil: a case-control study. *Int. J. Cancer*, 39, 710-716

METHYLXANTHINES

CAFFEINE

1. Chemical and Physical Data

1.1 Synonyms

Chem. Abstr. Services Reg. No.: 58-08-2
Chem. Abstr. Name: 3,7-Dihydro-1,3,7-trimethyl-1*H*-purine-2,6-dione
Synonyms: Anhydrous caffeine; coffeine; coffeinum; guaranine; methyltheobromine; methyltheophylline; thein; theine; 1,3,7-trimethyl-2,6-dioxopurine; 1,3,7-trimethylxanthine

1.2 Structural and molecular formulae and molecular weight

$C_8H_{10}N_4O_2$ Mol. wt: 194.19

1.3 Chemical and physical properties of the pure substance

(a) *Description*: White, odourless powder with a slightly bitter taste (Gennaro, 1985; Macrae, 1985; McElvoy, 1989); glistening white crystals or a white crystalline powder (Moffat, 1986); glistening white needles (National Research Council, 1981; Gennaro, 1985; McElvoy, 1989)

(b) *Sublimation-point*: 178°C (Budavari, 1989); about 180°C (Moffat, 1986)

(c) *Melting-point*: 234-239°C (Moffat, 1986); 238°C (Budavari, 1989). When crystallized from water, caffeine was thought until recently to contain one molecule of water (monohydrate, CAS No. 5743-12-4); more recent studies indicated that it is in fact a 4/5 hydrate (Macrae, 1985); anhydrous when crystallized from ethanol, chloroform or diethyl ether (Moffat, 1986)

(d) *Density*: d_4^{18} 1.23 (Budavari, 1989)

(e) *Spectroscopy data*: Ultraviolet spectra: aqueous acid; 273 nm (A_1^1 = 504a); no alkaline shift; infrared spectra: principal peaks at wave numbers 1658,

1698, 747, 1548, 1242 and 760 nm (potassium bromide disc); mass spectra: principal peaks at m/z 194, 109, 55, 67, 82, 195, 24 and 110 (Moffat, 1986)

(f) *Solubility*: Soluble in water (1.0 g/46 ml at 20°C, 1.0 g/5.5 ml at 80°C, 1.0 g/1.5 ml at 100°C (Budavari, 1989)); 1.0 g/50 ml water (Gennaro, 1985), ethanol (1.0 g/130 ml; Moffat, 1986; 1.0 g/22 ml at 60°C), acetone (1.0 g/50 ml), chloroform (1.0 g/5.5 ml), diethyl ether (1.0 g/530 ml), benzene (1.0 g/100 ml at 20°C, 1.0 g/22 ml in boiling benzene) and ethyl acetate; slightly soluble in petroleum ether (Budavari, 1989)

(g) *Stability*: Decomposed by strong solutions of caustic alkalis (Moffat, 1986); salts decomposed by water

(h) *Equilibrium constants*: acidic (K_a), $< 1.0 \times 10^{-14}$ at 25°C; basic (K_b), 0.7×10^{-14} at 19°C (Windholz, 1983)

(i) *Octanol/water partition coefficient (P)*: log P, 0.0 at pH 7.4 (Moffat, 1986)

1.4 Technical products and impurities

Caffeine (anhydrous or containing one molecule of water of hydration) is available in a USP grade with the following specifications: it contains not less than 98.5% and not more than 101.0% of the above ingredient calculated on an anhydrous basis, not more than 0.1% residue on ignition; 0.5% max weight loss on drying the anhydrous form and not more than 8.5% of its weight when drying the hydrous form (US Pharmacopeial Convention, 1990).

Trade names: Caffeedrine; Dexitac; No Doz (Nodoz); Quick Pep; Tirend; Vivarin (Griffith, 1989; McElvoy, 1989)

2. Production, Use, Occurrence and Analysis

2.1 Production and use

(a) *Production*

Caffeine is produced commercially by both extraction and synthetic procedures. Extraction procedures involve three methods: direct decaffeination of green coffee beans with solvents, extraction from tea dusts and wastes and fragments of tea leaves, and extraction from cola nuts (McCutheon, 1969; Menthe, 1985; Halsey & Johnston, 1987). Caffeine has been obtained as a by-product from the manufacture of caffeine-free coffee (Budavari, 1989), initially by water and then by solvents, e.g., trichloroethylene (see IARC, 1979a, 1987), dichloromethane (see IARC, 1979b; Anon., 1986; IARC, 1987), ethyl acetate (Anon., 1986, 1987a), water-carbon dioxide processes (Anon., 1987a), and also using oil from spent coffee grounds to remove caffeine from green coffee beans (Anon., 1986). Refining processes are needed to provide the pure caffeine of commerce.

Pressurized carbon dioxide is employed to remove caffeine from tea in the production of decaffeinated tea (Anon., 1986). The extraction yields in the production of natural caffeine have declined significantly in recent years, following the increasing use of water-based as opposed to direct solvent-based extraction procedures.

Synthetic production of caffeine involves the methylation of various xanthines (primarily theobromine) (Halsey & Johnston, 1987) and theophylline (Stanovnik *et al.*, 1982; Nesterov *et al.*, 1985) or the reaction of theophylline with carbon monoxide and methanol (Bott, 1982); total synthesis can be achieved with dimethyl carbamide and malonic acid (Anon., 1987b). Most of the caffeine produced in the USA prior to 1945 was obtained by methylation of theobromine extracted from cocoa; the methylation agents used were dichloromethane and dimethyl sulfate. Contemporary figures for the production of caffeine in the USA could not be obtained; production in 1962 totalled 1 959 000 pounds (889 400 kg), while caffeine imports totalled 1 807 000 pounds (820 400 kg) (Huber, 1964).

The US International Trade Commission did not report domestic production from green coffee beans or of synthetic caffeine for 1986 (US International Trade Commission, 1987). US imports of caffeine in 1988 totalled 6 345 310 pounds (2900 thousand kg), while exports during this period were 753 515 pounds (342.1 thousand kg) (US Bureau of the Census, 1989). US imports of caffeine and its derivatives totalled 6.9 million pounds (3133 thousand kg) in 1987 (Anon., 1988), 5.3 million pounds (2406 thousand kg) in 1986, 5 million pounds (2270 thousand kg) in 1985 (Anon., 1987a) and 6.2 million pounds (2815 thousand kg) in 1980 (Hirsh, 1984). Estimates for the amount of caffeine sold in the USA ranged from 8 to 12 million pounds (3632-5448 thousand kg) in 1986, 80% of which was used in soft drinks (Anon., 1986). Caffeine is produced from green coffee by two companies in the USA (Anon., 1987a) and synthetic caffeine by one (Anon., 1989a). US synthetic production capacity was reported to have been expanded in 1989 by an additional 500 000 pounds (227 000 kg) (Anon., 1989a). It is estimated that 60% of caffeine used in the USA is synthetic (Anon., 1986).

Caffeine is also produced in China, the Federal Republic of Germany, Italy, Japan, the Netherlands and Switzerland (Anon., 1987a, 1988, 1989a; Stabilimento Farmaceutico 'Cau. G. Testa', 1989). In the Federal Republic of Germany, approximately 500 tonnes of caffeine are obtained annually from the decaffeination of coffee, while some 3000-3300 tonnes are produced synthetically (Menthe, 1985).

(b) Use

Approximately 80-90% of caffeine extracted from green coffee is used in the beverage industry and most of the remainder and synthetic caffeine are used in pharmaceutical applications (Anon., 1987a, 1988). Caffeine is permitted in the USA in nonalcoholic carbonated cola-type beverages at a content of up to 0.02% by weight of the finished product (Anon., 1987b; US Food and Drug Administration, 1988). It may be used as a flavour enhancer or synergist in foods as served at levels of up to 200 ppm (0.02%) and as a flavouring agent in baked goods, frozen dairy desserts, mixes, gelatins, puddings, fillings and soft candy at levels of up to 400 ppm (Anon., 1987b).

Caffeine is an ingredient in many prescription and nonprescription drugs including stimulant tablets, headache and cold remedies, tablets for the relief of menstrual pain, weight control aids and diuretics (US Food and Drug Administration, 1980). About 1000 prescription drugs and 2000 'over-the-counter' drugs available in the USA contain caffeine (US Food and Drug Administration, 1980; Barone & Roberts, 1984). Caffeine is widely used in a variety of over-the-counter oral drug preparations, often in combination with analgesics such as aspirin, paracetamol (see IARC, 1990), phenacetin (see IARC, 1987) and propoxyphene for the relief of headaches or menstrual tension, with ergotamine tartrate for the treatment of migraine and in combination with some antihistamines to overcome their soporific effects (Gennaro, 1985; Griffith, 1989; McElvoy, 1989; Consumers Union, 1990; US Pharmacopeial Convention, 1990). Caffeine (usually as caffeine citrate) has been used intravenously in the treatment of neonatal apnoea (McElvoy, 1989), to control asthmatic symptoms and to relieve bronchial spasms (Stavric, 1988). Injection of caffeine and sodium benzoate has been used for the symptomatic relief of headache following spinal puncture (McElvoy, 1989). Caffeine has been used in combination with cisplatin (see IARC, 1987) and cytarabine in phase I-II chemotherapy of advanced pancreatic cancer (Dougherty *et al.*, 1989).

Concentrations of caffeine are 100-200 mg/tablet in stimulants (US Food and Drug Administration, 1980; Gennaro, 1985; Huff, 1989a,b), 15-65 mg/tablet in analgesic combinations (US Food and Drug Administration, 1980; Huff, 1989a), 15-33 mg/tablet in cold and allergy relief formulations, 66-200 mg/capsule in weight control aids, 16-200 mg/tablet in diuretics (US Food and Drug Administration, 1980) and 33-65 mg/tablet in menstrual relief products (Huff, 1989a,b). Caffeine levels in over-the-counter drugs vary widely but are typically 15-200 mg/tablet or capsule, depending on both the type of product and the brand (Barone & Roberts, 1984).

2.2 Occurrence

(a) Natural occurrence

Caffeine occurs in more than 60 plant species throughout the world (Barone & Roberts, 1984; Gilbert, 1984). It occurs in dry green beans of arabica and robusta coffees at levels of 0.9-1.4% (average, 1.1%) and 1.5-2.6% (average, 2.2%; Macrae, 1985), respectively. Darkly roasted coffee beans may contain about 20% more caffeine by weight than green beans (Gilbert, 1981; see the monograph on coffee, p. 67). The level of caffeine in tea (*Camellia sinensis*) is affected by a wide variety of parameters, including seasonal variations, genetic origin and use of nitrogen in fertilizers; thus, only average values can be estimated. The caffeine content of tea can be as high as 5% (Graham, 1984a) but is usually around 3.5% (Gilbert, 1984). The weighted average caffeine level in tea sold in the USA is approximately 3.0% (Graham, 1984a); those in tea sold in the UK range from 2.7 to 3.2% (Kazi, 1985; see also the monograph on tea, p. 223).

Cacao is a major source of theobromine and contains only small amounts of caffeine; significant differences in the caffeine content of dried unfermented and fermented cotyledons have been found, as well as in the bark, beans, leaves, roots and pods of *Theobroma cacao*. The bean is the main caffeine storage site, and there are only traces in the leaves and pods (Somorin, 1974). Less caffeine (0.066% in original and 0.152% in fat-free material) is found in cotyledons of fermented West African cacao beans than in unfermented cotyledons (0.085 and 0.196%, respectively). The mean concentrations in fat-free samples of Amelonado and Amazonas cacao beans after five days' fermentation were: green beans, 0.06 and 0.19%; yellow beans, 0.09 and 0.18%; orange beans, 0.08 and 0.23%; and black beans, 0.10 and 0.22%. Concentrations of caffeine in 16 other samples of various origins were 0.07-1.70% (Shively & Tarka, 1984). Cocoa grown in Africa contains as much as 1.7% caffeine (Graham, 1978). The average caffeine content of 22 samples of various chocolate liquors was 0.214% (compared to 1.22% theobromine) (Zoumas *et al.*, 1980).

Caffeine occurs in the *Ilex paraguariensis* plant from which the South American beverage mate is prepared and in other plants of the holly species (see also the monograph on mate, p. 276). Caffeine levels in mate vary from 0.9 to 2.2%; the age of the leaf is an important determinant of the caffeine content: young, growing leaves, 2.0-2.2%; adult, one-year old leaves, 1.6%; two-year old leaves, 0.68% (Graham, 1984b).

(b) Occupational exposure

No data were available to the Working Group.

(c) *Air*

Caffeine has been detected in the air of New York City and in New Jersey, USA, mainly due to emissions from coffee roasting plants (Dong *et al.*, 1977).

(d) *Water sediments*

Caffeine was not found in US industrial effluents (Perry *et al.*, 1979) or drinking-water (National Research Council, 1977a).

(e) *Food and beverages*

The monographs on coffee, tea and mate contain extensive information on the methylxanthine content of these beverages. The occurrence in and consumption of caffeine in foods and beverages has been reviewed extensively (National Research Council, 1977b; Graham, 1978; National Soft Drink Association, 1982; Pao *et al.*, 1982; Barone & Roberts, 1984; Gilbert, 1984; Graham, 1984a; Hirsh, 1984; Shively & Tarka, 1984; Lelo *et al.*, 1986; National Soft Drink Association, 1986; Stavric & Klassen, 1987; Schrieber *et al.*, 1988; Stavric *et al.*, 1988; Debry, 1989; National Research Council, 1989).

One or more caffeine-containing foods or beverages (coffee, tea, cocoa and chocolate products, soft drinks and mate) is consumed by most adults and children, although 90% of caffeine consumed is in the form of coffee or tea (Gilbert, 1984). A wide variety of values for caffeine content have been reported, especially in coffee (Burg, 1975a; Barone & Roberts, 1984). The caffeine content of natural products varies according to the plant species, growing conditions, the amount used and the method of brewing (e.g., brewing time) and preparation (Barone & Roberts, 1984). Many early values were determined using a variety of analytical methods, often undocumented, and different volumes ('cup' size) (Burg, 1975a; Barone & Roberts, 1984; Stavric & Klassen, 1984). The caffeine contents of a variety of food products are given in Table 1.

In foods and beverages consumed in Australia, reported caffeine levels were 300 mg/100 g in cocoa beans, 6-42 mg/100 g in cocoa drinks, 6 mg/30 g in milk chocolate and 35 mg/30 g in cooking chocolate (Anon., 1983). [The Working Group estimated that the average caffeine level in cola drinks was 120 mg/l.]

In the UK, the average caffeine content per cup is estimated to be 48.2 mg in instant coffee, 100 mg in percolated filter coffee, 55.2 mg in tea (theobromine, 2.3 mg) and 10 mg in colas.

The caffeine content in 12-oz servings of 22 soft drinks in the USA ranged from 30 to 58.8 mg (US Food and Drug Administration, 1984). In some countries, the caffeine content of soft drinks is not indicated on the label, and it thus may be consumed unwittingly (Galasko *et al.*, 1989).

Table 1. Caffeine content of various beverages and food products

Product	Volume or weight	Caffeine content (mg) Range	Caffeine content (mg) Average	Reference
Roasted, ground coffee (percolated)[a]	5 oz	64–124	83	Burg (1975a)
	5 oz	40–170	80	US Food and Drug Administration (1984)
	5 oz	–	74	Gilbert (1981)
	5 oz	–	85	Barone & Roberts (1984)
Instant coffee	5 oz	40–108	59	Burg (1975a)
	5 oz	–	66	Gilbert (1981)
	5 oz	30–120	65	US Food and Drug Administration (1984)
	5 oz	–	60	Barone & Roberts (1984)
Roasted, ground coffee (decaffeinated)	5 oz	2–5	3	Burg (1975a)
	5 oz	2–5	3	US Food and Drug Administration (1984)
	5 oz	–	2	Gilbert (1981)
	5 oz	–	3	Barone & Roberts (1984)
Instant coffee (decaffeinated)	5 oz	2–8	3	Burg (1975a)
	5 oz	1–5	2	US Food and Drug Administration (1984)
Roasted, ground coffee (drip)[a]	5 oz	60–180	115	US Food and Drug Administration (1984)
	5 oz	–	112	Gilbert (1981)
Instant, percolated and drip coffees	5 oz	29–176	–	Gilbert (1981)
Tea				
Major US brands	5 oz	8–91	27	Gilbert (1981)
	5 oz	20–90	40	US Food and Drug Administration (1984)
	5 oz	–	40	Barone & Roberts (1984)
Imported brands	5 oz	25–110	60	US Food and Drug Administration (1984)
Bagged tea	5 oz	–	42	Burg (1975a)
	5 oz	28–44	–	US Food and Drug Administration (1980)
	5 oz	–	40	Barone & Roberts (1984)
Iced tea	12 oz	67–76	70	US Food and Drug Administration (1984)
Leaf tea	5 oz	30–48	41	Burg (1975a)
Instant tea	5 oz	24–31	28	Burg (1975a)
	5 oz	25–50	30	US Food and Drug Administration (1984)
	5 oz	–	30	Barone & Roberts (1984)
Cocoa				
– African	5 oz	–	6	Burg (1975a)
– South American	5 oz	–	42	Burg (1975a)
Cocoa	5 oz	2–20	4	US Food and Drug Administration (1984)
	5 oz	2–7	4	Zoumas et al. (1980)
	5 oz	< 40	–	Gilbert (1981)
	5 oz	–	4	Barone & Roberts (1984)

Table 1 (contd)

Product	Volume or weight	Caffeine content (mg)		Reference
		Range	Average	
Chocolate bar	30 g	-	20	Gilbert (1981)
Milk chocolate	1 oz	1-15	6	US Food and Drug Administration (1984)
	1 oz	1-15	6	Zoumas *et al.* (1980)
Sweet chocolate	1 oz	5-36	20	Zoumas *et al.* (1980)
Dark chocolate, semi-sweet	1 oz	5-35	20	US Food and Drug Administration (1984)
Chocolate milk	8 oz	2-7	5	US Food and Drug Administration (1984)
	8 oz	2-7	5	Zoumas *et al.* (1980)
	8 oz	-	5	Barones & Roberts (1984)
Baking chocolate	1 oz	-	35	US Food and Drug Administration (1980)
Chocolate-flavoured syrup	1 oz		4	US Food and Drug Administration (1984)
Soft drinks				
Regular cola	6 oz	15-23	-	National Soft Drinks Association (1982)
	6 oz	-	18	Barone & Roberts (1984)
Decaffeinated cola	6 oz	Trace	-	National Soft Drinks Association (1982)
Diet cola	6 oz	1-29	-	
Decaffeinated diet cola	6 oz	0-trace	-	
Orange, lemon-lime, root beer, tonic, ginger ale, club soda	6 oz	0	-	

*a*The US Food and Drug Administration cites a range of 75-155 mg caffeine per cup of coffee, noting that percolated coffee is in the lower part of this range and drip coffee in the upper part.

-, not given

The mean caffeine levels in 39 tinned 'regular' soft drinks in New York State, USA, and Ontario, Canada, in 1986 were analysed: those in cola drinks were 34.3 and 22 mg/tin (concentration range, 2.3-133.4 and 0.1-104.9 µg/ml), respectively. The range of caffeine contents in all products was 0.8-50.8 mg/tin (12-oz [355 ml]) in New York State and 0.03-29.4 mg/tin (280-ml) in Ontario. Comparison with earlier reports (47.3 mg/tin in the USA in 1979; 40 mg/tin in Ontario in 1976) indicated a general decrease in the amount of caffeine in all types of cola beverages over the seven-year period (Stavric & Klassen, 1987).

The caffeine content of 14 soft drinks sold in the USA in 1989 ranged from 36 to 54 mg/12-oz serving. Another soft drink contained 72.0 mg/12-oz serving (Anon., 1989b).

Data on human consumption of caffeine are generally based on overall product usage or on a relatively small number of dietary consumption surveys. A gross estimate of consumption of caffeine can be derived by considering per-caput intake (International Coffee Organization, 1981, 1982; Barone & Roberts, 1984; Gilbert, 1984; Hirsh, 1984; International Coffee Organization, 1989). In the USA and Canada, coffee is the most important source of caffeine, accounting for approximately 75 and 60% per-caput intake, respectively; tea accounts for 15 and 30% caffeine intake, respectively (Barone & Roberts, 1984).

Gross estimates of world caffeine consumption (in coffee, tea, cocoa and soft drinks) compared to that in the Canada, Sweden, the UK and the USA for 1981 or 1982 and based on total caffeine consumption and per-caput consumption are shown in Table 2. Estimates of world consumption were derived by taking production data for 1981, converting to caffeine by assuming a 75:25 mixture of arabica coffee at 1.1% and robusta coffee at 2.2%, and tea at 3.5%, and then deducting 20% for spoilage and waste. Estimates of 'other' consumption include cocoa (approximately 1350 tonnes of caffeine), mate (approximately 1250 tonnes), chewed cola nuts and miscellaneous sources. Total world caffeine consumption in 1981 was estimated to be approximately 120 000 tonnes, equivalent to 70 mg per day for each inhabitant. Approximately 95% of all caffeine consumed is contained in coffee and tea. The per-caput rate of caffeine use in the USA and Canada is approximately three times that in the world as a whole, but only half that of countries, such as the UK, with heavy tea consumption (Gilbert, 1984).

Daily caffeine intake in the USA has been estimated at 200 mg on the basis of total US consumption (Graham, 1978; Barone & Roberts, 1984). Specific studies have indicated levels as high as 334 (Barone & Roberts, 1984) and 1022 mg/day (Stavric et al., 1988). In the Nordic countries, nearly all caffeine is derived from coffee, and consumption is estimated at 340 mg per day (Kraft General Foods, 1989). Overall mean daily caffeine intake in the UK was estimated to be 359 mg (smokers, 421 mg; nonsmokers, 329 mg); coffee contributed 55% of the total intake of caffeine, and this percentage was higher in men than in women; tea contributed 44%, with no sex difference. In Australia, the average daily intake of caffeine from all sources was estimated to be 240 mg per person (coffee, 54%; tea, 41%; soft drinks, 5%) (Shizlow, 1983) with a maximal average of 6.8 mg/kg bw for adult men (Lelo et al., 1986). Assuming that the mate leaf yields 0.5% caffeine, the average daily consumption of caffeine in Paraguay and Uruguay from this source was estimated to be 85 mg (Gilbert, 1984).

Table 2. Estimates of caffeine consumption: world, North America, Sweden and UK, 1981 or 1982[a]

Region	Caffeine source	Total caffeine consumption (tonnes)	Per-caput consumption	
			g/year	mg/day
World	Coffee	64 500	14	38
	Tea	51 500	11	30
	Other	4 000	1	2
	All	120 000	26	70
USA	Coffee	10 300	46	125
	Tea	2 850	13	35
	Soft drinks	2 850	13	35
	Cocoa	300	2	4
	Other	1 000	5	12
	Total	17 300	79	211
Canada	Coffee	1 200	47	128
	Tea	700	29	79
	Soft drinks	150	6	16
	Cocoa	30	1	3
	Other	120	5	12
	Total	2 200	88	238
Sweden	Coffee	1 300	125	340
	Tea	100	13	34
	Other	150	20	51
	Total	1 550	158	425
UK	Coffee	1 700	32	84
	Tea	6 500	118	320
	Other	800	15	40
	Total	9 000	165	444

[a]From Gilbert (1984)

Per-caput consumption of coffee, tea, cocoa and soft drinks in the USA and Canada in selected years between 1960 and 1982 is shown in Table 3. Total caffeine consumption from coffee in 1982 in the USA was estimated to be 10 300 tonnes, equivalent to a per-caput consumption of 125 mg/day. Per-caput tea-leaf consumption in the USA in 1982 was 0.4 kg, giving an approximate caffeine consumption from tea of 2850 tonnes, which is equivalent to a per-caput consumption of 35 mg/day — the amount of caffeine in one cup of weak-to-medium strength tea. Table 3 shows a 231% increase in per-caput consumption of soft drinks in the USA during the period 1960-82 (Gilbert, 1984).

Table 3. Per-caput consumption of caffeine-containing beverages, Canada and the USA, in selected years[a]

Beverage	1960	1965	1970	1973	1974	1975	1976	1977	1978	1979	1980	1981	1982
USA													
Coffee (kg)	7.2	6.7	6.2	6.2	5.9	5.6	5.8	4.3	4.8	5.1	4.7	4.7	4.6
Tea (kg)	0.3	0.3	0.3	0.4	0.4	0.4	0.4	0.4	0.4	0.3	0.4	0.4	0.4
Cocoa (kg)	1.6	1.8	1.8	1.9	1.7	1.5	1.7	1.5	1.5	1.5	1.5	1.6	1.7
Soft drinks (l)	45	61	85	101	100	103	115	125	133	138	142	146	149
Canada													
Coffee (kg)	4.1	4.0	4.2	4.2	4.2	4.3	4.4	3.5	4.2	4.5	4.5	4.8	4.4
Tea (kg)	1.1	1.1	1.0	1.1	1.1	1.1	1.2	1.0	1.0	1.0	1.0	0.9	0.9
Cocoa (kg)	NA	NA	NA	1.7	1.5	1.3	1.3	1.4	1.4	1.2	1.4	1.5	1.3
Soft drinks (l)	41	48	57	63	62	63	65	65	67	75	67	69	68

[a]From Gilbert (1984); amounts of coffee, tea, cocoa and chocolate products are expressed as kg of fresh equivalent, i.e., green coffee bean, tea leaf and cocoa bean; the amounts of soft drinks are expressed as litres of beverage.

NA, not available

Table 4 gives the consumption of coffee, tea and soft drinks in the USA in 1962 and in 1985-89 and shows that coffee is now the second most popular beverage after soft drinks.

Table 4. Consumption of coffee, tea and soft drinks in the USA, 1962 and 1985-89[a]

Beverage	Consumption (% of population)						Change	
	1962	1985	1986	1987	1988	1989	1962-89	1986-88 to 1989
Coffee	74.7	54.9	52.1	52.0	50.0	52.5	-22.2	+1.1
Tea	24.7	30.9	30.9	29.3	29.4	32.1	+7.4	+2.2
Soft drinks	32.6	59.4	58.4	58.1	58.8	62.1	+29.5	+3.7

[a]From International Coffee Organization (1989)

Gilbert (1984) estimated that the total intake of caffeine-containing soft drinks in the USA in 1982 was 28.7 billion litres, giving a total caffeine yield of 2850 tonnes and a daily per-caput consumption of approximately 35 mg (see Table 2). The total soft drink sales for 1988 in the USA were estimated to be 7.5 billion 192-oz cases, equivalent to a per-caput consumption of 45.9 gallons [174 l]. Caffeine-free soft drinks accounted for about 4.5% of the market (Anon., 1989c).

Table 5 gives estimations of the consumption of methylxanthines (caffeine, theophylline and theobromine) from foods and beverages; estimates of per-caput consumption are based on the 1980 US census population of 226.5 million. Coffee accounted for the majority of caffeine consumption (72.3%; 140.7 mg/day), and tea accounted for 11.5%; all other sources combined accounted for 16.2%. Total per-caput intake of methylxanthines was estimated to be 233.79 mg/day, of which 194.6 mg (83.2%) were from caffeine, 39.05 mg (16.7%) from theobromine and 0.14 mg (0.1%) from theophylline (Hirsh, 1984).

Additional data on caffeine consumption come from a national household census covering a 14-day (Barone & Roberts, 1984) period in 1972-73 (Federation of American Societies for Experimental Biology, 1978); Table 6 gives mean daily consumption of caffeine by source, and Table 7 gives mean daily consumption of individuals in the 90th-100th percentiles of caffeine intake from all sources. Another survey (Morgan et al., 1982) gave daily caffeine consumption and that over a seven-day period, by age group (Table 8), and the mean daily caffeine consumption by source (Table 9). From these data, it was estimated that mean daily caffeine intake is approximately 3 mg/kg bw for all adults in the general population and approximately 4 mg/kg bw for consumers of caffeine. Among the 10% of adults who consumed the most caffeine, mean intake was approximately 7 mg/kg bw per

Table 5. Consumption of methylxanthines in foods and beverages, USA, 1980[a]

	Content (millions of kg)			Methylxanthines consumed[b] (millions of kg)			Daily per-caput consumption (mg)			Percentage total consumed		
	Caffeine	Theo-phylline	Theo-bromine	Caffeine	Theo-phylline	Theo-bromine	Caffeine	Theo-phylline	Theo-bromine	Caffeine	Theo-phylline	Theo-bromine
Coffee	15.23			11.65			140.7			72.3		
Tea	2.72	0.03	0.15	1.85	0.01	0.06	22.3	0.14	0.75	11.5	100	1.9
Cocoa	0.55		4.14	0.42		3.17	5.1		38.3	2.6		98.1
Kola nut and other	0.05			0.04			0.4			0.2		
Caffeine	2.86			2.16			26.1			13.4		
Total (each methylxanthine)	21.41	0.03	4.29	16.12	0.01	3.23	194.6	0.14	39.05	100	100	100
Total (all methyl-xanthines)	25.73			19.36			233.79			83.2	0.1	16.7

[a]From Hirsh (1984)

[b]Preparation and extraction losses were estimated as 10% for caffeine from coffee; 25%, 50% and 50% for caffeine, theophylline and theobromine, respectively, from tea; 10% for both caffeine and theobromine from cocoa; 10% for caffeine from kola nut; and 10% for caffeine alkaloid. In each case, an additional loss totalling 15% was assumed as waste from all causes.

Table 6. Mean daily consumption of caffeine by source for subjects in a US national household census[a]

Age (years)	Consumption (mg/kg bw)				
	All sources	Coffee	Tea	Soft drinks	Chocolate
<1	0.18	0.009	0.13	0.02	0.02
1–5	1.20	0.11	0.57	0.34	0.16
6–11	0.85	0.10	0.41	0.21	0.13
12–17	0.74	0.16	0.34	0.16	0.08
≥18	2.60	2.1	0.41	0.10	0.03

[a]From Barone & Roberts (1984)

Table 7. Mean daily consumption of caffeine by subjects in a US national household census in the 90th to 100th percentiles of caffeine intake from all sources[a]

Age (years)	Consumption (mg/kg bw)				
	All sources	Coffee	Tea	Soft drinks	Chocolate
1–5	4.7	0.49	3.2	0.79	0.22
6–11	3.2	0.43	2.1	0.52	0.19
12–17	2.9	0.96	1.5	0.33	0.092
≥18	7.0	6.55	0.35	0.069	0.036

[a]From Barone & Roberts (1984)

Table 8. Mean daily caffeine consumption by respondents in a US survey[a]

Age group (years)	No. of subjects	Consumption (mg/kg bw)	
		per day	per 7 days
All	966	1.1	0.9
5–6	141	1.3	1.1
7–8	147	0.9	0.7
9–10	151	1.0	0.8
11–12	140	1.2	1.0
13–14	148	1.0	0.8
15–16	136	1.1	0.8
17–18	103	1.2	0.9

[a]From Morgan et al. (1982)

Table 9. Mean daily caffeine consumption by source for respondents in a US survey and for caffeine consumers on days of consumption[a]

Source	No. of subjects	Consumption (mg) per day	Consumption (mg) per 7 days	Proportion of total caffeine consumed: all subjects (%)
Soft drinks	825	33.3	9.8	26.4
Tea	457	59.5	12.8	34.2
Coffee	134	193.4	8.3	22.1
Chocolate and chocolate-containing foods and beverages	1053	11.7	6.4	17.3

[a]From Morgan et al. (1982)

day; for children under 18 years of age, the mean daily intake was approximately 1 mg/kg bw; and the 10% of children who consumed the most caffeine had a mean intake of approximately 3-5 mg/kg bw (Barone & Roberts, 1984).

In the US National Food Consumption Survey, 1977-78 (Pao et al., 1982), the average daily caffeine consumption from coffee, tea and cola was estimated for those respondents who consumed the particular beverage for at least three days (Barone & Roberts, 1984; Table 10). Average caffeine consumption among US tea drinkers was 76.2 mg/day. For cocoa and hot chocolate drinkers, caffeine intakes ranged from 0.06 to 0.22 mg/kg bw for children and averaged about 0.05 mg/kg bw for adults. Chocolate milk consumption gave caffeine intakes of 0.02-0.06 mg/kg bw for adults and 0.05-0.19 mg/kg bw for children. Children who consumed coffee and tea had similar caffeine intakes; adult consumers of coffee had a higher intake of caffeine than tea drinkers. Using caffeine contents of 85, 60 and 3 mg per cup for ground roasted, instant and decaffeinated coffee, respectively, the daily caffeine intake for all coffee drinkers was estimated to be 233 mg. From these data, which cover only consumers of caffeine-containing products rather than all individuals, it was estimated that, depending on age and sex, the mean daily caffeine intake from coffee for adult ($\geq$19 years) coffee drinkers ranged from 2.7 to 4.0 mg/kg bw, that from tea, 0.9-1.4 mg/kg bw, and that from colas, 0.23-0.47 mg/kg bw (Barone & Roberts, 1984).

2.3 Analysis

Analytical procedures for the determination of caffeine and its metabolites and other xanthines in biological fluids (Christensen & Whitsett, 1979; Tobias, 1982; Christensen & Neims, 1984; Hurst et al., 1984) and in foods (Hurst et al., 1984) have been reviewed. Until the mid 1970s, the usual technique for determining caffeine in biological fluids was ultraviolet spectroscopy (Axelrod & Reichenthal, 1953; Routh

Table 10. Average daily caffeine consumption from different beverages in the US National Food Consumption Survey[a]

Age group (years)	Sex	Total no. of subjects	Coffee drinkers (%)	Caffeine from coffee mg/day	Caffeine from coffee mg/kg bw	Tea drinkers (%)	Caffeine from tea mg/day	Caffeine from tea mg/kg bw	Cola drinkers (%)	Caffeine from cola mg/day	Caffeine from cola mg/kg bw
<1	M + F	498	0.0	0.0	0.0	4.9	28.3	5.2	2.2	7.5	1.4
1–2	M + F	1 045	1.0	46.9	4.2	19.9	32.7	2.9	31.0	11.4	1.0
3–5	M + F	1 719	1.2	38.9	2.4	22.4	42.1	2.6	37.8	14.4	0.88
6–8	M + F	1 841	2.0	48.2	2.1	24.5	45.7	2.0	38.2	16.5	0.71
9–14	M	2 089	4.7	63.0	1.6	27.4	62.4	1.6	44.9	21.9	0.55
9–14	F	2 158	4.1	57.6	1.6	29.3	55.9	1.6	44.4	21.3	0.59
15–18	M	1 394	16.4	108.5	1.7	30.1	80.6	1.2	54.8	31.5	0.48
15–18	F	1 473	17.1	119.3	2.2	33.5	66.1	1.2	54.8	27.9	0.51
19–34	M	3 928	53.9	211.7	2.7	38.3	87.1	1.1	57.3	33.9	0.44
19–34	F	5 346	53.0	202.3	3.4	46.8	80.6	1.4	46.1	27.9	0.47
35–64	M	4 929	84.2	282.7	3.6	41.0	87.1	1.1	30.3	25.5	0.32
35–64	F	7 069	82.4	253.3	4.0	48.4	81.3	1.3	26.4	21.9	0.34
65–74	M	1 118	84.7	237.2	3.2	39.5	79.9	1.1	12.8	20.4	0.27
65–74	F	1 738	85.0	198.3	3.0	50.5	74.8	1.1	10.4	17.1	0.26
≥75	M	536	85.1	215.7	2.9	32.6	69.0	0.9	9.2	21.9	0.29
≥75	F	993	81.7	187.6	2.9	47.3	71.9	1.1	8.2	15.3	0.23
All	M + F	37 874	51.1	233.2	–	38.5	76.2	–	36.1	25.2	–

[a] From Pao et al. (1982); Barone & Roberts (1984)

et al., 1969). Use of thin-layer chromatography (Welch *et al.*, 1977; Riechert, 1978; Bradbrook *et al.*, 1979), gas chromatography (Grab & Reinstein, 1968; Demas & Statland, 1977; Bradbrook *et al.*, 1979) and gas chromatography-mass spectrometry (Merriman *et al.*, 1978) for the analysis of caffeine in plasma has been described. The minimal level of caffeine detected in plasma by thin-layer chromatography was 0.1 µg/ml (Bradbrook *et al.*, 1979) and that in serum, saliva or urine was 1 µg/ml (Riechert, 1978); the level of detection of caffeine in plasma by gas chromatography was 0.05 µg/ml (Bradbrook *et al.*, 1979).

High-performance liquid chromatography is currently the most frequently used procedure for determining caffeine and its metabolites and for separating caffeine from other xanthines and drugs in biological fluids; detection techniques range from fixed-wavelength ultraviolet and variable ultraviolet to electrochemical methods, and separation techniques range from normal and reverse-phase to ion pairing (Sved & Wilson, 1977; Aldridge & Neims, 1979, 1980; Christensen & Whitsett, 1979; Tin *et al.*, 1979; Foenander *et al.*, 1980; Van der Meer & Haas, 1980; Christensen & Isernhagen, 1981; Haughey *et al.*, 1982; Muir *et al.*, 1982; Klassen & Stavric, 1983; O'Connell & Zurzola, 1984; Stavric & Klassen, 1984; Kapke & Franklin, 1987; Papadoyannis & Caddy, 1987; Wong *et al.*, 1987; Meatherall & Ford, 1988).

Additional procedures for the determination of caffeine in biological fluids include chromatography on ion-exchange resins (Walton *et al.*, 1979), radioimmunoassays (Cook *et al.*, 1976) and enzyme immunoassay techniques (Aranda *et al.*, 1987).

Caffeine has been determined and separated from theobromine and theophylline in foods and beverages, including coffee, tea and cocoa, and in drug formulations by a variety of techniques (Hurst *et al.*, 1984). Earlier procedures utilized spectrophotometry (Fincke, 1963; Ferren & Shane, 1968; Somorin, 1973, 1974; Horwitz, 1980a), titrimetry (Mayanna & Jayaram, 1981), column chromatography (Levine, 1962; Johnson, 1967) and Kjeldahl nitrogen determination (Moores & Campbell, 1948). These were followed by paper chromatography (Jalal & Collin, 1976), thin-layer chromatography (Senanayake & Wijesekera, 1968, 1971; Somorin, 1974; Jalal & Collin, 1976) and gas chromatography (Horwitz, 1980b). High-performance liquid chromatography is most widely used at present for determining caffeine and other methylxanthines in foods and beverages (Madison *et al.*, 1976; Kreiser & Martin, 1978; Timbie *et al.*, 1978; Horwitz, 1980c; Zoumas *et al.*, 1980; De Vries *et al.*, 1981; Reid & Good, 1982; Blauch & Tarka, 1983; Craig & Nguyen, 1984; Vergnes & Alary, 1986).

Methods used for determining caffeine in green, roasted and instant coffee have been reviewed by Macrae (1985).

3. Biological Data Relevant to the Evaluation of Carcinogenic Risk to Humans

3.1 Carcinogenicity studies in animals

The Working Group was aware of experiments (e.g., by Macklin & Szot, 1980) that were parts of studies on the modifying effects of caffeine on the activity of known carcinogens, in which a group given caffeine was frequently incorporated as a control group. Only a few of these studies were included here, since the experimental design of most of them was inadequate to reveal a possible carcinogenic effect of caffeine: i.e., short duration of exposure to caffeine and/or the histopathological examination was limited to the target organ of the carcinogen used.

(a) Oral administration

Mouse: In a series of experiments (Welsch *et al.*, 1988a) (see also p. 316), groups of 37-43 female C3H *mice*, eight weeks of age, received caffeine [purity unspecified] at 0 (control), 250 or 500 mg/l drinking-water for 43 weeks. At termination of the study all mammary tumours were excised, fixed in Bouin's fluid (Welsh *et al.*, 1988b) and examined histologically. The incidence of mammary carcinomas, mean time to tumour appearance and body weight gain were not significantly affected by caffeine treatment; however, the number of mammary adenocarcinomas per animal had significantly increased ($p < 0.05$) among those given 500 mg/l caffeine. [The Working Group noted the short treatment period and that histopathological examination was limited to the mammary gland.]

Rat: Three groups each of 50 male and 50 female Wistar rats, eight weeks of age, were maintained on basal diet and given tap-water (controls) or a 0.1% [1000 mg/l] solution of synthetic caffeine (purity 100%; total amount consumed, 14.5 g for males and 13.9 g for females) or a 0.2% caffeine solution (total amount consumed, 26.6 g for males and 21.7 g for females) as the drinking fluid for 78 weeks. Surviving rats were then given tap-water for a further 26 weeks. The numbers of tumour-bearing animals were 24/46 in control males and 41/50 in females; 31/48 in males given 0.1% caffeine and 44/48 in females; and 18/44 in males given 0.2% caffeine and 37/50 in females. The numbers of tumours at specific sites were not significantly different in treated and control rats (Takayama & Kuwabara, 1982).

Groups of 50 male and 50 female Sprague-Dawley rats, 28 days of age, received food-grade natural caffeine (containing less than 0.01% theobromine) at 200, 430,

930 or 2000 mg/l drinking-water for 104 weeks. Mean daily intakes were 12, 26, 49 and 102 mg/kg bw in males and 15, 37, 80 and 170 mg/kg bw in females. Two control groups of 50 male and 50 female rats received tap-water only. No significant increase in the numbers of tumour-bearing rats or of tumours at specific sites was observed in treated as compared to control groups (see Table 11). A slight increase in mortality was seen in males at the highest dose; a decrease in body weight was seen in males and females at the higher doses; decreased numbers of tumour-bearing animals and of tumours per animal were observed in males and females treated with the highest dose (Mohr et al., 1984). [The Working Group noted that the reduced number of tumours per animal might have been due partly to impaired growth.]

Table 11. Overall tumour response in rats treated with caffeine at different doses in the drinking-water[a]

Caffeine (mg/l)	Tumour incidence		No. of tumours per animal	
	Males	Females	Males	Females
0	37/50	46/50	1.41	1.46
0	32/50	38/50	1.56	1.63
200	35/50	40/50	1.37	1.68
430	29/50	40/50	1.24	1.60
930	27/50	36/50	1.48	1.61
2000	22/50	31/50	1.05	1.23

[a]From Mohr et al. (1984)

A group of 40 female Wistar rats, four weeks of age, was given 0.2% [2000 mg/l] caffeine solution [purity unspecified] as the drinking fluid *ad libitum* for 12 months (mean total dose of caffeine, 13.5 g per rat). A group of 40 controls (reduced to 30 at the end of the study) was given tap-water only. The number of pituitary adenomas (22/40) in the caffeine-treated group was significantly ($p < 0.02$) greater than that in controls (8/30). Pituitary hyperplasia was seen in 5/40 rats given caffeine and in 1/30 controls (Yamagami et al., 1983). [The Working Group noted the short duration of the study, that evaluation was limited to the pituitary gland and to one sex, and that ten control rats were not evaluated since they died before the end of the study.]

As part of a study of the carcinogenicity of analgesics, 30 male Sprague-Dawley rats, six weeks of age, were given 0.102% caffeine (purity, 99.6-99.9%) in the diet for up to 117 weeks; caffeine consumption was 21.4 g per rat. A control group of 30 males received basal diet alone. The mean survival times were 78 weeks in the treated group and 94 weeks in the controls. No difference in tumour incidence was found between the treated group (8/28) and controls (6/30) (Johansson, 1981). [The

Working Group noted that only one sex was used and the high mortality in the treated group.]

Groups of 40 male and 40 female Sprague-Dawley rats, weighing approximately 100 g, were fed diets containing 6% instant coffee (13 samples of coffee, including seven from which caffeine had been removed by extraction with dichloromethane; in three of these, caffeine has been restored to the coffee) for 24 months, at which time all survivors were killed. A control group of 40 males and 40 females was available. In general, survival was similar in all groups (males given decaffeinated coffees had a slightly lower death rate), but body weights of treated males were lower than those of controls. No increase in the number of tumour-bearing animals or of tumours at specific sites was observed in the group receiving decaffeinated coffee with added caffeine as compared to animals receiving decaffeinated coffee or left untreated. The incidence of tumours (benign and malignant combined) was significantly lowered ($p < 0.05$) in males in two of the six groups given coffee and in one of the three groups given decaffeinated coffee with added caffeine; in females, the decrease was not significant (Würzner et al., 1977a,b). [The Working Group noted that comparisons of numbers of tumours per animals were made and that the reduced number of tumours found might have been due partly to impaired growth.]

As part of a study on modifying effects (see p. 314), 32 male and 32 female Sprague-Dawley rats, ten weeks of age, were administered caffeine [purity unspecified] at 100 mg/kg bw (annual dose, 27 g/kg bw) by intragastric instillation five times a week for life. Mean survival time was 102 weeks in treated and 129 weeks in control animals. The number of tumour at distant organ sites was lower in the caffeine-treated group than in the controls; local tumours were seen in six caffeine-treated rats and in three controls (Brune et al., 1981). [The Working Group noted the limited reporting of the data and that the difference in survival times may have influenced the results.]

(b) *Intraperitoneal administration*

Mouse: In a screening assay based on the accelerated induction of lung adenomas in a strain highly susceptible to development of this neoplasm, groups of 40 male strain A mice, six weeks old, were given intraperitoneal injections of caffeine [purity unspecified] at 8, 20 or 40 mg/kg bw in saline, three times a week for eight weeks. A group of controls was given injections of saline only. Twenty-four weeks after the first injection, the mice were sacrificed. The number of surface adenomas was counted macroscopically. All three doses of caffeine decreased the incidence of lung tumours, but this effect was significant ($p < 0.05$) only with the highest dose (Theiss & Shimkin, 1978). [The Working Group noted that only lung tumours were examined.]

(c) *Administration with known carcinogens*

These studies are summarized in Table 12 on p. 318.

(i) *Morpholine plus sodium nitrite*

Groups of 33-34 male strain A *mice*, ten weeks of age, were fed 6.35 g/kg of diet morpholine and received 2.0 g/l sodium nitrite in the drinking-water either alone (controls) or in combination with 1 g/kg of diet caffeine [purity unspecified] on five days a week for 20 weeks. Mice were killed when 40 weeks old. The number of surface adenomas in the lungs of the group treated with caffeine (6.0 ± 0.7) was significantly ($p < 0.001$) lower than that in the control group (17.1 ± 1.3) (Mirvish *et al.*, 1975).

(ii) *N-Nitrosodiethylamine*

Groups of 25 and 30 male BDVI and Wistar *rats* received 0 or 600 mg/l caffeine in the drinking-water followed three days later by weekly intraperitoneal injections of 80 mg/kg bw *N*-nitrosodiethylamine (NDEA) for 10 weeks. Treatment with caffeine was continued for a further two weeks, and all animals were killed 24 weeks after the beginning of NDEA treatment. There was high mortality (40%) in the caffeine-treated group. Addition of caffeine to the drinking-water decreased the number of liver tumours induced by NDEA ($p < 0.05$): the average numbers of tumours were 1.17 ± 0.225 in the group treated with NDEA and caffeine and 3.23 ± 0.667 in the group treated with NDEA alone (Balansky *et al.*, 1983). [The Working Group noted that the reduction could be attributed to the high mortality in the caffeine-treated group.]

(iii) *4-Nitroquinoline-1-oxide*

A total of 339 male and 285 female ICR/Jcl *mice*, 21 days of age, were divided into five groups and received a single subcutaneous injection in the right flank of 12.5 µg/g bw 4-nitroquinoline-1-oxide (4NQO) dissolved in propylene glycol and five subcutaneous injections of 100 µg/g bw caffeine [purity unspecified] dissolved in water at intervals of 6-12 h: Groups 1 and 2 received caffeine 0-36 h or 120-156 h after 4NQO treatment; group 3 received caffeine 12-18 h before 4NQO treatment; group 4 received an equal volume of water instead of caffeine solution during the 0-36 h after 4NQO treatment; and group 5 received an equal volume of propylene glycol instead of 4NQO solution and caffeine during the following 0-36 h. The doses were the maximum tolerated doses. The mice were killed 20 weeks after 4NQO treatment and examined for the presence of lung tumours. The numbers of tumours were as follows: group 1, 26/57 males and 24/54 females ($p < 0.05$); group 2, 8/26 males and 15/28 females; group 3, 10/22 males and 17/28 females; group 4, 41/98 males and 37/57 females (Nomura, 1976). Similar results were obtained by Nomura (1980).

Two groups of 100 female ICR-Jcl *mice*, six weeks of age, received a single irradiation with a surface dose of 3 krad β-rays on an area of skin 2 cm in diameter followed 10 days later by skin applications of 0.1 mg 4NQO in benzene three times a week for a total of 20 applications. One of these groups received 0.8 mg caffeine [purity unspecified] in benzene painted onto the same site on alternate days from the 4NQO applications. The study was terminated after 94 weeks. Caffeine significantly ($p < 0.01$) increased the incidence of squamous-cell carcinomas of the skin: 21/96 in the group treated with β-rays and 4NQO; 43/94 in the group treated with β-rays, 4NQO and caffeine (Hoshino & Tanooka, 1979). [The Working Group noted the limited reporting of the experiment.]

(iv) *4-Hydroxyaminoquinoline-1-oxide*

Groups of 9-18 male Wistar *rats*, six weeks of age, received a single intravenous injection of 7 mg/kg bw 4-hydroxyaminoquinoline-1-oxide (4HAQO) in hydrochloric acid three days after partial pancreatectomy; they then received 6 or 12 subcutaneous injections of 120 mg/kg bw caffeine in saline (maximum tolerated dose) at 12-h intervals from 0 to 72 h (group 3), 72 to 132 h (group 4) and 0 to 132 h (group 5). Control rats received hydrochloric acid instead of 4HAQO (group 1) or 4HAQO plus saline instead of caffeine from 0 to 132 h (group 2). The animals were sacrificed 52 weeks after 4HAQO treatment. Growth retardation of 10-20% was observed in groups 3, 4 and 5 compared to groups 1 and 2, but surviving rats recovered growth after the last treatment with caffeine. The numbers of acinar-cell adenomas of the pancreas were not significantly different in the various groups; the total number of macroscopic nodules per pancreas was 16.8 ± 6.5 in group 2 and significantly lower ($p < 0.01$) in groups 3, 4 and 5 (3.5 ± 2.0, 3.3 ± 1.2 and 2.9 ± 2.3). No tumour was identified as an adenocarcinoma. In another experiment, rats received six subcutaneous injections of 120 mg/kg bw caffeine before the 4HAQO treatment (7 mg/kg) (group 2), and three other groups of rats received 12 subcutaneous injections of caffeine from 0 to 132 h after the 4HAQO treatment at doses of 120 (group 3), 60 (group 4) and 30 mg/kg bw (group 5). The animals were sacrificed at 52 weeks. The incidence of acinar-cell adenomas was 100% in all of the groups, and the numbers of pancreatic nodules in groups 4 and 5 were higher (significant only in group 5) than in group 1, which received saline instead of caffeine (Denda *et al.*, 1983).

(v) *Urethane*

Groups of 30 female ICR *mice*, six to eight weeks of age, received a single subcutaneous injection of 25 mg/ml urethane in saline [exact dose unspecified], followed two weeks later by a topical application of anthranil twice a week on clipped dorsal skin. Single subcutaneous injections of 100 μg/g bw (maximum tolerated dose) caffeine [purity unspecified] were given at various times between

24 h before and 6 h after injection of urethane. All animals were sacrificed 45 weeks after the beginning of anthranil treatment. Caffeine significantly ($p < 0.05$) enhanced the incidence of papillomas of the skin when given 6 h before urethane treatment but had no significant effect when given at any other time tested (Armuth & Berenblum, 1981). [The Working Group noted the use of the inadequate promotor.]

Groups of 20 male strain A *mice*, six weeks of age, were given a single subcutaneous injection of 0.25 or 1.0 mg/g bw urethane in saline solution. Intraperitoneal injections of 20 or 40 mg/kg bw caffeine [purity unspecified] were given three times a week for eight weeks beginning either seven days before, seven days after or on the same day as (3 h before and 3 h after) urethane injection. All mice were sacrificed 16 weeks after the urethane injection. Caffeine treatment beginning seven days before the high dose of urethane resulted in a significant ($p < 0.01$) suppression of the lung tumour response within the experimental period. Similarly, when caffeine treatment was given on the same day as the urethane injection, the lung tumour response was significantly ($p < 0.01$) suppressed at both doses of urethane (Theiss & Shimkin, 1978).

Groups of female ICR/Jcl *mice* [initial numbers unspecified], 25 days of age, received a single subcutaneous injection of 0.1 mg/g bw urethane followed immediately by seven intraperitoneal injections of caffeine [purity unspecified] at 0.05 μmol[10 μg]/g bw at 6-h intervals up to 36 h after urethane treatment. Mice were killed five months after urethane treatment. The incidence of lung tumours was 7/32 in the group given caffeine and 31/59 in those given only urethane ($p < 0.01$) (Nomura, 1983). [The Working Group noted that the effective numbers of mice varied considerably among the groups.]

(vi) *2-Acetylaminofluorene*

Groups of 15 or 20 male ACI *rats*, six weeks of age, were given 0.02% 2-acetylaminofluorene (2AAF) (purity, > 95%) in the diet and 0 or 0.2% caffeine (purity, > 98%) in the drinking-water (total caffeine intake, 3.26 ± 0.34 g/rat) for 18 weeks and were maintained on basal diet and caffeine-free water until 33 weeks, at which time the experiment was terminated. The number of tumours per animals but not the incidence of liver tumours was significantly ($p < 0.001$) lower in the group treated with 2AAF and caffeine (3.8 ± 2.3 tumours per rat) as compared to the group treated with 2AAF alone (13.5 ± 5.3 tumours per rat). The authors noted that the total intake of 2AAF in the group also treated with caffeine (277 ± 13 mg/rat) was significantly ($p < 0.01$) lower than that of the group treated with 2AAF alone (302 ± 24 mg/rat) (Hosaka *et al.*, 1984). [The Working Group noted that the finding may be due to different intakes of the carcinogen.]

(vii) *Benzo[a]pyrene*

Groups of 32 male and 32 female Sprague-Dawley *rats*, ten weeks of age, were either fed benzo[*a*]pyrene (BP) in the diet (average annual dose, 6 or 39 mg/kg bw) or administered BP by gavage in an aqueous 1.5% solution of caffeine [purity unspecified] (average annual dose, 6, 18 or 39 mg/kg bw) for life. The median survival time of rats given BP in caffeine was slightly shorter than that in the groups given BP in the diet (about 100 *versus* about 128 weeks). Groups given BP in caffeine developed more papillomas of the forestomach than groups given BP in the diet; this difference was statistically significant (chi-square test modified according to Peto) for the groups given 18 mg/kg bw ($p < 0.01$) and 39 mg/kg bw ($p < 0.05$) compared to untreated controls (Brune *et al.*, 1981). [The Working Group noted the difference in routes of administration between the groups.]

(viii) *Diethylstilboestrol*

Groups of 24-30 ACI female *rats*, four months of age, received a subcutaneous implantation of pellets containing 5 mg diethylstilboestrol (DES) one week after the start of treament with caffeine [purity not specified] at 0, 1 mg/ml (approximately 60 mg/kg bw per day) or 2 mg/ml (approximately 120 mg/kg bw per day) in the drinking-water for 10.5 months, at which time all animals were killed. The average body weight of treated animals was 157.7 g at the end of the experiment, compared to 179 g in controls. Mammary tumours were excised surgically when 1 cm in diameter [and the animals were put back in the experiment]. Increasing caffeine dosage significantly ($p < 0.05$) lengthened the time to appearance of mammary tumours and decreased their incidence (DES alone, 12/24; DES and low-dose caffeine, 10/24; DES and high-dose caffeine, 3/30) and the number of tumours per animal (DES alone, 12 rats with 92 tumours; DES and low-dose caffeine, 10 rats with 29 tumours; DES and high-dose caffeine, three rats with three tumours; $p < 0.05$ for the high-dose group). The histological pattern of the tumours was not influenced by caffeine (Petrek *et al.*, 1985). [The Working Group noted that the decrease in the number of mammary tumours per animal and their incidence in the high-caffeine group may have been related, at least in part, to the decrease in body weight.]

(ix) N-*Nitroso*-N-*butyl(4-hydroxybutyl)amine*

Six groups of 36 male Wistar *rats*, weighing on average 194 g, were given 0.01% or 0.05% *N*-nitroso-*N*-butyl(4-hydroxybutyl)amine (NBHBA) in the drinking-water for four weeks. One high-dose and one low-dose group received 0.1% (w/v) caffeine [purity unspecified] in the drinking-water for 32 weeks; a second pair of high-dose and low-dose groups received phenacetin at 2.5% in the diet for 30 weeks. Additional groups of 24 rats received either caffeine or phenacetin alone. Surviving rats were killed 36 weeks after the start of the experiment. Treatment with 0.05% NBHBA and caffeine did not change the incidence of bladder carcinomas (5/31 versus 4/27 with NBHBA alone), papillomas (15/31 versus 8/27) or papillary or nodular hyperplasia (22/31 versus 23/27). Similar results were obtained in animals treated with 0.01% NBHBA and caffeine (carcinomas, 0/28 versus 0/23; papillomas, 6/28 versus 3/23; papillary hyperplasia, 12/28 versus 6/23). Phenacetin, used as a positive control, significantly increased the incidences of tumours and of hyperplasia in the group receiving 0.05% NBHBA and of hyperplasia in those receiving 0.01%. No bladder lesion was found in caffeine controls (Nakanishi et al., 1978).

Groups of 40 male Wistar rats, eight weeks of age, were given 0.01% NBHBA in the drinking-water for four weeks followed by 0.1% caffeine [purity unspecified] for 32 weeks or were treated simultaneously with 0.001% NBHBA and 0.1% caffeine in the drinking-water for 40 weeks; similarly, NBHBA-treated groups received sodium saccharin alone (5.0% in the diet) or saccharin plus caffeine for the same length of time. At the end of the treatment period, all surviving animals were killed. Simultaneous administration of caffeine with 0.001% NBHBA did not modulate urinary bladder carcinogenesis, since no tumour was noted, whereas rats given saccharin or saccharin plus caffeine had papillomas (10/24 or 9/32 versus none in NBHBA controls) and carcinomas (2/24 and 1/32 versus none). When NBHBA (0.01%) and caffeine were given sequentially, only papillomas were seen in the caffeine-treated group (6/28 versus 3/23 in NBHBA controls). Treatment with saccharin or saccharin plus caffeine increased the incidences of hyperplasia significantly, but no increase was noted for papillomas (NBHBA plus saccharin, 9/31; NBHBA plus saccharin plus caffeine, 4/30; NBHBA controls, 3/23) or carcinomas (NBHBA plus saccharin, 1/31; none in the others) (Nakanishi et al., 1980).

Eight groups of 45 female Wistar rats, weighing 180-200 g, received three consecutive administrations of 100 mg/kg bw NBHBA by gavage at 24-h intervals with continuous administration of either 110 mg/kg bw per day caffeine (purity, 100%) in the drinking-water or 500 mg/kg bw phenacetin in the diet. Four groups (those receiving NBHBA, NBHBA plus caffeine, NBHBA plus phenacetin or NBHBA plus caffeine plus phenacetin) were terminated after 15 months and the other four groups after 21 months. Neither caffeine nor phenacetin nor caffeine plus phenacetin influenced the incidence of bladder tumours significantly. At 15 months, the numbers of tumour-bearing rats were: NBHBA, 8/31; NBHBA plus phenacetin, 9/40; NBHBA plus caffeine, 15/39; and NBHBA plus caffeine plus phenacetin, 15/40. After 21 months, these numbers were 16/36, 16/34, 17/39 and 15/31, respectively (Kunze et al., 1987).

(x) *7,12-Dimethylbenz[a]anthracene*

Groups of 54-55 female C57Bl x DBA/2fF$_1$ (BD2F$_1$) *mice*, eight weeks of age, received weekly intragastric intubations of 1 mg 7,12-dimethylbenz[*a*]anthracene (DMBA) for six weeks. One week after the last intubation the animals received 0 (controls), 250 or 500 mg/l caffeine [purity unspecified] in the drinking-water for 20 weeks, at which time the study was terminated. The number of mammary carcinomas per mouse was significantly ($p < 0.05$) increased in the group given 500 mg/l caffeine in drinking-water (0.7 *versus* 0.5 in controls). Caffeine did not significantly affect the number of mice with mammary carcinomas or the time to tumour appearance (Welsch *et al.*, 1988a).

Four groups of 20 female Sprague-Dawley *rats*, 50 days of age, received a single gastric intubation of 20 mg DMBA. One group was then given standard rat chow and tap-water *ad libitum*; a second group received standard chow and 10 mg/kg bw caffeine in the drinking-water; a third group received tap-water with a diet of 20% vegetable fat; and a fourth group received vegetable fat diet plus the caffeine solution. Nine months after DMBA administration, the animals were killed and mammary tumours were examined histologically. The mean latency of mammary tumour development was significantly ($p < 0.05$) reduced in the groups given caffeine and fat, whereas in the group given caffeine alone the latency period was significantly ($p < 0.05$) lengthened. In the groups maintained on high fat alone, the latency was similar to that of animals on standard chow. The combination of caffeine and fat resulted in a larger number of tumours per rat than in the other three groups (Minton *et al.*, 1983). [The Working Group noted, as did Pike and Bernstein (1985), that the analysis was based only on animals that developed tumours and may have been biased by differential survival in the various groups.]

Three groups of 30 female Sprague-Dawley *rats*, 30 days of age, were given 0 (control), 250 or 500 mg/l caffeine [purity unspecified] in the drinking-water for 30 consecutive days; at 57 days of age, all rats received single intragastric intubations of 5 mg DMBA in 1 ml sesame oil. Mammary tumours were excised surgically when they reached 2 cm in diameter, and the animals were put back in the experiment. The study was terminated 20 weeks after DMBA treatment. Three other groups of 30 females received single intragastric intubations of 5 mg DMBA in 1 ml sesame oil at 53 days of age followed three days later by 0 (control), 250 or 500 mg/l caffeine in the drinking-water. This study was terminated 21 weeks after DMBA treatment. Caffeine treatment of rats before or during DMBA treatment had no significant effect on the incidence of mammary carcinomas, the number of tumours per animal or the latency; caffeine treatment after DMBA treatment increased the incidence of mammary carcinoma (Welsch *et al.*, 1983).

Groups of 40-41 female Sprague-Dawley *rats* were administered 20 mg/kg bw DMBA intravenously at 53-55 days of age; treatment with 100-860 mg/l caffeine [purity unspecified] in the drinking-water began 29 days before and ended three days after DMBA treatment. Mammary tumours were excised surgically when they reached 2 cm in diameter, and the animals were put back in the experiment. The study was terminated 12-18 weeks after DMBA treatment. Administration of caffeine before DMBA treatment did not significantly affect the incidence of mammary carcinomas, but the number of mammary tumours per rat was reduced. Further groups of 40-41 females received a single intragastric administration of 5 mg DMBA followed three days later by 100-800 mg/l caffeine in the drinking-water until 12 or 18 weeks after DMBA treatment. An increase in the number of mammary gland carcinomas per animal was observed ($p < 0.05$) when caffeine was administered after DMBA treatment for 12 weeks but not after treatment for 18 weeks. In neither instance did caffeine influence the incidence of mammary carcinomas or the time to appearance of tumours (Welsch et al., 1988b).

In a subsequent study with the same experimental design, a chemically defined diet containing standard (5%) or high (20%) levels of corn oil was used instead of commercial laboratory animal chow. Caffeine (430-500 mg/l) consumption before and during the DMBA treatment significantly ($p < 0.05$) reduced the number of mammary carcinomas per animal, whereas no effect was found on the number of carcinomas per animal when caffeine was administered after DMBA treatment. No effect on incidence or latency was seen in either case (Welsch & DeHoog, 1988).

(xi) *Ultraviolet light*

Groups of 54-57 female, nonhomozygous Swiss *mice*, 10-12 weeks old, were exposed to light from an Ellipiol mercury vapour lamp (irradiation time, 90 min), five times a week for a total of 133 exposures in 27 weeks (total dose, 1×10^7 ergs/mm2). Before each irradiation, 40 µl of a 0.2% solution of caffeine [purity unspecified] in acetone/chloroform was applied to the right ears. The same amount of solvent was applied to the left ears as a control. The first tumours appeared on the ears five months after and the last 11 months after the onset of irradiation. The incidence of tumours of ears treated with caffeine (47-54%) was significantly ($p < 0.0001$) lower than that on the left ear (consistently varying from 84-89%) (Zajdela & Latarjet, 1973, 1975, 1978a,b).

(xii) *Cigarette-smoke condensate*

Groups of 51 *mice* [strain unspecified], four to six weeks of age, received skin applications of 100 or 200 mg of two different fractions of cigarette-smoke condensate dissolved in isopropanol:acetone (20:80) three times a week alone or in combination with 0.04 and 0.2 mg caffeine or 0.08 and 0.4 mg caffeine, respectively. Reduced incidences of skin tumour-bearing animals were found in all caffeine-treated groups, except with the low dose of one condensate fraction (Rothwell, 1974).

Table 12. Summary of results of studies with caffeine in combination with known carcinogens

Carcinogen	Animal	Site	Caffeine	Results	Comments
Morpholine and sodium nitrite (Mirvish et al., 1975)	Mice	Lung	1 g/kg in diet	Decrease in number of adenomas	$p < 0.001$
N-Nitrosodiethylamine (Balansky et al., 1983)	Rats	Liver	600 mg/l in drinking-water	Decrease in average number of tumours	Effect might be due to lower survival in the caffeine group
4-Nitroquinoline-1-oxide (Nomura, 1976, 1980)	Mice	Lung	100 µg/g bw subcutaneously	Decrease in numbers of tumours	$p < 0.05$
4-Nitroquinoline-1-oxide (Hoshino & Tanooka, 1979)	Mice	Skin	0.8 mg painted on skin	Increase in number of tumours	$p < 0.01$; limited reporting
4-Hydroxyaminoquinoline-1-oxide (Denda et al., 1983)	Rats	Pancreas	120 mg/kg bw subcutaneously	Decrease in number of pancreatic nodules when caffeine given after agent	$p < 0.01$
				Increase in number of pancreatic nodules when caffeine given before agent	$p < 0.01$
Urethane (Armuth & Berenblum, 1981)	Mice	Skin	100 µg/g bw single subcutaneous injection	Essentially no effect, except enhanced incidence of papillomas when caffeine given 6 h before initiation	Inadequate promotor
Urethane (Theiss & Shimkin, 1978)	Mice	Lung	20 or 40 mg/kg bw intraperitoneally	Number of tumours per animal decreased in both dose groups when caffeine given before or at the same time as agent	$p < 0.01$
Urethane (Nomura, 1983)	Mice	Lung	0.05 µmol/g bw intraperitoneally	Decreased incidence of tumours	$p < 0.01$

Table 12 (cont)

Carcinogen	Animal	Site	Caffeine	Results	Comments
2-Acetylaminofluorene (Hosaka et al., 1984)	Rats	Liver	0.2% in the diet	Decrease in number of tumours per animal	$p < 0.001$; differences in intake of the carcinogen
Benzo[a]pyrene (Brune et al., 1981)	Rats	Stomach	1.5% aqueous solution	Increase in number of tumours	$p < 0.05$; different routes for treated and control animals
Diethylstilboestrol (Petrek et al., 1985)	Rats	Mammary gland	1 or 2 mg/ml in drinking-water (60 or 120 mg/kg bw per day)	Time to tumour appearance lengthened; decrease in incidence and number of tumours per animal	$p < 0.05$; decrease may be due partly to decrease in body weight
N-Nitroso-N-butyl(4-hydroxybutyl)amine (Nakanishi et al., 1978)	Rats	Urinary bladder	0.1% (w/v) in drinking-water	No effect	
N-Nitroso-N-butyl(4-hydroxybutyl)amine (Nakanishi et al., 1980)	Rats	Urinary bladder	0.1% in drinking-water	No effect	
N-Nitroso-N-butyl(4-hydroxybutyl)amine (Kunze et al., 1987)	Rats	Urinary bladder	110 mg/kg bw per day in drinking-water	No effect	
7,12-Dimethylbenz[a]anthracene (Welsch et al., 1988a)	Mice	Mammary gland	250 or 500 mg/l in drinking-water	No effect on incidence or time to tumour appearance; increase in number of tumours per mouse at the high dose	

Table 12 (cont)

Carcinogen	Animal	Site	Caffeine	Results	Comments
7,12-Dimethylbenz[a]-anthracene (Minton et al., 1983)	Rats	Mammary gland	10 mg/kg bw in drinking-water	Decrease in latency and increase in the number of tumours per animal. Caffeine alone increased latency	Analysis based only on animals developing tumours; differential survival among groups
7,12-Dimethylbenz[a]-anthracene (Welsch et al., 1983)	Rats	Mammary gland	250–500 mg/l in drinking-water	No effect on incidence, number of tumours per animal or latency when given before or with carcinogen; increase in tumour incidence when given after carcinogen	
7,12-Dimethylbenz[a]-anthracene (Welsch et al., 1988b)	Rats	Mammary gland	100–860 mg/l in drinking-water	No effect on incidence or latency. Increase in number of tumours per animal when given for 12 weeks after carcinogen	
7,12-Dimethylbenz[a]-anthracene (Welsch & DeHoog, 1988)	Rats	Mammary gland	430–500 mg/l in drinking-water	No effect on incidence or latency. Decrease in number of tumours per animal when given before and with carcinogen	
Ultraviolet light (Zajdela & Latarjet, 1973, 1975, 1978a,b)	Mice	Skin (ear)	40 µl of a 0.2% solution	Decrease in ear tumour incidence	$p < 0.0001$
Cigarette smoke condensate (Rothwell, 1974)	Mice	Skin	0.04 and 0.2 or 0.08 and 0.4 mg	Decrease in incidence except with low dose of one condensate	Significant

3.2 Other relevant data

(a) *Experimental systems*

(i) *Absorption, distribution, metabolism and excretion*

The metabolism and pharmacokinetics of caffeine in animal species have been reviewed (Burg, 1975b; Lachance, 1982; Tarka, 1982; Arnaud, 1984; Bonati & Garattini, 1984; Bonati *et al.*, 1984-85; Arnaud, 1987; Bonati & Garattini, 1988).

Animal experiments using radiolabelled caffeine showed its rapid and complete gastrointestinal absorption and distribution (Bonati & Garattini, 1984; Arnaud, 1985a). Caffeine is distributed to all body fluids (Bonati & Garattini, 1984) and appeared in all tissues within 5 min (Burg & Werner, 1972). There was no accumulation of caffeine or its metabolites in specific organs, even after high doses (Bonati & Garattini, 1984). No blood-brain barrier or placental barrier for caffeine was observed in adult or fetal animals (Maickel & Snodgrass, 1973; Bonati & Garattini, 1984; Kimmel *et al.*, 1984; Tanaka *et al.*, 1984). Using an experimental protocol established to study a single passage through the cerebral circulation, caffeine at very high blood levels (K_i = 9.8 mM) may restrict the availability of circulating purines to the brain (McCall *et al.*, 1982).

The fraction of caffeine bound to plasma albumin varies from 10 to 30%. No significant first-pass effect occurs after oral administration. Caffeine is eliminated by various species by apparent first-order kinetics, described by a one-compartment open model system (Bonati & Garattini, 1984). The half-time for caffeine is 0.7-1.0 h in rats and mice, 1-1.6 h in rabbits, 3-5 h in monkeys, 4-4.3 h in dogs and 11-12 h in baboons (Christensen *et al.*, 1981; Bonati & Garattini, 1984; Bonati *et al.*, 1984-85; Bonati & Garattini, 1988). A mean volume of distribution of 0.8 l/kg has been reported for different species (Bonati & Garattini, 1984; Bonati *et al.*, 1984-85).

Non-linear kinetics, shown in rats by disproportionate increases in the dose-concentration relationship, indicate a limited capacity to absorb and metabolize caffeine at doses of 10-25 mg/kg bw (Aldridge *et al.*, 1977; Latini *et al.*, 1978).

A decreased half-time was reported when 10 mg/kg bw caffeine were administered to pregnant rats in drinking-water on day 18 of gestation (Nakazawa *et al.*, 1985); however a 25% decrease in mean total demethylation was demonstrated in rats between 19 and 21 days of pregnancy, with a breath test using [^{14}C-1,3,7-methyl]caffeine at a dose of 4 mg/kg, with an immediate return to normal values one day after birth (Arnaud & Getaz, 1986). Rabbits receiving 8-22 mg/kg bw per day caffeine through 29 days of gestation exibited increased plasma concentrations in the last half of gestation, demonstrating that there is an increased half-time (Dorrbecker *et al.*, 1988).

Caffeine is metabolized by liver microsomal mixed-function oxidases (Arnaud & Welsch, 1980a). It can increase drug-metabolizing enzyme activity at high doses (75 mg/kg bw) (Mitoma *et al.*, 1969); however, in-vitro studies showed no induction or inhibition of microsomal enzyme activity after a six-day treatment with oral doses of 37.5 mg/kg bw caffeine (Aeschbacher & Würzner, 1975). Enzyme induction was observed with doses of 100-150 mg/kg bw (Thithapandha *et al.*, 1974; Aeschbacher & Würzner, 1975; Govindwar *et al.*, 1984), while, with lower doses (30-50 mg/kg bw), inhibition (Khanna & Cornish, 1973) or the absence of an effect (Ahokas *et al.*, 1981) were reported. Inducers of cytochrome P450, such as 3-methylcholanthrene but not phenobarbital, increased caffeine clearance and shortened its half-time (Aldridge *et al.*, 1977; Welch *et al.*, 1977; Aldridge & Neims, 1979; Wietholtz *et al.*, 1981).

In-vivo and in-vitro experiments showed a progressive increase in the activity of the hepatic microsomal enzymes that metabolize caffeine during neonatal development (Warszawski *et al.*, 1981, 1982). In beagle puppies, change in caffeine clearance was determined by the rate of maturation of caffeine-7-demethylase (Aldridge & Neims, 1980). Caffeine is eliminated in animals by biotransformation in the liver to dimethylxanthines, dimethyl- and monomethyluric acids and uracil derivatives; important quantitative differences have been demonstrated in the formation and elimination of metabolites in rats, mice and Chinese hamsters (Arnaud, 1985b). These differences are even more important in monkeys, where caffeine is almost completely metabolized to theophylline (Gilbert *et al.*, 1985, 1986). In addition to the metabolites shown in Figure 1, some species-dependent metabolites have been identified. Trimethylallantoin was first reported in rats in 1973 (Rao *et al.*, 1973), and its chemical structure has now been reported (Arnaud *et al.*, 1986a). A new derivative of paraxanthine was found in mice and identified as the 3-β-D-glucuronide of paraxanthine (Arnaud, 1985b; Arnaud *et al.*, 1986b). Methylated ureas (Arnaud, 1976) and sulfur-containing derivatives (Kamei *et al.*, 1975; Rafter & Nilsson, 1981) found in urine in trace amounts are produced by the intestinal flora. In contrast, the acetylated uracil derivative, 5-acetylamino-6-formylamino-3-methyluracil, one of the most important caffeine metabolites in humans, has not been identified in rodents or other animal species. Other uracil derivatives produced from caffeine, theobromine and paraxanthine in rats were found in human urine (Arnaud, 1984). In rats, the hepatic demethylation of caffeine shows an age-related decline, resulting in a greatly increased elimination half-time in older adult rats (Latini *et al.*, 1980; Feely *et al.*, 1987).

The effects of dietary factors on methylxanthine metabolism have been reviewed (Anderson *et al.*, 1982).

Pharmacokinetic differences have been observed in mice after oral administration of caffeine, which may account for interstrain variation in toxicity

Fig. 1. Caffeine metabolites found in animal species

Name	Chemical formula	Reference
1,3,8-Trimethylallantoin	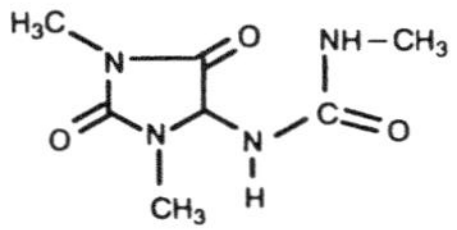	Rao et al. (1973); Arnaud et al. (1986a)
1,3-Dimethylxanthine; 1,8-Dimethylxanthine; 3,8-Dimethylxanthine		Arnaud et al. (1986a)
N-Methylurea	$NH_2-CO-NH-CH_3$	Arnaud et al. (1976)
N,N'-Dimethylurea	$H_3C-NH-CO-NH-CH_3$	Arnaud et al. (1976)
α-[7-(1,3-Dimethylxanthinyl)]methyl methyl sulfide	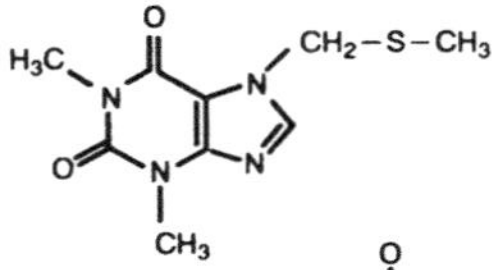	Kamei et al., 1975; Rafter & Nilsson (1981)
α-[7-(1,3-Dimethylxanthinyl)]methyl methyl sulfoxide	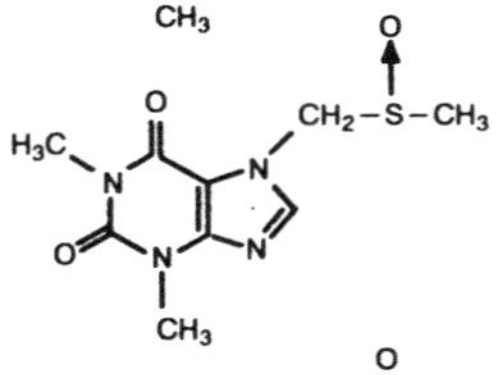	Kamei et al., 1975; Rafter & Nilsson (1981)
α-[7-(1,3-Dimethylxanthinyl)]methyl methyl sulfone	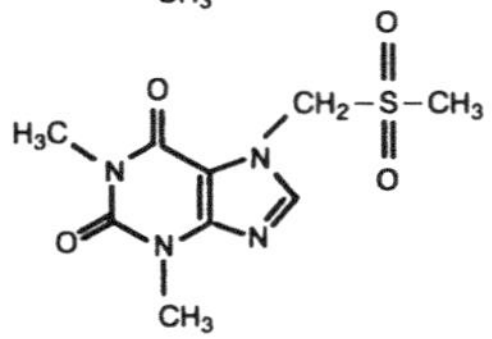	Kamei et al., 1975; Rafter & Nilsson (1981)
3-β-D-Paraxanthine glucuronide	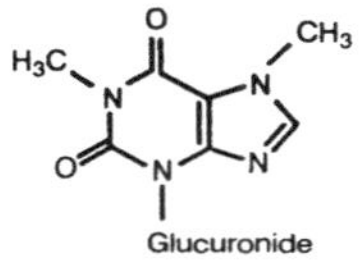	Arnaud (1985b); Arnaud et al. (1986b)

studies (Arnaud *et al.*, 1989). In rabbits, two subpopulations could be described, with slow or rapid caffeine metabolizing capacity. Animals with slow metabolism exhibited saturation kinetics with high doses of caffeine and inhibition of caffeine metabolism by paraxanthine. Rabbits appear to be the best model to study the inter- and intrasubject variability in caffeine disposition observed in man (Dorrbecker *et al.*, 1987).

Drug interactions with caffeine are known. Co-administration of caffeine was found to increase acetaminophen-induced hepatotoxicity by enhancing the production of a reactive metabolite (Sato & Izumi, 1989).

(ii) *Toxic effects*

The toxicity of caffeine has been reviewed extensively (Dews, 1982; Lachance, 1982; Tarka, 1982; Arnaud, 1987; Strubelt, 1987).

The acute oral LD_{50} of caffeine is 200 mg/kg bw in rats, 127 mg/kg bw in mice, 230 mg/kg bw in hamsters and in guinea-pigs and 246 mg/kg bw in rabbits; the intraperitoneal LD_{50}s of caffeine are 200 mg/kg bw in rats and 235 mg/kg bw in guinea-pigs; and the intravenous LD_{50}s of caffeine are 105 mg/kg bw in rats, 100 mg/kg bw in mice and 175 mg/kg bw in dogs. The toxicity of caffeine was determined after daily administration *via* intragastric cannula to female albino rats over 100 days (equivalent to 1/10 of the animals' life span). Rats given daily doses slightly above the maximal LD_{50} (110 mg/kg bw) exhibited a stressor reaction in the form of hypertrophy of the adrenal cortex and atrophy of the adrenal cortex and thymus gland. Some animals manifested a psychotic-like mutilation, gastric ulcers, hypertrophy of the salivary glands, liver, heart, kidneys and lungs, inhibition of oogenesis, minor changes in organ water levels, and an occasional death apparently from bronchopneumonia. Although no major change in growth rates or eating and drinking habits was apparent, some polydypsia and diuresis, thyroiditis, occasional dermatitis, some degree of nephritis, and loss of red pulp in the spleen were seen (Tarka, 1982).

The sensitivity of rats to the lethal effects of caffeine increased with age; caffeine was more toxic in male than in female rats (Tarka, 1982).

The effects of caffeine on the rodent testis are reviewed in detail below and are not covered here. Caffeine also induced thymic atrophy at a dietary level of 0.5% (approximately 150 mg/kg bw) when fed for eight weeks to rats (Gans, 1984).

(iii) *Effects on reproduction and prenatal toxicity*

The effects of caffeine on reproduction and development in experimental animals have been reviewed (Mulvihill, 1973; Tarka, 1982; Wilson & Scott, 1984; Nash & Persaud, 1988; Nolen, 1988; Al-Hachim, 1989).

Reproductive effects: CD-1 mice were administered 0.012, 0.025 or 0.05% caffeine in the drinking-water (daily caffeine intake, 21.9, 43.8 or 87.5 mg/kg bw) for seven days prior to mating and during a subsequent 100-day cohabitation period. Offspring were removed when one-day old. The last set of litters from the high-dose group and the F_1 generation of untreated controls were maintained on caffeine to 90 days of age and mated within their respective groups. Following treatment of the F_0 mice, no effect on pregnancy rate was observed but there was a decrease in the number of live pups per litter at the high dose. There was no effect on any parameter in a cross-mated trial between control and high dose animals. Among the F_1 males at termination of the study, there was no effect of caffeine on the weight of the testis or epididymus relative to body weight; there was a significant decrease in sperm motility, an increase in sperm density and no change in the proportion of abnormal sperm (Gulati *et al.*, 1984).

In a similar study, no effect on pregnancy rate was observed in F_0 and F_1 mice, but among F_0 groups there was a significant decrease in the number of live pups per litter at the two highest dose levels. There was no significant change in reproductive organ weight, sperm motility or density or in the frequency of sperm abnormalities (Reel *et al.*, 1984).

Groups of male and female Wistar rats were administered 10 mg/kg bw caffeine in the drinking-water daily through five successive sets of litters. Progressively reduced growth and increased neonatal mortality (significant) were observed in the offspring over sequential pregnancies (Dunlop & Court, 1981).

As reported in an abstract, female rats [strain unspecified] in a two-generation reproduction study received daily oral administrations of 4, 20 or 126 mg/kg bw caffeine for seven days before mating and through to 20 days of lactation. The F_1 offspring received the same treatment. When mature, F_1 offspring were mated with untreated animals. Pregnancy rate and reproduction were normal in F_0 females and F_1 males; among F_1 females, however, the pregnancy rate was normal, but there were decreases in the numbers of corpora lutea, implants and fetuses at the high dose. F_2 fetuses of these high-dose females were small and oedematous (Bradford *et al.*, 1983a).

Male and female Sprague-Dawley rats were given cocoa powder (containing 2.50-2.58% theobromine and 0.19% caffeine) in the diet at concentrations of 0, 1.5, 3.5 and 5.0% for three generations (Hostetler *et al.*, 1990, see p. 430 of the monograph on theobromine). No consistent dose-related effect was observed in any reproductive index; nonreproductive toxicity was observed at the two highest dose levels.

Female monkeys (*Macaca fascicularis*), 12-14 per group, received 0, 10-15 or 25-35 mg/kg bw caffeine in the drinking-water daily on seven days a week for a minimum of eight weeks prior to mating with untreated males. Miscarriages and some stillbirths were reported during two cycles of pregnancy in the caffeine-treated groups, and birthweights of male infants was also significantly lower in these groups in comparison to controls. The effects were dose-related but occurred with both levels of caffeine. No malformation was observed in any of the offspring (Gilbert *et al.*, 1988). [The Working Group noted that the exclusion criteria for stillbirths were not unequivocal.]

Ax *et al.* (1976) reported that when roosters were fed 0.1% caffeine [about 100 mg/kg bw per day] in a standard ration, hens inseminated with sperm from the roosters had significantly reduced numbers of fertile eggs. Semen and sperm counts were markedly reduced 17-21 days after treatment, and no semen could be collected after 30 days. These effects were reversible on removal of dietary caffeine.

Friedman *et al.* (1979) found that feeding caffeine in the diet to immature Osborne-Mendel rats at levels of 1% for three weeks and 0.5% [approximately 300 mg/kg bw per day] for 14-75 weeks produced severe testicular atrophy and aspermatogenesis. Analogous results were observed in Holtzman rats. [The Working Group noted the excessive doses used in the study.]

Developmental toxicity: Teratogenicity was reported in SMA mice given single intraperitoneal injections of 250 mg/kg bw caffeine on one of days 7-14 of gestation. Significant increases in the incidence of fetal resorptions, cleft palate and digital defects were observed, depending on the day of treatment (Nishimura & Nakai, 1960).

Subsequently, caffeine was shown to be teratogenic in rats and mice by oral intubation (Bertrand *et al.*, 1965, 1970; Palm *et al.*, 1978), by administration in the diet (Knoche & König, 1964; Fujii & Nishimura, 1972) and by administration in drinking-water (Knoche & König, 1964; Palm *et al.*, 1978; Elmazar *et al.*, 1982). The most common effects observed were digital defects, resorptions and cleft palate. Six out of 64 offspring of rabbits administered 100 mg/kg bw caffeine on days 1-25 of gestation were reported to have ectrodactyly (Bertrand *et al.*, 1970). [The Working Group noted that no control group was used in this study; however, this is the only study in rabbits reported.]

In order to establish a no-effect level, caffeine was administered to Osborne-Mendel rats by gavage; offspring had dose-related increases in the frequency of ectrodactyly and delayed ossification. A no-effect level for terata was 40 mg/kg bw caffeine per day, although a significant increase in the frequency of delayed sternebral ossification was observed with 6 mg/kg bw per day (Collins *et al.*, 1981). When administered in the drinking-water at a wider dose range (10-204 mg/kg bw per day), caffeine did not induce dose-related gross anomalies. Sternebral ossification was seen less frequently in all treated groups than in controls, except with the lowest dose (Collins *et al.*, 1983). [The Working Group concluded that caffeine was less toxic to the developing embryo and fetus when given in drinking-water than by gavage; this pattern of exposure to caffeine — small doses throughout the day — is closely similar to human exposure to caffeine.]

In another study by Collins *et al.* (1987), the previously reported delay in sternebral ossification was confirmed in day-20 fetuses of rats drinking caffeine-containing water from gestation day 0 to day 20. Among offspring that were raised to postnatal day 6, the delay in ossification was nearly reversed. The authors concluded that the reversal would have been complete if a longer postnatal period had been studied.

Wistar rats received total daily administrations of 10 or 100 mg/kg bw caffeine by gavage, either as a single dose or as four doses every three hours, on days 6-20 of gestation. While a dose-related decrease in fetal weight and an increase in the delay in ossification were observed with both modes of administration, the major malformation, ectrodactyly, was observed only in the group given 100 mg/kg bw as a single dose (Smith *et al.*, 1987).

When CD-COBS rats were administered 80 mg/kg bw caffeine orally as a single dose or as four doses every three hours on day 12 of gestation, the peak blood levels of caffeine and the area under the blood concentration-time curve were doubled with the single-dose as compared to multiple-dose regime (Jiritano *et al.*, 1985). [The Working Group noted that this finding is consistent with that of the preceding study.]

Sprague-Dawley rats were administered 5-75 mg/kg bw caffeine daily by gavage on days 3-19 of gestation and their offspring were observed for behavioural and developmental effects for nine weeks after birth. Dose-related developmental effects included delayed incisor eruption, delayed vaginal opening and decreased body weight. Active avoidance behaviour was also significantly decreased with the highest doses of caffeine (West *et al.*, 1986).

Many other developmental neurotoxicology studies, mostly in rats, have evaluated the effect of prenatal administration of caffeine on behavioural and neurochemical measures in neonates. These studies were reviewed by Sobotka *et al.* (1979). The effects are not consistent across studies: thus, caffeine may cause subtle changes in discrete neuronal subsystems but is not a neurotoxicant in the sense of disrupting primary neuronal systems.

(iv) *Genetic and related effects*

The genetic and related effects of caffeine have been reviewed (Bateman, 1969; Adler, 1970; Fishbein *et al.*, 1970; Anon., 1973; Mulvihill, 1973; Kihlman, 1974; Thayer & Palm, 1975; von Kreybig & Czok, 1976; Kihlman, 1977; Timson, 1977; Legator & Zimmering, 1979; Lachance, 1982; Tarka, 1982; Haynes & Collins, 1984;

Dalvi, 1986; Grice, 1987; Rosenkranz & Ennever, 1987), as have its antimutagenic effects (Clarke & Shankel, 1975).

The results described in this section are listed in Table 13 on p. 336, with the evaluation of the Working Group, as positive, negative or inconclusive, as defined in the footnotes. The results are tabulated separately for the presence and absence of an exogenous metabolic system. The lowest effective dose (LED), in the case of positive results, or the highest ineffective dose (HID), in the case of negative results, are shown, together with the appropriate reference. The studies are summarized briefly below.

Effects on DNA structure and DNA synthesis: Caffeine interacts in different ways with DNA structure and metabolism. There is some evidence of intercalation of caffeine in double-stranded DNA (Richardson *et al.*, 1981; Tornaletti *et al.*, 1989). Caffeine impairs the helical structure of DNA (T'so *et al.*, 1962), causes a slight increase in the rate of its elongation (Bowden *et al.*, 1979) and lowers its melting-point. There may be local unwinding of DNA, as suggested by susceptibility to single-strand-specific nuclease digestion (Chetsanga *et al.*, 1976).

It has been known since 1964 that caffeine interacts with DNA primarily at single-stranded regions; however, in the initial studies very high concentrations of methylxanthine were used (Byfield *et al.*, 1981). In ultraviolet-irradiated DNA treated with low concentrations of caffeine, the caffeine molecules bind to the DNA near the region of the radiation-induced conformational changes. Caffeine binds to single-stranded (denatured) DNA regions, and it seems to bind preferentially to A-T-rich regions. This might be due to costacking, particularly with adenine (Kihlman, 1977).

Co-incubation of caffeine with single-strand-specific endonuclease induced some breakage, whereas no breakage occurred when DNA was incubated with either caffeine or endonuclease alone (Sleigh & Grigg, 1974; Chetsanga *et al.*, 1976). Denatured (single-stranded) DNA has a higher affinity for caffeine than does native (double-stranded) DNA (Ts'o & Lu, 1964). In human lymphocytes, 3H-labelled caffeine did not bind *in situ* to chromosome preparations after heat or alkali denaturation (Brøgger, 1974).

There are many studies on the effects of caffeine on enzymes involved in DNA metabolism and on nucleotide pools. The RNA-dependent DNA polymerase activity of murine and avian oncogenic viruses was inhibited by caffeine (Srinivasan *et al.*, 1979). There were conflicting reports of inhibition of *Escherichia coli* polymerase I polymerizing activity (Solberg *et al.*, 1978; Balachandran & Srinivasan, 1982); however, caffeine inhibited nuclease activities of *E. coli* DNA polymerase (Solberg *et al.*, 1978). DNA polymerase activity in human embryonic lung cells was inhibited by caffeine (Wragg *et al.*, 1967). Caffeine inhibited three different exonucleases of *E. coli* (Roulland-Dussoix, 1967), thymidine kinase (at high concentrations; Sandlie et al., 1980) and some, but not all, of the purine nucleoside phosphorylases of both the ribose and deoxyribose series (Koch & Lamont, 1956); thymidine phosphorylase was not affected (Sandlie et al., 1980). Effects on nucleotide pools are discussed below (p. 335).

In E. coli, caffeine did not behave like a purine analogue in the purine biosynthesis pathway (Delvaux & Devoret, 1969). The effects of caffeine on DNA synthesis differed according to the assay system used. Caffeine did not inhibit DNA synthesis in vitro (Grigg, 1968), but DNA synthesis was inhibited in cell-free extracts of cultured human embryonic lung cells (Wragg et al., 1967), in Paramoecium aurelia (Smith-Sonneborn, 1974) and in Saccharomyces cerevisiae (Tsuboi & Yanagishima, 1975), but not in Tetrahymena pyriformis (Lakhanisky et al., 1981).

In Drosophila melanogaster larvae, caffeine strongly inhibited semi-conservative DNA synthesis but had no effect on repair replication (Boyd & Presley, 1974). Post-replication repair-deficient mutants were affected only minimally by caffeine (Boyd & Shaw, 1982).

In a study with partially hepatectomized mice in vivo, caffeine (given intraperitoneally at 50 mg/kg per day for four days) depressed the synthesis of DNA (as measured by 3H-thymidine incorporation) but not of RNA in the liver (Mitznegg et al., 1971). 3H-Thymidine incorporation into DNA was also depressed in mouse bone-marrow cells (Singh et al., 1984).

Caffeine increased the number of replication sites in the DNA of Chinese hamster V79 cells and in HeLa cells (Painter, 1980) and slightly increased the rate of DNA elongation in V79 cells, which qualitatively and reproducibly correlated with an increased cloning efficiency (Bowden et al., 1979). The pattern of condensation in DNA in chicken fibroblasts was changed by caffeine (Ghosh & Ghosh, 1972), which also partially inhibited cell-cycle progression from G_1 through to M phase in mouse S-180 ascites cells (Boynton et al., 1974). Caffeine inhibited DNA synthesis in Chinese hamster CHO-K_1 cells (Waldren & Patterson, 1979), V79 cells, mouse lymphoma L5178Y cells and mouse LS929 cells (Lehmann, 1973). An important element in this inhibition of DNA synthesis is reduced precursor uptake by cells: there were large reductions in the uptake of uridine and thymidine in Chinese hamster ovary (CHO)-K_1 cells (Waldren, 1973) and that of thymidine in L5178Y-UK cells (Lehmann & Kirk-Bell, 1974). In CHO-K_1 cells treated with caffeine, one complete cell cycle was possible, but in the second cycle there was a block near the G_2/S interface (Waldren, 1973).

In a test for differential cytotoxicity using wild-type and DNA repair-deficient strains of CHO cells, it was concluded that caffeine was probably not a DNA damaging agent, because no differential retardation of growth was observed (Hoy *et al.*, 1984).

In human HeLa cells, caffeine inhibited RNA but not DNA synthesis (Kuhlmann *et al.*, 1968). ^{14}C-Caffeine was not incorporated into the DNA of human lymphocytes (Brøgger, 1974), but it reduced the size of DNA segments synthesized by excision repair-defective xeroderma cells (Buhl & Regan, 1974).

Prokaryotes: Evidence of caffeine-induced DNA damage was observed in the *Bacillus subtilis rec* assay (weak responses) and in the *E. coli* repair test.

The mutagenic activity of caffeine was first observed in a streptomycin-dependent strain of *E. coli* in the 1940s (see Table 13); however, other studies in *E. coli* gave positive and negative results. Its mutagenic activity was confirmed using phage-resistance and a reverse mutation assay. Caffeine was shown to induce frameshift mutations (Clarke & Wade, 1975). In most cases, the mutation rate was directly proportional to the growth rate (Kubitscheck & Bendigkeit, 1964), and this is consistent with the hypothesis that a mutational event occurs as a mistake during DNA replication (Webb, 1970). Caffeine may also act as an antimutagen in *E. coli* (Grigg & Stuckey, 1966), perhaps by reducing growth rate (Barfknecht & Shankel, 1975).

Caffeine was consistently nonmutagenic in many studies in all the *Salmonella typhimurium* his⁻ reversion tester strains and in *S. typhimurium* forward mutation assays. It was, however, mutagenic to *Xanthomonas phaseoli*, *Klebsiella pneumoniae* and *Bacillus subtilis*.

Lower eukaryotes (including fungi): Caffeine was generally mutagenic in algae (*Plectonema boryanum*) and fungi (*Physarum polycephalum*, *Dictyostelium discoideum*, *Ophiostoma multiannulatum*). Some negative findings were observed in fungi (*Ophiostoma* reverse mutation) and yeast (*Schizosaccharomyces pombe*).

Caffeine induced aneuploidy (monosomics) in *Saccharomyces cerevisiae*.

Studies in the yeast *S. pombe* revealed a significant decrease in the frequency of meiotic recombination and an increase in that of mitotic gene conversion between closely linked heteroallelic markers. It was suggested that the reduction of meiotic crossing-over may be caused by an interaction of caffeine with DNA, which inhibits DNA degradation (Ahmad & Leupold, 1973; Loprieno *et al.*, 1974). As a result of this interaction, more stable pairing might occur at the level of mismatched bases, thereby generating an increase in mitotic gene conversion.

Plants: Caffeine increased the rate of point mutations in plants (*Glycine max*). It also induced chromosomal aberrations in many studies in plants (e.g., *Allium*, *Hordeum* and *Vicia* species), with only a few exceptions. The incidence of aberrations was modified by ATP (Kihlman *et al.*, 1971a) and low temperature (Osiecka, 1976). Sister chromatid exchange was induced in *Vicia faba*, and mitotic recombination was induced in a number of studies in plants (e.g., *Glycine max* and *Nicotiana tabacum*).

Insects: Results of tests for sex-linked recessive lethal mutation in *Drosophila melanogaster* were equivocal, but chromosomal aberrations were induced when the exposed cells were in G_2 or early mitosis, and there was evidence of recombinogenic effects. Predominantly positive responses were induced in tests for aneuploidy in *D. melanogaster*, although the frequencies were low. Dominant lethal responses were not observed in *Bombyx mori*.

Mammalian cells in vitro: DNA strand breakage was not induced by caffeine.

In V79 cells, mutation was not induced at the *hprt* locus, and there was no increase in the frequency of ouabain-resistant mutants. Also, caffeine failed to induce forward mutations either to auxotrophy at a variety of loci in CHO-K_1 cells or at the *tk* locus in mouse lymphoma L5178Y cells. Caffeine has been reported to be antimutagenic to V79 cells, in which it reduces the fractions of both induced and spontaneous mutations.

Sister chromatid exchange was induced in some studies but not in others. Its induction may well be related to an inhibition of the poly(ADP-ribose) polymerase; this inhibition could delay the rejoining of DNA strand breaks induced by bromodeoxyuridine (Natarajan *et al.*, 1981). Inhibition of this enzyme is associated with the induction of sister chromatid exchange (Levi *et al.*, 1978; Morgan & Cleaver, 1982).

Micronuclei have been induced by caffeine in a cell line and in cultured mouse preimplantation embryos. The sensitivity of different cell lines to the induction of chromosomal aberrations by caffeine clearly varies widely. When treated with caffeine, CHO cells responded with large increases in the frequency of chromosomal aberrations that were dependent upon treatment during S-phase (Kihlman *et al.*, 1971a,b; Kihlman, 1977). In mice deficient in folate, caffeine strongly increased the frequency of micronucleated cells (MacGregor, 1990).

Caffeine enhanced the frequency of cell transformation in several virus-induced systems but not in an assay for colony morphology in primary Syrian hamster embryo cells.

Human cells in vitro: The growth of HeLa cells was inhibited by concentrations of caffeine above 300 μg/ml (Ostertag *et al.*, 1965); exposure of these cells for 2 h to 1% caffeine had virtually no effect on cell cycle time (Kuhlmann *et al.*, 1968).

Caffeine did not induce unscheduled DNA synthesis or *hprt* locus mutations in human cells.

Caffeine weakly induced sister chromatid exchange in most of eight studies with human leukocytes and in all three published studies with leukocytes or lymphoblastoid cells from patients with xeroderma pigmentosum. Dose-dependent increases were obtained in only two of the studies (Ishii & Bender, 1978; Guglielmi *et al.*, 1982).

In contrast, numerous reports have described the induction of chromosomal aberrations in human leukocytes and in HeLa cell lines. In cultured human lymphocytes from people with the heritable fragility condition, caffeine enhanced the expression of fragile sites (Ledbetter *et al.*, 1986; Smeets *et al.*, 1989).

Mammals in vivo: In a large number of studies in mammals *in vivo*, caffeine usually failed to induce significant responses. While single-strand breaks were induced in mouse liver and kidney, there was no significant effect in host-mediated assays (incubation of bacteria in the intraperitoneal cavity or in-vitro testing against bacteria from the urine of dosed rats), in an assay for specific locus in a mouse germ-line cell or in a mouse spot test.

Variable responses were obtained, however, with respect to sister chromatid exchange: of seven reports, two gave negative results, one gave a weak positive result and four a significant positive response.

In a large number of studies on the possible clastogenic effects of caffeine, almost uniformly negative responses were obtained in tests for micronuclei, bone-marrow metaphases and dominant lethal mutation. Negative results were also seen in a translocation test, and chromosomal aberrations were not induced in metaphase-I cells of mouse spermatogenesis. In addition, no sperm abnormality was induced in mice. Among this wealth of negative data, three significant positive responses were seen in the micronucleus test; in each case, the doses were in the toxic range.

Effects of methylxanthines on relevant targets other than DNA: In this section, we consider the effects of the methylxanthines, caffeine, theophylline and theobromine, on non-DNA targets but which potentially lead indirectly to DNA damage, mutation and modification of the activities of xenobiotics (including carcinogens) co-administered with methylxanthines. These aspects have been reviewed (Kihlman, 1977; Roberts, 1978; Byfield *et al.*, 1981; Haynes & Collins, 1984; Roberts, 1984; Althaus & Richter, 1987; Boothman *et al.*, 1988).

Non-DNA targets that are important to the genotoxic and related effects of methylxanthines are (i) cytochrome P450s (see p. 322 *et seq.*), (ii) cAMP metabolism, (iii) DNA metabolism, chromatin structure and function and (iv) nucleotide pools.

(1) **cAMP metabolism**

It is well established that methylxanthines can inhibit the phosphodiesterase involved in the degradation of cyclic nucleotides (Leonard *et al.*, 1987), i.e., the intracellular messengers that control a wide variety of phenomena not related to survival *per se*. The majority of the studies were performed *in vitro* with caffeine concentrations higher than levels encountered by humans *in vivo*.

In mouse B-16 melanoma cells, Kolb and Mansfield (1980) found that theophylline inhibited DNA synthesis, reduced cell growth rate, elevated intracellular cAMP levels and changed cell morphology. Since these effects are also caused by cAMP and its potentiators in other cell lines, the inhibition of DNA synthesis is assumed to be a secondary effect of the increased level of cAMP resulting from inhibition of cAMP phosphodiesterase by theophylline. cAMP is known to inhibit cell growth and the transport of metabolites; it also mediates contact inhibition, the formation of cytoskeletal structures and increases cell adhesiveness (Rajaraman & Faulkner, 1984). Therefore, the reduced uptake of 3H-thymidine by L5178Y cells observed by Lehmann and Kirk-Bell (1974) may also, in part, be mediated by the increased cAMP concentration (Kolb & Mansfield, 1980).

cAMP does not, however, mimic the effects of caffeine on chromosomal structure nor on the gap filling process in radiation-damaged DNA. Furthermore, in some plant cells in which methylxanthines induce chromosome damage, the presence of cAMP is equivocal (Kihlman, 1977). Therefore, the effects of caffeine on cAMP levels appear not to be involved in the induction of chromosomal aberrations.

(2) DNA metabolism, chromatin structure and function

The effects of methylxanthines in cells treated with mutagenic agents can be summarized as follows (Roberts, 1984):

- (i) reversal of agent-induced depression of DNA synthesis;
- (ii) reversal of agent-induced inhibition of replicon initiation;
- (iii) decrease in size of replicons (also in the absence of DNA damage);
- (iv) inhibition of elongation of nascent DNA (to high-molecular-weight, template-sized DNA);
- (v) time-dependent incision of template DNA;
- (vi) time-dependent formation of DNA double-strand breaks;
- (vii) inhibition of excision of base damage;
- (viii) induction of protein synthesis; and
- (ix) prevention of S phase delay and G_2 arrest (induction of premature mitosis).

These aspects are considered together because they appear to result from two interrelated actions of methylxanthines affecting chromatin: interaction with single-stranded DNA and inhibition of poly(ADP-ribosyl)ation reactions.

Methylxanthines, in particular caffeine, interact with DNA primarily at single-stranded regions. In living cells, there is only indirect evidence for such interaction (Althaus & Richter, 1987). The finding that the production of chromosomal aberrations by methylxanthines in bean root tips is strongly dependent on temperature, with a sharp maximum around 12°C, led to the suggestion that chromosomal aberrations may be the result of an influence of the methylated oxypurines on macromolecular hydration structures (Kihlman, 1977).

Inhibition of poly(ADP-ribose)polymerase was determined in nucleotide-permeable human lymphocytes following three days of stimulation with 2 µg/ml L-phytohaemagglutinin: theophylline (2 mM) gave 89% inhibition, theobromine (1 mM), 81%, and caffeine (2 mM), 35% (Althaus & Richter, 1987). This is an important finding because poly(ADP-ribosyl)ation reactions are distributed ubiquitously among higher eukaryotes and have been demonstrated in a number of plants and lower eukaryotes. Various lines of evidence indicate an involvement of poly(ADP-ribosyl)ation in the normal cell cycle of mammalian cells and, in particular, in the molecular events occurring during S phase. Distinct changes in the levels of biosynthetic activity of poly(ADP-ribose) were observed in cellular differentiation processes. The presence of poly(ADP-ribosyl)ation in yeast is controversial. No activity has so far been found in prokaryotic organisms. An inhibition of poly(ADP-ribosyl)ation reactions by methylxanthines may result in genetic effects and in the modulation of genetic effects induced by other agents (ionizing radiation, ultraviolet light, and mutagenic and carcinogenic chemicals), because these reactions are involved in all major chromatin functions, i.e., DNA repair, DNA replication and transcriptional activity. They influence the local organization of chromatin and, in particular, the architecture of active chromatin domains as a consequence of altered protein interactions.

Important acceptor proteins for poly(ADP-ribose) are histone H2B and histone H1, which are involved in the nucleosomal organization of chromatin and of polynucleosome structures, respectively. The production of DNA strand breaks, either directly (ionizing radiation) or enzymatically in the process of DNA-excision repair, is required for the stimulation of poly(ADP-ribose) biosynthesis. In excision repair, several steps have been shown to be affected by poly(ADP-ribose)polymerase inhibitors: incision and ligation are inhibited, excision is reduced and repair synthesis is usually stimulated. Inhibition by methylxanthines of poly(ADP-ribose) synthesis usually results in reduced repair. Many unrepaired lesions are lethal, and reduced survival of damaged cells is observed.

There is a positive correlation between the sister chromatid exchange-inducing potential and the inhibitory effects of chemicals that reduce the activity of poly(ADP-ribose)polymerase. There is no concomitant increase in the frequency of chromosomal aberrations or point mutations (e.g., *hprt* mutants). In contrast, in cells with damaged DNA, ADP-ribosylation inhibitors significantly increased the frequency of chromosomal aberrations induced by alkylating agents and other types of chemical mutagens, and also by ultraviolet or ionizing radiation, and raised the incidence of *hprt* mutants (which can result from deletions) but not of ouabain-resistant mutants (resulting mostly from amino acid substitutions). Overall, an altered poly(ADP-ribose) metabolism can have specific effects on genetic phenomena such as DNA excision repair (Roberts, 1978), clastogenicity and mutagenicity (Roberts, 1984; Althaus & Richter, 1987), but also on neoplastic transformation (Roberts, 1984; Boothman *et al.*, 1988). In the last case, controversial results have been reported.

(3) **Nucleotide pools**

It has been established that genetic effects can be produced not only by radiation and chemical attack upon DNA, but also by disturbances in deoxyribonucleotide precursor pools. Some studies indicate that the purine analogue, caffeine, may affect DNA precursor metabolism (Haynes & Collins, 1984). Caffeine is known to inhibit enzymes of purine metabolism and may thereby alter the normal base ratio in the DNA precursor pool, thus causing errors in pairing. Caffeine doses enhance the killing action of ultraviolet light. It inhibits both de-novo synthesis and the utilization of exogenous purines in cultured CHO cells. Furthermore, caffeine inhibited incorporation of thymidine into DNA both in prokaryotic and eukaryotic cells. In *E. coli*, it has been suggested that this inhibition could be caused by a caffeine-induced inhibition of thymidine kinase or, more likely, an effect of caffeine on the DNA synthesis process itself. It was shown that, although thymidine kinase is inhibited by caffeine in *E. coli* cells, intracellular concentrations of thymidine triphosphate which one would consequently expect to decrease, actually increased significantly. Thus, the major effect of caffeine on the nucleotide pool appears to be the result of inhibition of processes that involve thymidine triphosphate. In these experiments, intracellular concentrations of the other nucleoside triphosphate pools were only slightly increased by caffeine. The finding that chronic exposure to caffeine led to sister chromatid exchange in human peripheral blood lymphocytes (Guglielmi *et al.*, 1982) was interpreted to be a result of inhibition of DNA synthesis brought about by inhibition of de-novo synthesis of endogenous purines and also the transport and use of exogenous purines.

(b) *Humans*

(i) *Absorption, distribution, metabolism and excretion*

Caffeine absorption from the gastrointestinal tract is rapid, virtually complete and directly dependent on pH (Chvasta & Cooke, 1971; Marks & Kelly, 1973; Robertson *et al.*, 1978; Bonati *et al.*, 1982; Blanchard & Sawers, 1983a,b). Plasma

Table 13. Genetic and related effects of caffeine

Test system	Results		Dose LED/HID	Reference
	Without exogenous metabolic activation	With exogenous metabolic activation		
ERD, Escherichia coli differential toxicity	+		935.0000	De Flora et al. (1984a)
BSD, Bacillus subtilis rec- assay (spore)	(+)		1000.0000	Kada et al. (1972)
SAF, Salmonella typhimurium, forward mutation	–		0.0000	Furth & Thilly (1978)
SAF, Salmonella typhimurium TM677, forward mutation, ara test	–	–	15000.0000	Ariza et al. (1988)
SA0, Salmonella typhimurium TA100, reverse mutation	–	–	3000.0000	McCann et al. (1975)
SA0, Salmonella typhimurium TA100, reverse mutation	–	–	0.0000	Heddle & Bruce (1977)
SA0, Salmonella typhimurium TA100, reverse mutation	–		1.0000	King et al. (1979)
SA0, Salmonella typhimurium TA100, reverse mutation	–	0	1000.0000	Aeschbacher et al. (1980)
SA0, Salmonella typhimurium TA100, reverse mutation	–	–	0.0000	De Flora et al. (1984a)
SA0, Salmonella typhimurium TA100, reverse mutation	–	–	1667.0000	Dunkel et al. (1985)
SA0, Salmonella typhimurium TA100, reverse mutation	–	–	5000.0000	Mortelmans et al. (1986)
SA2, Salmonella typhimurium TA102, reverse mutation	–	–	0.0000	De Flora et al. (1984b)
SA5, Salmonella typhimurium TA1535, reverse mutation	–	–	3000.0000	McCann et al. (1975)
SA5, Salmonella typhimurium TA1535, reverse mutation	–	–	0.0000	Heddle & Bruce (1977)
SA5, Salmonella typhimurium TA1535, reverse mutation	–		1.0000	King et al. (1979)
SA5, Salmonella typhimurium TA1535, reverse mutation	–	–	0.0000	De Flora et al. (1984a)
SA5, Salmonella typhimurium TA1535, reverse mutation	–	–	1667.0000	Dunkel et al. (1985)
SA5, Salmonella typhimurium TA1535, reverse mutation	–	–	5000.0000	Mortelmans et al. (1986)
SA7, Salmonella typhimurium TA1537, reverse mutation	–	–	3000.0000	McCann et al. (1975)
SA7, Salmonella typhimurium TA1537, reverse mutation	–		1.0000	King et al. (1979)
SA7, Salmonella typhimurium TA1537, reverse mutation	–	–	0.0000	De Flora et al. (1984a)
SA7, Salmonella typhimurium TA1537, reverse mutation	–	–	1667.0000	Dunkel et al. (1985)
SA7, Salmonella typhimurium TA1537, reverse mutation	–	–	5000.0000	Mortelmans et al. (1986)
SA8, Salmonella typhimurium TA1538, reverse mutation	–		1.0000	King et al. (1979)
SA8, Salmonella typhimurium TA1538, reverse mutation	–	–	0.0000	De Flora et al. (1984a)
SA8, Salmonella typhimurium TA1538, reverse mutation	–	–	1667.0000	Dunkel et al. (1985)
SA9, Salmonella typhimurium TA98, reverse mutation	–	–	3000.0000	McCann et al. (1975)
SA9, Salmonella typhimurium TA98, reverse mutation	–	–	0.0000	Heddle & Bruce (1977)
SA9, Salmonella typhimurium TA98, reverse mutation	–		1.0000	King et al. (1979)
SA9, Salmonella typhimurium TA98, reverse mutation	–	–	0.0000	De Flora et al. (1984a)
SA9, Salmonella typhimurium TA98, reverse mutation	–	–	1667.0000	Dunkel et al. (1985)
SA9, Salmonella typhimurium TA98, reverse mutation	–	–	5000.0000	Mortelmans et al. (1986)
SAS, Salmonella typhimurium TA97, reverse mutation	–	–	0.0000	De Flora et al. (1984b)
SAS, Salmonella typhimurium TA92, reverse mutation	–?	0	1000.0000	Kim & Levin (1986)
ECK, Escherichia coli K12 ND160, lac- reversion	+	0	1940.0000	Clarke & Wade (1975)
ECK, Escherichia coli K12 (343/113), forward mutation	–		10000.0000	King et al. (1979)
ECF, Escherichia coli B/Sd-4/, forward mutation	–	–	1667.0000	Demerec et al. (1951)
ECW, Escherichia coli WP2 uvrA, trp- reverse mutation	–	0		Dunkel et al. (1985)

Table 13 (contd)

Test system	Results		Dose LED/HID	Reference
	Without exogenous metabolic activation	With exogenous metabolic activation		
ECR, Escherichia coli, phage T5-resistance	+	0	150.0000	Novick & Szilard (1951)
ECR, Escherichia coli B, phage resistance	+	0	20000.0000	Gezelius & Fries (1952)
ECR, Escherichia coli, phage resistance	+	0	200.0000	Glass & Novick (1959)
ECR, Escherichia coli, methionine independence	(+)	0	250.0000	Greer (1958)
ECR, Escherichia coli, tryptophan independence	+	0	500.0000	Greer (1958)
ECR, Escherichia coli, streptomycin dependence	−	0	25.0000	Iyer & Szybalski (1958)[{HNT}]
ECR, Escherichia coli, phage T5-resistance	+	0	150.0000	Kubitschek & Bendigkeit (1958)
ECR, Escherichia coli, trp, pro, his reversions	−	0	0.0000	Paribock et al. (1967)
BSM, Bacillus subtilis, multigene sporulation test	+	0	2500.0000	Sacks & Mihara (1983)
KP2, Klebsiella pneumoniae, streptomycin resistance	+	0	2000.0000	Voogd & Vet (1969)
??F, Ophiostoma multiannulatum, forward mutation	+	0	0.0000	Fries & Kihlman (1948)
??R, Ophiostoma multiannulatum, reverse mutation	−	0	0.0000	Zetterberg (1960)
??R, Xanthomonas phaseoli, streptomycin resistance	+	0	0.0000	Györffy (1960)
??R, Plectonema boryanum (blue-green alga) cyanophage/streptomycin^R	+	0	0.0000	Singh & Kashyap (1977)
???, Physarum polycephalum, plaque size	+	0	0.0000	Haugli & Dove (1972)
???, Dictostelium discoideum, aggregateless mutants	+	0	0.0000	Liverant & Pereira Da Silva (1975)
???, Schizosaccharomyces pombe, intergenic recombination	+	0	0.0000	Loprieno & Schüpbach (1971)
SZG, Schizosaccharomyces pombe, gene conversion	+	0	1000.0000	Loprieno et al. (1974)
SZG, Schizosaccharomyces pombe, meiotic recombination	+	0	0.0000	Loprieno et al. (1974)
SCF, Saccharomyces cerevisiae, mitochondrial rho−	+	0	1500.0000	Wolf & Kaudewitz (1976)
SCF, Saccharomyces cerevisiae, mitochondrial rho−	+	0	100.0000	Bien et al. (1989)
SZR, Schizosaccharomyces pombe, ade and his revertants	−	0	2000.0000	Loprieno & Schüpbach (1971)
SCN, Saccharomyces cerevisiae, aneuploidy	+	0	125.0000	Parry et al. (1979)
PLM, Glycine max, gene mutation (point mutation)	+	0	625.0000	Vig (1973)
ACC, Allium cepa root tips, chromosomal aberrations	+	0	400.0000	Kihlman (1949)
ACC, Allium cepa root meristem bridges, fragments in ana-telophase	+	0	580.0000	González-Fernandez et al. (1985)
PLC, Allium sativum root tips, chromosomal aberrations	+	0	1000.0000	Koertting-Keiffer & Mickey (1969)
PLC, Allium proliferum root tips, chromosomal aberrations	+	0	1940.0000	Kihlman et al. (1971a)
HSC, Hordeum vulgare, chromatid aberrations	+	0	600.0000	Yamamoto & Yamaguchi (1969)
HSC, Hordeum vulgare, chromosomal aberrations	+	0	750.0000	Kesavan et al. (1973)
VFC, Vicia faba roots, chromosomal aberrations	−	0	3880.0000	Schöneich et al. (1970)
VFC, Vicia faba root tips, chromosomal breaks	+	0	1000.0000	Swietlin'ska (1971)
VFC, Vicia faba roots, chromosomal breaks and subchromatid exchanges	+	0	300.0000	Kaul & Zutshi (1973)
VFC, Vicia faba root tips, interchanges	−	0	1000.0000	Swietlin'ska et al. (1973)
VFC, Vicia faba, chromosomal aberrations	−	0	3880.0000	Kihlman & Sturelid (1975)
VFC, Vicia faba root tips, chromosomal aberrations	+	0	1000.0000	Osiecka (1976)
PLC, Coreopsis tinctoria, chromosomal aberrations	+	0	3000.0000	Batikjan & Pogosjan (1976)
PL?, Ustilago maydis, mitotic crossing-over	+	0	0.0000	Holliday (1961)

Table 13 (contd)

Test system	Results without exogenous metabolic activation	Results with exogenous metabolic activation	Dose LED/HID	Reference
PL?, Glycine max, mitotic recombination	+	0	0.0000	Vig (1973)
PL?, Nicotiana tabacum cell cultures, mitotic recombination	+	0	0.0000	Carlson (1974)
DMG, Drosophila melanogaster, meiotic crossing over, oogonia	–	0	0.0000	Yefremova & Filippova (1974)
DMG, Drosophila melanogaster, meiotic crossing over, oocytes & stem cells	–	0	0.0000	Yefremova & Filippova (1974)
DMM, Drosophila melanogaster, somatic mutation and recombination	–	0	3000.0000	Graf & Würgler (1986)
DMM, Drosophila melanogaster, somatic mutation and recombination	–	0	5000.0000	Graf & Würgler (1986)
DMX, Drosophila melanogaster, sex-linked recessive lethals, larval	(+)	0	2500.0000	Andrew (1959)
DMX, Drosophila melanogaster, sex-linked recessive lethals, adult	(+)	0	5000.0000	Andrew (1959)
DMX, Drosophila melanogaster, sex-linked recessive lethals, larval	–	0	5000.0000	Yanders & Seaton (1962)
DMX, Drosophila melanogaster, sex-linked recessive lethals, adult	–	0	5000.0000	Yanders & Seaton (1962)
DMX, Drosophila melanogaster, sex-linked recessive lethals, larval	+	0	10000.0000	Ostertag & Haake (1966)
DMX, Drosophila melanogaster, sex-linked recessive lethals	–	0	750.0000	Alderson & Khan (1967)
DMX, Drosophila melanogaster, sex-linked recessive lethals, injection	–	0	1940.0000	Clark & Clark (1968)
DMX, Drosophila melanogaster, sex-linked recessive lethals, fed	–	0	1940.0000	Clark & Clark (1968)
DMX, Drosophila melanogaster, sex-linked recessive lethals	+	0	1150.0000	Shakarnis (1970)
DMX, Drosophila melanogaster, sex-linked recessive lethals, fem.fed	–	0	970.0000	King et al. (1979)
DMX, Drosophila melanogaster, sex-linked recessive lethals, fed	–	0	2500.0000	Reguly & Marques (1988)
DMC, Drosophila melanogaster, larval ganglia cells, chromosomal aberration	–	0	194.0000	De Marco & Cozzi (1980)
DMC, Drosophila melanogaster, ganglia cells, chromosomal aberrations	+	0	1940.0000	De Marco & Polani (1981)
DMH, Drosophila melanogaster, translocations	–	0	1230.0000	Mittler et al. (1967b)
DMN, Drosophila melanogaster, aneuploidy (chromosoal loss XO males)	+	0	10000.0000	Ostertag & Haake (1966)
DMN, Drosophila melanogaster, aneuploidy (nondisjunction XXY females)	–	0	10000.0000	Ostertag & Haake (1966)
DMN, Drosophila melanogaster, aneuploidy (chromosoal loss XO males)	+	0	1230.0000	Mittler et al. (1967a,b)
DMN, Drosophila melanogaster, aneuploidy (nondisjunction XXY females)	+	0	1230.0000	Mittler et al. (1967a,b)
DMN, Drosophila melanogaster, aneuploidy (chromosomal loss XO males)	+	0	1940.0000	Clark & Clark (1968)
DMN, Drosophila melanogaster, aneuploidy (nondisjunction XXY females)	+	0	1940.0000	Clark & Clark (1968)
DMN, Drosophila melanogaster, aneuploidy (nondisjunction XXY males)	+	0	10000.0000	Kuhlman et al. (1968)
DMN, Drosophila melanogaster, aneuploidy (nondisjunction XXY females)	–	0	10000.0000	Kuhlman et al. (1968)
DMN, Drosophila melanogaster, aneuploidy (X-chromosome nondisjunction)	+	0	1150.0000	Shakarnis (1970)
DMN, Drosophila melanogaster, aneuploidy (chromosomal loss)	–	0	5000.0000	Zettle & Murnick (1973)
DMN, Drosophila melanogaster, aneuploidy (nondisjunction)	–	0	5000.0000	Zettle & Murnick (1973)
DMN, Drosophila melanogaster, aneuploidy (chromosomal loss, males)	+	0	0.0000	Arisimova (1975)
DMN, Drosophila melanogaster, aneuploidy (chromosomal loss, females)	–	0	0.0000	Arisimova (1975)
??L, Bombyx mori, dominant lethal test	+	0	388.0000	Murota & Murakami (1976)
DIA, DNA strand breaks, Chinese hamster ovary cells in vitro	+	0	5800.0000	Ishida et al. (1985)
DIA, DNA strand breaks, Chinese hamster V79 cells in vitro	–	0	1000.0000	Swenberg (1981)
DIA, DNA strand breaks, Syrian hamster embryo cells in vitro	–	0	1000.0000	Casto et al. (1976)
UIA, Unscheduled DNA synthesis, Syrian hamster embryo cells	–	0	1000.0000	Casto et al. (1976)

Table 13 (contd)

Test system	Results without exogenous metabolic activation	Results with exogenous metabolic activation	Dose LED/HID	Reference
GCO, Gene mutation, Chinese hamster ovary cells in vitro	−	0	6000.0000	Kao & Puck (1969)
GCO, Gene mutation, Chinese hamster ovary cells in vitro, hprt locus	−[a]	0	0.0000	Arlett & Harcourt (1972)
GCO, Gene mutation, Chinese hamster ovary cells in vitro	−[a]	0	8000.0000	Amacher & Zelljadt (1984)
G9H, Gene mutation, Chinese hamster V79 cells, hprt locus	−[a]	0	194.0000	Trosko & Chu (1971)
G9O, Gene mutation, Chinese hamster V79 cells, ouabain resistance	−	0	175.0000	Chang et al. (1977)
G9O, Gene mutation, Chinese hamster V79 cells, ouabain resistance	−	0	194.0000	Bowden et al. (1979)
G5T, Gene mutation, mouse lymphoma L5178Y cells, tk locus	−	0	9000.0000	Amacher et al. (1980)
SIC, Sister chromatid exchange, Chinese hamster Don cells	−	0	194.0000	Kato (1973)
SIC, Sister chromatid exchange, Chinese hamster Cl-1 cells	−	0	194.0000	Palitti & Becchetti (1977)
SIC, Sister chromatid exchange, Chinese hamster V79 cells	−	0	194.0000	Bowden et al. (1979)
SIC, Sister chromatid exchange, Chinese hamster V79 cells	−	0	3100.0000	Speit (1986)
SIM, Sister chromatid exchange, mouse blastocysts	+	0	19.0000	Spindle & Wu (1985)
MIA, Micronucleus test, rat kidney cell line NRK-49F in vitro	+	0	1940.0000	Dunn et al. (1987)
CIC, Chromosomal aberrations (rearrangements) Chinese hamster CHO cells	+	0	0.0000	Kao & Puck (1969)
CIC, Chromosomal aberrations, Chinese hamster cells	+	0	970.0000	Kihlman et al. (1971a)
CIC, Chromosomal aberrations, Chinese hamster endoreduplicated cells	+	0	5000.0000	Palitti et al. (1974)
CIC, Chromosomal aberrations, Chinese hamster Cl 1 lung cells	+	0	97.0000	Sturelid (1976)
CIC, Chromosomal aberrations, Chinese hamster Cl 1 cells	+	0	194.0000	Palitti & Becchetti (1977)
CIC, Chromosomal aberrations, Chinese hamster CHL cells	+	0	500.0000	Ishidate et al. (1984)
CIR, Chromosomal aberrations (breaks/rearrangements), rat MCT1 cells	−	0	160.0000	Bishun et al. (1974)
TCS, Cell transformation, Syrian hamster embryo cells	+	0	250.0000	Pienta (1980)[(HNT)]
T7S, Cell transformation, SA7/Syrian hamster embryo cells	+	0	125.0000	Casto et al. (1976)
TEV, Cell transformation, adenovirus/hamster embryo cells	+	0	150.0000	Ledinko & Evans (1973)
TEV, Cell transformation, SV40/mouse C3H2K cells	+	0	194.0000	Ide et al. (1975)
UHL, Unscheduled DNA synthesis, normal human lymphocytes	−	0	388.0000	Apfelzweig & Teplitz (1979)
UIH, Unscheduled DNA synthesis, human lupus erythematosus cells	−	0	388.0000	Apfelzweig & Teplitz (1979)
GIH, Gene mutation, human lymphoblast MIT-2 and HH-4 cells, HPR	−	0	0.0000	Furth & Thilly (1978)
SHF, Sister chromatid exchange, human fibroblasts in vitro	+	0	100.0000	Sasaki (1977)
SHL, Sister chromatid exchange, human lymphocytes in vitro	−	0	250.0000	Pant et al. (1976)
SHL, sister chromatid exchange, human lymphocytes in vitro	−	0	194.0000	Waksvik et al. (1977)
SHL, Sister chromatid exchange, human lymphocytes in vitro	(+)	0	100.0000	Faed & Mourelatos (1978)
SHL, Sister chromatid exchange, human lymphocytes in vitro	(+)	0	100.0000	Ishii & Bender (1978)
SHL, Sister chromatid exchange, human lymphocytes in vitro	+	0	50.0000	Guglielmi et al. (1982)
SHT, Sister chromatid exchange, human XP2LE lymphocytes	+	0	0.0000	Andriadzee et al. (1986)
SHT, Sister chromatid exchange, human XP3LE lymphocytes	+	0	0.0000	Andriadzee et al. (1986)
SHT, Sister chromatid exchange, human XP lymphoblastoid cells	(+)	0	194.0000	Tohida & Oikawa (1988)

Table 13 (contd)

Test system	Results without exogenous metabolic activation	Results with exogenous metabolic activation	Dose LED/HID	Reference
CHL, Chromosomal aberrations (gaps/breaks), human lymphocytes	+	0	50.0000	Lee (1971)
CHL, Chromosomal aberrations (gaps/breaks), human lymphocytes	+	0	250.0000	Weinstein et al. (1972)
CHL, Chromosomal aberrations (deletions, exchanges), human lymphocytes	+	0	388.0000	Ceccherini et al. (1988)
CHT, Chromosomal aberrations (breaks), human HeLa cells	+	0	500.0000	Ostertag et al. (1965)
CHT, Chromosomal aberrations, human HeLa cells	–	0	20.0000	Thayer et al. (1971)
CHT, Chromosomal aberrations (breaks/rearrangments), human HeLa	+	0	80.0000	Bishun et al. (1974)
CHL, Chromosomal aberrations, Fanconi's anaemia lymphocytes	+	0	50.0000	Sasaki & Tonomura (1973)
CHT, Chromosomal aberrations (breaks), human leukocytes + HeLa cells	+	0	10000.0000	Ostertag (1966)
CHF, Chromosomal aberrations (gaps/breaks), human embryonic tissue	–	0	50.0000	Lee (1971)
BFA, Urine of female rats, Salmonella typhimurium mutagenicity	–	0	126.0000	Bradford et al. (1983b) (Abstr.)
HMM, Host-mediated assay, Salmonella typhimurium G46 in mice	–	0	150.0000 i.p.	Gabridge & Legator (1969)
HMM, Host-mediated assay, Escherichia coli K12 in mice	–	–	194.0000 i.p.	King et al. (1979)
DVA, Single-strand DNA breakage, Swiss mouse liver/kidney in vivo	+	0	100.0000 i.p.	Cesarone et al. (1982)
MST, PrxHTf1 mouse spot test	–	0	50.0000 i.p.	Nomura (1983)
SLO, Mouse specific locus test (C3H/HCH female x 101/H male) F$_1$ female x DCT male	–	0	250.0000 d.w. x 70 d	Lyon et al. (1962)
SVA, Sister chromatid exchange, Chinese hamster bone marrow	+	0	100.0000 oral	Basler et al. (1979)
SVA, Sister chromatid exchange, C57Bl/6J mouse bone marrow	(+)	0	50.0000 i.v.	Nakanishi & Schneider (1979)
SVA, Sister chromatid exchange, Chinese hamster bone marrow	–	0	200.0000 i.p.	Tsuchimoto & Matter (1979)
SVA, Sister chromatid exchange, Sprague-Dawley rat blood	+	0	1000.0000 diet	Granberg-Öhman et al. (1980)
SVA, Sister chromatid exchange, Chinese hamster bone marrow	+	0	300.0000 oral	Renner (1982)
SVA, Sister chromatid exchange, Swiss albino mice bone marrow	+	0	830.0000 oral	Panigrahi & Rao (1983)
SVA, Sister chromatid exchange, Chinese hamster bone marrow	+	0	300.0000 oral	Aeschbacher et al. (1986)
MVM, Micronucleus test, C3HxC57 mouse bone marrow	–	0	250.0000 i.p.	Matter & Grauwiler (1974)
MVM, Micronucleus test, CBA male mouse bone marrow	–	0	0.0000 inj.	Heddle & Bruce (1977)
MVM, Micronucleus test, NMRI mouse bone marrow	–	0	100.0000 oral	Jenssen & Ramel (1978)
MVM, Micronucleus test, CD-1 mouse bone marrow	–	0	97.0000 i.p.	King et al. (1979)
MVM, Micronucleus test, CD-1 mouse bone marrow	–	0	250.0000 i.p.	Tsuchimoto & Matter (1979)
MVM, Micronucleus test, outbred Swiss CD-1 mouse bone marrow	+	0	100.0000 oral	Aeschbacher et al. (1986)
MVM, Micronucleus test, MS/Ae inbred mouse bone marrow	–	0	100.0000 oral	Aeschbacher et al. (1986)
MVR, Micronucleus test, rat bone marrow and peripheral blood	–	0	126.0000 oral	Bradford et al. (1983b) (Abstr.)
MVC, Micronucleus test, Chinese hamster bone marrow	–	0	250.0000 i.p.	Tsuchimoto & Matter (1979)
MVC, Micronucleus test, Chinese hamster bone marrow	+	0	300.0000 oral	Aeschbacher et al. (1986)
MIA, Micronucleus test, mouse pre-implantation embryo ex vivo	+	0	388.0000	Müller et al. (1985)
CBA, Chromosomal aberrations, C57Bl mouse bone marrow	+	0	4000.0000 d.w.	Frei & Venitt (1975)
CBA, Chromosomal aberrations, Chinese hamster bone marrow	–	0	200.0000 i.p.	Röhrborn & Buckel (1976)
CBA, Chromosomal aberrations, C57Bl/6J mouse bone marrow	(+)	0	50.0000 i.v.	Nakanishi & Schneider (1979)
CBA, Chromosomal aberrations, Chinese hamster bone marrow	–	0	200.0000 i.p.	Tsuchimoto & Matter (1979)
CBA, Chromosomal aberrations, BALB/c mouse bone marrow	+	0	50.0000 i.p.	Dulout et al. (1981)

Table 13 (contd)

Test system	Results		Dose LED/HID	Reference
	Without exogenous metabolic activation	With exogenous metabolic activation		
CLA, Chromosomal aberrations, Sprague-Dawley rat blood	–	0	40.0000 diet	Granberg-Öhman et al. (1980)
CGC, Chromosomal aberrations, C3H mouse meiotic metaphase spermatogenesis	–	0	300.0000 d.w. x 351 d	Adler & Röhrborn (1969)
CVA, Chromosomal aberrations (translocations), male JU mice	–	0	500.0000 d.w. x 90 d	Cattanach (1962)
CGC, Chromosomal aberrations, C3H mouse testes	–	0	250.0000 i.p. x 21 d	Adler (1966)
CVA, Chromosomal aberrations, mouse ascites S2-sarcoma cells	–	0	250.0000 i.p. x 1 d	Adler & Schöneich (1967)
CVA, Chromosomal aberrations, rat Guérin ascites tumour cells	+	0	5.0000 i.v.	Georgian et al. (1980)
DLM, Dominant lethal test, male C3Hx101 mice	–	0	250.0000 d.w.	Lyon et al. (1962)
DLM, Dominant lethal test, male mice	–	0	500.0000 d.w. x 42 d	Cattanach (1964)
DLM, Dominant lethal test, male Swiss CD-1 mice	(+)	0	168.0000 i.p.	Epstein & Shafner (1968)
DLM, Dominant lethal test, male C57Bl mice	–	0	850.0000 oral	Kuhlmann et al. (1968)
DLM, Dominant lethal test, male C3H mice	–	0	250.0000 i.p.	Adler (1969)
DLM, Dominant lethal test, male ICR mice	–	0	140.0000 oral	Epstein et al. (1970)
DLM, Dominant lethal test, male ICR mice	–	0	240.0000 i.p.	Epstein et al. (1970)
DLM, Dominant lethal test, male C3H mice	–	0	15.0000 d.w. x 550 d	Röhrborn (1972)
DLM, Dominant lethal test, male 101 x C3H	–	0	250.0000 i.p. x 1	Röhrborn (1972)
DLM, Dominant lethal test, male 101 x C3H mice	–	0	17.0000 d.w. x 550 d	Röhrborn (1972)
DLM, Dominant lethal test, male C57Bl mice	–	0	515.0000 d.w. x 245 d	Röhrborn (1972)
DLM, Dominant lethal test, male C3H mice	–	0	300.0000 d.w. x 351 d	Röhrborn (1972)
DLM, Dominant lethal test, male 101xC3H mice	–	0	17.0000 d.w. x 246 d	Röhrborn (1972)
DLM, Dominant lethal test, mice	–	0	122.0000 d.w.	Thayer & Kensler (1973)
DLM, Dominant lethal test, mice	–	0	15.0000 i.p.	Thayer & Kensler (1973)
DLM, Dominant lethal test, male Swiss CD-1 mice	–	0	112.0000 d.w. x 8 wk	Aeschbacher et al. (1978)
DLM, Dominant lethal test, male Swiss CD-1 mice	–	0	90.0000 oral x 5 d	Aeschbacher et al. (1978)
SPF, Sperm morphology, (C3HxC57)F1 mice	–	0	0.0000 inj.	Heddle & Bruce (1977)
CLH, Chromosomal aberrations, human lymphocytes in vivo	–	0	11.0000 d.w. x 4 wk	Weinstein et al. (1972)
MVH, Micronuclei, human (splenectomized) erythrocytes/reticulocytes in vivo	+	0	0.0000	Smith et al. (1990)

[a]Antimutagenic effect
i.p., intraperitoneal; s.c., subcutaneous; inj., injection (route not specified); i.v., intravenous; d.w., drinking water; oral, by gavage; d, day; wk, week

concentration curves following oral and intravenous doses were superimposable, suggesting that there is no pronounced first-pass effect (Axelrod & Reichenthal, 1953); after oral doses of 5-8 mg/kg bw, peak plasma concentrations of 8-10 μg/ml were observed (Arnaud & Welsch, 1980b, 1982; Bonati et al., 1982; Blanchard & Sawers, 1983a,b; Arnaud, 1987). After oral ingestion, the time to reach peak plasma concentration exhibits wide variations, ranging from 15 to 120 min (Robertson et al., 1978; Bonati et al., 1982; Arnaud, 1987). These variations can be explained by the effect of gastric emptying (Chvasta & Cooke, 1971; Arnaud, 1987) and also by the presence of dietary constituents (Arnaud, 1987).

After absorption, caffeine is rapidly and uniformly distributed into body fluids (Bonati & Garattini, 1984). The volume of distribution of caffeine in man ranges from 0.5 to 0.8 l/kg bw, but the value most often reported is close to 0.7 l/kg bw (Arnaud, 1987). In newborns, the levels of caffeine in plasma and cerebrospinal fluid are virtually identical (Turmen et al., 1979; Somani et al., 1980). In-vivo and in-vitro studies have shown that caffeine is bound at 10-35% to plasma proteins, mainly albumins, over a wide range of concentrations (1-100 μg/ml) (Bonati & Garattini, 1984; Yesair et al. 1984). The binding capacity of caffeine to breast milk proteins is about 3.2% (Tyrala & Dodson, 1979).

Caffeine is eliminated by apparent first-order kinetics, described by a one-compartment open model system. A study of a limited number of patients with a small range of doses ($\leq$10 mg/kg bw) excluded the existence of dose-dependent kinetics in man at the levels at which people are normally exposed to caffeine (Bonati et al., 1982).

The half-time of caffeine decreases gradually after birth and reaches adult values (2.5-4.5 h) at about the age of six months (Aldridge et al., 1979; Aranda et al., 1979a,b; Parsons & Neims, 1981; Gorodischer & Karplus, 1982). A serum clearance of 31.5 ml/kg bw per h in 1-2.5-month-old infants increased to a mean maximum value of 331.7 ml/kg bw per h in 5-6-month-old infants, while values of 155 and 94 ml/kg bw per h were observed in adult smokers and nonsmokers, respectively (Aranda et al., 1979a). No significant difference in the elimination of caffeine in young and elderly subjects has been found, although a slight decrease in plasma caffeine binding was observed in the older group (Blanchard & Sawers, 1983b).

Caffeine clearance is stimulated by smoking (Parsons & Neims, 1978; Wietholtz et al., 1981; Kotake et al., 1982; May et al., 1982; Arnaud, 1987; Joeres et al., 1988); after stopping smoking for only three or four days, the rate of caffeine metabolism is substantially slower (Brown et al., 1988; Murphy et al., 1988). The metabolic disposition or volume of distribution of caffeine does not differ between men and women (Callahan et al., 1983; Arnaud, 1987). In women, the use of oral contraceptives was shown to double the half-time of caffeine (Patwardhan et al., 1980; Callahan et al., 1983). A gradual prolongation of the half-time was also shown during pregnancy (Neims *et al.*, 1979; Aldridge *et al.*, 1981; Knutti *et al.*, 1981, 1982; Parsons & Pelletier, 1982; Brazier *et al.*, 1983), and caffeine clearance had increased by more than three fold at 2-12 weeks *postpartum* (Parsons & Pelletier, 1982).

Caffeine concentrations in human and fetal gonads were similar to those in plasma (Goldstein & Warren, 1962). A small percentage (0.5-4%) of an ingested dose of caffeine is excreted unchanged in urine (Arnaud, 1987). Caffeine is also excreted in bile (Arnaud, 1987) and is found in saliva (Cook *et al.*, 1976; Parsons & Neims, 1978; Newton *et al.*, 1981), semen (Beach *et al.*, 1982, 1984) and breast milk (Tyrala & Dodson, 1979; Findlay *et al.*, 1981; Bailey *et al.*, 1982; Ryu, 1985); it was also detected in umbilical cord blood (Parsons *et al.*, 1976; van't Hoff, 1982). As salivary concentrations correspond to 65-85% of plasma concentrations, they can be used to predict serum concentrations (Khanna *et al.*, 1980; Callahan *et al.*, 1982). An average milk to serum concentration ratio of 0.52 was observed (Tyrala & Dodson, 1979).

The metabolism of caffeine is the rate-limiting factor for its plasma clearance (Arnaud, 1987). It is transformed by hepatic microsomal enzymes (Grant *et al.*, 1987; Berthou *et al.*, 1989), and no significant metabolism occurs in other organs (Arnaud, 1987). The initial major step in caffeine biotransformation in humans is selective catalysis by cytochrome P450PA (P450IA2) in human liver microsomes, which is also responsible for the *N*-oxidation of aryl amines (Butler *et al.* 1989). The major role of the liver is demonstrated by the impaired clearance of caffeine in subjects with liver disease, in whom serum half-times of 60-168 h were reported (Statland *et al.*, 1976; Desmond *et al.*, 1980; Statland & Demas, 1980; Renner *et al.*, 1984). Many drug interactions have been reported to lead to impaired caffeine elimination, explained by competitive inhibition at the enzymatic level (Reynolds, 1989). Allopurinol causes dose-dependent inhibition of the conversion of 1-methylxanthine to 1-methyluric acid (Grygiel *et al.*, 1979; Grant *et al.*, 1986). Alcohol has been shown to impair caffeine elimination (Mitchell *et al.*, 1983; George *et al.*, 1986). Ingestion of 480 mg/day of caffeine for one week by healthy male volunteers failed to alter its pharmacokinetics (George *et al.*, 1986).

Caffeine metabolism has been reviewed extensively (Arnaud, 1984, 1987) (see Figure 2). After oral administration of caffeine, plasma concentrations of theobromine and theophylline showed a small and similar increase, while a ten-fold higher paraxanthine concentration was observed. In most of the subjects studied, caffeine plasma concentrations decreased more rapidly than those of paraxanthine, so that paraxanthine concentrations became higher than those of caffeine from 8 to 10 h after administration (Bonati *et al.*, 1982). The amount of urinary caffeine metabolites depends on the rate of each biotransformation step, the body distribution of metabolites, their plasma concentrations and their renal excretion (Arnaud, 1987). All the metabolic transformations shown in Figure 2 include

Fig. 2. Metabolism of caffeine in humans[a]

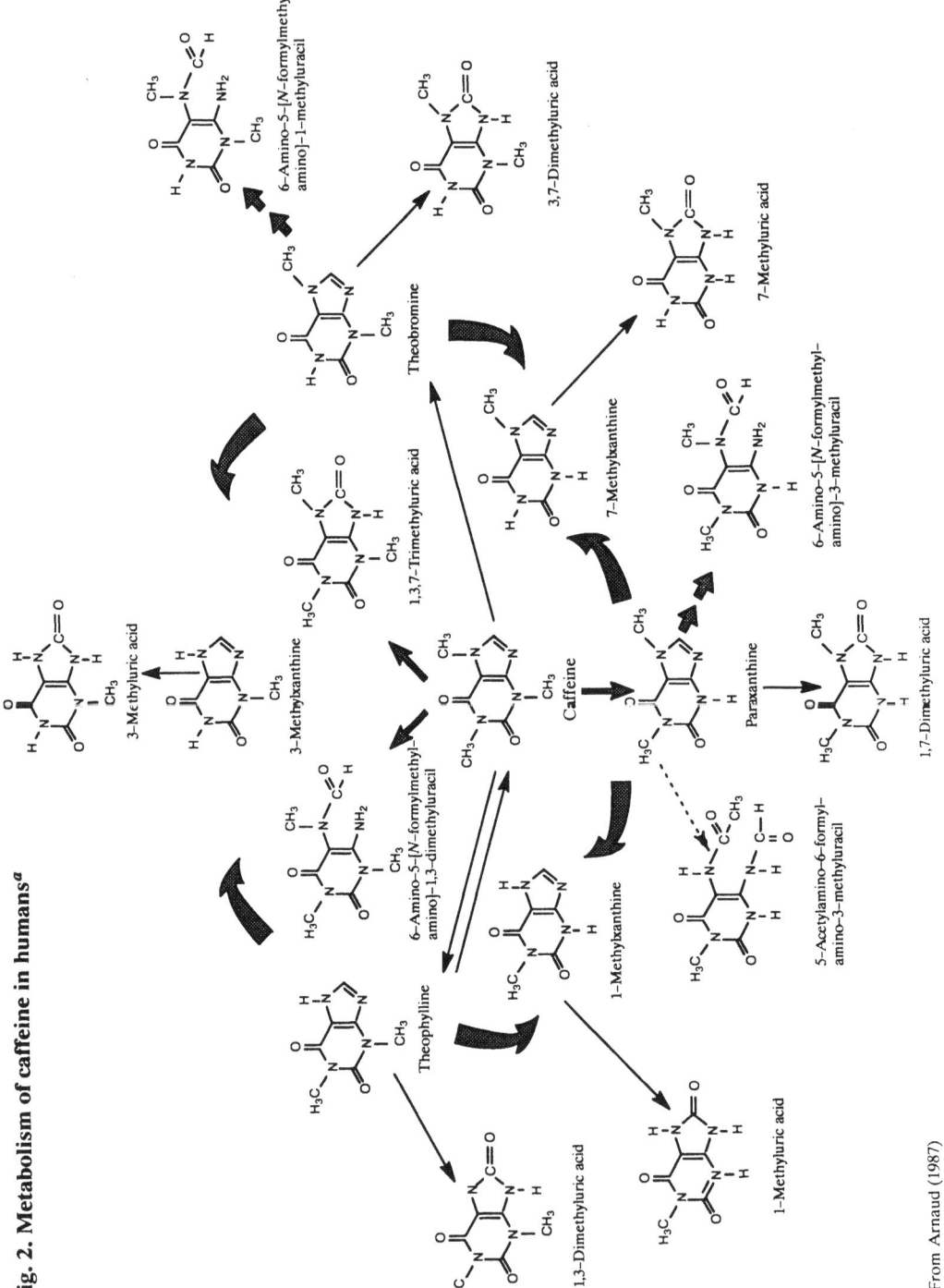

[a]From Arnaud (1987)

multiple and separate pathways with demethylation, C-8 oxidation and perhaps, associated with this transformation, the formation of uracil derivatives. In contrast to these biotransformations, the C-8 oxidation of 1-methylxanthine into 1-methyluric acid is not a microsomal transformation but was shown to be performed by xanthine oxidase (Bergmann & Dikstein, 1956; Grygiel et al., 1979; Grant et al., 1986; Arnaud, 1987).

Although in women who used oral contraceptives, the half-time of caffeine was doubled, only minor changes in the proportion of the formed metabolites have been reported (Callahan et al., 1983). Compared to controls, pregnant women produced smaller amounts of 1-methylxanthine and 1-methyluric acid (Scott et al., 1986).

The most important metabolic pathway in humans is demethylation of caffeine (95%), only 5% giving trimethyl derivatives, whereas in rodents 40% trimethyl derivatives are found (Arnaud & Welsch, 1980b; Arnaud, 1987). Therefore, collection of labelled carbon dioxide after demethylation of [14C- or 13C-methyl]-caffeine constitutes a breath test used in clinical studies to detect impaired liver function (Wietholtz et al., 1981; Kotake et al., 1982; Renner et al., 1984; Arnaud, 1987).

The 5-acetylamino-6-formylamino-3-methyluracil metabolite of caffeine is found only in humans; paraxanthine was shown to be its precursor (Grant et al., 1983a; Arnaud, 1984). Although its estimated rate of production (3-35%) approximates those of 1-methylxanthine (18%) and 1-methyluric acid (15%) (Callahan et al., 1982; Yesair et al., 1984), however, its metabolic formation is not yet understood. The variability in the production and excretion rates of acetylated urinary metabolites (Callahan et al., 1982; Tang et al., 1983) was related to acetylation polymorphism (Grant et al., 1983b). The demonstration that the general population could be divided into fast and slow acetylators (Evans & White, 1964) explains some of the variability observed in caffeine metabolism. A simple marker for acetylator status in man is the ratio 5-acetylamino-6-formylamino-3-methyluracil:1-methylxanthine in urine (El-Yazigi et al., 1989). The ratios of the urinary concentrations of 1-methyluric acid:1-methylxanthine, of 1,7-dimethyluric acid:1,7-dimethylxanthine and of 5-acetylamino-6-formylamino-3-methyluracil plus 1-methyluric acid plus 1-methylxanthine:1,7-dimethylxanthine represent indices of xanthine oxidase, 8-hydroxylation and 7-demethylation activities, respectively (Kalow, 1984).

After oral administration of labelled caffeine, 2-5% was excreted in the faeces. The most important products identified were 1,7-dimethyluric acid at 44%, 1-methyluric acid at 38%, 1,3-dimethyluric acid at 14%, 1,3,7-trimethyluric acid at 6% and caffeine at 2% of faecal radioactivity (Callahan et al., 1982).

(ii) *Toxic effects*

General toxicity: The toxicity of caffeine in humans has been reviewed (Lachance, 1982; Rall, 1985; Arnaud, 1987; Ashton, 1987; Leonard *et al.*, 1987; Stavric, 1988).

At low doses (up to 2 μg/ml in blood), caffeine stimulates the central nervous system, and this effect is perceived by many caffeine users as beneficial. High blood concentration (10-30 μg/ml) of caffeine may produce restlessness, excitement, tremor, tinnitus, headache and insomnia (Lachance, 1982; Ashton, 1987; Stavric, 1988).

Caffeine can induce alterations in mood and sleep patterns, increase urine production and gastric acid secretion, alter myocardial function, induce hypertension and arrhythmia, and increase plasma catecholamine levels and plasma renin activity, especially when administered to non-users or recent abstainers (Leonard *et al.*, 1987; Stavric, 1988). Excessive consumption of caffeine may lead to an anxiety neurosis known as 'caffeinism'. Similar symptoms have been described after withdrawal of caffeine (Greden, 1979; Griffiths & Woodson, 1988).

Acute toxicity due to caffeine is not very common, although some adverse effects (e.g., gastric symptoms, insomnia, diuresis) have been observed as a result of overdoses (Lachance, 1982; Rall, 1985; Stavric, 1988). Caffeine poisoning can be especially hazardous to persons with impaired liver function. Patients with liver cirrhosis may accumulate up to 40 times more caffeine and its metabolites than healthy controls (Wahlländer *et al.*, 1985).

The effects of coffee and tea on plasma lipid levels and on morbidity and mortality from cardiovascular disease are discussed in detail in the respective monographs.

The effect of caffeine consumption (86.8% from coffee) on mortality from cardiovascular disease was evaluated in a cohort study of more than 10 000 hypertensive people from 14 communities in the USA over four years. No evidence was found to support an association between increased caffeine consumption and increased mortality due to cardiovascular disease (Martin *et al.*, 1988).

Blood pressure: The effects of caffeine on blood pressure have been reviewed (Myers, 1988; Robertson & Curatolo, 1984).

In volunteers who abstained from caffeine-containing products, a bolus dose of 250 mg led to a 5-10% increase in both systolic and diastolic blood pressure for 1-3 h. Tolerance to this effect developed, however, when caffeine was given three times a day for seven days (Robertson *et al.*, 1978, 1981; Arnaud, 1987). Increases in systolic and diastolic blood pressure (by 5.1 and 11.5 mm Hg, respectively) were observed in 10 volunteers who drank coffee corresponding to about 240 mg caffeine (Smits *et al.*, 1986). In another study, daily use of decaffeinated coffee (40 mg caffeine) instead of five cups of regular coffee (445 mg caffeine) for six weeks led to a small but significant decrease in systolic (by 1.5 mm Hg) and diastolic (by 1.0 mm Hg) blood pressure in 45 healthy volunteers (van Dusseldorp et al., 1989).

Several epidemiological studies have investigated the association between coffee drinking and blood pressure. One showed that only systolic blood pressure was related to coffee intake, and the overall increase before adjustment for other variables was 2.5 mm Hg (Lang et al., 1983). In another study (Birkett & Logan, 1988) caffeine intake was positively related to an increase in diastolic blood pressure, but the effect was small — less than 1 mm Hg at usual caffeine intake. A longitudinal study with more than 51 000 participants found no relationship between either systolic or diastolic blood pressure and the number of cups of coffee consumed (Bertrand et al., 1978). A significant decrease in blood pressure with increased coffee consumption was found in an epidemiological investigation involving 500 persons (Periti et al., 1987).

The available data indicate that consumption of caffeine in moderate amounts does not cause a persistent increase in blood pressure in normotensive subjects. Caffeine can, however, acutely raise blood pressure in non-users of caffeine-containing beverages, but after one to four days of regular consumption a tolerance develops, with blood pressure returning to previous levels.

Cardiac arrhythmias: Caffeine and caffeine-containing beverages have long been implicated in the etiology of cardiac arrhythmias, but only a few well-designed studies have been carried out in humans (for a review, see Dobmeyer et al., 1983). An association between premature ventricular beats and consumption of large amounts of coffee or tea was found in a large cross-sectional study reported by Prineas et al. (1980).

Contrary to several earlier authors (for reviews, see Dobmeyer et al., 1983; Robertson & Curatolo, 1984), Myers et al. (1987) found no increase in the severity or frequency of ventricular arrhythmia after intake of caffeine (300 mg) in a placebo-controlled study of patients with previous myocardial infarction. These results are in contrast to those of another study (Sutherland et al., 1985) in which 200 mg caffeine induced a considerable increase in the frequency of extrasystoles in subjects with a high incidence of spontaneous ventricular ectopic beats. Thus, the traditional clinical view that caffeine induces cardiac arrhythmias in humans still remains open, both in healthy subjects and in patients with existing heart disease.

Benign breast disease:

(1) *Case series and intervention trials*: A clinical association between fibrocystic breast disease and caffeine consumption was suggested in 1979, when Minton et al. (1979a,b) reported differences in the levels of cAMP and cGMP in normal, fibrotic, fibroadenomatous, fibrocystic and carcinomatous breast tissues. They also found

an improvement in signs of the disease among women who eliminated methylxanthines from their diet. Similar findings were reported in a subsequent study by the same group (Minton *et al.*, 1981). Several concerns about the studies have been raised. They were not randomized, information on the extent of disease at baseline was not always provided, caffeine consumption and the course of the disease were not monitored during the study, and outcome was ascertained by people who were aware of the caffeine consumption status of the subject.

Several clinical case series were subsequently studied. Brooks *et al.* (1981) found an improvement in signs of fibrocystic breast disease after restricting methylxanthine consumption. Heyden and Muhlbaier (1984; reported again by Heyden & Fodor, 1986) found that the mean change in total methylxanthine consumption in women who experienced a total or transient disappearance of nodules was similar to that in women who did not experience such changes. Hindi-Alexander *et al.* (1985) found that the severity of fibrocystic breast disease was greater with greater intake of caffeine, theophylline and total methylxanthines. Three randomized studies were conducted: Ernster *et al.* (1982) found a reduction in clinically palpable breast nodes in women on the methylxanthine-free diet but found no relation between changes in caffeine levels in breast fluid and degree of improvement in breast findings score. Parazzini *et al.* (1986) observed no difference among the methylxanthine-abstention groups in respect of change in size, clinical characteristics or mean scores at follow-up. Data from Allen and Froberg (1987) did not support the hypothesis of decreasing nodularity in the caffeine-free group relative to that in the group with no dietary restriction group or in a placebo group.

[The Working Group noted that studies of case series and intervention trials were concerned mainly with the effect of caffeine consumption on the symptoms of benign breast disease; they have little, if any, bearing on the occurrence of this condition.]

(2) *Etiological studies*: Lawson *et al.* (1981) analysed data obtained from the Boston Collaborative Drug Surveillance Program (January-September 1972) and from a collaborative study conducted in the USA, Scotland and New Zealand (from 1977 to present). Coffee and tea drinking were grouped as 'hot beverage consumption'. When cases of fibrocystic disease were compared to controls who did not drink coffee or tea, the relative risks (RRs) were 1.4, 1.5 and 1.3 for increasing levels of intake.

Marshall *et al.* (1982) analysed a series of patients admitted to the Roswell Park Memorial Institute, Buffalo, NY, USA, between 1957 and 1965. When data were analysed by number of cups per day, no relation was found between the occurrence of fibrocystic breast disease and coffee consumption (age-adjusted RR, 0.9 for more than three cups per day *versus* non-coffee drinker); a nonsignificant reduction in risk was associated with tea consumption (RR, 0.8 for more than three cups per day), and no relation was seen when results for the two beverages were combined.

Boyle et al. (1984) conducted a hospital-based case-control study in Connecticut, USA, from 1979 to 1981. The study showed a clear, significant dose-response relationship between the occurrence of fibrocystic breast disease and the amount of caffeine that had been consumed daily five years previously. When patients were compared with women who consumed fewer than 30 mg caffeine per day, the RRs were 1.5, 2.0 and 2.3 for those who consumed 31-250, 251-500 and >500 mg per day ($p < 0.0001$ test for trend). The increase in risk was greater among women with those subtypes of benign breast disease that are thought to be most closely related to an increased risk for breast cancer. The data were based on patient recall of caffeine consumption.

Odenheimer et al. (1984) studied female twins from the Kaiser-Permanente Twin Registry (USA) in 1977-79. For the 90 pairs in which one twin had biopsy-confirmed benign breast disease, the RR was 1.6 (95% confidence interval (CI), 1.0-2.4) for each cup of coffee consumed per day. For the 48 pairs in which cases were determined by clinical examination, the RR was 4.2 (1.1-15.6) for different categories of consumption. Fifteen pairs were in both groups.

Lubin et al. (1984, 1985a) conducted a hospital-based case-control study in Israel between 1977 and 1980. No significant association between the occurrence of benign breast disease and coffee consumption was found: in comparison with surgical controls, the adjusted RRs were 1.0, 1.1, 0.95 and 0.80 for four categories of consumption (0, 1, 2-3, >4 cups/day); compared to neighbourhood controls they were 1.0, 0.85, 0.83 and 0.70. No association between total methylxanthine intake and benign breast disease was found. Similarly, no association was found when women with different histological types or women with different degrees of ductal atypia were examined separately.

La Vecchia et al. (1985) conducted a hospital-based case-control study of benign breast disease in Milan, Italy, between 1981 and 1983. Categorizing coffee consumption in three levels (0, 1-2 and >3 cups/day), the RRs by multivariate analysis were 1.0, 3.0 (95% CI, 1.7-5.3) and 3.8 (2.2-6.7) compared to the inpatient controls, and 1.0, 1.4 (0.8-2.5) and 2.1 (1.2-3.8) compared to outpatient controls for all benign breast disease together. For benign tumours (85 cases), the RRs were 1.0, 2.3 (1.0-4.8) and 1.6 (0.7-3.5) compared to the inpatient controls, and 1.0, 1.0 (0.5-2.2) and 1.0 (0.4-2.1) compared to outpatient controls. For dysplasia (203 cases), the RRs were 1.0, 4.1 (2.0-8.4) and 6.4 (3.1-13.1) compared to inpatient controls and 1.0, 2.0 (1.0-4.1) and 3.7 (1.8-7.7) when compared to outpatient controls.

Schairer et al. (1986) conducted a case-control study on participants in the Breast Cancer Detection Demonstration Project in the USA. For all benign breast disease cases, the RRs were 1.0, 1.0 (95% CI, 0.8-1.2), 1.0 (0.8-1.2), 1.0 (0.7-1.2) and

1.1 (0.8-1.5) for five increasing levels of methylxanthine consumption (< 125, 126-250, 251-500, 501-750, > 750 mg/day). When analysed specifically for cases of fibrocystic disease, cases of unknown type and cases of benign neoplasms, the RRs were all near unity. When cases with fibrocystic disease were subdivided by the presence of atypia, hyperplasia, sclerosing adenosis and cyst, RRs near unity were again observed.

Rohan *et al.* (1989) conducted a case-control study in Adelaide, Australia, between 1983 and 1985 which included both biopsy-confirmed controls (women whose biopsy did not show epithelial proliferation) and community controls. Total methylxanthine intake (caffeine, theobromine and theophylline) was not related to the risk of benign proliferative epithelial disorders: adjusted RRs for increased quintiles of intake (< 173.2, 173.2-270.0, 270.1-344.0, 344.1-429.3, > 429.3 mg/day) were 1.0, 0.8 (0.5-1.3), 0.8 (0.5-1.5), 0.8 (0.4-1.3) and 1.2 (0.7-2.1) using community controls, and 1.0, 0.7 (0.4-1.2), 0.7 (0.5-1.7), 0.7 (0.4-1.3) and 1.0 (0.6-1.9) using biopsy controls. Separate analyses for theophylline, theobromine and caffeine and for degree of atypia generally showed no association; however, theobromine intake was associated with an increased risk when biopsy controls were used as the comparison group. Total methylxanthine intake was associated with an increased risk of severe atypia when community controls were used.

[The Working Group noted that the positive association between coffee intake and benign breast disease found in some etiological studies could be due to the difference in the likelihood of disease detection between consumers and nonconsumers of methylxanthines. The one study in which biopsy-confirmed controls were used found no association.]

(iii) *Effects on reproduction and prenatal toxicity*

Malformations: A case-control study was carried out in Scotland by Nelson and Forfar (1971) of 458 mothers who gave birth to infants with congenital abnormalities and two control groups; the first was composed of the mothers of the next 500 normal babies delivered in the same maternity units as the patients, and the second were 411 mothers matched to the mothers of cases by age, parity and babies' sex. Mothers were interviewed on the use of pharmaceuticals during pregnancy. This information was confirmed by doctors' or pharmacists' records; 11.3% of the reports were rejected due to lack of confirmation. Caffeine-containing drugs had been used by 2.4% of the mothers of cases and 1.5% of those of controls (nonsignificant). Few data are provided on losses and refusals. [The Working Group noted the restricted use of caffeine-containing drugs; other sources of caffeine were not considered.]

A large North American study followed 5378 women exposed during pregnancy to caffeine-containing drugs for possible malformations in their offspring (Heinonen, 1982). For all malformations considered together (n = 350), the RR was 0.98. For malformations at individual sites, the RRs ranged from 0.70 to 1.2 (nonsignificant). [The Working Group noted that non-medicinal sources of caffeine were not accounted for.]

Several studies have reported congenital malformations in relation to consumption of caffeine in beverages (Borlée et al., 1978; Linn et al., 1982; Rosenberg et al., 1982; Tohnai et al., 1984, Furuhashi et al., 1985). These are discussed in the monograph on coffee (pp. 104-106).

Rosenberg et al. (1982) estimated total caffeine intake from coffee, tea and cola for 2030 mothers of malformed infants and 712 controls. Total caffeine intake was related neither to all malformations nor to those at invididual sites.

Low birthweight and/or preterm birth: Studies relating coffee intake and low birthweight (Mau & Netter, 1974; van den Berg, 1977; Arnandova & Kaculov, 1978; Kuzma & Sokol, 1982; Linn et al., 1982; Berkowitz et al., 1982; Watkinson & Fried, 1985; Furuhashi et al., 1985; Martin & Bracken, 1987; Muñoz et al., 1988; Brooke et al., 1989; Caan & Goldhaber, 1989) are described on pp. 106-112. In several of these studies sources of caffeine other than coffee were considered.

Total caffeine intake, as determined from various sources including coffee, tea, cola and drugs, was positively associated with the proportion of low-birthweight babies after controlling for smoking and other potential confounders (RR, 4.6 for consumption of >300 mg/day *versus* no consumption; $p < 0.001$) (Martin & Bracken, 1987). A significant increase in the frequency of low birthweight was found by Caan and Goldhaber (1989) among women with heavy consumption of caffeine from coffee and cola as compared to women with none (odds ratio, 3.5; $p < 0.05$). [The Working Group was concerned that cola and coffee were considered to be equivalent sources of caffeine per drink.]

Effects on sperm and fertility: The addition of caffeine to human sperm increased sperm mobility (Hommonai et al., 1976; Traub et al., 1982; Aitken et al., 1983). Barkay et al. (1984) reported that women undergoing artificial insemination were twice as likely to become pregnant if their husband's semen had been treated with caffeine than if it had not. Scanning electron microscopic examination of fresh semen showed no morphological change caused by in-vitro treatment with caffeine.

(iv) *Genetic and related effects*

Vogel et al. (1966) published results of an epidemiological study in which the sex ratios of children in German families were examined relative to the parents' coffee-drinking habits. Using multiple regression techniques, no evidence was found that caffeine induced sex-linked recessive lethal mutations in women or sex-linked dominant mutations in men. The authors suggested that since the questionnaires on coffee drinking were completed by the children and their parents, there might be uncontrolled biases in the study. [The Working Group noted that others have pointed out that during the years in which many of the children involved were conceived, 'coffee' consumption may not necessarily have been synonymous with caffeine consumption because of wartime substitutions.]

The urine of coffee drinkers was not mutagenic to *S. typhimurium* TA100 or TA98 (Aeschbacher & Chappuis, 1981) (see the monograph on coffee, p. 112).

Drinking coffee or tea to result in a total caffeine intake corresponding to that in five cups of coffee per day [exact amount not stated] was associated by multiple regression analysis with a roughly two-fold higher frequency of both micronucleated reticulocytes and micronucleated mature erythrocytes in splenectomized but otherwise healthy individuals after adjustment for smoking. Drinking decaffeinated coffee was not associated with an increase in the number of micronucleated cells (Smith *et al.*, 1990).

Cultured human lymphocytes from volunteers on a regime of 800 mg caffeine daily for four weeks, resulting in caffeine blood levels as high as 29.6 µg/ml after four weeks showed no significant increase in the frequency of chromosomal damage (Weinstein *et al.*, 1972, 1973a,b, 1975).

In one study of caffeine ingestion during pregnancy, an elevated frequency of chromosomal anomalies was reported (Furuhashi *et al.*, 1985). [The Working Group noted that the laboratory and the epidemiological methods, as well as the data, were so inadequately reported that the study was not suitable for evaluation.]

3.3 Epidemiological studies of cancer in humans

The epidemiological studies considered are those in which the effect of caffeine was examined as well as those in which the effects of methylxanthines (caffeine, theophylline and theobromine) were looked at.

(a) Cohort studies

(i) *All sites*

The effect of caffeine consumption on mortality from cancer at all sites among the 10 064 participants in the Hypertension Detection and Follow-up Program in the USA was examined after four years of follow-up (Martin *et al.*, 1988). Exposure to caffeine was estimated on the basis of data obtained at interview concerning coffee and tea consumption and use of caffeine-containing medications; no data were collected on consumption of caffeine-containing soft drinks. The unadjusted RRs showed no association between caffeine consumption and mortality from cancer or any other cause, although in all of these analyses, the confidence intervals were very wide.

(ii) *Breast cancer*

Phelps and Phelps (1988) conducted an ecological study, which did not distinguish between tea and coffee consumption, and reported a correlation of 0.004 with breast cancer mortality ratios after adjusting for dietary fat intake.

(b) *Case-control studies*

(i) *Breast*

Case-control studies of breast cancer and methylxanthine consumption are summarized in Table 14.

In the hospital-based case-control study of Lubin *et al.* (1984, 1985b), described on p. 145, methylxanthine intake was quantified on the basis of caffeine in coffee, tea and cola and theobromine in chocolate and in cocoa. No association was found, even after stratification for ethnic group, age or consumption of total, saturated or polyunsaturated fats.

In the study of Schairer *et al.* (1987), described on p. 146, on participants in a five-year screening programme for the detection of breast cancer in the USA, information on methylxanthine consumption was derived from information about consumption of brewed coffee, instant coffee, decaffeinated coffee, hot non-herbal tea, hot cocoa, iced tea, chocolate milk, cola soft drinks and diet cola drinks. The results for total caffeine alone were similar to those for total methylxanthines consumed, so only the latter were given. No association was found.

Rohan and McMichael (1988) conducted a population-based case-control study of breast cancer in Adelaide, South Australia. A total of 559 cases were diagnosed between April 1982 and July 1984; 451 were included in the study. Controls were matched to the age of the cases at diagnosis and selected at random from the electoral roll. A total of 648 individuals were approached in order to enroll the 451 controls included in this study. Methylxanthine intake was measured by means of a self-administered, quantitative food frequency questionnaire, and daily intake of caffeine was calculated in instant coffee, decaffeinated coffee, percolated coffee, drip coffee, tea, cocoa, chocolate drink, solid chocolate and cola; daily intake of theobromine in cocoa, chocolate drink and solid chocolate was also calculated. No increased risk for breast cancer was found in postmenopausal women in association with total caffeine and total methylxanthine intake. However, premenopausal women had an increase in risk at mid-third of intake (caffeine: RR, 2.0; 95% CI, 1.0-4.2; methylxanthines: 2.0, 1.0-4.1) and a smaller increase in risk at the upper third of intake (caffeine: 1.4; 0.6-3.0; methylxanthines: 1.6; 0.7-3.3). None of the RRs deviated markedly from unity and none was statistically significant. The patterns of RR provided little support for an interaction between methylxanthine and fat in determining breast cancer risk.

Iscovich *et al.* (1989) conducted a case-control study in La Plata, Argentina in 1984-85. Of the 153 cases of breast cancer identified, only three were not interviewed. Two matched controls were selected for each case: one from a hospital and the other from the neighbourhood of the case. Caffeine-containing beverages were one of 147 dietary items on the questionnaire, along with questions on demographic and socioeconomic characteristics, reproductive history and smoking. Multivariate analysis, adjusting for known risk factors, showed no effect of caffeine-containing beverages, analysed in quartiles, on breast cancer risk. Smoking was not adjusted for.

In the study by Pozner *et al.* (1986), described on p. 146, caffeine and coffee intake were examined in women with breast cancer to determine whether their consumption influenced cell differentiation in tumours. Caffeine consumption was calculated for coffee, instant coffee, decaffeinated coffee, tea, cola and cocoa. Women with moderately or well-differentiated tumours had higher intakes of all coffee, caffeinated coffee, decaffeinated coffee, cola and tea.

Table 14. Summary of results of case-control studies of breast cancer and methylxanthine consumption

Reference and location	Subjects (cases, controls)	Methylxanthine consumption (mg/day)	Relative risk (95% confidence interval)	Comments
Lubin *et al.* (1984, 1985b) Israel	724, 724 surgical controls	0-126 127-213 214-316 317-1008	1.0 0.6 (0.4-0.9) 0.8 (0.5-1.2) 0.8 (0.5-1.4)	Matched on age, country of origin, length of residence in Israel
	794, 794 neighbourhood controls	0-129 130-215 216-311 312-877	1.0 0.7 (0.5-1.0) 0.5 (0.3-0.8) 0.8 (0.5-1.3)	
Schairer *et al.* (1987) USA	1510, 1882	≤125 126-250 251-500 501-750 751-1000 >1000	1.0 0.8 (0.7-1.0) 0.8 (0.7-1.0) 0.7 (0.6-1.0) 1.1 (0.7-1.6) 0.7 (0.4-1.0)	Crude unmatched analysis; similar results obtained after adjustment for other risk factors
Rohan & McMichael (1988) Australia	451, 451	0-179.3 179.4-255.0 255.1-317.8 37.9-415.0 ≥415.1	1.0 0.9 (0.6-1.3) 1.0 (0.6-1.4) 1.1 (0.7-1.6) 1.1 (0.7-1.7)	Matched on age

Table 14 (contd)

Reference and location	Subjects (cases, controls)	Methylxanthine consumption (mg/day)	Relative risk (95% confidence interval)	Comments
Iscovich et al. (1989) Argentina	150, 150 hospital controls	1 2 3 4	1.0 0.7 0.99 1.1	Quartiles of caffeine-containing beverage consumption; multivariate analysis
	150, 150 neighbourhood controls	1 2 3 4	1.0 0.9 0.9 0.5	

(ii) *Urinary bladder*

In a case-control study in Copenhagen, Denmark (Jensen et al., 1986), described on p. 126, a weak association was found between cancer of the urinary bladder and caffeine intake from coffee and tea. This association was significant in men ($p < 0.05$) after adjustment for consumption of beer and soft drinks, in addition to age and smoking.

4. Summary of Data Reported and Evaluation

4.1 Exposure data

Caffeine is a methylxanthine and occurs naturally in more than 60 plant species throughout the world. It is prepared on an industrial scale by methylation of theobromine.

Global per-caput consumption of caffeine from all sources was estimated to be 70 mg per day in 1981-82.

Caffeine is consumed in beverages such as coffee, tea and mate and in soft drinks to which caffeine is added. Coffee is the main source of dietary caffeine consumption. The caffeine content of beverages varies widely. Caffeine is also used in numerous prescription and non-prescription pharmaceutical preparations.

4.2 Experimental carcinogenicity data

Caffeine was tested for carcinogenicity in five studies in rats by oral administration. In two of these studies, no significant difference in the incidence of tumours at any site was found. The other three studies were found to be inadequate for evaluation.

Studies on oral and intraperitoneal administration of caffeine to mice were found to be inadequate for evaluation.

In one study, decaffeinated coffee to which caffeine was added was tested by oral administration to rats; overall, no increase in the incidence of tumours at any site was observed as compared to appropriate controls.

Administration of caffeine in combination with known carcinogens resulted in decreased incidences of lung tumours in mice treated with urethane, of mammary tumours in rats treated with diethylstilboestrol and of skin tumours in mice treated with either ultraviolet light or cigarette-smoke condensate. Caffeine did not influence the incidence of bladder tumours induced in rats by N-nitroso-N-butyl(4-hydroxybutyl)amine in three experiments or of pancreatic tumours induced in rats by 4-hydroxyaminoquinoline-1-oxide in another study.

4.3 Human carcinogenicity data

A cohort study with a short follow-up period showed no association between caffeine consumption and mortality from cancers at all sites, although there were few deaths on which to base an analysis.

Four case-control studies of breast cancer in which an attempt was made to measure methylxanthine intake showed no association. A slight increase in risk was seen in premenopausal women in one study, but in general the relative risks were below unity.

One case-control study of bladder cancer showed a weak association with caffeine consumption.

Caffeine and coffee consumption are highly correlated in most of the populations studied; thus, it is very difficult to separate the two exposures in epidemiological studies. It was therefore not possible to evaluate adequately the effect of caffeine *per se*.

4.4 Other relevant data

Caffeine intake from pharmaceutical sources has not been related to teratogenic effects in humans. High levels of either coffee or caffeine consumption were related to an increased frequency of low birthweight.

Quantitative and qualitative differences in the metabolism of caffeine are seen between humans and experimental animals.

On the basis of the available evidence, caffeine consumed in moderate amounts does not cause any persistent increase in blood pressure in normotensive subjects. Whether caffeine consumed in amounts present in coffee or tea causes cardiac arrhythmia in healthy subjects or in patients with heart disease remains an open question.

Caffeine has been shown to cause adverse reproductive and developmental effects in mice, rats, rabbits and monkeys. Testicular atrophy was observed at high dose levels in rats. Reproductive studies in mice showed no effect on pregnancy, but there was a decrease in litter size at birth. Teratogenic effects were usually associated with high, single, daily doses that were also associated with other signs of maternal toxicity. High daily levels given as divided doses were less toxic to the conceptus than when given as a single dose. Reduced fetal body weight was observed in rats. A reversible delay in ossification of the sternum was observed in rats at a relatively low dose given by gavage. With administration in drinking-water, similar effects were seen, but at higher doses.

One epidemiological study revealed no effect of caffeine (in coffee-drinking subjects) on the sex ratio of their children. In lymphocytes of normal, caffeine-exposed people, chromosomal aberrations were not observed. An increased frequency of micronucleated blood cells was observed in otherwise healthy splenectomized people exposed to caffeine. Urine of caffeine-exposed persons was not mutagenic to *Salmonella typhimurium*.

Although it has been suggested that caffeine may induce gene mutations in mammals and man, direct evidence *in vivo* is limited and the indirect evidence is based largely on extrapolation from results in lower organisms, in which there is no doubt about the mutagenic action of caffeine, and from cultured mammalian cells, in which caffeine is clastogenic at high concentrations.

Overall, caffeine affects photoreactivation, excision repair and postreplication repair. The antagonistic effect of caffeine on mutations induced by ultraviolet radiation has been explained on the basis of inhibition of an error-prone, postreplicative, recombination repair process. Caffeine can modulate the effects of xenobiotics by acting on (i) cytochrome P450, (ii) cAMP metabolism, (iii) DNA metabolism, chromatin structure and function and (iv) nucleotide pools.

4.5 Evaluation[1]

There is *inadequate evidence* for the carcinogenicity in humans of caffeine.

There is *inadequate evidence* for the carcinogenicity in experimental animals of caffeine.

Overall evaluation

Caffeine is *not classifiable as to its carcinogenicity to humans (Group 3)*.

---

[1]For description of the italicized terms, see Preamble, pp. 27–31.

5. References

Adler, I.-D. (1966) Cytogenetic investigations of mutagenic action of caffeine in premeiotic spermiogenesis in mice. *Humangenetik*, *3*, 82-83

Adler, I.-D. (1969) Does caffeine induce dominant lethal mutations in mice? *Humangenetik*, *7*, 137-148

Adler, I.-D. (1970) The problems of caffeine mutagenicity. In: Vogel, F. & Röhrborn, G., eds, *Chemical Mutagenesis in Mammals and Man*, Berlin, Springer, pp. 383-403

Adler, I.-D. & Röhrborn, G. (1969) Cytogenetic investigation of meiotic chromosomes of male mice after chronic caffeine treatment. *Humangenetik*, *8*, 81-85

Adler, I.-D. & Schöneich, J. (1967) Mutagenic action of caffeine in an ascites tumour strain of mice: cytogenetic investigation. *Humangenetik*, *4*, 374-376

Aeschbacher, H.U. & Chappuis, C. (1981) Non-mutagenicity of urine from coffee drinkers compared with that from cigarette smokers. *Mutat. Res.*, *89*, 161-177

Aeschbacher, H.U. & Würzner, H.P. (1975) Effect of methylxanthines on hepatic microsomal enzymes in the rat. *Toxicol. appl. Pharmacol.*, *33*, 575-581

Aeschbacher, H.U., Milon, H. & Würzner, H.P. (1978) Caffeine concentrations in mice plasma and testicular tissue and the effect of caffeine on the dominant lethal test. *Mutat. Res.*, *57*, 193-200

Aeschbacher, H.U., Chappuis, C. & Würzner, H.P. (1980) Mutagenicity testing of coffee: a study of problems encountered with the Ames *Salmonella* test system. *Food Cosmet. Toxicol.*, *18*, 605-613

Aeschbacher, H.U., Meier, H. & Jaccaud, E. (1986) The effect of caffeine in the in vivo SCE and micronucleus mutagenicity tests. *Mutat. Res.*, *174*, 53-58

Ahmad, A. & Leupold, U. (1973) On a possible correlation between fine-structure map expansion and reciprocal recombination based on crossing-over. *Mol. gen. Genet.*, *123*, 143-158

Ahnström, G. & Natarajan, A.T. (1971) Repair of gamma-ray and neutron-induced lesions in germinating barley seeds. *Int. J. Radiat. Biol.*, *19*, 433-443

Ahokas, J.T., Pelkonen, O., Ravenscroft, P.J. & Emmerson, B.T. (1981) Effects of theophylline and caffeine on liver microsomal drug metabolizing mono-oxygenase in genetically AHH-responsive and non-responsive mice. *Res. Commun. Subst. Abuse*, *2*, 277-290

Aitken, R.J., Best, F., Richardson, D.W., Schats, R. & Simm, G. (1983) Influence of caffeine on movement characteristics, fertilizing capacity and ability to penetrate cervical mucus of human spermatozoa. *J. Reprod. Fertil.*, *67*, 19-27

Alderson, T. & Khan, A.H. (1967) Caffeine-induced mutagenesis in *Drosophila*. *Nature*, *215*, 1080-1081

Aldridge, A. & Neims, A.H. (1979) The effects of phenobarbital and β-naphthoflavone on the elimination kinetics and metabolic pattern of caffeine in the beagle dog. *Drug Metab. Disposition*, *7*, 378-382

Aldridge, A. & Neims, A.H. (1980) Relationship between the clearance of caffeine and its 7-*N*-demethylation in developing beagle puppies. *Biochem. Pharmacol.*, *29*, 1909-1914

Aldridge, A., Parsons, W.D. & Neims, A.H. (1977) Stimulation of caffeine metabolism in the rat by 3-methylcholanthrene. *Life Sci.*, *21*, 967-974

Aldridge, A., Aranda, J.V. & Neims, A.H. (1979) Caffeine metabolism in the newborn. *Clin. Pharmacol. Ther.*, *25*, 447-453

Aldridge, A., Bailey, J. & Neims, A.H. (1981) The disposition of caffeine during and after pregnancy. *Semin. Perinatol.*, *5*, 310-314

Al-Hachim, G.M. (1989) Teratogenicity of caffeine: a review. *Eur. J. Obstet. Gynecol. reprod. Biol.*, *31*, 237-247

Allen, S.S. & Froberg, D.G. (1987) The effect of decreased caffeine consumption on benign proliferative breast disease: a randomized clinical trial. *Surgery*, *101*, 720-730

Althaus, F.R. & Richter, C. (1987) *ADP-Ribosylation of Proteins*, Berlin, Springer

Amacher, D.E. & Zelljadt, I. (1984) Mutagenic activity of some clastogenic chemicals at the hypoxanthine guanine phosphoribosyl transferase locus of Chinese hamster ovary cells. *Mutat. Res.*, *136*, 137-145

Amacher, D.E., Paillet, S.C., Turner, G.N., Ray, V.A. & Salsburg, D.S. (1980) Point mutations at the thymidine kinase locus in L5178Y mouse lymphoma cells. II. Test validation and interpretation. *Mutat. Res.*, *72*, 447-474

Anderson, K.E., Conney, A.H. & Kappas, A. (1982) Nutritional influences on chemical biotransformations in humans. *Nutr. Rev.*, *40*, 161-171

Andersson, H.C. (1982) G2 repair and the formation of chromosomal aberrations. III. The effect of hydroxyurea, 5-fluorodeoxyuridine and caffeine on X-ray-induced chromosome damage in *Vicia faba*. *Hereditas*, *97*, 193-209

Andrew, L.E. (1959) The mutagenic activity of caffeine in *Drosophila*. *Am. Nat.*, *43*, 135-138

Andriadzee, M.I., Pleskach, N.M., Mikhelson, V.M. & Zhestyanikov, V.D. (1986) Spontaneous and induced sister chromatid exchanges in blood lymphocytes of healthy donors and a xeroderma pigmentosum patient under the action of inhibitors of DNA synthesis and repair: novobiocin, 3-methoxybenzamide and caffeine (Russ.). *Tsitologia*, *28*, 69-85

Anon. (1973) Caffeine, coffee, and cancer. *Br. med. J.*, *281*, 1031-1032

Anon. (1983) Caffeine levels in Australian foods. *Food Technol. Austr.*, *35*, 87

Anon. (1986) Caffeine's no wide-awake market. *Chem. Bus.*, *8*, 44

Anon. (1987a) Caffeine prices skyrocketing as total supplies tighten. *Chem. Mark. Rep.*, 6 April, 201

Anon. (1987b) Caffeine. *Food Chem. News Guide*, 25 May, 78.1

Anon. (1988) Caffeine prices strengthened as coffee consumption slides. *Chem. Mark. Rep.*, 28 November, pp. 17-18

Anon. (1989a) Caffeine seen as stable despite Chinese imports. *Chem. Mark. Rep.*, 7 August, 20-21

Anon. (1989b) Caffeine content for various sodas. *Beverage Ind.*, June, 57

Anon. (1989c) Annual soft drink report. *Beverage Ind.*, March

Apfelzweig, R.A. & Teplitz, R.L. (1979) A study of the effect of caffeine upon excision repair of damaged DNA. *Mutat. Res.*, 62, 151-158

Aranda, J.V., Collinge, J.M., Zinman, R. & Watters, G. (1979a) Maturation of caffeine elimination in infancy. *Arch. Dis. Child.*, 54, 946-949

Aranda, J.V., Cook, C.E., Gorman, W., Collinge, J.M., Loughnan, P.M., Outerbridge, E.W., Aldridge, A. & Neims, A.H. (1979b) Pharmacokinetic profile of caffeine in the premature newborn infant with apnea. *J. Pediatr.*, 94, 663-668

Aranda, J.V., Beharry, K., Rex, J., Johannes, R.J. & Charest-Boule, L. (1987) Caffeine enzyme immunoassay in neonatal and pediatric drug monitoring. *Ther. Drug Monit.*, 9, 97-103

Arisimova, L.E. (1975) Comparative study of sex chromosome nondisjunction and loss frequencies in female and male *Drosophila melanogaster* under the combined action of caffeine and X-rays (Russ.). *Vestn. Leningr. Univ. Biol.*, 2, 145-147

Ariza, R.R., Dorado, G., Barbancho, M. & Pueyo, C. (1988) Study of the causes of direct-acting mutagenicity in coffee and tea using the ara test in *Salmonella typhimurium*. *Mutat. Res.*, 201, 89-96

Arlett, C.F. & Harcourt, S.A. (1972) The induction of 8-azaguanine-resistant mutants in cultured Chinese hamster cells by ultraviolet light. The effect of changes in post-irradiation conditions. *Mutat. Res.*, 14, 431-437

Armuth, V. & Berenblum, I. (1981) The effect of caffeine on two-stage skin carcinogenesis and on complete systemic carcinogenesis. *Carcinogenesis*, 2, 977-979

Arnandova, R. & Kaculov, A. (1978) Coffee and pregnancy (Russ.). *Akush. Ginekol. (Sofia)*, 17, 57-61

Arnaud, M.J. (1976) Identification, kinetic and quantitative study of [$2\text{-}^{14}C$] and [$1\text{-Me}^{14}C$] caffeine metabolites in rat's urine by chromatographic separations. *Biochem. Med.*, 16, 67-76

Arnaud, M.J. (1984) Products of metabolism of caffeine. In: Dews, P.B., ed., *Caffeine. Perspectives from Recent Research*, Berlin, Springer, pp. 3-38

Arnaud, M.J. (1985a) Pharmacokinetics in animal chronic toxicological studies, *J. Pharm. clin.*, 4, 259-268

Arnaud, M.J. (1985b) Comparative metabolic disposition of [$1\text{-Me}^{14}C$]caffeine in rats, mice, and chinese hamsters. *Drug Metab. Disposition*, 13, 471-478

Arnaud, M.J. (1987) The pharmacology of caffeine. *Progr. Drug Res.*, 31, 273-313

Arnaud, M.J. & Getaz, F. (1986) Effect of pregnancy on [$1,3,7\text{-Me}^{14}C$]caffeine breath test in the rat. *Acta pharmacol. toxicol.*, Suppl. 5, Abstract 859

Arnaud, M.J. & Welsch, C. (1980a) Comparison of caffeine metabolism by perfused rat liver and isolated microsomes. In: Coon, M.J., Conney, A.H., Estabrook, R.W., Gelboin, H.V., Gillette, J.R. & O'Brien, P.J., eds, *Microsomes, Drug Oxidations and Chemical Carcinogenesis*, Vol. II, New York, Academic Press, pp. 813-816

Arnaud, M.J. & Welsch, C. (1980b) Caffeine metabolism in human subjects. In: *9e Colloque Scientifique International sur le Café, London, 1980*, Paris, Association Scientifique Internationale du Café, pp. 385-396

Arnaud, M.J. & Welsch, C. (1982) Theophylline and caffeine metabolism in man. In: Rietbrock, N., Woodcock, B.G. & Staib, A.H., eds, *Theophylline and Other Methylxanthines*, Braunschweig, Wiesbaden, Friedr. Vieweg and Sohn, pp. 135-148

Arnaud, M.J., Ben-Zvi, Z., Yaari, A. & Gorodischer, R. (1986a) 1,3,8-Trimethylallantoin: a major caffeine metabolite formed by rat liver. *Res. Commun. chem. Pathol. Pharmacol.*, 52, 407-410

Arnaud, M.J., Richli, U. & Philippossian, G. (1986b) Isolation and identification of paraxanthine (Px) glucuronide as the major caffeine metabolite in mice (Abstract). *Experientia*, 42, 696

Arnaud, M.J., Bracco, I. & Getaz, F. (1989) Synthesis of ring labelled caffeine for the study of metabolic and pharmacokinetics. Mouse interstrain differences in relation to pharmacologic and toxic effects. In: Baillie, T.A. & Jones, J.R., eds, *Synthesis and Applications of Isotopically Labelled Compounds*, Amsterdam, Elsevier, pp. 645-648

Ashton, C.H. (1987) Caffeine and health. *Br. med. J.*, 295, 1293-1294

Ax, R.L., Collier, R.J. & Lodge, J.R. (1976) Effects of dietary caffeine on the testis of domestic fowl, *Gallus domesticus*. *J. Reprod. Fertil.*, 47, 235-238

Axelrod, J. & Reichenthal, J. (1953) The fate of caffeine in man and a method for its estimation in biological material. *J. Pharmacol. exp. Ther.*, 107, 519-523

Bailey, D.N., Weibert, R.T., Naylor, A.J. & Shaw, R.F. (1982) A study of salicylate and caffeine excretion in the breast milk of two nursing mothers. *J. anal. Toxicol.*, 6, 64-68

Balachandran, R. & Srinivasan, A. (1982) Caffeine inhibits DNA polymerase I from *Escherichia coli*: studies *in vitro*. *Carcinogenesis*, 3, 151-153

Balansky, R.M., Blagoeva, P.M. & Mirtcheva, Z. (1983) The influence of selenium and caffeine on chemical carcinogenesis in rats, mutagenesis in bacteria, and unscheduled DNA synthesis in human lymphocytes. *Biol. Trace Element Res.*, 5, 331-343

Barfknecht, T.R. & Shankel, D.M. (1975) The effect of streptomycin resistance, caffeine and acriflavine on ultraviolet light-induced reversion to tryptophan independence in strains of *Escherichia coli* B/r. *Mutat. Res.*, 30, 163-176

Barkay, J., Bartoov, B., Ben-Ezra, S., Langsam, J., Feldman, E., Gordon, S. & Zuckerman, H. (1984) The influence of in vitro caffeine treatment on human sperm morphology and fertilizing capacity. *Fertil. Steril.*, 41, 913-918

Barone, J.J. & Roberts, H. (1984) Human consumption of caffeine. In: Dews, P.B., ed., *Caffeine: Perspectives from Recent Research*, Berlin, Springer, pp. 59-73

Basler, A., Bachmann, U., Roszinsky-Köcher, G. & Röhrborn, G. (1979) Effects of caffeine on sister-chromatid exchanges (SCE) *in vivo*. *Mutat. Res.*, 59, 209-214

Bateman, A.J. (1969) A storm in a coffee cup. *Mutat. Res.*, 7, 475-478

Batikjan, G.G. & Pogosjan, V.S. (1976) Investigation of caffeine action in different tissues of *Coreopsis tinctoria* Nutt (Russ.). *Tsitol. Genet.*, 10, 240-243

Beach, C.A., Bianchine, J.R. & Gerber, N. (1982) The excretion of caffeine in the semen of men: comparison of the concentrations in blood and semen. *Proc. west. Pharmacol. Soc.*, 25, 377-380

Beach, C.A., Bianchine, J.R. & Gerber, N. (1984) The excretion of caffeine in the semen of men: pharmacokinetics and comparison of the concentrations in blood and semen. *J. clin. Pharmacol.*, 24, 120-126

van den Berg, B.J. (1977) Epidemiologic observations of prematurity: effects of tobacco, coffee and alcohol. In: Reed, D.M. & Stanley, F.J., eds, *The Epidemiology of Prematurity*, Baltimore, Urban & Schwarzenberg, pp. 157-176

Bergmann, F. & Dikstein, S. (1956) Studies on uric acid and related compounds. III. Observations on the specificity of mammalian xanthine oxidases. *J. biol. Chem.*, 223, 765-780

Berkowitz, G.S., Holford, T.R. & Berkowitz, R.L. (1982) Effects of cigarette smoking, alcohol, coffee and tea consumption on preterm delivery. *Early Hum. Dev.*, 7, 239-250

Berthou, F., Ratanasavanh, D., Riche, C., Picart, D., Voirin, T. & Guillouzo, A. (1989) Comparison of caffeine metabolism by slices, microsomes and hepatocyte cultures from adult human liver. *Xenobiotica*, 19, 401-417

Bertrand, M., Schwam, E., Frandon, A., Vagne, A. & Alary, J. (1965) The systematic and specific teratogenic effect of caffeine in rodents (Fr.). *C.R. Soc. Biol. (Paris)*, 159, 2199-2202

Bertrand, M., Girod, J. & Rigaud, M.F. (1970) Ectrodactyly induced by caffeine in rodents: role of specific and genetic factors (Fr.). *C.R. Soc. Biol. (Paris)*, 164, 1488-1489

Bertrand, C.A., Pomper, I., Hillman, G., Duffy, J.C. & Michell, I. (1978) No relation between coffee and blood pressure (Letter to the Editor). *New Engl. J. Med.*, 299, 315-316

Bień, M., Piatkowski, J. & Lachowicz, T.M. (1989) Inhibition of mating process by caffeine and its effect on antibiotic marker segregation in yeast *Saccharomyces cerevisiae*. In: Martini, A. & Vaughan Martini, A., eds, *Yeast as a Main Protagonist of Biotechnology*, Vol. 2, London, John Wiley & Sons, pp. S267-S271

Birkett, N.J. & Logan, A.G. (1988) Caffeine-containing beverages and the prevalence of hypertension. *J. Hypertension*, 6 (Suppl. 4), S620-S622

Bishun, N., Williams, D. & Mills, J. (1974) The cytogenetic effects of caffeine on two tumour cell lines. *Mutat. Res.*, 26, 151-155

Blanchard, J. & Sawers, S.J.A. (1983a) The absolute bioavailability of caffeine in man. *Eur. J. clin. Pharmacol.*, 24, 93-98

Blanchard, J. & Sawers, S.J.A. (1983b) Comparative pharmacokinetics of caffeine in young and elderly men. *J. Pharmacokin. Biopharm.*, 11, 109-126

Blauch, J.L. & Tarka, S.M., Jr (1983) HPLC determination of caffeine and theobromine in coffee, tea and instant hot cocoa mixes. *J. Food Sci.*, 48, 745-750

Bonati, M. & Garattini, S. (1984) Interspecies comparison of caffeine disposition. In: Dews, P.B., ed., *Caffeine. Perspectives from Recent Research*, Berlin, Springer, pp. 48-56

Bonati, M. & Garattini, S. (1988) Pharmacokinetics of caffeine. *ISI Atlas Sci. Pharmacol.*, 2, 33-39

Bonati, M., Latini, R., Galletti, F., Young, J.F., Tognoni, G. & Garattini, S. (1982) Caffeine disposition after oral doses. *Clin. Pharmacol. Ther.*, 32, 98-106

Bonati, M., Latini, R., Tognoni, G., Young, J.F. & Garattini, S. (1984-85) Interspecies comparison of in vivo caffeine pharmacokinetics in man, monkey, rabbit, rat, and mouse. *Drug Metab. Rev.*, *15*, 1355-1383

Boothman, D.A., Schlegel, R. & Pardee, A.B. (1988) Anticarcinogenic potential of DNA-repair modulators. *Mutat. Res.*, *202*, 393-411

Borlée, I., Lechat, M.F., Bouckaert, A. & Misson, C. (1978) Coffee, risk factor during pregnancy (Fr.). *Louvain Méd.*, *97*, 279-284

Bott, K. (1982) *Caffeine from Theophylline, Carbon Monoxide and Methanol*, German Patent 3,113,880 (BASF A.-G.) [*Chem. Abstr.*, *98*, 53545m]

Bowden, G.T., Hsu, I.C. & Harris, C.C. (1979) The effect of caffeine on cytotoxicity, mutagenesis, and sister-chromatid exchanges in Chinese hamster cells treated with dihydrodiol epoxide derivatives of benzo[*a*]pyrene. *Mutat. Res.*, *63*, 361-370

Boyd, J.B. & Presley, J.M. (1974) Repair replication and photorepair of DNA in larvae of *Drosophila melanogaster*. *Genetics*, *77*, 687-700

Boyd, J.B. & Shaw, K.E.S. (1982) Postreplication repair defects in mutants of *Drosophila melanogaster*. *Mol. gen. Genet.*, *186*, 289-294

Boyle, C.A., Berkowitz, G.S., LiVolsi, V.A., Ort, S., Merino, M.J., White, C. & Kelsey, J.L. (1984) Caffeine consumption and fibrocystic breast disease: a case-control epidemiologic study. *J. natl Cancer Inst.*, *72*, 1015-1019

Boynton, A.L., Evans, T.C. & Crouse, D.A. (1974) Effects of caffeine on radiation-induced mitotic inhibition in S-180 ascites tumor cells. *Radiat. Res.*, *60*, 89-97

Bradbrook, I.D., James, C.A., Morrison, P.J. & Rogers, H.J. (1979) Comparison of thin-layer and gas chromatographic assays for caffeine in plasma. *J. Chromatogr.*, *163*, 118-122

Bradford, J.C., Caldwell, J.A., Barbolt, T.A. & Drobeck, H.P. (1983a) Chronic administration of caffeine to two generations of rats (Abstract). *Teratology*, *27*, 32A

Bradford, J.C., Naismith, R.W., Sorg, R.M., Godek, E.G., Matthews, R.J., Caldwell, J.A. & Drobreck, H.P. (1983b) Micronucleus test and body fluid analysis of rats exposed to caffeine in a reproductive study (Abstract No. Cb-10). *Environ. Mutagenesis*, *5*, 402

Brazier, J.L., Ritter, J., Berland, M., Khenfer, D. & Faucon, G. (1983) Pharmacokinetics of caffeine during and after pregnancy. *Dev. Pharmacol. Ther.*, *6*, 315-322

Brøgger, A. (1974) Caffeine-induced enhancement of chromosome damage in human lymphocytes treated with methyl methanesulfonate, mitomycin C and X-rays. *Mutat. Res.*, *23*, 353-360

Brooke, O.G., Anderson, H.R., Bland, J.M., Peacock, J.L. & Stewart, C.M. (1989) Effects on birth weight of smoking, alcohol, caffeine, socioeconomic factors, and psychosocial stress. *Br. med. J.*, *298*, 795-801

Brooks, P.G., Gart, S., Heldfond, A.J., Margolin, M.L. & Allen, A.S. (1981) Measuring the effect of caffeine restriction on fibrocystic breast disease: the role of graphic stress telethermometry as an objective monitor of disease. *J. reprod. Med.*, *26*, 279-282

Brown, C.R., Jacob, P., III, Wilson, M. & Benowitz, N.L. (1988) Changes in rate and pattern of caffeine metabolism after cigarette abstinence. *Clin. Pharmacol. Ther.*, *43*, 488-491

Brune, H., Deutsch-Wenzel, R.P., Habs, M., Ivankovic, S. & Schmähl, D. (1981) Investigation of the tumorigenic response to benzo(a)pyrene in aqueous caffeine solution applied orally to Sprague-Dawley rats. *J. Cancer Res. clin. Oncol.*, *102*, 153-157

Budavari, S., ed. (1989) *The Merck Index*, 11th ed., Rahway, NJ, Merck & Co., p. 248

Buhl, S.N. & Regan, J.D. (1974) Effect of caffeine on postreplication repair in human cells. *Biophys. J.*, *14*, 519-527

Burg, A.W. (1975a) Effects of caffeine on the human system. *Tea Coffee Trade J.*, *147*, 40-42

Burg, A.W. (1975b) Physiological disposition of caffeine. *Drug Metab. Rev.*, *4*, 199-228

Burg, A.W. & Werner, E. (1972) Tissue distribution of caffeine and its metabolites in the mouse. *Biochem. Pharmacol.*, *21*, 923-936

Butler, M.A., Iwasaki, M., Guengerich, F.P. & Kadlubar, F.F. (1989) Human cytochrome P-450PA (P-450IA2), the phenacetin O-deethylase, is primarily responsible for the hepatic 3-demethylation of caffeine and N-oxidation of carcinogenic arylamines. *Proc. natl Acad. Sci. USA*, *86*, 7696-7700

Byfield, J.E., Murnane, J., Ward, J.F., Calabro-Jones, P., Lynch, M. & Kulhanian, F. (1981) Mice, men, mustards and methylated xanthines: the potential role of caffeine and related drugs in the sensitization of human tumours to alkylating agents. *Br. J. Cancer*, *43*, 669-683

Caan, B.J. & Goldhaber, M.K. (1989) Caffeinated beverages and low birthweight: a case-control study. *Am. J. public Health*, *79*, 1299-1300

Callahan, M.M., Robertson, R.S., Arnaud, M.J., Branfman, A.R., McComish, M.F. & Yesair, D.W. (1982) Human metabolism of [1-methyl-^{14}C]- and [2-^{14}C]caffeine after oral administration. *Drug Metab. Disposition*, *10*, 417-423

Callahan, M.M., Robertson, R.S., Branfman, A.R., McComish, M.F. & Yesair, D.W. (1983) Comparison of caffeine metabolism in three nonsmoking populations after oral administration of radiolabeled caffeine. *Drug Metab. Disposition*, *11*, 211-217

Carlson, P.S. (1974) Mitotic crossing-over in a higher plant. *Genet. Res.*, *24*, 109-112

Casto, B.C., Pieczynski, W.J., Janosko, N. & DiPaolo, J.A. (1976) Significance of treatment interval and DNA repair in the enhancement of viral transformation by chemical carcinogens and mutagens. *Chem.-biol. Interact.*, *13*, 105-125

Cattanach, B.M. (1962) Genetical effects of caffeine in mice. *Z. Vererbungsl.*, *93*, 215-219

Cattanach, B.M. (1964) A genetical approach to the effects of radiomimetic chemicals on fertility in mice. In: Carlson, W.D. & Gassner, F.X., eds, *Effects of Ionizing Radiation on the Reproductive System*, Oxford, Pergamon, pp. 415-426

Ceccherini, I., Loprieno, N. & Sbrana, I. (1988) Caffeine post-treatment causes a shift in the chromosome aberration types induced by mitomycin C, suggesting a caffeine-sensitive mechanism of DNA repair in G2. *Mutagenesis*, *3*, 39-44

Cesarone, C.F., Bolognesi, C. & Santi, L. (1982) Evaluation of damage to DNA after in vivo exposure to different classes of chemicals. *Arch. Toxicol.*, Suppl. *5*, 355-359

Chang, C.-C., Philipps, C., Trosko, J.E. & Hart, R.W. (1977) Mutagenic and epigenetic influence of caffeine on the frequencies of UV-induced ouabain-resistant Chinese hamster cells. *Mutat. Res.*, *45*, 125-136

Chetsanga, C.J., Rushlow, K. & Boyd, V. (1976) Caffeine enhancement of digestion of DNA by nuclease S_1. *Mutat. Res., 34*, 11-20

Christensen, H.D. & Isernhagen, R. (1981) The application of the radial compression separation system for biological materials. In: Hawk, G.L., ed., *Biological/Biomedical Applications of Liquid Chromatography*, Vol. 3, New York, Marcel Dekker, pp. 71-93

Christensen, H.D. & Neims, A.H. (1984) Measurement of caffeine and its metabolites. In: Dews, P.B., ed., *Caffeine. Perspectives from Recent Research*, Berlin, Springer, pp. 39-47

Christensen, H.D. & Whitsett, T.L. (1979) Measurements of xanthines and their metabolites by means of high pressure liquid chromatography. *Chromatogr. Sci., 10*, 507-537

Christensen, H.D., Manion, C.V. & Kling, O.R. (1981) Caffeine kinetics during late pregnancy. In: Soyka, L.F. & Redmond, G.P., eds, *Drug Metabolism in the Immature Human*, New York, Raven Press, pp. 163-181

Chvasta, T.E. & Cooke, A.R. (1971) Emptying and absorption of caffeine from the human stomach. *Gastroenterology, 61*, 838-843

Clark, A.M. & Clark, E.G. (1968) The genetic effects of caffeine in *Drosophila melanogaster*. *Mutat. Res., 6*, 227-234

Clarke, C.H. & Shankel, D.M. (1975) Antimutagenesis in microbial systems. *Bacteriol. Rev., 39*, 33-53

Clarke, C.H. & Wade, M.J. (1975) Evidence that caffeine, 8-methoxypsoralene and steroidal diamines are frameshift mutagens for *E. coli* K-12. *Mutat. Res., 28*, 123-125

Collins, T.F.X., Welsh, J.J., Black, T.N. & Collins, E.V. (1981) A study of the teratogenic potential of caffeine given by oral intubation to rats. *Regul. Toxicol. Pharmacol., 1*, 355-378

Collins, T.F.X., Welsh, J.J., Black, T.N. & Ruggles, D.I. (1983) A study of the teratogenic potential of caffeine ingested in drinking water. *Food chem. Toxicol., 21*, 763-777

Collins, T.F.X., Welsh, J.J., Black, T.N., Whitby, K.E. & O'Donnell, M.W., Jr (1987) Potential reversibility of skeletal effects in rats exposed *in utero* to caffeine. *Food chem. Toxicol., 25*, 647-662

Consumers Union (1990) *US Pharmacopeia. Drug Information for the Consumer*, Easton, PA, Mack Publishing, pp. 274-277, 287-289

Cook C.E., Tallent, C.R., Amerson, E.W., Myers, M.W., Kepler, J.A., Taylor, G.F. & Christensen, H.D. (1976) Caffeine in plasma and saliva by a radioimmunoassay procedure. *J. Pharmacol. exp. Ther., 199*, 679-686

Craig, W.J. & Nguyen, T.T. (1984) Caffeine and theobromine levels in cocoa and carob products. *J. Food Sci., 49*, 302-305

Dalvi, R.R. (1986) Acute and chronic toxicity of caffeine: a review. *Vet. hum. Toxicol., 28*, 144-150

Debry, G. (1989) *Le Café* [Coffee], Nancy, Centre de Nutrition Humaine

De Flora, S., Zanacchi, P., Camoirano, A., Bennicelli, C. & Badolati, G.S. (1984a) Genotoxic activity and potency of 135 compounds in the Ames reversion test and in a bacterial DNA-repair test. *Mutat. Res., 133*, 161-198

De Flora, S., Camoirano, A., Zanacchi, P. & Bennicelli, C. (1984b) Mutagenicity testing with TA97 and TA102 of 30 DNA-damaging compounds, negative with other *Salmonella* strains. *Mutat. Res.*, *134*, 159-165

Delvaux, A.-M. & Devoret, R. (1969) The occurrence of suppressors in caffeine-resistant mutants from *E. coli* K12. *Mutat. Res.*, *7*, 273-285

De Marco, A. & Cozzi, R. (1980) Chromosomal aberrations induced by caffeine in somatic ganglia of *Drosophila melanogaster*. *Mutat. Res.*, *69*, 55-69

De Marco, A. & Polani, S. (1981) Cell-stage-specific enhancement by caffeine of the frequency of chromatid aberrations induced by X-rays in neural ganglia of *Drosophila melanogaster*. *Mutat. Res.*, *84*, 91-99

Demas, T. & Statland, B.E. (1977) Prolonged half-life of serum caffeine in patients with hepatic insufficiency (Abstract No. 203). *Clin. Chem.*, *23*, 1156

Demerec, M., Bertani, G. & Flint, J. (1951) A survey of chemicals for mutagenic action on E. coli. *Am. Naturalist*, *85*, 119-136

Denda, A., Yokose, Y., Emi, Y., Murata, Y., Ohara, T., Sunagawa, M., Mikami, S., Takahashi, S. & Konishi, Y. (1983) Effects of caffeine on pancreatic tumorigenesis by 4-hydroxyaminoquinoline 1-oxide in partially pancreatectomized rats. *Carcinogenesis*, *4*, 17-22

Desmond, P.V., Patwardhan, R.V., Johnson, R.F. & Schenker, S. (1980) Impaired elimination of caffeine in cirrhosis. *Dig. Dis. Sci.*, *25*, 193-197

De Vries, J.W., Johnson, K.D. & Heroff, J.C. (1981) HPLC determination of caffeine and theobromine content of various natural and red dutched cocoas. *J. Food Sci.*, *46*, 1968-1969

Dews, P.B. (1982) Caffeine. *Ann. Rev. Nutr.*, *2*, 323-341

Dobmeyer, D.J., Stine, R.A., Leier, C.V., Greenberg, R. & Schaal, S.F. (1983) The arrhythmogenic effects of caffeine in human beings. *New Engl. J. Med.*, *308*, 814-816

Dong, M., Hoffmann, D., Locke, D.C. & Ferrand, E. (1977) The occurrence of caffeine in the air of New York City. *Atmos. Environ.*, *11*, 651-653

Dorrbecker, S.H., Ferraina, R.A., Dorrbecker, B.R. & Kramer, P.A. (1987) Caffeine and paraxanthine pharmacokinetics in the rabbit: concentration and product inhibition effects. *J. Pharmacokinet. Biopharmacol.*, *15*, 117-132

Dorrbecker, S.H., Raye, J.R., Dorrbecker, B.R. & Kramer, P.A. (1988) Caffeine disposition in the pregnant rabbit. I. Pharmacokinetics following administration by intravenous bolus and continuous zero-order infusion. *Dev. Pharmacol. Ther.*, *11*, 109-117

Dougherty, J.B., Kelsen, D., Kemeny, N., Magill, G., Botet, J. & Niedzwiecki, D. (1989) Advanced pancreatic cancer: a phase I-II trial of cisplatin, high-dose cytarabine and caffeine. *J. natl Cancer Inst.*, *81*, 1735-1738

Dulout, F.N., Larramendy, M.L. & Olivero, O.A. (1981) Effect of caffeine on the frequency of chromosome aberrations induced *in vivo* by triethylenemelamine (TEM) and adriamycin (ADR) in mice. *Mutat. Res.*, *82*, 295-304

Dunkel, V.C., Zeiger, E., Brusick, D., McCoy, E., McGregor, D., Mortelmans, K., Rosenkranz, H.S. & Simmon, V.F. (1985) Reproducibility of microbial mutagenicity assays: II. Testing of carcinogens and noncarcinogens in *Salmonella typhimurium* and *Escherichia coli*. *Environ. Mutagenesis*, 7 *(Suppl. 5)*, 1-248

Dunlop, M. & Court, J.M. (1981) Effects of maternal caffeine ingestion on neonatal growth in rats. *Biol. Neonat.*, *39*, 178-184

Dunn, T.L., Gardiner, R.A., Seymour, G.J. & Lavin, M.F. (1987) Genotoxicity of analgesic compounds assessed by an in vitro micronucleus assay. *Mutat. Res.*, *189*, 299-306

van Dusseldorp, M., Smits, P., Thien, T. & Katan, M.B. (1989) Effect of decaffeinated *versus* regular coffee on blood pressure. A 12-week, double-blind trial. *Hypertension*, *14*, 563-569

Elmazar, M.M.A., McElhatton, P.R. & Sullivan, F.M. (1982) Studies on the teratogenic effects of different oral preparations of caffeine in mice. *Toxicology*, *23*, 57-71

El-Yazigi, A., Chaleby, K. & Martin, C.R. (1989) A simplified and rapid test for acetylator phenotyping by use of the peak height ratio of two urinary caffeine metabolites. *Clin. Chem.*, *35*, 848-851

Epstein, S.S. & Shafner, H. (1968) Chemical mutagens in the human environment. *Nature*, *219*, 385-387

Epstein, S.S., Bass, W., Arnold, E. & Bishop, Y. (1970) The failure of caffeine to induce mutagenic effects or to synergize the effects of known mutagens in mice. *Food Cosmet. Toxicol.*, *8*, 381-401

Ernster, V.L., Mason, L., Goodson, W.H., Sickles, E.A., Sacks, S.T., Selvin, S., Dupuy, M.E., Hawkinson, J. & Hunt, T.K. (1982) Effects of caffeine-free diet on benign breast disease: a randomized trial. *Surgery*, *91*, 263-267

Evans, D.A.P. & White, T.A. (1964) Human acetylation polymorphism. *J. Lab. clin. Med.*, *63*, 394-403

Faed, M.J.W. & Mourelatos, D. (1978) Enhancement by caffeine of sister-chromatid exchange frequency in lymphocytes from normal subjects after treatment by mutagens. *Mutat. Res.*, *49*, 437-440

Federation of American Societies for Experimental Biology (1978) *Evaluation of the Health Aspects of Caffeine as a Food Ingredient. A Report to the Food and Drug Administration by the Select Committee on GRAS Substances* (Contract No. FDA 223-75-2004; SCOGS-89), Bethesda, MD

Feely, J., Kelleher, P. & Odumosu, A. (1987) The effects of ageing on aminopyrine and caffeine breath tests in the rat . *Fundam. clin. Pharmacol.*, *1*, 409-412

Ferren, W.P. & Shane, N.A. (1968) Differential spectrometric determination of caffeine in soluble coffee and in drug combinations. *J. Assoc. off. anal. Chem.*, *51*, 573-577

Fincke, A. (1963) The occurrence of caffeine and theobromine in chocolate fats (Ger.). *Fet. Seif. Anstrichmitt.*, *65*, 647-650

Findlay, J.W.A., DeAngelis, R.L., Kearney, M.F., Welch, R.M. & Findlay, J.M. (1981) Analgesic drugs in breast milk and plasma. *Clin. Pharmacol. Ther.*, *29*, 625-633

Fishbein, L., Flamm, W.G. & Falk, H.L. (1970) *Chemical Mutagens*, New York, Academic Press

Foenander, T., Birkett, D.J., Miners, J.O. & Wing, L.M.H. (1980) The simultaneous determination of theophylline, theobromine and caffeine in plasma by high performance liquid chromatography. *Clin. Biochem.*, 13, 132-134

Frei, J.V. & Venitt, S. (1975) Chromosome damage in the bone marrow of mice treated with the methylating agents methyl methanesulphonate and *N*-methyl-*N*-nitrosourea in the presence or absence of caffeine, and its relationship with thymoma induction. *Mutat. Res.*, 29, 89-96

Friedman, L., Weinberger, M.A., Farber, T.M., Moreland, F.M., Peters, E.L., Gilmore, C.E. & Khan, M.A. (1979) Testicular atrophy and impaired spermatogenesis in rats fed high levels of the methylxanthines caffeine, theobromine, or theophylline. *J. environ. Pathol. Toxicol.*, 2, 687-706

Fries, N. & Kihlman, B. (1948) Fungal mutations obtained with methyl xanthines. *Nature*, 162, 573-574

Fujii, T. & Nishimura, H. (1972) Adverse effects of prolonged administration of caffeine on rat fetus. *Toxicol. appl. Pharmacol.*, 22, 449-457

Furth, E.E. & Thilly, W.G. (1978) Caffeine is non-mutagenic to *Salmonella typhimurium* and human cells in culture. *J. Food Saf.*, 1, 222-237

Furuhashi, N., Sato, S., Suzuki, M., Hiruta, M., Tanaka, M. & Takahashi, T. (1985) Effects of caffeine ingestion during pregnancy. *Gynecol. obstet. Invest.*, 19, 187-191

Gabridge, M.G. & Legator, M.S. (1979) A host-mediated microbial assay for the detection of mutagenic compounds. *Proc. Soc. exp. Biol. Med.*, 130, 831-834

Galasko, G.T.F., Furman, K.I. & Alberts, E. (1989) Brief communication. The caffeine contents of non-alcoholic beverages. *Food chem. Toxicol.*, 27, 49-51

Gans, J.H. (1984) Comparative toxicities of dietary caffeine and theobromine in the rat. *Food chem. Toxicol.*, 22, 365-369

Gennaro, A.R., ed. (1985) *Remington's Pharmaceutical Sciences*, 17th ed., Easton, PA, Mack Publishing, pp. 1133-1135

George, J., Murphy, T., Roberts, R., Cooksley, W.G.E., Halliday, J.W. & Powell, L.W. (1986) Influence of alcohol and caffeine consumption on caffeine elimination. *Clin. exp. Pharmacol. Physiol.*, 13, 731-736

Georgian, L., Moraru, I. & Comisel, V. (1980) Caffeine effects on the chromosomal aberrations induced *in vivo* by sarcolysine and methotrexate. *Rev. roum. Morphol. Embryol. Physiol.*, 26, 179-183

Gezelius, K. & Fries, N. (1952) Phage resistant mutants induced in *Escherichia coli* by caffeine. *Hereditas*, 38, 112-114

Ghosh, S. & Ghosh, I. (1972) Condensation of interphase chromatin in caffeine-treated cells. *Naturwissenschaften*, 59, 277-278

Gilbert, R.M. (1981) Caffeine: overview and anthology. In: Miller, S.A., ed., *Nutrition and Behavior*, Philadelphia, The Franklin Institute Press, pp. 145-166

Gilbert, R.M. (1984) Caffeine consumption. In: Spiller, G.A., ed., *The Methylxanthine Beverages and Foods: Chemistry, Consumption, and Health Effects*, New York, Alan R. Liss, pp. 185-213

Gilbert, S.G., Stavric, B., Klassen, R.D. & Rice, D.C. (1985) The fate of chronically consumed caffeine in the monkey (*Macaca fascicularis*). *Fundam. appl. Toxicol.*, 5, 578-587

Gilbert, S.G., So, Y., Klassen, R.D., Geoffroy, S., Stavric, B. & Rice, D.C. (1986) Elimination of chronically consumed caffeine in the pregnant monkey (*Macaca fascicularis*). *J. Pharmacol. exp. Ther.*, 239, 891-897

Gilbert, S.G., Rice, D.C., Reuhl, K.R. & Stavric, B. (1988) Adverse pregnancy outcome in the monkey (*Macaca fascicularis*) after chronic caffeine exposure. *J. Pharmacol. exp. Ther.*, 245, 1048-1053

Glass, E.A. & Novick, A. (1959) Induction of mutation in chloramphenicol-inhibited bacteria. *J. Bacteriol.*, 77, 10-16

Goldstein, A. & Warren, R. (1962) Passage of caffeine into human gonadal and fetal tissue. *Biochem. Pharmacol.*, 11, 166-168

González-Fernández, A., Hernández, P. & López-Sáez, J.F. (1985) Effect of caffeine and adenosine on G2 repair: mitotic delay and chromosome damage. *Mutat. Res.*, 149, 275-281

Gorodischer, R. & Karplus, M. (1982) Pharmacokinetic aspects of caffeine in premature infants with apnoea. *Eur. J. clin. Pharmacol.*, 22, 47-52

Govindwar, S.P., Kachole, M.S. & Pawar, S.S. (1984) In vivo and in vitro effects of caffeine on hepatic mixed-function oxidases in rodents and chicks. *Food chem. Toxicol.*, 22, 371-375

Grab, F.L. & Reinstein, J.A. (1968) Determination of caffeine in plasma by gas chromatography. *J. pharm. Sci.*, 57, 1703-1706

Graf, U. & Würgler, F.E. (1986) Investigation of coffee in *Drosophila* genotoxicity tests. *Food chem. Toxicol.*, 24, 835-842

Graham, D.M. (1978) Caffeine — its identity, dietary sources, intake and biological effects. *Nutr. Rev.*, 36, 97-102

Graham, H.N. (1984a) Tea: the plant and its manufacture, chemistry and consumption of the beverage. In: Spiller, G.A., ed., *The Methylxanthine Beverages and Foods: Chemistry, Consumption, and Health Effects*, New York, Alan R. Liss, pp. 29-74

Graham, H.N. (1984b) Mate. In: Spiller, G.A., ed., *The Methylxanthine Beverages and Foods: Chemistry, Consumption, and Health Effects*, New York, Alan R. Liss, pp. 179-183

Granberg-Öhman, I., Johansson, S. & Hjerpe, A. (1980) Sister-chromatid exchanges and chromosomal aberrations in rats treated with phenacetin, phenazone and caffeine. *Mutat. Res.*, 79, 13-18

Grant, D.M., Tang, B.K. & Kalow, W. (1983a) Variability in caffeine metabolism. *Clin. Pharmacol. Ther.*, 33, 591-602

Grant, D.M., Tang, B.K. & Kalow, W. (1983b) Polymorphic N-acetylation of a caffeine metabolite. *Clin. Pharmacol. Ther.*, 33, 355-359

Grant, D.M., Tang, B.K., Campbell, M.E. & Kalow, W. (1986) Effect of allopurinol on caffeine disposition in man. *Br. J. clin. Pharmacol.*, 21, 454-458

Grant, D.M., Campbell, M.E., Tang, B.K. & Kalow, W. (1987) Biotransformation of caffeine by microsomes from human liver. Kinetics and inhibition studies. *Biochem. Pharmacol.*, 36, 1251-1260

Greden, J.F. (1979) Coffee, tea and you. *Sciences, 19,* 6-11

Greer, S.B. (1958) Growth inhibitors and their antagonists as mutagens and antimutagens in *Escherichia coli. J. gen. Microbiol., 18,* 543-564

Grice, H.C. (1987) Genotoxicity and carcinogenicity assessment of caffeine and theobromine (Letter to the Editor). *Food chem. Toxicol., 25,* 295

Griffith, H.W. (1989) *Complete Guide to Prescription and Non-prescription Drugs,* Los Angeles, The Body Press, pp. 1044-1045

Griffiths, R.R. & Woodson, P.P. (1988) Caffeine physical dependence: a review of human and laboratory animal studies. *Psychopharmacology, 94,* 437-451

Grigg, G.W. (1968) Caffeine-death in *Escherichia coli. Mol. gen. Genet., 102,* 316-335

Grigg, G.W. & Stuckey, J. (1966) The reversible suppression of stationary phase mutation in *Escherichia coli* by caffeine. *Genetics, 53,* 823-834

Grygiel, J.J., Wing, L.M.H., Farkas, J. & Birkett, D.J. (1979) Effects of allopurinol on theophylline metabolism and clearance. *Clin. Pharmacol. Ther., 26,* 660-667

Guglielmi, G.E., Vogt, T.F. & Tice, R.R. (1982) Induction of sister chromatid exchanges and inhibition of cellular proliferation *in vitro.* I. Caffeine. *Environ. Mutagenesis, 4,* 191-200

Gulati, D.K., Russell, V.S., Hommel, L.M., Poonacha, K.B., Sabharwal, P.S. & Lamb, J.C. (1984) *Caffeine: Reproduction and Fertility Assessment in CD-1 Mice When Administered in Drinking Water* (NTP-85-097), Research Triangle Park, NC, National Institute of Environmental Health Sciences

Györffy, B. (1960) The effect of some chemical mutagens on *Xanthomonas phaseoli* var. *fuscans* (Ger.). In: *Abteilung Deutsches Akademie Wissenschaft Berlin, Klinisches Medizin,* pp. 110-115

Halsey, W.D. & Johnston, B., eds (1987) Caffeine. In: *Collier's Encyclopedia,* Vol. 5, New York, MacMillan-Collier, p. 110

Haughey, D.B., Greenberg, R., Schaal, S.F. & Lima, J.J. (1982) Liquid chromatographic determination of caffeine in biological fluids. *J. Chromatogr., 229,* 387-395

Haugli, F.B. & Dove, W.F. (1972) Mutagenesis and mutant selection in *Physarum polycephalum. Mol. gen. Genet., 118,* 109-124

Haynes, R.H. & Collins, J.D.B. (1984) The mutagenic potential of caffeine. In: Dews, P.B., ed., *Caffeine. Perspectives from Recent Research,* Berlin, Springer, pp. 221-238

Heddle, J.A. & Bruce, W.R. (1977) Comparison of tests for mutagenicity or carcinogenicity using assays for sperm abnormality, formation of micronuclei, and mutation in *Salmonella.* In: Hiatt, H.H., Watson, J.D. & Winsten, J.A., eds, *Origins of Human Cancer,* Cold Spring Harbor, NY, CSH Press, pp. 1549-1557

Heinonen, O.P. (1982) *Birth Defects and Drugs in Pregnancy,* Littleton, MA, Publishing Sciences

Heyden, S. & Fodor, J.G. (1986) Coffee consumption and fibrocystic breasts: an unlikely association. *Can. J. Surg., 29,* 208-211

Heyden, S. & Muhlbaier, L.H. (1984) Prospective study of 'fibrocystic breast disease' and caffeine consumption. *Surgery, 96,* 479-484

Hindi-Alexander, M.C., Zielezny, M.A., Montes, N., Bullough, B., Middleton, E., Jr, Rosner, D.H. & London, W.M. (1985) Theophylline and fibrocystic breast disease. *J. Allergy clin. Immunol.*, 75, 709-715

Hirsh, K. (1984) Central nervous system pharmacology of the dietary methylxanthines. In: Spiller, G.A., ed., *The Methylxanthine Beverages and Foods: Chemistry, Consumption, and Health Effects*, New York, Alan R. Liss, pp. 235-301

van't Hoff, W. (1982) Caffeine in pregnancy. *Lancet, i*, 1020

Holliday, R. (1961) Induced mitotic crossing-over in *Ustilago maydis*. *Genet. Res.*, 2, 231-248

Homonnai, Z.T., Paz, G., Sofer, A., Kraicer, P.F. & Harell, A. (1976) Effect of caffeine on the motility, viability, oxygen consumption and glycolytic rate of ejaculated human normokinetic and hypokinetic spermatozoa. *Int. J. Fertil.*, 21, 163-170

Horwitz, W., ed. (1980a) Coffee and tea, spectrophotometric and chromatographic methods. In: *Official Methods of Analysis of the Association of Official Analytical Chemists*, 13th ed., Washington DC, Association of the Official Analytical Chemists, p. 234

Horwitz, W., ed. (1980b) Coffee and tea, GLC method. In: *Official Methods of Analysis of the Association of Official Analytical Chemists*, 13th ed., Washington DC, Association of the Official Analytical Chemists, p. 234

Horwitz, W., ed. (1980c) Coca bean and its product, HPLC method. In: *Official Methods of Analysis of the Association of Official Analytical Chemists*, 13th ed., Washington DC, Association of the Official Analytical Chemists, p. 382

Hosaka, S., Nagayama, H. & Hirono, I. (1984) Suppressive effect of caffeine on the development of hepatic tumors induced by 2-acetylaminofluorene in ACI rats. *Gann*, 75, 1058-1061

Hoshino, H. & Tanooka, H. (1979) Caffeine enhances skin tumor induction in mice. *Toxicol. Lett.*, 4, 83-85

Hostetler, K.A., Morrissey, R.B., Tarka, S.M., Jr, Apgar, J.L. & Shively, C.A. (1990) Three-generation reproductive studies of cocoa powder in rats. *Food chem. Toxicol.*, 28, 483-490

Hoy, C.A., Salazar, E.P. & Thompson, L.H. (1984) Rapid detection of DNA-damaging agents using repair-deficient CHO cells. *Mutat. Res.*, 130, 321-332

Huber, J., Jr (1964) Caffeine. In: Kirk, R.E. & Othmer, D.F., eds, *Kirk-Othmer Encyclopedia of Chemical Technology*, 2nd ed., Vol. 3, New York, John Wiley & Sons, pp. 911-917

Huff, B.B., ed. (1989a) *Physicians' Desk Reference*, 43rd, Oradell, NJ, Medical Economics, pp. 407, 415, 756, 2226

Huff, B.B., ed. (1989b) *Physicians' Desk Reference for Non-prescription Drugs*, 10th ed., Oradell, NJ, Medical Economics, pp. 516, 527, 529, 556

Hurst, W.J., Martin, R.A. & Tarka, S.M., Jr (1984) Analytical methods for quantitation of methylxanthines. In: Spiller, G.A., ed., *The Methylxanthine Beverages and Foods: Chemistry, Consumption and Health Effects*, New York, Alan R. Liss, pp. 17-28

IARC (1979a) *IARC Monographs on the Evaluation of the Carcinogenic Risk of Chemicals to Humans*, Vol. 20, *Some Halogenated Hydrocarbons*, Lyon, pp. 545-572

IARC (1979b) *IARC Monographs on the Evaluation of the Carcinogenic Risk of Chemicals to Humans*, Vol. 20, *Some Halogenated Hydrocarbons*, Lyon, pp. 449-465

IARC (1987) *IARC Monographs on the Evaluation of Carcinogenic Risks to Humans*, Suppl. 7, *Overall Evaluations of Carcinogenicity: An Updating of* IARC Monographs *Volumes 1 to 42*, Lyon

IARC (1990) *IARC Monographs on the Evaluation of Carcinogenic Risks to Humans*, Vol. 50, *Pharmaceutical Drugs*, Lyon, pp. 307-332

Ide, T., Anzai, K. & Andoh, T. (1975) Enhancement of SV40 transformation by treatment of C3H2K cells with UV light and caffeine. I. Combined effect of UV light and caffeine. *Virology*, 66, 568-578

International Coffee Organization (1981) *Robusta Coffee: Study of World Production and Consumption* (Publ. No. EB 1860810(E)), London

International Coffee Organization (1982) *United States of America. Coffee Drinking Study*, London

International Coffee Organization (1989) *United States of America. Coffee Drinking Study. Winter 1989* (Rep. PC-585/89), London

Iscovich, J.M., Iscovich, R.B., Howe, G., Shiboski, S. & Kaldor, J.M. (1989) A case-control study of diet and breast cancer in Argentina. *Int. J. Cancer*, 44, 770-776

Ishida, R., Kozaki, M. & Takahashi, T. (1985) Caffeine alone causes DNA damage in Chinese hamster ovary cells. *Cell Struct. Function*, 10, 405-409

Ishidate, M., Jr (1988) *Data Book of Chromosomal Aberration Tests In Vitro*, rev. ed., Amsterdam, Elsevier, p. 69

Ishii, Y. & Bender, M.A. (1978) Caffeine inhibition of prereplication repair of mytomycin C-induced DNA damage in human peripheral lymphocytes. *Mutat. Res.*, 51, 419-425

Iyer, V.N. & Szybalski, W. (1958) Two simple methods for the detection of chemical mutagens. *Appl. Microbiol.*, 6, 23-29

Jalal, M.A.F. & Collin, H.A. (1976) Estimation of caffeine, theophylline and theobromine in plant material. *New Phytol.*, 76, 277-281

Jensen, O.M., Wahrendorf, J., Knudsen, J.B. & Sørensen, B.L. (1986) The Copenhagen case-control study of bladder cancer. II. Effect of coffee and other beverages. *Int. J. Cancer*, 37, 651-657

Jenssen, D. & Ramel, C. (1978) Factors affecting the induction of micronuclei at low doses of X-rays, MMS and dimethylnitrosamine in mouse erythroblasts. *Mutat. Res.*, 58, 51-65

Jiritano, L., Bortolotti, A., Gaspari, F. & Bonati, M. (1985) Caffeine disposition after oral administration to pregnant rats. *Xenobiotica*, 15, 1045-1051

Joeres, R., Klinker, H., Heusler, H., Epping, J., Zilly, W. & Richter, E. (1988) Influence of smoking on caffeine elimination in healthy volunteers and in patients with alcoholic liver cirrhosis. *Hepatology*, 8, 575-579

Johansson, S.L. (1981) Carcinogenicity of analgesics: long-term treatment of Sprague-Dawley rats with phenacetin, phenazone, caffeine and paracetamol (acetamidophen). *Int. J. Cancer*, 27, 521-529

Johnson, A.R. (1967) Collaborative study of a method for the determination of caffeine in nonalcoholic beverages. *J. Assoc. off. anal. Chem.*, 50, 857-858

Kada, T., Tutikawa, K. & Sadaie, Y. (1972) In vitro and host-mediated 'rec-assay' procedures for screening chemical mutagens and phloxine, a mutagenic red dye detected. *Mutat. Res.*, *16*, 165-174

Kalow, W. (1984) Pharmacoanthropology: drug metabolism. *Fed. Proc.*, *43*, 2326-2331

Kamei, K., Matsuda, M. & Momose, A. (1975) New sulfur-containing metabolites of caffeine. *Chem. pharm. Bull. (Tokyo)*, *23*, 683-685

Kao, F.-T. & Puck, T.T. (1969) Genetics of somatic mammalian cells. IX. Quantitation of mutagenesis by physical and chemical agents. *J. Cell Physiol.*, *74*, 245-258

Kapke, G.F. & Franklin, R.B. (1987) A direct liquid chromatography method for serum caffeine analysis. *J. liquid Chromatogr.*, *10*, 451-463

Kato, H. (1973) Induction of sister chromatid exchanges by UV light and its inhibition by caffeine. *Exp. Cell Res.*, *82*, 383-390

Kaul, B.L. & Zutshi, U. (1973) On the production of chromosome breakage in *Vicia faba* by caffeine. *Cytobios*, *7*, 261-264

Kazi, T. (1985) Determination of caffeine and other purine alkaloids in coffee and tea products by high performance liquid chromatography. In: *11e Colloque Scientifique Internationale sur le Café, Lomé, 1985*, Paris, Association Scientifique Internationale du Café, pp. 227-244

Kesavan, P.C., Trasi, S. & Ahmad, A. (1973) Modification of barley seed sensitivity by post-treatment with caffeine. I. Effect of post-irradiation heat shock and nature of hydration. *Int. J. Radiat. Biol.*, *24*, 581-587

Khanna, K.L. & Cornish, H.H. (1973) The effect of daily ingestion of caffeine on the microsomal enzymes of rat liver. *Food Cosmet. Toxicol.*, *11*, 11-17

Khanna, N.N., Bada, H.S. & Somani, S.M. (1980) Use of salivary concentrations in the prediction of serum caffeine and theophylline concentrations in premature infants. *J. Pediatr.*, *96*, 494-499

Kihlman, B.A. (1949) The effect of purine derivatives on chromosomes (Abstract). *Hereditas*, *35*, 393

Kihlman, B.A. (1974) Effects of caffeine on the genetic material. *Mutat. Res.*, *26*, 53-71

Kihlman, B.A. (1977) *Caffeine and Chromosomes*, Amsterdam, Elsevier

Kihlman, B.A. & Sturelid, S. (1975) Enhancement by methylated oxypurines of the frequency of induced chromosomal aberrations. III. The effect in combination with X-rays in root tips of *Vicia faba*. *Hereditas*, *80*, 247-254

Kihlman, B.A., Sturelid, S., Norlén, K. & Tidriks, D. (1971a) Caffeine, caffeine derivatives and chromosomal aberrations. II. Different responses of *Allium* root tips and Chinese hamster cells to treatments with caffeine, 8-ethoxycaffeine and 6-methylcoumarin. *Hereditas*, *69*, 35-50

Kihlman, B.A., Norlén, K., Sturelid, S. & Odmark, G. (1971b) Caffeine and 8-ethoxycaffeine produce different types of chromosome-breaking effects depending on the treatment temperature. *Mutat. Res.*, *12*, 463-468

Kihlman, B.A., Sturelid, S., Palitti, F. & Becchetti, A. (1977) Effect of caffeine, an inhibitor of post-replication repair in mammalian cells, on the frequencies of chromosomal aberrations and sister chromatid exchanges induced by mutagenic agents (Abstract No. 36). *Mutat. Res.*, 46, 130

Kim, J. & Levin, R.E. (1986) Influence of caffeine on mitomycin C induced mutagenesis. *Microbios*, 46, 15-20

Kimmel, C.A., Kimmel, G.L., White, C.G., Grafton, T.F., Young, J.F. & Nelson, C.J. (1984) Blood flow changes and conceptal development in pregnant rats in response to caffeine. *Fundam. appl. Toxicol.*, 4, 240-247

King, M.-T., Beikirch, H., Eckhardt, K., Gocke, E. & Wild, D. (1979) Mutagenicity studies with X-ray-contrast media, analgesics, antipyretics, antirheumatics and some other pharmaceutical drugs in bacterial, *Drosophila* and mammalian test systems. *Mutat. Res.*, 66, 33-43

Klassen, R. & Stavric, B. (1983) HPLC separation of theophylline, paraxanthine, theobromine, caffeine and other metabolites in biological fluids. *J. liquid Chromatogr.*, 6, 895-906

Knoche, C. & König, J. (1964) Prenatal toxicity of diphenylpyraline-8-chlorotheophyllinate, having regard to experience with thalidomine and caffeine (Ger.). *Arzneimittel-Forsch.*, 14, 415-424

Knutti, R., Rothweiler, H. & Schlatter, C. (1981) Effect of pregnancy on the pharmacokinetics of caffeine. *Eur. J. clin. Pharmacol.*, 21, 121-126

Knutti, R., Rothweiler, H. & Schlatter, C. (1982) The effect of pregnancy on the pharmacokinetics of caffeine. *Arch. Toxicol.*, Suppl. 5, 187-192

Koch, A.L. & Lamont, W.A. (1956) The metabolism of methylpurines by *Escherichia coli*. II. Enzymatic studies. *J. biol. Chem.*, 219, 189-201

Koerting-Keiffer, L.E. & Mickey, G.H. (1969) Influence of caffeine on chromosomes (Ger.). *Z. Pflanzenzucht*, 61, 244-251

Kolb, C.A. & Mansfield, J.M. (1980) Effect of theophylline treatment of mouse B-16 melanoma cells *in vitro*. *Oncology*, 37, 343-352

Kotake, A.N., Schoeller, D.A., Lambert, G.H., Baker, A.L., Schaffer, D.D. & Josephs, H. (1982) The caffeine CO_2 breath test: dose response and route of *N*-demethylation in smokers and nonsmokers. *Clin. Pharmacol. Ther.*, 32, 261-269

Kraft General Foods (1989) *Coffee Consumption*, White Plains, NY

Kreiser, W.R. & Martin, R.A., Jr (1978) High pressure liquid chromatographic determination of theobromine and caffeine in cocoa and chocolate products. *J. Assoc. off. anal. Chem.*, 61, 1424-1427

von Kreybig, T. & Czok, G. (1976) Teratogenic and mutagenic studies with caffeine in animal experiment (Ger.). *Z. Ernährungswiss.*, 15, 64-70

Kubitschek, E.H. & Bendigkeit, H.E. (1958) Delay in the appearance of caffeine-induced T5 resistance in *Escherichia coli*. *Genetics*, 43, 647-661

Kubitschek, H.E. & Bendigkeit, H.E. (1964) Mutation in continuous cultures. I. Dependence of mutational response upon growth-limiting factors. *Mutat. Res.*, 1, 113-120

Kuhlmann, W., Fromme, H.-G., Heege, E.-M. & Ostertag, W. (1968) The mutagenic action of caffeine in higher organisms. *Cancer Res.*, 28, 2375-2389

Kunze, E., Rath, G. & Graewe, T. (1987) Effect of phenacetin and caffeine on N-butyl-N-(4-hydroxybutyl)nitrosamine-initiated urothelial carcinogenesis in rats. *Urol. int.*, 42, 108-114

Kuzma, J.W. & Sokol, R.J. (1982) Maternal drinking behavior and decreased intrauterine growth. *Alcohol. clin. exp. Res.*, 6, 396-402

Lachance, M.P. (1982) The pharmacology and toxicology of caffeine. *J. Food Saf.*, 4, 71-112

Lakhanisky, T., Hendrickx, B. & Mouton, R.F. (1981) Chemical induction of DNA damage and its repair in *T. pyriformis*. Influence of caffeine, quinacrine and chloroquine (Abstract). *Mutat. Res.*, 85, 275

Lang, T., Degoulet, P., Aime, F., Fouriaud, C., Jacquinet-Salord, M.-C., Laprugne, J., Main, J., Oeconomos, J., Phalente, J. & Prades, A. (1983) Relation between coffee drinking and blood pressure: analysis of 6,321 subjects in the Paris region. *Am. J. Cardiol.*, 52, 1238-1242

Latini, R., Bonati, M., Castelli, D. & Garattini, S. (1978) Dose-dependent kinetics of caffeine in rats. *Toxicol. Lett.*, 2, 267-270

Latini, R., Bonati, M., Marzi, E., Tacconi, M.T., Sadurska, B. & Bizzi, A. (1980) Caffeine disposition and effects in young and one-year old rats. *J. Pharm. Pharmacol.*, 32, 596-599

La Vecchia, C., Franceschi, S., Parazzini, F., Regallo, M., Decarli, A., Gallus, G., Di Pietro, S. & Tognoni, G. (1985) Benign breast disease and consumption of beverages containing methylxanthines. *J. natl Cancer Inst.*, 74, 995-1000

Lawson, D.H., Jick, H. & Rothman, K.J. (1981) Coffee and tea consumption and breast disease. *Surgery*, 90, 801-803

Ledbetter, D.H., Airhart, S.D. & Nussbaum, R.L. (1986) Caffeine enhances fragile (X) expression in somatic cell hybrids. *Am. J. med. Genet.*, 23, 445-455

Ledinko, N. & Evans, M. (1973) Enhancement of adenovirus transformation of hamster cells by *N*-methyl-*N'*-nitro-*N*-nitrosoguanidine, caffeine, and hydroxylamine. *Cancer Res.*, 33, 2936-2938

Lee, S. (1971) Chromosome aberrations induced in cultured human cells by caffeine. *Jpn. J. Genet.*, 46, 337-344

Legator, M.S. & Zimmering, S. (1979) Review of the genetic effects of caffeine. *J. environ. Sci. Health*, C13, 135-188

Lehmann, A.R. (1973) Effects of caffeine and theophylline on DNA synthesis in untreated and UV-irradiated mammalian cells (Abstract No. 15). *Mutat. Res.*, 21, 192-193

Lehmann, A.R. & Kirk-Bell, S. (1974) Effects of caffeine and theophylline on DNA synthesis in unirradiated and UV-irradiated mammalian cells. *Mutat. Res.*, 26, 73-82

Lelo, A., Miners, J.O., Robson, R. & Birkett, D.J. (1986) Assessment of caffeine exposure: caffeine content of beverages, caffeine intake, and plasma concentration of methylxanthines. *Clin. Pharmacol. Ther.*, 39, 54-59

Leonard, T.K., Watson, R.R. & Mohs, M.E. (1987) The effects of caffeine on various body systems: a review. *J. Am. diet. Assoc.*, 87, 1048-1053

Levi, V., Jacobson, E.L. & Jacobson, M.K. (1978) Inhibition of poly(ADP-ribose)polymerase by methylated xanthines and cytokinins. *FEBS Lett.*, *88*, 144-146

Levine, J. (1962) Determination of caffeine in coffee products, beverages and tablets. *J. Assoc. off. anal. Chem.*, *45*, 254-255

Lieb, M. (1961) Enhancement of ultraviolet-induced mutation in bacteria by caffeine. *Z. Vererbungsl.*, *92*, 416-429

Linn, S., Schoenbaum, S.C., Monson, R.R., Rosner, B., Stubblefield, P.G. & Ryan, K.J. (1982) No association between coffee consumption and adverse outcomes of pregnancy. *New Engl. J. Med.*, *306*, 141-145

Liwerant, I.J. & Pereira Da Silva, L.H. (1975) Comparative mutagenic effects of ethyl methanesulfonate, *N*-methyl-*N'*-nitro-*N*-nitrosoguanidine, ultraviolet radiation and caffeine on *Dictyostelium discoideum*. *Mutat. Res.*, *33*, 135-146

Loprieno, N. & Schüpbach, M. (1971) On the effect of caffeine on mutation and recombination in *Schizosaccharomyces pombe*. *Mol. gen. Genet.*, *110*, 348-354

Loprieno, N., Barale, R. & Baroncelli, S. (1974) Genetic effects of caffeine. *Mutat. Res.*, *26*, 83-87

Lubin, F., Ron, E., Wax, Y., Funaro, M., Shitrit, A., Black, M. & Modan, B. (1984) Coffee and methylxanthine in benign and malignant breast diseases. In: MacMahon, B. & Sugimura, T., eds, *Coffee and Health* (Banbury Report 17), Cold Spring Harbor, NY, CSH Press, pp. 177-187

Lubin, F., Ron, E., Wax, Y., Black, M., Funaro, M. & Shitrit, A. (1985a) A case-control study of caffeine and methylxanthines in benign breast disease. *J. Am. med. Assoc.*, *253*, 2388-2392

Lubin, F., Ron, E., Wax, Y. & Modan, B. (1985b) Coffee and methylxanthines and breast cancer: a case-control study. *J. natl Cancer Inst.*, *74*, 569-573

Lyon, M.F., Phillips, R.J.S. & Searle, A.G. (1962) A test for mutagenicity of caffeine in mice. *Z. Verebungsl.*, *93*, 7-13

Macklin, A.W. & Szot, R.J. (1980) Eighteen month oral study of aspirin, phenacetin and caffeine in C57Bl/6 mice. *Drug Chem. Toxicol.*, *3*, 135-163

Macrae, R. (1985) Nitrogenous components. In: Clarke, R.Y. & Macrae, R., eds, *Coffee*, Vol. 1, *Chemistry*, London, Elsevier Applied Science, pp. 115-152

Madison, B.L., Kozarek, W.J. & Damo, C.P. (1976) High-pressure liquid chromatography of caffeine in coffee. *J. Assoc. off. anal. Chem.*, *59*, 1258-1261

Maher, V.M., Quellette, L.M., Curren, R.D. & McCormick, J.J. (1976) Caffeine enhancement of the cytotoxic and mutagenic effect of ultraviolet irradiation in a xeroderma pigmentosum variant strain of human cells. *Biochem. biophys. Res. Comm.*, *71*, 228-234

Maickel, R. & Snodgrass, W.R. (1973) Physicochemical factors in maternal-fetal distribution of drugs. *Toxicol. appl. Pharmacol.*, *26*, 218-230

Marks, V. & Kelly, J.F. (1973) Absorption of caffeine from tea, coffee, and Coca Cola. *Lancet*, *i*, 827

Marshall, J., Graham, S. & Swanson, M. (1982) Caffeine consumption and benign breast disease: a case-control comparison. *Am. J. public Health*, *72*, 610-612

Martin, T.R. & Bracken, M.B. (1987) The association between low birth weight and caffeine consumption during pregnancy. *Am. J. Epidemiol.*, *126*, 813-821

Martin, J.B., Annegers, J.F., Curb, J.D., Heyden, S., Howson, C., Lee, E.S. & Lee, M. (1988) Mortality patterns among hypertensives by reported level of caffeine consumption. *Prev. Med.*, *17*, 310-320

Matter, B.E. & Grauwiler, J. (1974) Micronuclei in mouse bone-marrow cells. A simple in vivo model for the evaluation of drug-induced chromosomal aberrations. *Mutat. Res.*, *23*, 239-249

Mau, G. & Netter, P. (1974) Coffee and alcohol consumption. Risk factors in pregnancy? (Ger.). *Geburtsh. Frauenheilk.*, *34*, 1018-1022

May, D.C., Jarboe, C.H., VanBakel, A.B. & Williams, W.M. (1982) Effects of cimetidine on caffeine disposition in smokers and nonsmokers. *Clin. Pharmacol. Ther.*, *31*, 656-661

Mayanna, S.M. & Jayaram, B. (1981) Determination of caffeine using sodium N-chloro-p-toluenesulfonamide. *Analyst*, *106*, 729-732

McCall, A.L., Millington, W.R. & Wurtman, R.J. (1982) Blood-brain barrier transport of caffeine: dose-related restriction of adenine transport. *Life Sci.*, *31*, 2709-2715

McCann, J., Choi, E., Yamasaki, E. & Ames, B.N. (1975) Detection of carcinogens as mutagens in the *Salmonella*/microsome test: assay of 300 chemicals. *Proc. natl Acad. Sci. USA*, *72*, 5135-5139

McCutheon, G.F. (1969) Caffeine. In: Snell, F.D. & Ettre, L.S., eds, *Encyclopedia of Industrial Chemical Analysis*, Vol. 8, New York, Interscience, pp. 55-71

McElvoy, G.K. (1989) *American Health Formulary Service (AHFS) Drug Information*, Bethesda, MD, American Society of Hospial Pharmacists, pp. 1179-1181

McMillan, S. & Fox, M. (1979) Failure of caffeine to influence induced mutation frequencies and the independence of cell killing and mutation induction in V79 Chinese hamster cells. *Mutat. Res.*, *60*, 91-107

Meatherall, R. & Ford, D. (1988) Isocratic liquid chromatographic determination of theophylline, acetaminophen, chloramphenicol, caffeine, anticonvulsants, and barbiturates in serum. *Ther. Drug Monit.*, *10*, 101-115

Menthe, J. (1985) Caffeine — a commodity in demand. *Tea Coffee Trade J.*, *February*, 18

Merriman, R.L., Swanson, A., Anders, M.W. & Sladek, N.E. (1978) Micro-determination of caffeine in blood by gas chromatography-mass spectrometry. *J. Chromatogr.*, *146*, 85-90

Minton, J.P., Foecking, M.K., Webster, D.J.T. & Matthews, R.H. (1979a) Response of fibrocystic disease to caffeine withdrawal and correlation of cyclic nucleotides with breast disease. *Am. J. Obstet. Gynecol.*, *135*, 157-158

Minton, J.P., Foecking, M.K., Webster, D.J.T. & Matthews, R.H. (1979b) Caffeine, cyclic nucleotides, and breast disease. *Surgery*, *86*, 105-109

Minton, J.P., Abou-Issa, H., Reiches, N. & Roseman, J.M. (1981) Clinical and biochemical studies on methylxanthine-related fibrocystic breast disease. *Surgery*, *90*, 299-304

Minton, J.P., Abou-Issa, H., Foecking, M.K. & Sriram, M.G. (1983) Caffeine and unsaturated fat diet significantly promotes DMBA-induced breast cancer in rats. *Cancer*, *51*, 1249-1253

Mirvish, S.S., Cardesa, A., Wallcave, L. & Shubik, P. (1975) Induction of mouse lung adenomas by amines or ureas plus nitrite and by N-nitroso compounds: effects of ascorbate, gallic acid, thiocyanate, and caffeine. *J. natl Cancer Inst.*, *55*, 633-636

Mitchell, M.C., Hoyumpa, A.M., Schenker, S., Johnson, R.F., Nichols, S. & Patwardhan, R.V. (1983) Inhibition of caffeine elimination by short-term ethanol administration. *J. Lab. clin. Med.*, *101*, 826-834

Mitoma, C., Lombrozo, L., LeValley, S.E. & Dehn, F. (1969) Nature of the effect of caffeine on the drug-metabolizing enzymes. *Arch. Biochem. Biophys.*, *134*, 434-441

Mittler, S., Mittler, J.E., Tonetti, A.M. & Szymczak, M.E. (1967a) The effect of caffeine on chromosome loss and nondisjunction in *Drosophila*. *Mutat. Res.*, *4*, 708-710

Mittler, S., Mittler, J.E. & Owens, S.L. (1967b) Loss of chromosomes and nondisjunction induced by caffeine in *Drosophila*. *Nature*, *214*, 424

Mitznegg, P., Heim, F., Hach, B. & Säbel, M. (1971) The effect of ageing, caffeine-treatment, and ionising-radiation on nucleic acid synthesis in the mouse liver. *Life Sci.*, *10*, 1281-1292

Moffat, A.C., ed. (1986) *Clarke's Isolation and Identification of Drugs*, 2nd ed., London, The Pharmaceutical Press, pp. 420-422

Mohr, U., Althoff, J., Ketkar, M.B., Conradt, P. & Morgareidge, K. (1984) The influence of caffeine on tumour incidence in Sprague-Dawley rats. *Food chem. Toxicol.*, *22*, 377-382

Moores, R.G. & Campbell, H.A. (1948) Determination of theobromine and caffeine in cocoa materials. *Anal. Chem.*, *20*, 40-47

Morgan, W.F. & Cleaver, J.E. (1982) 3-Aminobenzamide synergistically increases sister-chromatid exchanges in cells exposed to methyl methanesulfonate but not to ultraviolet light. *Mutat. Res.*, *104*, 361-366

Morgan, K.J., Stults, V.J. & Zabik, M.E. (1982) Amount and dietary sources of caffeine and saccharin intake by individuals aged 5 to 18 years. *Regul. Toxicol. Pharmacol.*, *2*, 296-307

Mortelmans, K., Haworth, S., Lawlor, T., Speck, W., Tainer, B. & Zeiger, E. (1986) *Salmonella* mutagenicity tests: II. Results from the testing of 270 chemicals. *Environ. Mutagenesis*, *8 (Suppl. 7)*, 1-119

Muir, K.T., Kunitani, M. & Riegelman, S. (1982) Improved high-performance liquid chromatographic assay for theophylline in plasma and saliva in the presence of caffeine and its metabolites and comparisons with three other assays. *J. Chromatogr.*, *231*, 73-82

Müller, W.-U., Streffer, C. & Wurm, R. (1985) Supraadditive formation of micronuclei in preimplantation mouse embryos *in vitro* after combined treatment with X-rays and caffeine. *Teratog. Carcinog. Mutagenesis*, *5*, 123-131

Mulvihill, J.J. (1973) Caffeine as teratogen and mutagen. *Teratology*, *8*, 69-72

Muñoz, L.M., Lönnerdal, B., Keen, C.L. & Dewey, K.G. (1988) Coffee consumption as a factor in iron deficiency anemia among pregnant women and their infants in Costa Rica. *Am. J. clin. Nutr.*, *48*, 645-651

Murota, T. & Murakami, A. (1976) Induction of dominant lethal mutation by alkylating agents in germ cells of the silkworm, *Bombyx mori* (Abstract No. 14). *Mutat. Res.*, *38*, 343-344

Murphy, T.L., McIvor, C., Yap, A., Cooksley, W.G.E., Halliday, J.W. & Powell, L.W. (1988) The effect of smoking on caffeine elimination: implications for its use as a semiquantitative test of liver function. *Clin. exp. Pharmacol. Physiol.*, *15*, 9-13

Myers, M.G. (1988) Effects of caffeine on blood pressure. *Arch. intern. Med.*, *148*, 1189-1193

Myers, M.G., Harris, L., Leenen, F.H.H. & Grant, D.M. (1987) Caffeine as a possible cause of ventricular arrhythmias during the healing phase of acute myocardial infarction. *Am. J. Cardiol.*, *59*, 1024-1028

Nakanishi, Y. & Schneider, E.L. (1979) In vivo sister-chromatid exchange: a sensitive measure of DNA damage. *Mutat. Res.*, *60*, 329-337

Nakanishi, K., Fukushima, S., Shibata, M., Shirai, T., Ogiso, T. & Ito, N. (1978) Effect of phenacetin and caffeine on the urinary bladder of rats treated with N-butyl-N-(4-hydroxybutyl)nitrosamine. *Gann*, *69*, 395-400

Nakanishi, K., Hirose, M., Ogiso, T., Hasegawa, R., Arai, M. & Ito, N. (1980) Effects of sodium saccharin and caffeine on the urinary bladder of rats treated with N-butyl-N-(4-hydroxybutyl)nitrosamine. *Gann*, *71*, 490-500

Nakazawa, K., Tanaka, H. & Arima, M. (1985) The effect of caffeine ingestion on pharmacokinetics of caffeine and its metabolites after a single administration in pregnant rats. *J. Pharmacobio-Dyn.*, *8*, 151-160

Nash, J. & Persaud, T.V.N. (1988) Reproductive and teratological risks of caffeine. *Anat. Anz. (Jena)*, *167*, 265-270

Natarajan, A.T., Csukás, I. & van Zeeland, A.A. (1981) Contribution of incorporated 5-bromodeoxyuridine in DNA to the frequencies of sister-chromatid exchanges induced by inhibitors of poly-(ADP-ribose)-polymerase. *Mutat. Res.*, *84*, 125-132

National Research Council (1977a) *Drinking Water and Health*, Washington DC, National Academy of Sciences

National Research Council (1977b) *Estimating Distribution of Daily Intakes of Caffeine. Committee on GRAS List Survey — Phase III Food and Nutrition Board*, Washington DC, National Academy of Sciences

National Research Council (1981) *Food Chemicals Codex*, 3rd ed., Washington DC, National Academy Press, p. 44

National Research Council (1989) *Diet and Health — Implications for Reducing Chronic Disease Risk*, Washington DC, National Academy Press, pp. 465-471

National Soft Drink Association (1982) *What's in Soft Drinks*, 2nd ed., Washington DC

National Soft Drink Association (1986) *Sales Survey of the Soft Drink Industry*, Washington DC

Neims, A.H., Bailey, J. & Aldridge, A. (1979) Disposition of caffeine during and after pregnancy (Abstract). *Clin. Res.*, *27*, 236A

Nelson, M.M. & Forfar, J.O. (1971) Associations between drugs administered during pregnancy and congenital abnormalities of the fetus. *Br. med. J.*, *i*, 523-527

Nesterov, M., Kucherya, L.A., Zaval'nyuk, R.G. & Alibaeva, T.D. (1985) Improvement of caffeine synthesis (Russ.). *Khim.-Farm. Zh.*, *19*, 1389-1390

Newton, R., Broughton, L.J., Lind, M.J., Morrison, P.J., Rogers, H.J. & Bradbrook, I.D. (1981) Plasma and salivary pharmacokinetics of caffeine in man. *Eur. J. clin. Pharmacol.*, *21*, 45-52

Nishimura, H. & Nakai, K. (1960) Congenital malformations in offspring of mice treated with caffeine. *Proc. Soc. exp. biol. Med.*, *104*, 140-142

Nolen, G.A. (1988) The developmental toxicology of caffeine. In: Kalter, H., ed., *Issues and Reviews in Teratology*, New York, Plenum Press, pp. 305-350

Nomura, T. (1976) Diminution of tumorigenesis initiated by 4-nitroquinoline-1-oxide by post-treatment with caffeine in mice. *Nature*, *260*, 547-549

Nomura, T. (1980) Timing of chemically induced neoplasia in mice revealed by the antineoplastic action of caffeine. *Cancer Res.*, *40*, 1332-1340

Nomura, T. (1983) Comparative inhibiting effects of methylxanthines on urethan-induced tumors, malformations, and presumed somatic mutations in mice. *Cancer Res.*, *43*, 1342-1346

Novick, A. & Szilard, L. (1951) Experiments on spontaneous and chemically induced mutations of bacteria growing in the chemostat. *Cold Spring Harbor Symp. Quant. Biol.*, *16*, 337-343

O'Connell, S.E. & Zurzola, F.J. (1984) Rapid quantitative liquid chromatographic determination of caffeine levels in plasma after oral dosing. *J. pharm. Sci.*, *73*, 1009-1011

Odenheimer, D.J., Zunzunegui, M.V., King, M.C., Shipler, C.P. & Friedman, G.D. (1984) Risk factors for benign breast disease: a case-control study of discordant twins. *Am. J. Epidemiol.*, *120*, 565-571

Osiecka, R. (1976) Effect of the treatment-temperature on induction of chromosome aberrations by caffeine in *Vicia faba*. *Genet. Pol.*, *17*, 159-163

Ostertag, W. (1966) Caffeine and theophylline mutagenicity in cell and leucocyte cultures of man (Ger.). *Mutat. Res.*, *3*, 249-267

Ostertag, W. & Haake, J. (1966) The mutagenicity in *Drosophila melanogaster* of caffeine and other compounds which produce chromosome breakage in human cells in culture. *Z. Vererbungsl.*, *98*, 299-308

Ostertag, W., Duisberg, E. & Stürmann, M. (1965) The mutagenic activity of caffeine in man. *Mutat. Res.*, *2*, 293-296

Painter, R.B. (1980) Effect of caffeine on DNA synthesis in irradiated and unirradiated mammalian cells. *J. mol. Biol.*, *143*, 289-301

Palitti, F. & Becchetti, A. (1977) Effect of caffeine on sister chromatid exchanges and chromosomal aberrations induced by mutagens in Chinese hamster cells. *Mutat. Res.*, *45*, 157-159

Palitti, F., Rizzoni, M., Gatti, M. & Olivieri, G. (1974) Chromosomal aberrations induced by caffeine in endoreduplicated Chinese hamster cells. *Mutat. Res.*, *26*, 145-150

Palm, P.E., Arnold, E.P., Rachwall, P.C., Leyczek, J.C., Teague, K.W. & Kensler, C.J. (1978) Evaluation of the teratogenic potential of fresh-brewed coffee and caffeine in the rat. *Toxicol. appl. Pharmacol.*, *44*, 1-16

Panigrahi, G.B. & Rao, A.R. (1983) Influence of caffeine on arecoline-induced SCE in mouse bone-marrow cells *in vivo*. *Mutat. Res.*, *122*, 347-353

Pant, G.S., Kamada, N. & Tanaka, R. (1976) Sister chromatid exchanges in peripheral lymphocytes of atomic bomb survivors and of normal individuals exposed to radiation and chemical agents. *Hiroshima J. med. Sci.*, 25, 99-105

Pao, E.M., Fleming, K.H., Guenther, P.M. & Mickle, S.J. (1982) *Foods Commonly Eaten by Individuals: Amount Per Day and Per Eating Occasion* (Home Economics Research Report No. 44), Hyattsville, MD, US Department of Agriculture

Papadoyannis, I.N. & Caddy, B. (1987) Application of high-performance liquid chromatography for the simultaneous determination of morphine, codeine and caffeine. *Microchem. J.*, 36, 182-191

Parazzini, F., La Vecchia, C., Riundi, R., Pampallona, S., Regallo, M. & Scanni, A. (1986) Methylxanthine, alcohol-free diet and fibrocystic breast disease: a factorial clinical trial. *Surgery*, 99, 576-580

Paribok, V.P., Kassinova, G.V. & Bandas. E.L. (1967) Effects of repair inhibitors on the reversion frequency in the polyauxotrophic strain of *Escherichia coli* during ultraviolet light radiation (Russ.). *Tsitologiya*, 9, 1496-1502

Parry, J.M., Sharp, D., Tippins, R.S. & Parry, E.M. (1979) Radiation-induced mitotic and meiotic aneuploidy in the yeast *Saccharomyces cerevisiae*. *Mutat. Res.*, 61, 37-55

Parsons, W.D. & Neims, A.H. (1978) Effect of smoking on caffeine clearance. *Clin. Pharmacol. Ther.*, 24, 40-45

Parsons, W.D. & Neims, A.H. (1981) Prolonged half-life of caffeine in healthy term newborn infants. *J. Pediatr.*, 98, 640-641

Parsons, W.D. & Pelletier, J.G. (1982) Delayed elimination of caffeine by women in the last 2 weeks of pregnancy. *Can. med. Assoc. J.*, 127, 377-380

Parsons, W.D., Aranda, J.V. & Neims, A.H. (1976) Elimination of transplacentally acquired caffeine in fullterm neonates (Abstract No. 195). *Pediatr. Res.*, 10, 333

Patwardhan, R.V., Desmond, P.V., Johnson, R.F. & Schenker, S. (1980) Impaired elimination of caffeine by oral contraceptive steroids. *J. Lab. clin. Med.*, 95, 603-608

Periti, M., Salvaggio, A., Quaglia, G. & Di Marzio, L. (1987) Coffee consumption and blood pressure: an Italian study. *Clin. Sci.*, 72, 443-447

Perry, D.L., Chuang, C.C., Jungclaus, G.A. & Warner, J.S. (1979) *Identification of Organic Compounds in Industrial Effluent Discharges* (EPA-600/4-79-016), Athens, GA, US Environmental Protection Agency

Petrek, J.A., Sandberg, W.A., Cole, M.N., Silberman, M.S. & Collins, D.C. (1985) The inhibitory effect of caffeine on hormone-induced rat breast cancer. *Cancer*, 56, 1977-1981

Phelps, H.M. & Phelps, C.E. (1988) Caffeine ingestion and breast cancer. A negative correlation. *Cancer*, 61, 1051-1054

Pienta, R.J. (1980) Evaluation and relevance of the Syrian hamster embryo cell system. In: Williams, G.M., Kroes, R., Waaijers, H.W. & Van de Poll, K.W., eds, *The Predictive Value of Short-term Screening Tests in Carcinogenicity*, Amsterdam, Elsevier, pp. 149-169

Pike, M.C. & Bernstein, L. (1985) Statistical errors invalidate conclusions in 'caffeine and unsaturated fat diet significantly promotes DMBA-induced breast cancer in rats'. *Cancer*, 55, 1855-1858

Pozner, J., Papatestas, A.E., Fagerstrom, R., Schwartz, I., Saevitz, J., Feinberg, M. & Aufses, A.H., Jr (1986) Association of tumor differentiation with caffeine and coffee intake in women with breast cancer. *Surgery*, *100*, 482-488

Prineas, R.J., Jacobs, D.R., Jr, Crow, R.S. & Blackburn, H. (1980) Coffee, tea and VPB. *J. chron. Dis.*, *33*, 67-72

Rafter, J.J. & Nilsson, L. (1981) Involvement of the intestinal microflora in the formation of sulfur-containing metabolites of caffeine. *Xenobiotica*, *11*, 771-778

Rajaraman, R. & Faulkner, G. (1984) Reverse transformation of Chinese hamster ovary cells by methyl xanthines. *Exp. Cell Res.*, *154*, 342-356

Rall, T.W. (1985) The methylxanthines. In: Gilman, A.G., Goodman, L.S., Rall, T.W. & Murad, F., eds, *Goodman and Gilman's The Pharmacological Basis of Therapeutics*, 7th ed., New York, MacMillan, pp. 589-603

Rao, G.S., Khanna, K.L. & Cornish, H.H. (1973) Identification of two new metabolites of caffeine in the rat urine. *Experientia*, *29*, 953-955

Reel, J.R., Wolkowski-Tyl, R., Lawton, A.D., Feldman, D.B. & Lamb, J.C. (1984) *Caffeine: Reproduction and Fertility Assessment in CD-1 Mice When Administered in the Drinking Water* (NTP-84-158), Research Triangle Park, NC, National Institute of Environmental Health Sciences

Reguly, M.L. & Marques, E.K. (1988) Effect of caffeine on the radioresistance and radiosensitivity of *Drosophila melanogaster*. *Rev. Brasil. Genet.*, *11*, 1-11

Reid, S.J. & Good, T.J. (1982) Use of chromatographic mode sequencing for sample preparation in the analysis of caffeine and theobromine from beverages. *J. agric. Food Chem.*, *30*, 775-778

Renner, H.W. (1982) Sister chromatid exchanges induced by methylxanthines contained in coffee, tea and cocoa. *Experientia*, *38*, 600

Renner, E., Wietholtz, H., Huguenin, P., Arnaud, M.J. & Preisig, R. (1984) Caffeine: a model compound for measuring liver function. *Hepatology*, *4*, 38-46

Reynolds, J.E.F., ed. (1989) *Martindale. The Extra Pharmacopoeia*, 29th ed., London, The Pharmaceutical Press, pp. 1522-1524

Richardson, C.L., Grant, A.D. & Schulman, G.E. (1981) The interaction of caffeine and other xanthine analogs with DNA as measured by competitive fluorescence polarization (Abstract No. AC-5). *Environ. Mutagenesis*, *3*, 343

Riechert, M. (1978) Micromethod for the determination of caffeine and theophylline allowing direct application of biological fluids to thin-layer chromatography plates. *J. Chromatogr.*, *146*, 175-180

Roberts, J.J. (1978) The repair of DNA modified by cytotoxic, mutagenic, and carcinogenic chemicals. *Adv. Radiat. Biol.*, *7*, 211-436

Roberts, J.J. (1984) Mechanism of potentiation by caffeine of genotoxic damage induced by physical and chemical agents: possible relevance to carcinogenesis. In: Dews, P.B., ed., *Caffeine. Perspectives from Recent Research*, Berlin, Springer, pp. 239-253

Robertson, D. & Curatolo, P.W. (1984) The cardiovascular effects of caffeine. In: Dews, P.B., ed., *Caffeine. Perspectives from Recent Research*, Berlin, Springer, pp. 77-85

Robertson, D., Frölich, J.C., Carr, R.K., Watson, J.T., Hollifield, J.W., Shand, D.G. & Oates, J.A. (1978) Effects of caffeine on plasma renin activity, catecholamines and blood pressure. *New Engl. J. Med.*, 298, 181-186

Robertson, D., Wade, D., Workman, R., Woosley, R.L. & Oates, J.A. (1981) Tolerance to the humoral and hemodynamic effects of caffeine in man. *J. clin. Invest.*, 67, 1111-1117

Rohan, T.E. & McMichael, A.J. (1988) Methylxanthines and breast cancer. *Int. J. Cancer*, 41, 390-393

Rohan, T.E., Cook, M.G. & McMichael, A.J. (1989) Methylxanthines and benign proliferative epithelial disorders of the breast in women. *Int. J. Epidemiol.*, 18, 626-633

Röhrborn, G. (1972) Mutagenicity studies on mouse after chronic administration of caffeine (Ger.). *Z. Ernährungswiss.*, Suppl. 14, 54-67

Röhrborn, G. & Buckel, U. (1976) Investigations on the frequency of chromosome aberrations in bone marrow cells of Chinese hamster after simultaneous application of caffeine and cyclophosphamide. *Hum. Genet.*, 33, 113-119

Rosenberg, L., Mitchell, A.A., Shapiro, S. & Slone, D. (1982) Selected birth defects in relation to caffeine-containing beverages. *J. Am. med. Assoc.*, 247, 1429-1432

Rosenkranz, H.S. & Ennever, F.K. (1987) Genotoxicity and carcinogenicity assessment of caffeine and theobromine (Letter to the Editor). *Food chem. Toxicol.*, 25, 795-796

Rothwell, K. (1974) Dose-related inhibition of chemical carcinogenesis in mouse skin by caffeine. *Nature*, 252, 69-70

Roulland-Dussoix, D. (1967) Degradation of ultraviolet-irradiated lambda bacteriophage DNA by the host cell (Fr.). *Mutat. Res.*, 4, 241-252

Routh, J.I., Shane, N.A., Arredondo, E.G. & Paul, W.D. (1969) Determination of caffeine in serum and urine. *Clin. Chem.*, 15, 661-668

Ryu, J.E. (1985) Caffeine in human milk and in serum of breast-fed infants. *Dev. Pharmacol. Ther.*, 8, 329-337

Sacks, L.E. & Mihara, K. (1983) Induction at high frequency of a unique phenotypic class of *Bacillus subtilis* mutants by methylxanthines. *Mutat. Res.*, 117, 55-65

Sandlie, I., Solberg, K. & Kleppe, K. (1980) The effect of caffeine on cell growth and metabolism of thymidine in *Escherichia coli*. *Mutat. Res.*, 73, 29-41

Sasaki, M.S. (1977) Sister chromatid exchange and chromatid interchange as possible manifestation of different DNA repair processes. *Nature*, 269, 623-625

Sasaki, M.S. & Tonomura, A. (1973) A high susceptibility of Fanconi's anemia to chromosome breakage by DNA cross-linking agents. *Cancer Res.*, 33, 1829-1836

Sato, C. & Izumi, N. (1989) Mechanism of increased hepatotoxicity of acetaminophen by the simultaneous administration of caffeine in the rat. *J. Pharmacol. exp. Ther.*, 248, 1243-1247

Schairer, C., Brinton, L.A. & Hoover, R.N. (1986) Methylxanthines and benign breast disease. *Am. J. Epidemiol.*, 124, 603-611

Schairer, C., Brinton, L.A. & Hoover, R.N. (1987) Methylxanthines and breast cancer. *Int. J. Cancer*, 40, 469-473

Schöneich, J., Michaelis, A. & Rieger, R. (1970) Caffeine and chemical induction of chromatid aberrations in *Vicia faba* and ascites tumours of the mouse (Ger.). *Biol. Zentralbl.*, *88*, 49-63

Schrieber, G.B., Maffeo, C.E., Robins, M., Masters, M.N. & Bond, A.P. (1988) Measurement of coffee and caffeine intake: implications for epidemiologic research. *Prev. Med.*, *17*, 280-294

Scott, N.R., Chakraborty, J. & Marks, V. (1986) Urinary metabolites of caffeine in pregnant women. *Br. J. clin. Pharmacol.*, *22*, 475-478

Senanayake, U.M. & Wijesekera, R.O.B. (1968) A rapid micro-method for the separation, identification and estimation of the purine bases: caffeine, theobromine and theophylline. *J. Chromatogr.*, *32*, 75-86

Senanayake, U.M. & Wijesekera, R.O.B. (1971) Theobromine and caffeine content of the cocoa bean during its growth. *J. Sci. Food Agric.*, *22*, 262-263

Shakarnis, V.F. (1970) A comparative study on the action of caffeine on the X-chromosome nondisjunction and recessive sex-linked lethal mutation of different *Drosophila melanogaster* stocks (Russ.). *Genetica*, *6*, 83-87

Shankel, D.M. (1962) 'Mutational synergism' of ultraviolet light and caffeine in *Escherichia coli*. *J. Bacteriol.*, *84*, 410-415

Shirlow, M.J. (1983) Patterns of caffeine consumption. *Human Nutr. appl. Nutr.*, *37A*, 307-313

Shively, C.A. & Tarka, S.M., Jr (1984) Methylxanthine composition and consumption patterns of cocoa and chocolate products. In: Spiller, G.A., ed., *The Methylxanthine Beverages and Foods: Chemistry, Consumption, and Health Effects*, New York, Alan R. Liss, pp. 149-178

Singh, R.N. & Kashyap, A.K. (1977) Induction of mutations in the blue-green alga *Plectonema boryanum* Gomont. *Mutat. Res.*, *43*, 37-44

Singh, K.P., Saxena, A.K., Srivastava, S.N. & Shanker, R. (1984) Effect of caffeine (1,3,7-trimethylxanthine) on bone marrow cells of mice. *Indian J. exp. Biol.*, *22*, 608-611

Sleigh, M.J. & Grigg, G.W. (1974) Induction of local denaturation in DNA *in vitro* by phleomycin and caffeine. *FEBS Lett.*, *39*, 35-38

Smeets, D., Verhagen, A. & Hustinx, T. (1989) Familial and individual variation in chromosome fragility. *Mutat. Res.*, *212*, 223-229

Smith, S.E., McElhatton, P.R. & Sullivan, F.M. (1987) Effects of administering caffeine to pregnant rats either as a single daily dose or as divided doses four times a day. *Food chem. Toxicol.*, *25*, 125-133

Smith, D.F., MacGregor, J.T., Hiatt, R.A., Hooper, N.K., Wehr, C.M., Peters, B., Goldman, L.R., Yuan, L.A., Smith, P.A. & Becker, C.E. (1990) Micronucleated erythrocytes as an index of cytogenetic damage in humans: demographic and dietary factors associated with micronucleated erythrocytes in splenectomized subjects. *Cancer Res.*, *50*, 5049-5054

Smith-Sonneborn, J. (1974) Age-correlated effects of caffeine on non-irradiated and UV-irradiated *Paramecium aurelia*. *J. Gerontol.*, *29*, 256-260

Smits, P., Pieters, G. & Thien, T. (1986) The role of epinephrine in the circulatory effects of coffee. *Clin. Pharmacol. Ther.*, *40*, 431-437

Sobotka, T.J., Spaid, S.L. & Brodie, R.E. (1979) Neurobehavioral teratology of caffeine exposure in rats. *Neurotoxicology*, *1*, 403-416

Solberg, K.A., Øvrebø, S., Kleppe, R.K. & Kleppe, K. (1978) Effect of caffeine on DNA polymerase I from *Escherichia coli*. Studies *in vitro* and *in vivo*. *Mutat. Res.*, *51*, 1-10

Somani, S.M., Khanna, N.N. & Bada, H.S. (1980) Caffeine and theophylline: serum/CSF correlation in premature infants. *J. Pediatr.*, *96*, 1091-1093

Somorin, O. (1973) Spectrophotometric determination of caffeine in Nigerian kola nuts. *J. Food Sci.*, *38*, 911-912

Somorin, O. (1974) Caffeine distribution in *C. acuminata*, *T. cacao* and *C. arabica*. *J. Food Sci.*, *39*, 1055-1056

Speit, G. (1986) The relationship between the induction of SCEs and mutations in Chinese hamster cells. I. Experiments with hydrogen peroxide and caffeine. *Mutat. Res.*, *174*, 21-26

Spindle, A. & Wu, K. (1985) Development and cytogenetic effects of caffeine on mouse blastocysts, alone or in combination with benzo[*a*]pyrene. *Teratology*, *32*, 213-218

Srinivasan, A., Reddy, E.P., Sarma, P.S. & Schultz, R.A. (1979) Inhibition of RNA-dependent DNA polymerase activity of oncornaviruses by caffeine. *Biochem. biophys. Res. Commun.*, *91*, 239-246

Stabilimento Farmaceutico 'Cau. G. Testa' (1989) *Caffeine Production*, Albenga

Stanovnik, B., Mirtič, T., Koren, B., Tišler, M. & Belčič, B. (1982) Methylation of some oxopurines and 1,2,4-triazoles with *N,N*-dimethylformamide dimethyl acetal. *Vestn. Slov. Kem. Drus.*, *29*, 331-343

Statland, B.E. & Demas, T.J. (1980) Serum caffeine half-lives. Healthy subjects *vs* patients having alcoholic hepatic disease. *Am. J. clin. Pathol.*, *73*, 390-393

Statland, B.E., Demas, T.J. & Danis, M. (1976) Caffeine accumulation associated with alcoholic liver disease. *New Engl. J. Med.*, *295*, 110-111

Stavric, B. (1988) Methylxanthines: toxicity to humans. 2. Caffeine. *Food chem. Toxicol.*, *26*, 645-662

Stavric, B. & Klassen, R. (1984) Automated high-performance liquid chromatographic assay for monitoring caffeine and its metabolites in biological fluids of monkeys consuming caffeine. *J. Chromatogr.*, *310*, 107-118

Stavric, B. & Klassen, R. (1987) Caffeine content in colas from New York State and Ontario. *J. Food Saf.*, *8*, 179-185

Stavric, B., Klassen, R., Watkinson, B., Karpinski, K., Stapley, R. & Fried, P. (1988) Variability in caffeine consumption from coffee and tea: possible significance for epidemiological studies. *Food chem. Toxicol.*, *26*, 111-118

Strubelt, O. (1987) Toxicity of coffee and caffeine (Ger.). *Dtsch. med. Wochenschr.*, *112*, 852-858

Sturelid, S. (1976) Enhancement by caffeine of cell killing and chromosome damage in Chinese hamster cells treated with thiotepa. *Hereditas*, *84*, 157-162

Sutherland, D.J., McPherson, D.D., Renton, K.W., Spencer, C.A. & Montague, T.J. (1985) The effect of caffeine on cardiac rate, rhythm, and ventricular repolarization. Analysis of 18 normal subjects and 18 patients with primary ventricular dysrhythmia. *Chest*, *87*, 319-324

Sved, S. & Wilson, D.L. (1977) Simultaneous assay of the methylxanthine metabolites of caffeine in plasma by high performance liquid chromatography. *Res. Commun. chem. Pathol. Pharmacol.*, *17*, 319-331

Swenberg, J.A. (1981) Utilization of the alkaline elution assay as a short-term test for chemical carcinogens. In: Stich, H.F. & San, R.H.C., eds, *Short-term Tests for Chemical Carcinogens*, New York, Springer, pp. 48-58

Swietlińska, Z. (1971) High frequency of chromosome aberrations induced by DEB with caffeine posttreatment in *Vicia faba* var. Minor. *Mol. gen. Genet.*, *112*, 87-90

Swietlińska, Z., Zaborowska, D. & Zuk, J. (1973) Induction of chromosome aberrations by diepoxybutane and caffeine in root meristems and germinating seeds of *Vicia faba*. *Mutat. Res.*, *17*, 199-205

Takayama, S. & Kuwabara, N. (1982) Long-term study on the effect of caffeine in Wistar rats. *Gann*, *73*, 365-371

Tanaka, H., Nakazawa, K., Arima, M. & Iwasaki, S. (1984) Caffeine and its dimethylxanthines in fetal cerebral development in rat. *Brain Dev.*, *6*, 355-361

Tang, B.K., Grant, D.M. & Kalow, W. (1983) Isolation and identification of 5-acetylamino-6-formylamino-3-methyluracil as a major metabolite of caffeine in man. *Drug Metab. Dispos.*, *11*, 218-220

Tarka, S.M., Jr (1982) The toxicology of cocoa and dimethylxanthines: a review of the literature. *CRC crit. Rev. Toxicol.*, *9*, 275-312

Thayer, P.S. & Kensler, C.J. (1973) Genetic tests in mice of caffeine alone and in combination with mutagens. *Toxicol. appl. Pharmacol.*, *25*, 157-168

Thayer, P.S. & Palm, P.E. (1975) A current assessment of the mutagenic and teratogenic effects of caffeine. *CRC crit. Rev. Toxicol.*, *3*, 345-369

Thayer, P.S., Himmelfarb, P., Liss, R.H. & Carlson, B.L. (1971) Continuous exposure of HeLa cells to caffeine. *Mutat. Res.*, *12*, 197-203

Theiss, J.C. & Shimkin, M.B. (1978) Inhibiting effect of caffeine on spontaneous and urethan-induced lung tumors in strain A mice. *Cancer Res.*, *38*, 1757-1761

Thithapandha, A., Chaturapit, S., Limlomwongse, L. & Sobhon, P. (1974) The effects of xanthines on mouse liver cell. *Arch. Biochem. Biophys.*, *161*, 178-186

Timbie, D.J., Sechrist, L. & Keeney, P.G. (1978) Application of high-pressure liquid chromatography to the study of variables affecting theobromine and caffeine concentrations in cocoa beans. *J. Food Sci.*, *43*, 560-565

Timson, J. (1977) Caffeine. *Mutat. Res.*, *47*, 1-52

Tin, A.A., Somani, S.M., Bada, H.S. & Khanna, N.N. (1979) Caffeine, theophylline and theobromine determinations in serum, saliva and spinal fluid. *J. anal. Toxicol.*, *3*, 26-29

Tobias, D.Y. (1982) *Current Methods of Caffeine Determination: Review of the Literature, 1975-1980*. *FDA By Lines*, *3*, 129-156

Tohda, H. & Oikawa, A. (1988) Characterization of the enhancing effect of caffeine on sister-chromatid exchanges induced by ultraviolet radiation in excision-proficient xeroderma pigmentosum lymphoblastoid cells. *Mutat. Res.*, *201*, 1-8

Tohnai, I., Oka, T. & Ohno, Y. (1984) A case-control study on cleft lip and/or palate: maternal dietary practices in early pregnancy (Abstract). *Teratology*, *30*, 23A

Tornaletti, S., Russo, P., Parodi, S. & Pedrini, A.M. (1989) Studies on DNA binding of caffeine and derivatives: evidence of intercalation by DNA-unwinding experiments. *Biochem. biophys. Acta*, *1007*, 112-115

Traub, A.I., Earnshaw, J.C., Brannigan, P.D. & Thompson, W. (1982) A critical assessment of the response to caffeine of human sperm motility. *Fertil. Steril.*, *37*, 436-437

Trosko, J.E. & Chu, E.H.Y. (1971) Effects of caffeine on the induction of mutations in Chinese hamster cells by ultraviolet light. *Mutat. Res.*, *12*, 337-340

Ts'o, P.O. & Lu, P. (1964) Interaction of nucleic acids. I. Physical binding of thymidine, adenine, steroids, and aromatic hydrocarbons to nucleic acids. *Proc. natl Acad. Sci. USA*, *51*, 17-24

Ts'o, P.O.P., Helmkamp, G.K. & Sander, C. (1962) Interaction of nucleosides and related compounds with nucleic acids as indicated by the change of helix-coil transition temperature. *Proc. natl Acad. Sci. USA*, *48*, 686-698

Tsuboi, M. & Yanagishima, N. (1975) Comparative studies on sporulation-promotive actions of cyclic AMP, theophylline and caffeine in *Saccharomyces cerevisiae*. *Arch. Mikrobiol.*, *105*, 83-86

Tsuchimoto, T. & Matter, B.E. (1979) In vivo cytogenetic screening methods for mutagens, with special reference to the micronucleus test. *Arch. Toxicol.*, *42*, 239-248

Turmen, T., Louridas, T.A. & Aranda, J.V. (1979) Relationship of plasma and CSF concentrations of caffeine in neonates with apnea. *J. Pediatr.*, *95*, 644-646

Tyrala, E.E. & Dodson, W.E. (1979) Caffeine secretion into breast milk. *Arch. Dis. Child.*, *54*, 787-789

US Bureau of the Census (1989) *US Exports and US Imports for Consumption* (Customs Values) (Reports EM 522 and IM146), Washington DC, Foreign Trade Commission, pp. 5161-5162, 5179-5180

US Food and Drug Administration (1980) *Caffeine Content of Various Products* (FDA Talk Paper T80-45), Rockville, MD

US Food and Drug Administration (1984) The latest caffeine scorecard. *FDA Consumer*, *March*, 14-16

US Food and Drug Administration (1988) Caffeine. *US Code fed. Regul.*, *182.1180*, 392

US International Trade Commission (1987) *Synthetic Organic Chemicals, US Production and Sales 1986* (USITC Publ. No. 2009), Washington DC, US Government Printing Office

US Pharmacopeial Convention (1990) *US Pharmacopeia — The National Formulary*, 22nd ed., Rockville, MD, pp. 204-205

Van der Meer, C. & Haas, R.E. (1980) Determination of caffeine in serum by straight-phase high-performance liquid chromatography. *J. Chromatogr.*, *182*, 121-124

Vergnes, M.F. & Alary, J. (1986) Determination of natural xanthines by HPLC (Fr.). *Talanta*, *33*, 997-1000

Vig, B.K. (1973) Somatic crossing over in *Glycine max* (L.) Merrill: effect of some inhibitors of DNA synthesis on the induction of somatic crossing over and point mutations. *Genetics*, *73*, 583-596

Vogel, F., Krüger, J., Kurth, M. & Schroeder, T.M. (1966) On the lack of a relationship between coffee drinking by parents and the sex ratio of their children (Ger.). *Humangenetik*, *2*, 119-132

Voogd, C.E. & van der Vet, P. (1969) Mutagenic action of ethylene halogenhydrins. *Experientia*, *25*, 85-86

Wahlländer, A., Renner, E. & Karlaganis, G. (1985) High-performance liquid chromatographic determination of dimethylxanthine metabolites of caffeine in human plasma. *J. Chromatogr. (Biomed. Appl.)*, *338*, 369-375

Waksvik, H., Brøgger, A. & Stene, J. (1977) Psoralen/UVA treatment and chromosomes. I. Aberrations and sister chromatid exchange in human lymphocytes *in vitro* and synergism with caffeine. *Hum. Genet.*, *38*, 195-207

Waldren, C.A. (1973) The use of in vitro techniques in mammalian cell biology: some aspects of the action of caffeine and other agents on cells in culture. *Diss. Abstr. int. B*, *34*, 553-B — 554-B

Waldren, C.A. & Patterson, D. (1979) Effect of caffeine on purine metabolism and ultraviolet light-induced lethality in cultured mammalian cells. *Cancer Res.*, *39*, 4975-4982

Walton, H.F., Eiceman, G.A. & Otto, J.L. (1979) Chromatography of xanthines on ion-exchange resins. *J. Chromatogr.*, *180*, 145-156

Warszawski, D., Ben-Zvi, Z. & Gorodischer, R. (1981) Caffeine metabolism in liver slices during postnatal development in the rat. *Biochem. Pharmacol.*, *30*, 3145-3150

Warszawski, D., Ben-Zvi, Z., Gorodischer, R., Arnaud, M.J. & Bracco, I. (1982) Urinary metabolites of caffeine in young dogs. *Drug Metab. Disposition*, *10*, 424-428

Watkinson, B. & Fried, P.A. (1985) Maternal caffeine use before, during and after pregnancy and effects upon offspring. *Neurobehav. Toxicol. Teratol.*, *7*, 9-17

Webb, R.B. (1970) Continuous cultures in mutagen testing (Abstract). *Genetics*, *64*, S64-S65

Weinstein, D., Mauer, I. & Solomon, H.M. (1972) Effect of caffeine on chromosomes of human lymphocytes: in vivo and in vitro studies. *Mutat. Res.*, *16*, 391-399

Weinstein, D., Mauer, I., Katz, M.L. & Kazmer, S. (1973a) The effect of caffeine on chromosomes of human lymphocytes: a search for the mechanism of action. *Mutat. Res.*, *20*, 115-125

Weinstein, D., Mauer, I., Katz, M. & Kazmer, S. (1973b) The effect of caffeine on chromosomes of human lymphocytes: non-random distribution of damage. *Mutat. Res.*, *20*, 441-443

Weinstein, D., Mauer, I., Katz, M.L. & Kazmer, S. (1975) The effect of methylxanthines on chromosomes of human lymphocytes in culture. *Mutat. Res.*, *31*, 57-61

Welch, R.M., Hsu, S.-Y. & DeAngelis, R.L. (1977) Effect of Aroclor 1254, phenobarbital, and polycyclic aromatic hydrocarbons on the plasma clearance of caffeine in the rat. *Clin. Pharmacol. Ther.*, *22*, 791-798

Welsch, C.W. & DeHoog, J.V. (1988) Influence of caffeine consumption on 7,12-dimethylbenz(*a*)anthracene-induced mammary gland tumorigenesis in female rats fed a chemically defined diet containing standard and high levels of unsaturated fat. *Cancer Res.*, 48, 2074-2077

Welsch, C.W., Scieszka, K.M., Senn, E.R. & DeHoog, J.V. (1983) Caffeine (1,3,7-trimethylxanthine), a temperate promotor of DMBA-induced rat mammary gland carcinogenesis. *Int. J. Cancer*, 32, 479-484

Welsch, C.W., DeHoog, J.V. & O'Connor, D.H. (1988a) Influence of caffeine consumption on carcinomatous and normal mammary gland development in mice. *Cancer Res.*, 48, 2078-2082

Welsch, C.W., DeHoog, J.V. & O'Connor, D.H. (1988b) Influence of caffeine and/or coffee consumption on the initiation and promotion phases of 7,12-dimethylbenz(*a*)anthracene-induced rat mammary gland tumorigenesis. *Cancer Res.*, 48, 2068-2073

West, G.L., Sobotka, T.J., Brodie, R.E., Beier, J.M. & O'Connell, M.W., Jr (1986) Postnatal neurobehavioral development in rats exposed *in utero* to caffeine. *Neurobehav. Toxicol. Teratol.*, 8, 29-43

Wietholtz, H., Voegelin, M., Arnaud, M.J., Bircher, J. & Preisig, R. (1981) Assessment of the cytochrome P-448 dependent liver enzyme system by a caffeine breath test. *Eur. J. clin. Pharmacol.*, 21, 53-59

Wilson, J.G. & Scott, W.J., Jr (1984) The teratogenic potential of caffeine in laboratory animals. In: Dews, P.B., ed., *Caffeine. Perspectives from Recent Research*, Berlin, Springer, pp. 165-187

Windholz, M., ed. (1983) *The Merck Index*, 10th ed., Rahway, NJ, pp. 225-226

Wolf, K. & Kaudewitz, F. (1976) Effect of caffeine on the rho⁻-induction with ethidium bromide in *Saccharomyces cerevisiae*. *Mol. gen. Genet.*, 146, 89-93

Wong, S.H.Y., Marzouk, N., Aziz, O. & Sheeran, S. (1987) Microbore liquid chromatography for therapeutic drug monitoring and toxicology: clinical analyses of theophylline, caffeine, procainamide and N-acetyl procainamide. *J. liquid Chromatogr.*, 10, 491-506

Wragg, J.B., Carr, J.V. & Ross, V.C. (1967) Inhibition of DNA polymerase activity by caffeine in a mammalian cell line (Abstract No. 305). *J. Cell Biol.*, 35, 146A-147A

Würzner, H.-P., Lindström, E. & Vuataz, L. & Luginbühl, H. (1977a) A 2-year feeding study of instant coffees in rats. I. Body weight. Food consumption, haematological parameters and plasma chemistry. *Food Cosmet. Toxicol.*, 15, 7-16

Würzner, H.-P., Lindström, E. & Vuataz, L. & Luginbühl, H. (1977b) A 2-year feeding study of instant coffees in rats. II. Incidence and types of neoplasms. *Food Cosmet. Toxicol.*, 15, 289-296

Yamagami, T., Handa, H., Takeuchi, J., Munemitsu, H., Aoki, M. & Kato, Y. (1983) Rat pituitary adenoma and hyperplasia induced by caffeine administration. *Surg. Neurol.*, 20, 323-331

Yamamoto, K. & Yamaguchi, H. (1969) Inhibition by caffeine of the repair of γ-ray-induced chromosome breaks in barley. *Mutat. Res.*, 8, 428-430

Yanders, A.F. & Seaton, R.K. (1962) The lack of mutagenicity of caffeine in *Drosophila*. *Am. Nat.*, *96*, 277-280

Yefremova, G.I. & Filippova, L.M. (1974) Effect of caffeine on crossing-over in *Drosophila melanogaster*. *Mutat. Res.*, *23*, 347-352

Yesair, D.W., Branfman, A.R. & Callahan, M.M. (1984) Human disposition and some biochemical aspects of methylxanthines. In: Spiller, G.A., ed., *The Methylxanthine Beverages and Foods: Chemistry, Consumption and Health Effects*, New York, Alan R. Liss, pp. 215-233

Zajdela, F. & Latarjet, R. (1973) Inhibitory effect of caffeine on the induction of skin cancers by UV light in the mouse (Fr.). *C.R. Acad. Sci. (Paris)*, *277*, 1073-1076

Zajdela, F. & Latarjet, R. (1975) The inhibitory effect of caffeine on the induction of cutaneous tumors in mice by ultraviolet rays. In: Bucalossi, P., Veronesi, U. & Cascinelli, N., eds, *Proceedings of the XI International Cancer Congress, Florence, 20-26 October 1974*, Vol. 3, Amsterdam, Excerpta Medica, pp. 120-123

Zajdela, F. & Latarjet, R. (1978a) Ultraviolet light induction of skin carcinoma in the mouse; influence of cAMP modifying agents. *Bull. Cancer*, *65*, 305-314

Zajdela, F. & Latarjet, R. (1978b) Inhibition of skin carcinogenesis *in vivo* by caffeine and other agents. *Natl Cancer Inst. Monogr.*, *50*, 133-140

Zetterberg, G. (1960) The mutagenic effect of 8-ethoxycaffeine, caffeine and dimethylsulfate in the *Ophiostoma* back-mutation test. *Hereditas*, *46*, 279-311

Zettle, T.E. & Murnik, M.R. (1973) Effects of caffeine on chromosomal loss and nondisjunction in *Drosophila melanogaster*. *Genetica*, *44*, 146-153

Zoumas, B.L., Kreiser, W.R. & Martin, R.A. (1980) Theobromine and caffeine content of chocolate products. *J. Food Sci.*, *45*, 314-316

THEOPHYLLINE

1. Chemical and Physical Data

1.1 Synonyms

Chem. Abstr. Services Reg. No.: 58-55-9
Chem. Abstr. Name: 3,7-Dihydro-1,3-dimethyl-1H-purine-2,6-dione
Synonym: 1,3-Dimethylxanthine

1.2 Structural and molecular formulae and molecular weight

$C_7H_8N_4O_2$ Mol. wt: 180.17

1.3 Chemical and physical properties of the pure substance

(a) *Description*: White crystalline powder (Moffat, 1986)
(b) *Melting-point*: 270-274°C (Windholz, 1983)
(c) *Spectroscopy data*: Ultraviolet spectra: aqueous acid-270 nm (A_1^1 = 536a), aqueous alkali-275 nm (A_1^1 = 650a); infrared spectra: principal peaks at wave numbers 1670, 1717, 1567, 745, 980 and 1190 (potassium bromide disc); mass spectra: principal peaks at m/z 180, 95, 68, 41, 53, 181, 96, 40; 3-methylxanthine, 166, 68, 95, 41, 53, 123 (Moffat, 1986)
(d) *Solubility*: Soluble in water (1.0 g/120 ml), ethanol (1.0 g/80 ml), chloroform (1.0 g/110 ml), hot water, alkali hydroxides, ammonia and dilute hydrochloric and nitric acids; sparingly soluble in diethyl ether (Windholz, 1983)

(e) *Equilibrium constants*: acidic (Ka), 1.69×10^{-9}; basic (Kb), 1.9×10^{-14} at 25°C (Windholz, 1983)
(f) *Octanol/water partition coefficient (P)*: log P, 0.0 (Moffat, 1986)
(g) *Reactivity*: Solutions generally quite stable over the entire pH range; strongly alkaline solutions (pH > 12) show decomposition and apparent ring opening after several weeks (Cohen, 1975)

1.4 Technical products and impurities

Theophylline is available in a USP grade with the following specifications: 97.0-102.0% active ingredient calculated on a dried basis; 0.5% max weight loss on drying for the anhydrous form and 7.5-9.5% for the monohydrate form; 0.15% max residue on ignition; and melting-point, 270-274°C (US Pharmacopeial Convention, 1990). Theophylline should contain not less than 99.0% and not more than 101.0% active ingredient on a dried basis (Anon., 1988).

Trade names: Accurbron; Aerolate; Afonilum; Aquaphyllin; Armophylline; Asthmophylline; Bronchoretard; Bronkodyl; Duraphyl; Elixicon; LaBid; Lasma; Nuelin; Optiphyllin; Oralphyllin; Physpan; Primatene; Pro-vent; Quibron-T; Rona-Phyllin; Slixophylline; Slo-Bid; Slo-Phyllin; Somophyllin-T; Sustaire; Teofilina; Thealtabl; Theobid; Theocap; Theocin; Theoclear; Theocontin; Theocord; Theodel; Theodrine; Theo-Dur; Theofed; Theofedral; Theograd; Theolair; Theolate; Theolixir; Theoliz; Theon-300; Theophenyllin; Theophyl; Theophyl-SR; Theoral; Theosol; Theospan; Theostat; Theovent; Unicontin; Uniphyllin. It is also an ingredient of Franol; Franyl; Labophylline; Phyldrox; Quibron; Tancolin; Taumasthman; Tedral (Moffat, 1986)

2. Production, Use, Occurrence and Analysis

2.1 Production and use

(a) *Production*

Theophylline has been prepared from dimethylurea and ethyl cyanoacetate (Windholz, 1983).

The production of theophylline derivatives in the USA in 1977 amounted to 51 000 kg and total US imports of theophylline and its derivatives in 1978 were 590 000 kg (Haley, 1983a). Domestic production data were not reported for 1981-86; however, on the basis of the total imports of food and beverages containing methylxanthines into the USA in 1980, 185 million pounds (84 million kg) of tea containing 0.03% theophylline were imported, resulting in approximately 60 000 pounds (27 000 kg) of theophylline (Hirsh, 1984). Five companies in the USA were reported to produce theophylline or theophylline derivatives in 1986 (SRI, 1986). US imports of theophylline, theophylline ethylenediamine and their derivatives in January to June 1989 amounted to approximately 825 000 kg (US Bureau of the Census, 1989).

Data were not available from other parts of the world.

(b) Use

Theophylline and its monohydrate, aluminium hydroxide, choline (oxtriphylline), calcium salicylate, ethylenediamine (aminophylline), dihydroxypropyl (dyphylline), monoethanolamine and sodium glycinate derivatives (Weinberger, 1978) are used to control asthmatic symptoms, to relieve bronchial spasms, to alleviate neonatal apnoea (Stavric, 1988), in the treatment of respiratory diseases, such as bronchitis, obstructive pulmonary disease and emphysema, as a myocardial stimulant, to relieve biliary colic and in diuretics (Ritchie, 1975; Stavric, 1988; Barnhart, 1989). The doses used are 180-1000 mg per day (Moffat, 1986), which result in 10-20 µg/ml plasma.

Theophylline is also administered in combination with ephedrine, guaifenesin, butabarbital and phenobarbital (Gennaro, 1985; Moffat, 1986; Consumers Union, 1990). Sodium and potassium salts and a large number of less basic salts and/or complexes have been prepared in order to increase the water solubility of theophylline for parenteral administration (Cohen, 1975). More than 200 different theophylline preparations exist in the USA as prescription or over-the-counter drugs and fewer than 100 in Canada (Weinberger, 1978; Stavric, 1988). In the USA in 1986, over 11 million prescriptions were written for the theophylline drug, Theo-Dur (Anon., 1986). In 1985, over 25 million prescriptions were written for theophylline-containing medications in the USA (Collins, 1987). In the USA in 1980, theophylline was ranked twentieth among the 100 most prescribed drugs.

2.2 Occurrence

(a) Natural occurrence

Theophylline occurs in black tea (*Camellia sinensis*) at very low levels; values cited in the literature vary greatly, but the most reliable range is 0.02-0.04% dry weight (Jalal & Collin, 1976; Graham, 1984a). Theophylline has been found in green coffee beans at approximately 5 mg/kg (Spiller, 1984), and trace amounts were detected in cacao cotyledon (Shively & Tarka, 1984). Theophylline was detected at 0.004% in dried mate (Graham, 1984b).

(b) *Occupational exposure*

A national occupational hazard survey conducted in the USA in 1972-74 estimated that approximately 7500 people were exposed occupationally to theophylline (National Institute for Occupational Safety and Health, 1974). No occupational standard has been established for theophylline.

(c) *Water and sediments*

Theophylline was not found in US industrial effluents (Perry *et al.*, 1979) or drinking-water (National Research Council, 1977) or in European water supplies (Commission of the European Communities, 1976).

(d) *Foods and beverages* (see also the monograph on caffeine, pp. 296 *et seq.*)

Theophylline was detected in blended black tea beverages at a level of 0.25% of the extractable solids present (Graham, 1984a). In the USA in 1980, 26 000 pounds (11 800 kg) of theophylline were consumed, as estimated from an importation of 185 million pounds of tea containing an average of 0.03% theophylline, equal to 60 000 pounds and a preparation and extraction loss of 50%. The total daily per-caput intake of theophylline in the USA was estimated to be 0.14 mg (Hirsh, 1984).

2.3 Analysis

The techniques and analytical procedures for theophylline and other methylxanthines have been reviewed (Cohen, 1975; Christensen & Neims, 1984; Hurst *et al.*, 1984; Christensen & Neims, 1985; Stavric, 1988).

A large variety of analytical procedures, including spectrophotometry, fluorimetry, thin-layer chromatography, gas chromatography, high-performance liquid chromatography, radioimmunoassay, enzyme immunoassay and isotachophoresis have been employed for the determination of theophylline (and concomitant separation from other methylxanthines and metabolites) in biological fluids and dosage formulations. Earlier procedures primarily involved ultraviolet spectrophotometry with a sensitivity ranging from 1-10 µg/ml in plasma (Schack & Waxler, 1949; Gupta & Lundberg, 1973) and 2-15 µg/ml in dosage formulations (Kirichenko & Kagan, 1970); but these methods lacked specificity. Gas chromatographic procedures for the analysis of theophylline are more sensitive and more selective, in that interfering xanthines are separated from theophylline; in general, however, these methods require more sample preparation and derivatization. The sensitivity of detection is 1 µg/ml theophylline in plasma, serum or saliva (Chrzanowski *et al.*, 1974; Shah & Riegelman, 1974; Johnson *et al.*, 1975). High-performance liquid chromatography procedures are sensitive and specific and generally require smaller amounts of biological fluids; they are used extensively for monitoring theophylline levels (Hurst *et al.*, 1984; Christensen & Neims, 1985; Stavric, 1988) in serum or plasma (Adams *et al.*, 1976; Orcutt *et al.*, 1977; Soldin & Hill, 1977; Broussard *et al.*, 1981; Muir *et al.*, 1982; Matsumoto *et al.*, 1988; Meatherall & Ford, 1988) and urine (Muir *et al.*, 1980; Kester *et al.*, 1987) of treated patients. Sensitivities of 1 µg/ml (Adams *et al.*, 1976), 5 µg/ml (Broussard *et al.*, 1981), 8 µg/ml (Soldin & Hill, 1977), 20 µg/ml (Orcutt *et al.*, 1977) and 0.5 µg/ml plasma or saliva (Muir *et al.*, 1982) and 0.15 µg/ml urine (Kester *et al.*, 1987) have been obtained using high-performance liquid chromatography. In all of the commonly used clinical procedures, detection was accomplished by ultraviolet spectrophotometry at wavelengths of 254, 270-277 or 280 nm (Christensen & Neims, 1985).

Additional procedures for the determination of theophylline in biological fluids include fluorimetry (Meola *et al.*, 1979), substrate-labelled fluorescent immunoassay (Messenger *et al.*, 1980; Li *et al.*, 1981a,b; Lee & Liberti, 1987), enzyme multiplied immunoassay (Gushaw *et al.*, 1977; Eppel *et al.*, 1978; Chang *et al.*, 1982), automated fluoroimmunoassay (Allain *et al.*, 1989), homogeneous enzyme-inhibitor immunoassay (Chan *et al.*, 1987), radioimmunoassay (Neese & Soyka, 1977), nephelometric inhibition immunoassay (Nishikawa *et al.*, 1979), isotachophoresis (Moberg *et al.*, 1980) and ion-exchange chromatography (Walton *et al.*, 1979). Sensitivities ranged from 10 µg/ml by fluorimetry (Meola *et al.*, 1979) to 0.7 µg/ml by substrate-labelled fluorescent immunoassay (Li *et al.*, 1981a), 1 µg/ml by automated fluoroimmunoassay (Allain *et al.*, 1989) and 10 ng or less by ion-exchange chromatography (Walton *et al.*, 1979).

3. Biological Data Relevant to the Evaluation of Carcinogenic Risk to Humans

3.1 Carcinogenicity studies in animals

No data were available from studies on the carcinogenicity of theophylline.

Modifying effects on the activity of known carcinogens

(i) *Urethane*

Groups of female ICR/Jcl *mice* [initial numbers unspecified], 25 days of age, received a single subcutaneous injection of 0.1 mg/g bw urethane followed immediately by seven intraperitoneal injections (0.05 µmol/g bw) of theophylline [purity unspecified] at 6-h intervals up to 36 h after urethane treatment, to give a total dose of 63 μg/g bw theophylline. Mice were killed five months after urethane treatment. No significant difference was noted in the numbers of mice with lung tumours (31/59 controls compared to 25/43 mice that received theophylline) or in the numbers of tumours/lung (1.07 compared to 1.36) (Nomura, 1983). [The Working Group noted that the effective numbers of mice varied considerably among the different groups.]

(ii) *Ultraviolet light*

Groups of 54-56 female nonhomozygous Swiss *mice*, 10-12 weeks old, were exposed to the light from an Ellipiol mercury vapour lamp (irradiation time, 90 min) five times a week for a total of 133 exposures over 27 weeks (total dose, 1×10^7 ergs/mm^2). Before each irradiation, 40 μl of a 0.2% solution of theophylline [purity unspecified] in acetone/chloroform were applied to the right ear; the same amount of solvent was applied to the left ear as a control. The first tumours of the ears appeared five months after and the last 11 months after the onset of irradiation. The incidence of tumours on the ears treated with theophylline (48%) was significantly ($p < 0.0001$) lower than that of the control ears (85%) (Zajdela & Latarjet, 1973, 1974, 1978a,b).

3.2 Other relevant data

(*a*) *Experimental systems*

(i) *Absorption, distribution, metabolism and excretion*

The metabolism and pharmacokinetics of theophylline have been reviewed (Arnaud, 1984).

Theophylline was rapidly and completely absorbed from the digestive tract of dogs (McKiernan *et al.*, 1981; Tse & Szeto, 1982). Large variations in its bioavailability were reported in pigs (Koritz *et al.*, 1981) while complete bioavailability was found in cats and rats (Arnaud *et al.*, 1982; McKiernan *et al.*, 1983).

Transport of theophylline from blood to the intestinal lumen was demonstrated in rats (Arimori & Nakano, 1985). After intravenous administration, theophylline was distributed to all organs of rats except adipose tissue (Shum & Jusko, 1984). Whole-body autoradiographs showed no accumulation of radioactivity in any specific tissue 24 h after oral administration of [8-^{14}C]theophylline to rats. By 1 h after oral administration, theophylline had crossed the placenta and was distributed among the organs of fetuses and of pregnant rats, except for the brain of adults. Low theophylline concentrations were found in fetal brain; no blood-brain barrier was observed (Arnaud *et al.*, 1982).

Similar results were found after intravenous administration to rats (Gabrielsson *et al.*, 1984). In rabbits, transplacental transfer of theophylline from maternal to fetal circulation occurred within less than 1 h (Brashear *et al.*, 1982).

Mean serum protein binding of theophylline was lower in dogs (10%) than in man (60%) and rabbits (74%) (Brashear *et al.*, 1980; May & Jarboe, 1981; Munsiff *et al.*, 1988a), and less was bound in pregnant rats [6%] than in non-pregnant rats [20%] (Ramzan & DeDonato, 1988). Similarly, a significant increase in the half-time of theophylline was found in pregnant as compared to non-pregnant rabbits (Brashear *et al.*, 1982) and rats (Brandstetter *et al.*, 1986). The half-time in newborn rabbits was approximately 15 times longer than that in adult animals (Brashear *et al.*, 1982).

Theophylline is distributed rapidly within the body, and plasma half-times were 5.7-11.5 h in dogs (Barnhart & Combes, 1974; McKiernan *et al.*, 1981), 11 h in pigs (Koritz *et al.*, 1981), 7.8 h in cats (McKiernan *et al.*, 1983), 3.8-5.5 h in rabbits (Ng & Locock, 1979; May & Jarboe, 1981) and 1.2-4 h in rats. At higher doses (52-115 mg/kg bw), rats had longer half-times probably because of a combination of increased diuresis and saturation of the metabolism (Teunissen *et al.*, 1985).

Linear pharmacokinetics apply in rats only with intra-arterial doses not exceeding 10 mg/kg bw (Teunissen *et al.*, 1985); similar results were obtained in guinea-pigs (Madsen & Ribel, 1981a,b). In rabbits, there was no evidence of concentration-dependent clearance of theophylline at 15, 22.5 and 30 mg/kg bw (El-Yazigi & Sawchuk, 1981). The clearance and disposition were unchanged in rats with dietary induced obesity (Shum & Jusko 1984).

Theophylline is metabolized only in the liver, mainly by the microsomal system (Lohmann & Miech, 1976; McManus *et al.*, 1988). In rats, oral doses of 40 mg/kg bw per day for three days did not induce liver microsomal enzyme activity, as measured by aromatic ring hydroxylation of acetanilide (Mitoma *et al.*, 1968), while doses of 75-150 mg did.

The pathways of theophylline metabolism reported in rats are presented in Figure 1. Unchanged theophylline (35% of urinary radioactivity) and 1,3-dimethyluric acid (34%) are the main compounds excreted in urine, followed by 1-methyluric acid (18%), 3-methylxanthine (3%) and unidentified polar metabolites (4.8%). Theophylline metabolism was impaired in rats at day 18 of gestation, as shown by increased excretion of theophylline (73%); this was explained by a decreased formation of 1,3-dimethyluric acid (-68%) and 1-methyluric acid (-30%) (Arnaud *et al.*, 1982). Essentially similar results were obtained with pregnant baboons (Logan *et al.*, 1983). Each animal species is characterized by differences in

Fig. 1. Metabolism of theophylline

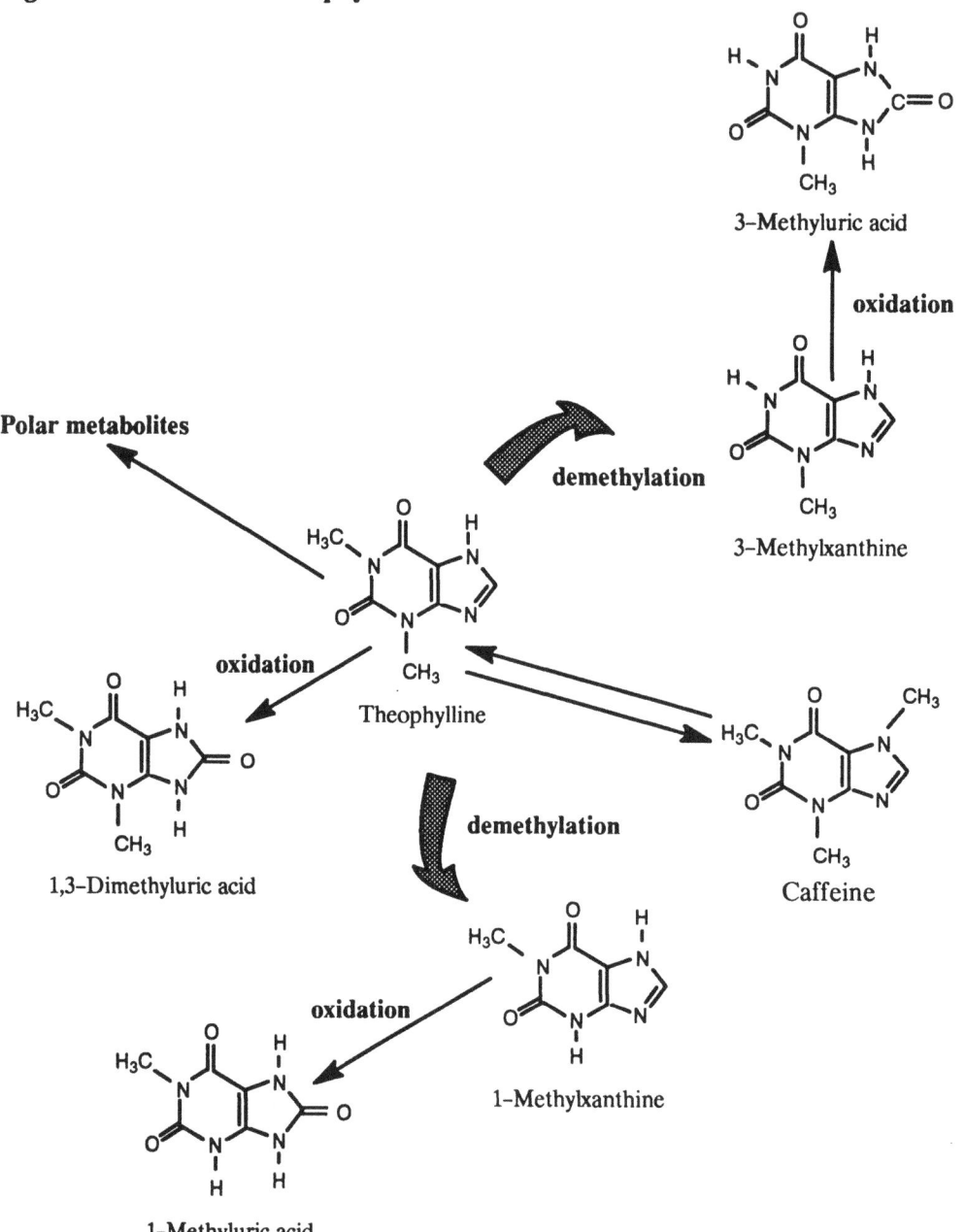

"From Arnaud (1984)

the profile of the metabolites recovered in urine; in addition, quantitative differences in theophylline metabolic pathways were seen even in different strains of mice (Betlach & Tozer, 1980).

Experiments in hepatectomized dogs have shown that the liver plays a central role in theophylline elimination (Brashear *et al.*, 1980). Theophylline and its metabolites are excreted into the bile; in rats, 0.2% (Arimori & Nakano, 1985) and in dogs, 2-4% (Barnhart & Combes, 1974) of the dose was recovered.

(ii) *Toxic effects*

The acute intraperitoneal LD_{50} of theophylline in rats was reported to be 206 mg/kg bw, and accompanying clinical signs were delayed convulsions and tetanic spasm. Acute studies in mice showed an oral LD_{50} of 332 mg/kg bw and an intraperitoneal LD_{50} of 217 mg/kg bw; clinical signs included convulsions, profuse salivation and emesis (Tarka, 1982).

A single oral dose of 400 mg/kg bw theophylline was acutely toxic to rats and mice. Administration of the same daily dose as two separate doses of 200 mg/kg bw was acutely toxic to rats but not to mice (Lindamood *et al.*, 1988). In dogs, the minimal oral toxic concentration of theophylline appears to be higher (37-60 µg/ml plasma) than in man (> 20 µg/ml) (Munsiff *et al.*, 1988b). Theophylline has been reported to be more toxic than caffeine or theobromine to the heart, bronchi and kidneys (Tarka, 1982).

Two weeks' feeding 800 ppm (mg/kg) theophylline in the diet to rats induced no significant toxicity except for dose-related uterus hypoplasia (Lindamood *et al.*, 1988).

(iii) *Effects on reproduction and prenatal toxicity*

Reproductive toxicity. Feeding theophylline to immature (five to six weeks old) Osborne-Mendel rats at 0.5% in the diet [approximately 300 mg/kg bw per day] for 75 weeks produced severe testicular atrophy in 50% of animals, oligo-spermatogenesis and aspermatogenesis. These results were confirmed in Holtzman rats fed 0.5% theophylline for 19 weeks: 86% showed testicular atrophy (Friedman *et al.*, 1979).

In 13-week toxicity studies, weanling $B6C3F_1$ mice and Fischer 344 rats were administered theophylline by gavage or in the diet. Gavage with 300 mg/kg bw per day led to a slight but significant decrease in testicular weight in mice, but 150 mg/kg bw or less had no effect. In rats, a significant decrease in testicular weight was observed after gavage with 150 mg/kg bw per day but not with 75 mg/kg bw or less. No effect on sperm motility, sperm density or the number of abnormal sperm was observed in male rats or mice, and no effect was seen on the mean length of the oestrous cycle in females. Daily administration of 184-793 mg/kg bw theophylline in the diet to mice had no effect on sperm, whereas abnormal sperm were seen in rats given 258 mg/kg in the diet but not at lower doses (Morrissey et al., 1988).

In a reproductive study, Swiss CD-1 mice were administered 0.075, 0.15 or 0.30% theophylline in the diet (average daily doses, 125, 265 or 530 mg/kg bw) for one week before mating and during 13 weeks of cohabitation. Litters were removed one day after birth, except for the last litter which was raised to 21 days of age. Among all treated groups, there was a dose-related decrease in the number of live pups per litter; in the high-dose groups, there was a significant decrease in the number of litters per breeding pair and a significant decrease in live pup weight. In the high- and mid-dose groups, a significant decrease in the percentage of pups born alive was observed. Only mild toxicity was observed in adults at these doses. In a cross-over mating trial at the end of a 19-week exposure to 0.3% theophylline, animals of each sex were found to be affected, although females were more severely affected than males. The decrease in reproductive capacity was considered by the authors to be related partially to embryotoxicity (Morrissey et al., 1988).

Developmental toxicity. IRC-JCL mice received a single intraperitoneal injection of 175, 200 or 225 mg/kg bw theophylline on day 12 of gestation. Subsequently, 40% of dams in the high-dose group died, and dyspnoea and convulsions were observed in those in the low- and mid-dose groups. Fetal body weight was decreased with the high and medium doses, and the incidence of resorptions was significantly increased with the high dose. Malformations were observed in all treated groups; these included cleft palate, digital defects and macrognathia. Subcutaneous haematomas were also seen (Fujii & Nishimura, 1969).

ICR mice received an intraperitoneal injection of 100, 150 or 200 mg/kg bw theophylline on one of gestation days 10-13. A dose-related increase in the incidence of resorptions and malformations — mostly cleft palate — was observed, with a peak embryotoxic response in fetuses treated on day 11 (Tucci & Skalko, 1978).

Sprague-Dawley rats were fed theophylline in the diet (average daily dose, 124, 218 or 259 mg/kg bw) on days 6-15 of gestation. In parallel, Swiss CD-1 mice received theophylline in the drinking-water (daily doses, 282, 372 or 396 mg/kg bw) on the same gestation days. Slight maternal toxicity (decreased weight gain) was observed in high-dose rats and in mid- and high-dose mice. In rats, fetal body weight was significantly decreased with the medium and high doses, and live litter size was decreased with the high dose; no malformation was observed. In mice, fetal body weight was significantly decreased in the mid- and high-dose groups, and the incidence of resorptions was increased in the mid-dose group (Lindström et al., 1990).

(iv) *Genetic and related effects*

The genetic effects of theophylline have been reviewed (Timson, 1975). Additional information on theophylline is included in reviews by Timson (1977) and Tarka (1982).

The results described below are listed in Table 1 on p. 403, with the evaluation of the Working Group, as positive, negative or inconclusive, as defined in the footnotes. The results are tabulated separately for the presence and absence of an exogenous metabolic sytem. The lowest effective dose (LED), in the case of positive results, or the highest ineffective dose (HID), in the case of negative results, are shown, together with the appropriate reference. The studies are summarized briefly below.

As reported in an abstract, theophylline at 3.2 mM displaced 50% of intercalated acridine orange from DNA *in vitro* (Richardson *et al.*, 1981). In extracts of *Escherichia coli*, theophylline selectively inhibited some purine nucleoside phosphorylases (Koch & Lamont, 1956). In *E. coli*, which may not demethylate the drug, theophylline was not incorporated to 'any great extent' into DNA (Koch, 1956) and, unlike other inhibitors of DNA synthesis, had little or no effect on λ prophage induction (Noack & Klaus, 1972). The effects of theophylline on relevant targets other than DNA are discussed in the monograph on caffeine (p. 332).

Theophylline gave negative results in the *Bacillus subtilis rec* assay [details not given]. It was mutagenic to *E. coli* chemostat cultures (Novick & Szilard, 1951; Novick, 1956), and this activity could be inhibited by guanosine (Novick & Szilard, 1952). It was also mutagenic to *E. coli* and in the *B. subtilis* multigene sporulation test, but not to *Salmonella typhimurium*.

In *Saccharomyces cerevisiae*, theophylline promoted sporulation in glucose-containing medium, where it increased the intracellular cAMP level. It had no effect on DNA, RNA or protein synthesis or in medium in which glucose was replaced by potassium acetate (Tsuboi & Yanagishima, 1975).

Theophylline induced mutation in *Ophiostoma multiannulatum* and *Euglena gracilis*. It induced chromosomal fragment formation and translocations in *Allium cepa* root tips, but no chromosomal aberration in *Vicia faba* root tips.

Theophylline was reported in an abstract to induce aneuploidy in *Drosophila melanogaster* (Mittler & Mittler, 1968).

Doses of theophylline greater than 0.3 mg/ml inhibited DNA synthesis in mouse L5178Y lymphoma cells, LS929 mouse fibroblasts and V79 Chinese hamster cells. Theophylline slightly reduced the size of newly synthesized DNA in both unirradiated and ultraviolet-irradiated cells and reversibly inhibited the DNA gap-filling process in ultraviolet-damaged cells (Lehmann, 1973, abstract; Lehmann & Kirk-Bell, 1974). Theophylline also inhibited DNA synthesis in human fibroblastoid EUE cells, and the shape of the dose-response curves and the absence of theophylline-induced DNA strand breaks indicated that theophylline does not directly damage the DNA but acts as a metabolic inhibitor (Slamenová et al., 1986). The results of a study with synchronized HeLa S3 cells exposed to theophylline indicate that the block in DNA replication results from inhibition of histone 1 phosphorylation, which prevents the normal release of chromatin structure between G_1 and S phases (Dolby et al., 1981).

The incidence of 6-thioguanine-resistant mutants in V79 cells was not increased by theophylline.

In the pseudodiploid Chinese hamster cell line, Don-6, theophylline induced a dose-related increase in sister chromatid exchange but did not induce micronuclei. It induced sister chromatid exchange in hamster lung fibroblasts *in vitro* [details not given]. The induction of sister chromatid exchange is not necessarily due to a directly damaging effect upon DNA, since theophylline can inhibit poly-(ADP-ribose)polymerase (Levi et al., 1978). This activity is associated with the induction of sister chromatid exchange (Morgan & Cleaver, 1982) and may even give rise to false-positive effects, the primary effect upon DNA being due to bromodeoxyuridine (Natarajan et al., 1981).

Theophylline induced sister chromatid exchange in human cells *in vitro*. Studies on the induction of chromosomal aberrations in human and mammalian cells is equivocal. The apparent lack of mutagenic activity of theophylline may be due to the antimitotic threshold being the same as the mutagenic threshold, so that any mutant cells produced are unable to reproduce (Timson, 1972).

Butcher and Sutherland (1962) reported that theophylline is the most potent naturally occurring phosphodiesterase inhibitor. Inhibition of cyclic $3',5'$-nucleotide phosphodiesterase from beef heart by theophylline is apparently competitive, with a K_i in the order of 0.1 mM. Since theophylline in combination with increasing concentrations of cAMP (up to 500 µg/ml) had no clastogenic effect, Weinstein et al. (1973) argued that inhibition of phosphodiesterase is not involved in clastogenicity in human lymphocytes in culture.

In Chinese hamster ovary CHO-R1 cells, theophylline reduced the expression of parameters associated with transformation, causing an increase in surface fibronectin, cell-substratum adhesive strength and anchorage dependence for growth and a reduction in cell population saturation density (Rajaraman & Faulkner, 1984).

Theophylline inhibited mitosis of mouse ear epidermal cells in the G_2 phase (Marks & Rebien, 1972). In the host-mediated assay with *S. typhimurium* (G46, nonsense mutation) in Swiss albino mice, theophylline gave negative results. It

Table 1. Genetic and related effects of theophylline

Test system	Results		Dose LED/HID	Reference
	Without exogenous metabolic activation	With exogenous metabolic activation		
BSD, Bacillus subtilis rec assay (spore)	–		0.0000	Kawachi et al. (1980)
SA0, Salmonella typhimurium TA100, reverse mutation	–	–	0.0000	Kawachi et al. (1980)
SA0, Salmonella typhimurium TA100, reverse mutation	–	–	0.0000	Ishidate et al. (1981)
SA0, Salmonella typhimurium TA100, reverse mutation	–	–	500.0000	Slameňová et al. (1986)
SA7, Salmonella typhimurium TA1537, reverse mutation	–	–	0.0000	Ishidate et al. (1981)
SA9, Salmonella typhimurium TA98, reverse mutation	–	–	0.0000	Kawachi et al. (1980)
SA9, Salmonella typhimurium TA98, reverse mutation	–	–	0.0000	Ishidate et al. (1981)
SA9, Salmonella typhimurium TA98, reverse mutation	–	–	500.0000	Slamenova et al. (1986)
ECR, Escherichia coli, phage T5-resistance	+		150.0000	Novick & Szilard (1951)
ECR, Escherichia coli Methionine auxotrophy to protrophy	+		500.0000	Greer (1958)
BSM, Bacillus subtilis, multigene sporulation test	+	0	7500.0000	Sacks & Mihara (1983)
???, Ophiostoma multiannulatum, ascomycete, auxotrophic mutations	+	0	0.0000	Fries & Kihlman (1948)
???, Euglena gracilis, auxotrophic mutations	+	0	0.0000	Come & Travis (1969)
???, Euglena gracilis, auxotrophic mutations	+	0	0.0000	Schiff et al. (1971)
ACC, Allium cepa, chromosomal aberrations	+	0	200.0000	Kihlman & Levan (1949)
VFC, Vicia faba, chromosomal aberrations	+	0	3600.0000	Kihlman & Sturelid (1975)
VFC, Vicia faba, chromosomal aberrations	–	0	900.0000	Kihlman & Sturelid (1975)
???, Silkworm, mutation	–	0	0.0000	Kawachi et al. (1980)
G9H, Gene mutation, Chinese hamster lung V79 cells, 6-thioguanine	–	0	9.0000	Slameňová et al. (1986)
SIA, Sister chromatid exchange, hamster lung fibroblasts	+	0	0.0000	Kawachi et al. (1980)
SIC, Sister chromatid exchange, Chinese hamster Don-6 cells	+	0	180.0000	Sasaki et al. (1980)
MIA, Micronucleus test, Chinese hamster Don-6 cells	+	0	900.0000	Sasaki et al. (1980)
CIA, Chromosomal aberrations, hamster lung fibroblasts	+	0	0.0000	Kawachi et al. (1980)
CIC, Chromosomal aberrations, Chinese hamster lung fibroblasts (CHL)	+	0	0.0000	Ishidate et al. (1981)
CIC, Chromosomal aberrations, Chinese hamster lung fibroblasts (CHL)	+	0	500.0000	Ishidate (1988)
CIC, Chromosomal aberrations, Chinese hamster lung fibroblasts (CHL)	–		2000.0000	Ishidate (1988)
SHF, Sister chromatid exchange, human embryo fibroblasts	+	0	0.0000	Kawachi et al. (1980)
SHF, Sister chromatid exchange, human diploid fibroblasts (HE2144)	+	0	180.0000	Sasaki et al. (1980)
MIH, Micronucleus test, human diploid fibroblasts (HE2144)	–	0	360.0000	Sasaki et al. (1980)
CHL, Chromosomal aberrations, human lymphocytes	+	0	500.0000	Weinstein et al. (1975)
CHL, Chromosomal aberrations, human lymphocytes	+	0	1800.0000	Timson (1972)
CHT, Chromosomal aberrations (chromatid breaks), HeLa cells	+	0	13000.0000	Ostertag (1966)
HMM, Host-mediated assay, Salmonella typhimurium in Swiss mice	–	0	150.0000 i.p.	Gabridge & Legator (1969)
SVA, Sister chromatid exchanges, Chinese hamster bone-marrow	+	0	0.0000 oral	Renner (1982)
CBA, Chromosomal aberrations, rat bone-marrow	–	0	0.0000 i.p.	Kawachi et al. (1980)
DLM, Dominant lethal test, male Swiss CD-1 mice	–	0	380.0000 i.p.	Epstein & Shafer (1968)

i.p., intraperitoneal; oral, by gavage

induced sister chromatid exchange in Chinese hamsters, but did not cause chromosomal aberrations in rat bone marrow *in vivo* (Renner, 1982). Theophylline did not induce dominant lethal mutations in male Swiss CD-1 mice.

(b) *Humans*

(i) *Absorption, distribution, metabolism and excretion*

The metabolism and pharmacokinetics of theophylline in humans have been reviewed (Haley, 1983b; Mungall, 1983; Arnaud, 1984; Stavric, 1988).

Theophylline is readily absorbed after an oral dose. The absorbed fraction of a dose of 7.5 mg/kg bw averaged 99% (Hendeles *et al.*, 1977); however, the absorption of oral theophylline can be delayed by food (Welling *et al.*, 1975; Heimann *et al.*, 1982). Ageing had no effect on the rate or extent of absorption (Cusack *et al.*, 1980; Shin *et al.*, 1988). Peak serum levels are generally achieved within 1.5-2 h (Hendeles *et al.*, 1977; Ogilvie, 1978).

At 17 µg/ml, 56% of theophylline was bound reversibly to adult plasma proteins compared to ~36% in cord plasma proteins from full-term infants (Aranda *et al.*, 1976; Ogilvie, 1978). Protein binding was also reduced to 11-13% during the last two trimesters of pregnancy (Frederiksen *et al.*, 1986). Theophylline is not accumulated in specific target organs: it was distributed in erythrocytes (Ogilvie, 1978), saliva (Culig *et al.*, 1982) and breast milk (milk:serum concentration ratio, 0.70; Yurchak & Jusko, 1976), but not extensively in adipose tissue (Rohrbaugh *et al.*, 1982). Theophylline also passed into the amniotic fluid (Sommer *et al.*, 1975; Arwood *et al.*, 1979; Labovitz & Spector, 1982). The presence of a blood-brain barrier reduces theophylline concentrations in the brain, and a cerebrospinal fluid:plasma ratio of 0.68 was reported (Kadlec *et al.*, 1978).

The elimination half-time of theophylline was 15-60 h in premature infants for at least the first two to four weeks postpartum compared to 3.4 h in children aged one to four years (Aranda *et al.*, 1976), while the corresponding values for adults exhibited large variations, between 3 and 11 h (Jenne *et al.*, 1972; Hunt *et al.*, 1976; Chrzanowski *et al.*, 1977). Theophylline clearance increased by 10% per year over the age range 1-15 years (Driscoll *et al.*, 1989). In subjects over 60 years, half-times of 5.4-9.0 h were reported (Nielsen-Kudsk *et al.*, 1978; Fox *et al.*, 1983).

The half-times were decreased from 7 h in nonsmokers to 4 h in smokers, possibly due to induction of theophylline metabolizing enzymes (Jenne *et al.*, 1975; Hunt *et al.*, 1976). Use of oral contraceptives lowered total plasma clearance and prolonged the half-time of theophylline (9-10 h *versus* 6-7 h), with no change in plasma binding or volume of distribution (Tornatore *et al.*, 1982; Roberts *et al.*, 1983). Cirrhotic patients and patients with acute pulmonary oedema have a prolonged half-time of theophylline (between 23 and 26 h) and decreased plasma clearance (Piafsky *et al.*, 1977a,b; Staib *et al.*, 1980). Plasma binding is also reduced in cirrhotic patients (37% *versus* 53% in normal subjects) (Piafsky *et al.*, 1977a). The half-time of theophylline was prolonged significantly during exercise (Schlaeffer *et al.*, 1984).

The apparent volumes of distribution of theophylline ranged from 0.44 to 0.51 l/kg bw in adults and children (Ogilvie, 1978), but a value of 0.69 was found in premature newborns (Aranda *et al.*, 1976). The distribution volume and elimination half-time of theophylline were increased in the third trimester of pregnancy (Frederiksen *et al.*, 1986).

Disproportionate increases and decreases in serum theophylline concentrations with changes in oral dosage in adults suggest that the rate of elimination is dose-dependent (Jenne *et al.*, 1972; Ogilvie, 1978; Tang-Liu *et al.*, 1982a). Several studies showed that linear pharmacokinetics is a valid model within the therapeutic range (Mungall *et al.*, 1982; Rovei *et al.*, 1982; Brown *et al.*, 1983). Dose-dependent pharmacokinetics seem to be more frequent in children and in some individual adult patients and are generally seen with plasma theophylline concentrations greater than 15 µg/ml (Weinberger & Ginchansky, 1977). Nonlinearity may be due to metabolic saturation or to the diuretic effect of theophylline (Lesko, 1979, 1986; Tang-Liu *et al.*, 1982b). There is also an age-dependent variation in the elimination of theophylline (Jusko *et al.*, 1979).

Experiments with human liver microsomes showed the involvement of at least two cytochrome P450 isozymes in the metabolism of theophylline (Robson *et al.*, 1988). The pathways were presented in Figure 1.

Only 7-12% of theophylline is excreted unchanged in the urine, while several parallel pathways produced 9-18% 3-methylxanthine, 0.3-4% 1-methylxanthine, traces of 3-methyluric acid, 13-26% 1-methyluric acid and the main metabolite, 1,3-dimethyluric acid, at 35-55% (Arnaud, 1984; Birkett *et al.*, 1985). Allopurinol, a xanthine oxidase inhibitor, increased 1-methylxanthine excretion and decreased 1-methyluric acid excretion, demonstrating that the conversion is mediated by xanthine oxidase (Grygiel *et al.*, 1979). Methylation of theophylline into caffeine is the predominant metabolic pathway in neonates because the other enzymatic systems are immature (Bory *et al.*, 1979). Methylation occurs to some extent in adults, but caffeine does not accumulate because it is metabolized further (Tang-Liu & Riegelman, 1981). Patients with decompensated liver cirrhosis have different patterns of urinary metabolites of theophylline than healthy subjects (Staib *et al.*, 1980).

Dietary factors have been shown to modify the elimination of theophylline in children (Feldman *et al.*, 1980) and adults (Anderson *et al.*, 1979). A high protein diet and diets containing charcoal-broiled beef resulted in accelerated elimination of theophylline (Kappas *et al.*, 1978; Feldman *et al.*, 1980). Serum theophylline levels follow a circadian rhythm (for review, see Smolensky & McGovern, 1985), but these effects are less pronounced than interindividual variations (Straughn et al., 1984).

Studies of twins demonstrated that the large interindividual variations in theophylline elimination observed in human subjects are predominantly under genetic control (Miller et al., 1985).

(ii) *Toxic effects*

The toxicology of theophylline has been reviewed (Ellis, 1983; Haley, 1983a,b; Bukowskyj et al., 1984; Stavric, 1988).

Toxicity can be produced easily owing to its narrow therapeutic index (Labovitz & Spector, 1982; Greenberg et al., 1984; Singer & Kolischenko, 1985). A small percentage of patients taking theophylline therapeutically to control asthma may develop toxicity at serum levels of 20-30 µg/ml. These effects are generally not seen at levels below 15 µg/ml (Stavric, 1988).

Administration of theophylline to premature babies in the preterm period caused sleep disturbances that persisted after the drug had been cleared from the body (Thoman et al., 1985). In a study on long-term effects of theophylline administration in the preterm period, no difference was found at one or two years of age as a function of drug treatment (Nelson et al., 1980). The question of whether theophylline affects learning ability in children remains open (Stavric, 1988).

'Mild' toxicity may include headache, gastrointestinal disturbances, hypotension, irritability and insomnia. Symptoms of 'severe toxicity' include tachycardia, arrhythmia, cardiac arrest and serious neurological symptoms. Seizures and death have occurred (Helliwell & Berry, 1979; Winek et al., 1980; Woo et al., 1980; Woodcock et al., 1983; Greenberg et al., 1984; Singer & Kolischenko, 1985; Stavric, 1988).

Studies of a possible association between consumption of methylxanthines and benign breast disease are discussed on pp. 347-350.

(iii) *Effects on reproduction and prenatal toxicity*

No association was seen between use of bronchodilators (theophylline being one of 11 preparations used) and congenital abnormalities in the offspring (Nelson & Forfar, 1971). This finding was corroborated by a study of 117 women who had used the drug (Heinonen, 1982).

(iv) *Genetic and related effects*

Lymphocytes from a mother given continuous treatment for asthma with theophylline-containing drugs and from her stillborn triploid child both showed increased frequencies of chromatid breaks (14 and 16%, respectively; Halbrecht et al., 1973). Timson (1975) suggested that theophylline may have been involved in the induction of the chromatid breaks. [The Working Group noted that the medication also contained ephedrine, phenobarbital and diphenylhydramine.]

The apparent lack of mutagenic activity of theophylline and other methylxanthines in man may be due to the fact that the antimitotic threshold is the same as the mutagenic threshold, so that any mutant cells produced are unable to reproduce; the net effect is therefore nonmutagenicity (Timson, 1972).

3.3 Epidemiological studies of carcinogenicity to humans

Studies on methylxanthines are summarized in the monograph on caffeine.

4. Summary of Data Reported and Evaluation

4.1 Exposure data

Theophylline is found in black tea and to a lesser extent in green coffee, cocoa cotyledon and dried mate. Theophylline is synthesized on an industrial scale and is used principally in pharmaceutical preparations.

Per-caput daily intake of theophylline from black tea in the USA has been estimated to be 0.14 mg.

4.2 Experimental carcinogenicity data

No data on the carcinogenicity of theophylline were available.

In the one adequate study, theophylline applied to the skin of female mice induced a significantly smaller number of ultraviolet light-induced tumours than in controls.

4.3 Human carcinogenicity data

No data were available to the Working Group to evaluate the carcinogenicity of theophylline *per se*.

For descriptions of studies on methylxanthines, see the monograph on caffeine.

4.4 Other relevant data

Limited data on mothers taking theophylline during pregnancy showed no excess in the frequency of malformations in their offspring.

Theophylline given by gavage at high doses decreased testicular weight in rats and mice, but there was no change in semen characteristics. Administration of theophylline in the diet at dose levels that were mildly toxic to adults caused decreased numbers of litters per breeding pair, decreased live litter size, an increased number of resorptions and decreased neonatal weight. Abnormal sperm were observed in rats but not in mice at high dose levels.

Theophylline induced sister chromatid exchange in Chinese hamsters *in vivo* but did not induce dominant lethal mutations in mice or chromosomal aberrations in the bone marrow of rats. Theophylline gave negative results in a host-mediated assay with *Salmonella typhimurium* in mice. In cultured human cells, theophylline induced sister chromatid exchange and chromosomal breaks but not micronuclei or chromosomal aberrations. It induced sister chromatid exchange and chromosomal aberrations but not micronuclei or gene mutation in animal cells *in vitro*. Results on the induction of chromosomal aberrations in plants are equivocal. In lower eukaryotes, it induced gene mutations. Theophylline gave negative results in the *Salmonella*/mammalian microsome assay but induced mutation in other bacteria.

4.5 Evaluation[1]

There is *inadequate evidence* for the carcinogenicity in humans of theophylline.

There is *inadequate evidence* for the carcinogenicity in experimental animals of theophylline.

Overall evaluation

Theophylline is *not classifiable as to its carcinogenicity to humans (Group 3)*.

5. References

Adams, R.F., Vandemark, F.L. & Schmidt, G.J. (1976) More sensitive high-pressure liquid-chromatographic determination of theophylline in serum. *Clin. Chem.*, 22, 1903-1906

Allain, P., Turcant, A. & Prémel-Cabic, A. (1989) Automated fluoroimmunoassay of theophylline and valproic acid by flow-injection analysis with use of HPLC instruments. *Clin. Chem.*, 35, 469-470

---

[1]For description of the italicized terms, see Preamble, pp. 27-31.

Anderson, K.E., Conney, A.H. & Kappas, A. (1979) Nutrition and oxidative drug metabolism in man: relative influence of dietary lipids, carbohydrate, and protein. *Clin. pharmacol. Ther.*, *26*, 493-501

Anon. (1986) *Scrip World Pharmaceutical News*, *1158*, 15

Anon. (1988) *British Pharmacopoeia*, Vol. 1, London, Her Majesty's Stationery Office, pp. 564-565

Aranda, J.V., Sitar, D.S., Parsons, W.D., Loughnan, P.M. & Neims, A.H. (1976) Pharmacokinetic aspects of theophylline in premature newborns. *New Engl. J. Med.*, *295*, 413-416

Arimori, K. & Nakano, M. (1985) Transport of theophylline from blood to the intestinal lumen following i.v. administration to rats. *J. Pharmacobio-Dyn.*, *8*, 324-327

Arnaud, M.J. (1984) Products of metabolism of caffeine. In: Dews, P.B., ed., *Caffeine. Perspectives from Recent Research*, Berlin, Springer, pp. 3-38

Arnaud, M.J., Bracco, I. & Welsch, C. (1982) Metabolism and distribution of labeled theophylline in the pregnant rat. Impairment of theophylline metabolism by pregnancy and absence of a blood-brain barrier in the fetus. *Pediatr. Res.*, *16*, 167-171

Arwood, L.L., Dasta, J.F. & Friedman, C. (1979) Placental transfer of theophylline: two case reports. *Pediatrics*, *63*, 844-846

Barnhart, E.R., ed. (1989) *Physicians' Desk Reference*, 43rd ed., Oradell, NJ, Medical Economics, pp. 404, 408, 412, 415, 423, 426, 428, 600, 944, 991, 1872, 2214, 2240

Barnhart, J.L. & Combes, B. (1974) Effect of theophylline on hepatic excretory function. *Am. J. Physiol.*, *227*, 194-199

Betlach, C.J. & Tozer, T.N. (1980) Biodisposition of theophylline. I. Genetic variation in inbred mice. *Drug Metab. Disposition*, *8*, 268-270

Birkett, D.J., Dahlqvist, R., Miners, J.O., Lelo, A. & Billing, B. (1985) Comparison of theophylline and theobromine metabolism in man. *Drug Metab. Disposition*, *13*, 725-728

Bory, C., Baltassat, P., Porthault, M., Bethenod, M., Frederich, A. & Aranda, J.V. (1979) Metabolism of theophylline to caffeine in premature newborn infants. *J. Pediatr.*, *94*, 988-993

Brandstetter, Y., Kaplanski, J., van Creveld, C. & Ben-Zvi, Z. (1986) Theophylline pharmacokinetics in pregnant and lactating rats. *Res. Commun. chem. Pathol. Pharmacol.*, *53*, 269-272

Brashear, R.E., Nelson, R.L., Glick, M.R., Oei, T.O. & DeAtley, R.E. (1980) The role of the liver in theophylline elimination. *Lung*, *158*, 101-109

Brashear, R.E., Veng-Pedersen, P., Rhodes, M.L. & Smith, C.N. (1982) Theophylline elimination in the pregnant and fetal rabbit. *J. Lab. clin. Med.*, *100*, 15-25

Broussard, L.A., Stearns, F.M., Tulley, R. & Frings, C.S. (1981) Theophylline determination by high-pressure liquid chromatography. *Clin. Chem.*, *27*, 1931-1933

Brown, P.J., Dusci, L.J. & Shenfield, G.M. (1983) Lack of dose dependent kinetics of theophylline. *Eur. J. clin. Pharmacol.*, *24*, 525-527

Bukowskyj, M., Nakatsu, K. & Munt, P.W. (1984) Theophylline reassessed. *Ann. intern. Med.*, *101*, 63-73

Butcher, R.W. & Sutherland, E.W. (1962) Adenosine 3',5'-phosphate in biological materials. I. Purification and properties of cyclic 3',5'-nucleotide phosphodiesterase and use of this enzyme to characterize adenosine 3',5'-phosphate in human urine. *J. biol. Chem.*, 237, 1244-1250

Chan, K.-M., Koenig, J., Walton, K.G., Francoeur, T.A., Lau, B.W.C. & Ladenson, J.H. (1987) The theophylline method of the Abbott 'vision' analyzer evaluated. *Clin. Chem.*, 33, 130-132

Chang, J., Gadsden, R.H., Bradley, C.A. & Stewart, T.C. (1982) Homogeneous enzyme immunoassay for theophylline in serum and plasma. *Clin. Chem.*, 28, 361-367

Christensen, H.D. & Neims, A.H. (1984) Measurement of caffeine and its metabolites in biological fluids. In: Dews, P.B., ed., *Caffeine. Perspectives from Recent Research*, Berlin, Springer, pp. 39-47

Christensen, H.D. & Neims, A.H. (1985) Antiasthmatics. *Chromatogr. Sci.*, 32, 237-267

Chrzanowski, F.A., Niebergall, P.J., Nikelly, J.G., Sugita, E.T. & Schnaare, R.L. (1974) Gas chromatographic analysis of theophylline in human serum. *Biochem. Med.*, 11, 26-31

Chrzanowski, F.A., Niebergall, P.J., Mayock, R.L., Taubin, J.M. & Sugita, E.T. (1977) Kinetics of intravenous theophylline. *Clin. pharmacol. Ther.*, 22, 188-195

Cohen, J.L. (1975) Theophylline. In: Florey, K., ed., *Analytical Profiles of Drug Substances*, Vol. 4, New York, Academic Press, pp. 466-493

Collins, J.J. (1987) *Theophylline — Review of Toxicity and Testing Recommendations — Protocol Outline for the NTP Chronic Toxicity/Carcinogenicity Testing*, Research Triangle Park, NC, National Toxicology Program

Come, T.V. & Travis, D.M. (1969) Induction of auxotrophic mutations in *Euglena gracilis*. *J. Hered.*, 60, 39-41

Commission of the European Communities (1976) *European Cooperation and Coordination in the Field of Scientific and Technical Research. Eurocop-Cost Project 64B. A Comprehensive List of Polluting Substances which Have Been Identified in Various Fresh Waters, Effluent Discharges, Aquatic Animals and Plants, and Bottom Sediments*, 2nd ed., Luxembourg

Consumers Union (1990) *US Pharmacopeia's Drug Information for the Consumer*, Easton, PA, Mack Publishing, pp. 1341-1352

Culig, J., Johnston, A. & Turner, P. (1982) Saliva theophylline concentrations after a single oral dose. *Br. J. clin. Pharmacol.*, 13, 243-245

Cusack, B., Kelly, J.G., Lavan, J., Noel, J. & O'Malley, K. (1980) Theophylline kinetics in relation to age: the importance of smoking. *Br. J. clin. Pharmacol.*, 10, 109-114

Dolby, T.W., Belmont, A., Borun, T.W. & Nicolini, C. (1981) DNA replication, chromatin structure, and histone phosphorylation altered by theophylline in synchronized HeLa S3 cells. *J. cell. Biol.*, 89, 78-85

Driscoll, M.S., Ludden, T.M., Casto, D.T. & Littlefield, L.C. (1989) Evaluation of theophylline pharmacokinetics in a pediatric population using mixed effects models. *J. Pharmacokin. Biopharm.*, 17, 141-168

Ellis, E.F. (1983) Theophylline. *Clin. Rev. Allergy*, 1, 73-85

El-Yazigi, A. & Sawchuk, R.J. (1981) Theophylline absorption and disposition in rabbits: oral, intravenous and concentration-dependent kinetic studies. *J. pharm. Sci.*, 70, 452-456

Eppel, M.L., Oliver, J.S., Smith, H., Mackay, A. & Samsay, L.E. (1978) Determination of theophylline in plasma: comparison of high-performance liquid chromatography and an enzyme multiplied immunoassay technique. *Analyst*, 103, 1061-1065

Epstein, S.S. & Shafner, H. (1968) Chemical mutagens in the human environment. *Nature*, 219, 385-387

Epstein, S.S., Arnold, E., Andrea, J., Bass, W. & Bishop, Y. (1972) Detection of chemical mutagens by the dominant lethal assay in the mouse. *Toxicol. appl. Pharmacol.*, 23, 288-325

Feldman, C.H., Hutchinson, V.E., Pippenger, C.E., Blumenfeld, T.A., Feldman, B.R. & Davis, W.J. (1980) Effect of dietary protein and carbohydrate on theophylline metabolism in children. *Pediatrics*, 66, 956-962

Fox, R.W., Samaan, S., Bukantz, S.C. & Lockey, R.F. (1983) Theophylline kinetics in a geriatric group. *Clin. pharmacol. Ther.*, 34, 60-67

Frederiksen, M.C., Ruo, T.I., Chow, M.J. & Atkinson, A.J. (1986) Theophylline pharmacokinetics in pregnancy. *Clin. pharmacol. Ther.*, 40, 321-328

Friedman, L., Weinberger, M.A., Farber, T.M., Moreland, F.M., Peters, E.L., Gilmore, C.E. & Khan, M.A. (1979) Testicular atrophy and impaired spermatogenesis in rats fed high levels of the methylxanthines caffeine, theobromine, or theophylline. *J. environ. Pathol. Toxicol.*, 2, 687-706

Fries, N. & Kihlman, B. (1948) Fungal mutations obtained with methyl xanthines. *Nature*, 162, 573-574

Fujii, T. & Nishimura, H. (1969) Teratogenic actions of some methylated xanthines in mice. *Okajimas Folia anat. jpn.*, 46, 167-175

Gabridge, M.G. & Legator, M.S. (1969) A host-mediated microbial assay for the detection of mutagenic compounds. *Proc. Soc. exp. Biol. Med.*, 130, 831-834

Gabrielsson, J.L., Paalzow, L.K. & Nordström, L. (1984) A physiologically based pharmacokinetic model for theophylline disposition in the pregnant and nonpregnant rat. *J. Pharmacokinet. Biopharmacol.*, 12, 149-165

Gennaro, A.R., ed. (1985) *Remington's Pharmaceutical Sciences*, 17th ed., Easton, PA, Mack Publishing, pp. 873-875

Graham, H.N. (1984a) Tea: the plant and its manufacture; chemistry and consumption of the beverage. In: Spiller, G.A., ed., *The Methylxanthine Beverages and Foods: Chemistry, Consumption and Health Effects*, New York, Alan R. Liss, pp. 29-74

Graham, H.N. (1984b) Mate. In: Spiller, G.A., ed., *The Methylxanthine Beverages and Foods: Chemistry, Consumption and Health Effects*, New York, Alan R. Liss, pp. 179-183

Greenberg, A., Piraino, B.H., Kroboth, P.D. & Weiss, J. (1984) Severe theophylline toxicity. Role of conservative measures, antiarrhythmic agents, and charcoal hemoperfusion. *Am. J. Med.*, 76, 854-860

Greer, S.B. (1958) Growth inhibitors and their antagonists as mutagens and antimutagens in *Escherichia coli*. *J. gen. Microbiol.*, 18, 543-564

Grygiel, J.J., Wing, L.M.H., Farkas, J. & Birkett, D.J. (1979) Effects of allopurinol on theophylline metabolism and clearance. *Clin. Pharmacol. Ther.*, 26, 660-667

Gupta, R.C. & Lundberg, G.D. (1973) Qualitative determination of theophylline in blood by differential spectrophotometry. *Anal. Chem.*, 45, 2403-2405

Gushaw, J.B., Hu, M.W., Singh, P., Miller, J.G. & Schneider, R.S. (1977) Homogeneous enzyme immunoassay for theophylline in serum (Abstract No. 138). *Clin. Chem.*, 23, 1144

Halbrecht, I., Komlos, L., Shabtay, F., Solomon, M. & Böck, J.A. (1973) Triploidy 69, XXX in a stillborn girl. *Clin. Genet.*, 4, 210-212

Haley, T.J. (1983a) Theophylline. *Dangerous Properties ind. Mater. Rep.*, July/August, 8-15

Haley, T.J. (1983b) Metabolism and pharmacokinetics of theophylline in human neonates, children, and adults. *Drug Metab. Rev.*, 14, 295-335

Heimann, G., Murgescu, J. & Bergt, U. (1982) Influence of food intake on bioavailability of theophylline in premature infants. *Eur. J. clin. Pharmacol.*, 22, 171-173

Heinonen, O.P. (1982) *Birth Defects and Drugs in Pregnancy*, Littleton, MA, Publishing Sciences Group

Helliwell, M. & Berry, D. (1979) Theophylline poisoning in adults. *Br. med. J.*, ii, 1114

Hendeles, L., Weinberger, M. & Bighley, L. (1977) Absolute bioavailability of oral theophylline. *Am. J. Hosp. Pharm.*, 34, 525-527

Hirsh, K. (1984) Central nervous system pharmacology of the dietary methylxanthines. In: Spiller, G.A., ed., *The Methylxanthine Beverages and Foods: Chemistry, Consumption and Health Effects*, New York, Alan R. Liss, pp. 235-301

Hunt, S.N., Jusko, W.J. & Yurchak, A.M. (1976) Effect of smoking on theophylline disposition. *Clin. pharmacol. Ther.*, 19, 546-551

Hurst, W.J., Martin, R.A. & Tarka, S.M., Jr (1984) Analytical methods for quantitation of methylxanthines. In: Spiller, G.A., ed., *The Methylxanthine Beverages and Foods: Chemistry, Consumption, and Health Effects*, New York, Alan R. Liss, pp. 17-28

Ishidate, M., Jr (1988) *Data Book of Chromosomal Aberration Tests* In Vitro, rev. ed., Amsterdam, Elsevier, p. 410

Ishidate, M., Jr, Sofuni, T. & Yoshikawa, K. (1981) Chromosomal aberration tests *in vitro* as a primary screening tool for environmental mutagens and/or carcinogens. *Gann Monogr. Cancer Res.*, 27, 95-108

Jalal, M.A.F. & Collin, H.A. (1976) Estimation of caffeine, theophylline and theobromine in plant material. *New Phytol.*, 76, 277-281

Jenne, J.W., Wyze, E., Rood, F.S. & MacDonald, F.M. (1972) Pharmacokinetics of theophylline. Application to adjustment of the clinical dose of aminophylline. *Clin. Pharmacol. Ther.*, 13, 349-360

Jenne, J., Nagasawa, H., McHugh, R., MacDonald, F. & Wyse, E. (1975) Decreased theophylline half-life in cigarette smokers. *Life Sci.*, 17, 195-198

Johnson, G.T., Dechtiaruk, W.A. & Solomon, H.M. (1975) Gas chromatographic determination of theophylline in human serum and saliva. *Clin. Chem.*, 21, 144-147

Jusko, W.J., Gardner, M.J., Mangione, A., Schentag, J.J., Koup, J.R. & Vance, J.W. (1979) Factors affecting theophylline clearances: age, tobacco, marijuana, cirrhosis, congestive heart failure, obesity, oral contraceptives, benzodiazepines, barbiturates, and ethanol. *J. pharm. Sci.*, 68, 1358-1366

Kadlec, G.J., Jarboe, C.H., Pollard, S.J. & Sublett, J.L. (1978) Acute theophylline intoxication. Biphasic first order elimination kinetics in a child. *Ann. Allergy*, 41, 337-339

Kappas, A., Alvares, A.P., Anderson, K.E., Pantuck, E.J., Pantuck, C.B., Chang, R. & Conney, A.H. (1978) Effect of charcoal-broiled beef on antipyrine and theophylline metabolism. *Clin. Pharmacol. Ther.*, 23, 445-450

Kawachi, T., Yahagi, T., Kada, T., Tazima, Y., Ishidate, M., Sasaki, M. & Sugimura, T. (1980) Cooperative programme on short-term assays for carcinogenicity in Japan. In: Montesano, R., Bartsch, H. & Tomatis, L., eds, *Molecular and Cellular Aspects of Carcinogen Screening Tests* (IARC Scientific Publications No. 27), Lyon, IARC, pp. 323-330

Kester, M.B., Saccar, C.L., Rocci, M.L., Jr & Mansmann, H.C., Jr (1987) A new simplified assay for the quantitation of theophylline and its major metabolites in urine by high-performance liquid chromatography. *J. pharm. Sci.*, 76, 238-241

Kihlman, B.A. & Levan, A. (1949) The cytological effects of caffeine. *Hereditas*, 35, 109-111

Kihlman, B.A. & Sturelid, S. (1975) Enhancement by methylated oxypurines of the frequency of induced chromosomal aberrations. III. The effect in combination with X-rays on root tips of *Vicia faba*. *Hereditas*, 80, 247-254

Kihlman, B.A., Sturelid, S., Hartley-Asp, B. & Nilsson, K. (1974) The enhancement by caffeine of the frequencies of chromosomal aberrations induced in plant and animal cells by chemical and physical agents. *Mutat. Res.*, 26, 105-122

Kirichenko, L.O. & Kagan, F.Y. (1970) Chromatospectrophotometric method for the quantitative estimation of theophylline, dimedrol and ephedrine hydrochloride in drugs. *Farm. Zh. (Kiev)*, 25, 42-47 [*Chem. Abstr.*, 73, 28951s]

Koch, A.L. (1956) The metabolism of methylpurines by *Escherichia coli*. I. Tracer studies. *J. biol. Chem.*, 219, 181-188

Koch, A.L. & Lamont, W.A. (1956) The metabolism of methylpurines by *Escherichia coli*. II. Enzymatic studies. *J. biol. Chem.*, 219, 189-201

Koritz, G.D., Bourne, D.W.A., Hunt, J.P., Prasad, V.I., Bevill, R.F. & Gautam, S.R. (1981) Pharmacokinetics of theophylline in swine: a potential model for human drug bioavailability studies. *J. vet. Pharmacol. Ther.*, 4, 233-239

Labovitz, E. & Spector, S. (1982) Placental theophylline transfer in pregnant asthmatics. *J. Am. med. Assoc.*, 247, 786-788

Lee, S.R. & Liberti, P.A. (1987) Quantitative immunochromatographic analysis: theory and application to theophylline immunoassay. *Anal. Biochem.*, 166, 41-48

Lehmann, A.R. (1973) Effects of caffeine and theophylline on DNA synthesis in untreated and UV-irradiated mammalian cells (Abstract No. 15). *Mutat. Res.*, 21, 192-193

Lehmann, A.R. & Kirk-Bell, S. (1974) Effects of caffeine and theophylline on DNA synthesis in unirradiated and UV-irradiated mammalian cells. *Mutat. Res.*, 26, 73-82

Lesko, L.J. (1979) Dose-dependent elimination kinetics of theophylline. *Clin. Pharmacokinet.*, *4*, 449-459

Lesko, L.J. (1986) Dose-dependent kinetics of theophylline. *J. Allergy clin. Immunol.*, *78*, 723-727

Levi, V., Jacobson, E.L. & Jacobson, M.K. (1978) Inhibition of poly(ADP-ribose)polymerase by methylated xanthines and cytokinins. *FEBS Lett.*, *88*, 144-146

Li, T.M., Benovic, J.L., Buckler, R.T. & Burd, J.F. (1981a) Homogenous substrate-labeled fluorescent immunoassay for theophylline in serum. *Clin. Chem.*, *27*, 22-26

Li, T.M., Benovic, J.L. & Burd, J.F. (1981b) Serum theophylline determination by fluorescence polarization immunoassay utilizing an imbelliferone derivative as a fluorescent label. *Anal. Biochem.*, *118*, 102-107

Lindamood, C., III, Lamb, J.C., IV, Bristol, D.W., Collins, J.J., Heath, J.E. & Prejean, J.D. (1988) Studies on the short-term toxicity of theophylline in rats and mice. *Fundam. appl. Toxicol.*, *10*, 477-489

Lindström, P., Morrissey, R.E., George, J.D., Price, C.J., Marr, M.C., Kimmel, C.A. & Schwetz, B.A. (1990) The developmental toxicity of orally administered theophylline in rats and mice. *Fundam. appl. Toxicol.*, *14*, 167-178

Logan, L., Kling, O.R. & Christensen, H.D. (1983) Xanthine metabolism in pregnant baboons (Abstract No. 5870). *Fed. Proc.*, *42*, 1293

Lohmann, S.M. & Miech, R.P. (1976) Theophylline metabolism by the rat liver microsomal system. *J. Pharmacol. exp. Ther.*, *196*, 213-225

Madsen, S.M. & Ribel, U. (1981a) Pharmacokinetics of theophylline and 3-methylxanthine in guinea pigs. I. Single dose administration. *Acta pharmacol. toxicol.*, *48*, 1-7

Madsen, S.M. & Ribel, U. (1981b) Pharmacokinetics of theophylline and 3-methylxanthine in guinea pigs. II. Multiple dose administration. *Acta pharmacol. toxicol.*, *48*, 8-12

Marks, F. & Rebien, W. (1972) Cyclic 3',5'-AMP and theophylline inhibit epidermal mitosis in G_2-phase. *Naturwissenschaften*, *59*, 41-42

Matsumoto, K., Kikuchi, H., Iri, H., Takahasi, H. & Umino, M. (1988) Automated determination of drugs in serum by column-switching high-performance liquid chromatography. II. Separation of theophylline and its metabolites. *J. Chromatogr.*, *425*, 323-330

May, D.C. & Jarboe, C.H. (1981) Elimination kinetics and protein binding of theophylline in the rabbit. *Life Sci.*, *29*, 473-476

McKiernan, B.C., Neff-Davis, C.A., Koritz, G.D., Davis, L.E. & Pheris, D.R. (1981) Pharmacokinetic studies of theophylline in dogs. *J. vet. Pharmacol. Ther.*, *4*, 103-110

McKiernan, B.C., Koritz, G.D., Davis, L.E., Neff-Davis, C.A. & Pheris, D.R. (1983) Pharmacokinetic studies of theophylline in cats. *J. vet. Pharmacol. Ther.*, *6*, 99-104

McManus, M.E., Miners, J.O., Gregor, D., Stupans, I. & Birkett, D.J. (1988) Theophylline metabolism by human, rabbit and rat liver microsomes and by purified forms of cytochrome P450. *J. pharm. Pharmacol.*, *40*, 388-391

Meatherall, R. & Ford, D. (1988) Isocratic liquid chromatographic determination of theophylline, acetaminophen, chloramphenicol, caffeine, anticonvulsants, and barbiturates in serum. *Ther. Drug Monit.*, *10*, 101-115

Meola, J.M., Brown, H.H. & Swift, T. (1979) Fluorometric measurement of theophylline. *Clin. Chem.*, 25, 1835-1837

Messenger, L.J., Li, T.M., Benovic, J.L. & Burd, J.F. (1980) Stat assay for theophylline concentrations in human serum using a modified substrate labeled fluorescent immunoassay (SLFIA) (Abstract No. 41). *J. Allergy clin. Immunol.*, 65, 175

Miller, C.A., Slusher, L.B. & Vesell, E.S. (1985) Polymorphism of theophylline metabolism in man. *J. clin. Invest.*, 75, 1415-1425

Mitoma, C., Sorich, T.J., II & Neubauer, S.E. (1968) The effect of caffeine on drug metabolism. *Life Sci.*, 7, 145-151

Mittler, S. & Mittler, J.E. (1968) Theobromine and theophylline and chromosome aberrations in *Drosophila melanogaster* (Abstract). *Genetics*, 60, 205

Moberg, U., Hjalmarsson, S.-G. & Mellstrand, T. (1980) New rapid assay of theophylline in plasma by isotachophoresis. *J. Chromatogr.*, 181, 147-152

Moffat, A.C., ed. (1986) *Clarke's Isolation and Identification of Drugs*, 2nd ed., London, The Pharmaceutical Press, pp. 1011-1012

Morgan, W.F. & Cleaver, J.E. (1982) 3-Aminobenzamide synergistically increases sister-chromatid exchanges in cells exposed to methyl methanesulfonate but not to ultraviolet light. *Mutat. Res.*, 104, 361-366

Morrissey, R.E., Collins, J.J., Lamb, J.C., IV, Manus, A.G. & Gulati, D.K. (1988) Reproductive effects of theophylline in mice and rats. *Fundam. appl. Toxicol.*, 10, 525-536

Muir, K.T., Jonkman, J.H.G., Tang, D.-S., Kunitani, M. & Riegelman, S. (1980) Simultaneous determination of theophylline and its major metabolites in urine by reversed-phase ion-pair high performance liquid chromatography. *J. Chromatogr.*, 221, 85-95

Muir, K.T., Kunitani, M. & Riegelman, S. (1982) Improved high-performance liquid chromatographic assay for theophylline in plasma and saliva in the presence of caffeine and its metabolites and comparisons with three other assays. *J. Chromatogr.*, 231, 73-82

Mungall, D. (1983) Theophylline. In: Mungall, D., ed., *Applied Clinical Pharmacokinetics*, New York, Raven Press, 127-152

Mungall, D., Bancroft, W. & Marshall, J. (1982) Computer-assisted oral and intravenous theophylline therapy. *Computers biomed. Res.*, 15, 18-28

Munsiff, I.J., Koritz, G.D., McKiernan, B.C. & Neff-Davis, C.A. (1988a) Plasma protein binding of theophylline in dogs. *J. vet. Pharmacol. Ther.*, 11, 112-114

Munsiff, I.J., McKiernan, B.C., Neff-Davis, C.A. & Koritz, G.D. (1988b) Determination of the acute oral toxicity of theophylline in conscious dogs. *J. vet. Pharmacol. Ther.*, 11, 381-389

Natarajan, A.T., Csukás, I. & van Zeeland, A.A. (1981) Contribution of incorporated 5-bromodeoxyuridine in DNA to the frequencies of sister-chromatid exchanges induced by inhibitors of poly-(ADP-ribose)-polymerase. *Mutat. Res.*, 84, 125-132

National Institute for Occupational Safety and Health (1974) *National Occupational Hazard Survey, 1972-1974*, Cincinnati, OH, p. 150

National Research Council (1977) *Drinking Water and Health*, Washington DC, National Academy of Sciences

Neese, A.L. & Soyka, L.F. (1977) Development of a radioimmunoassay for theophylline. Application to studies in premature infants. *Clin. pharmacol. Ther.*, 21, 633-641

Nelson, M.M. & Forfar, J.O. (1971) Associations between drugs administered during pregnancy and congenital abnormalities of the fetus. *Br. med. J.*, i, 523-527

Nelson, R.M., Resnick, M.B., Holstrum, W.J. & Eitzman, D.V. (1980) Developmental outcome of premature infants treated with theophylline. *Dev. Pharmacol. Ther.*, 1, 274-280

Ng, P.K. & Locok, R.A. (1979) Comparative pharmacokinetics of theophylline and dyphylline following intravenous injection in rabbits. *Res. Commun. chem. Pathol. Pharmacol.*, 26, 509-524

Nielsen-Kudsk, F., Magnussen, I. & Jakobsen, P. (1978) Pharmacokinetics of theophylline in ten elderly patients. *Acta pharmacol. toxicol.*, 42, 226-234

Nishikawa, T., Kubo, H. & Saito, M. (1979) Competitive nephelometric immunoassay of theophylline in plasma. *Clin. chim. Acta*, 91, 59-65

Noack, D. & Klaus, S. (1972) Efect of purine and pyrimidine derivatives on prophage induction in *Escherichia coli* C600 T44 (Ger.). *Z. allg. Mikrobiol.*, 12, 583-591

Nomura, T. (1983) Comparative inhibiting effects of methylxanthines on urethan-induced tumors, malformations, and presumed somatic mutations in mice. *Cancer Res.*, 43, 1342-1346

Novik, A. (1956) Mutagens and antimutagens. *Brookhaven Symp. Biol.*, 8, 201-215

Novick, A. & Szilard, L. (1951) Experiments on spontaneous and chemically induced mutations of bacteria growing in the chemostat. *Cold Spring Harbor Symp. quant. Biol.*, 16, 337-343

Novick, A. & Szilard, L. (1952) Anti-mutagens. *Nature*, 170, 926-927

Ogilvie, R.I. (1978) Clinical pharmacokinetics of theophylline. *Clin. Pharmacokinet.*, 3, 267-293

Orcutt, J.J., Kozak, P.P., Jr, Gillman, S.A. & Cummins, L.H. (1977) Micro-scale method for theophylline in body fluids by reversed-phase, high-pressure liquid chromatography. *Clin. chem.*, 23, 599-601

Ostertag, W. (1966) Caffeine and theophylline mutagenesis in cell and leukocyte cultures in humans (Ger.). *Mutat. Res.*, 3, 249-267

Perry, D.L., Chuang, C.C., Jungclaus, G.A. & Warner, J.S. (1979) *Identification of Organic Compounds in Industrial Effluent Discharges*, Athens, GA, US Environmental Protection Agency, Environmental Research Laboratory

Piafsky, K.M., Sitar, D.S., Rangno, R.E. & Ogilvie, R.I. (1977a) Theophylline disposition in patients with hepatic cirrhosis. *New Engl. J. Med.*, 296, 1495-1597

Piafsky, K.M., Sitar, D.S., Rangno, R.E. & Ogilvie, R.I. (1977b) Theophylline kinetics in acute pulmonary edema. *Clin. pharmacol. Ther.*, 21, 310-316

Rajaraman, R. & Faulkner, G. (1984) Reverse transformation of Chinese hamster ovary cells by methyl xanthines. *Exp. Cell Res.*, 154, 342-356

Ramzan, I. & DeDonato, V. (1988) Theophylline neurotoxicity in pregnant rats. *Life Sci.*, 42, 491-495

Renner, H.W. (1982) Sister chromatid exchanges induced by methylxanthines contained in coffee, tea and cocoa. *Experientia*, 38, 600

Richardson, C.L., Grant, A.D. & Schulman, G.E. (1981) The interaction of caffeine and other xanthine analogs with DNA as measured by competitive fluorescence polarization (Abstract No. AC-5). *Environ. Mutagenesis*, 3, 343

Ritchie, J.M. (1975) The xanthines. In: Goodman, L.S. & Gilman, A., eds, *The Pharmacological Basis of Therapeutics*, 5th ed., New York, MacMillan, pp. 367-378

Roberts, R.K., Grice, J., McGuffie, C. & Heilbronn, L. (1983) Oral contraceptive steroids impair the elimination of theophylline. *J. Lab. clin. Med.*, 101, 821-825

Robson, R.A., Miners, J.O., Matthews, A.P., Stupans, I., Meller, D., McManus, M.E. & Birkett, D.J. (1988) Characterisation of theophylline metabolism by human liver microsomes. Inhibition and immunochemical studies. *Biochem. Pharmacol.*, 37, 1651-1659

Rohrbaugh, T.M., Danish, M., Ragni, M.C. & Yaffe, S.J. (1982) The effect of obesity on apparent volume of distribution of theophylline. *Pediatr. Pharmacol.*, 2, 75-83

Rovei, V., Chanoine, F. & Strolin Benedetti, M. (1982) Pharmacokinetics of theophylline: a dose-range study. *Br. J. clin. Pharmacol.*, 14, 769-778

Sacks, L.E. & Mihara, K. (1983) Induction at high frequency of a unique phenotypic class of *Bacillus subtilis* mutants by methylxanthines. *Mutat. Res.*, 117, 55-65

Sasaki, M., Sugimura, K., Yoshida, M.A. & Abe, S. (1980) Cytogenetic effects of 60 chemicals on cultured human and Chinese hamster cells. *Kromosomo*, II-20, 574-584

Schack, J.A. & Waxler, S.H. (1949) An ultraviolet spectrophotometric method for the determination of theophylline and theobromine in blood and tissues. *J. Pharmacol. exp. Ther.*, 97, 283-291

Schiff, J.A., Lyman, H. & Russell, G.K. (1971) Isolation of mutants from *Euglena gracilis*. *Methods Enzymol. (Part A)*, 23, 143-162

Schlaeffer, F., Engelberg, I., Kaplanski, J. & Danon, A. (1984) Effect of exercise and environmental heat on theophylline kinetics. *Respiration*, 45, 438-442

Shah, V.P. & Riegelman, S. (1974) GLC determination of theophylline in biological fluids. *J. pharm. Sci.*, 63, 1283-1285

Shin, S.-G., Juan, D. & Rammohan, M. (1988) Theophylline pharmacokinetics in normal elderly subjects. *Clin. pharmacol. Ther.*, 44, 522-530

Shively, C.A. & Tarka, S.M., Jr (1984) Methylxanthine composition and consumption patterns of cocoa and chocolate products. In: Spiller, G.A., ed., *The Methylxanthine Beverages and Foods: Chemistry, Consumption and Health Effects*, New York, Alan R. Liss, pp. 149-178

Shum, L. & Jusko, W.J. (1984) Theophylline disposition in obese rats. *J. Pharmacol. exp. Ther.*, 228, 380-386

Singer, E.P. & Kolischenko, A. (1985) Seizures due to theophylline overdose. *Chest*, 87, 755-757

Slameňová, D., Budayová, E., Dušinská, M. & Gabelová, G. (1986) Results of genotoxicity testing of theophylline on bacteria and two lines of mammalian cells. *Neoplasma*, 33, 457-463

Smolensky, M.H. & McGovern, J.P. (1985) Circadian rhythms in theophylline disposition. *Curr. clin. Pract. Ser.*, 18, 75-92

Soldin, S.J. & Hill, J.G. (1977) A rapid micromethod for measuring theophylline in serum by reverse-phase high performance liquid chromatography. *Clin. Biochem.*, 10, 74-77

Sommer, K.R., Hill, R.M. & Horning, M.G. (1975) Identification and quantification of drugs in human amniotic fluid. *Res. Commun. chem. Pathol. Pharmacol.*, 12, 583-594

Spiller, M.A. (1984) The chemical components of coffee. In: Spiller, G.A., ed., *The Methylxanthine Beverages and Foods: Chemistry, Consumption, and Health Effects*, New York, Alan R. Liss, pp. 91-147

SRI (1986) *1986 Directory of Chemical Producers, United States of America*, Menlo Park, CA

Staib, A.H., Schuppan, D., Lissner, R., Zilly, W., von Bomhard, G. & Richter, E. (1980) Pharmacokinetics and metabolism of theophylline in patients with liver diseases. *Int. J. clin. Pharmacol. Ther. Toxicol.*, 18, 500-502

Stavric, B. (1988) Methylxanthines: toxicity to humans. 1. Theophylline. *Food chem. Toxicol.*, 26, 541-565

Straughn, A., Meyer, M., Golub, A. & Gonzalez, M. (1984) A chronopharmacokinetic model for controlled-release formulations. *Ann. Rev. Chronopharmacol.*, 1, 93-96

Sturelid, S. & Kihlman, B.A. (1975) Enhancement by methylated oxypurines of the frequency of induced chromosomal aberrations. I. The dependence of the effect on the molecular structure of the potentiating agent. *Hereditas*, 79, 29-42

Tang-Liu, D.D-S. & Riegelman, S. (1981) Metabolism of theophylline to caffeine in adults. *Res. Commun. chem. Pathol. Pharmacol.*, 34, 371-380

Tang-Liu, D.D.-S., Williams, R.L. & Riegelman, S. (1982a) Nonlinear theophylline elimination. *Clin. pharmacol. Ther.*, 31, 358-369

Tang-Liu, D.D.-S., Tozer, T.N. & Riegelman, S. (1982b) Urine flow-dependence of theophylline renal clearance in man. *J. Pharmacokinet. Biopharmacol.*, 10, 351-364

Tarka, S.M., Jr (1982) The toxicology of cocoa and methylxanthines: a review of the literature. *Crit. Rev. Toxicol.*, 9, 275-312

Teunissen, M.W.E., Brorens, I.O.N., Geerlings, J.M. & Breimer, D.D. (1985) Dose-dependent elimination of theophylline in rats. *Xenobiotica*, 15, 165-171

Thoman, E.B., Davis, D.H., Raye, J.R., Philipps, A.F., Rowe, J.C. & Denenberg, V.H. (1985) Theophylline affects sleep-wake state development in premature infants. *Neuropediatrics*, 16, 13-18

Timson, J. (1972) Effect of theobromine, theophylline and caffeine on the mitosis of human lymphocytes. *Mutat. Res.*, 15, 197-201

Timson, J. (1975) Theobromine and theophylline. *Mutat. Res.*, 32, 169-178

Timson, J. (1977) Caffeine. *Mutat. Res.*, 47, 1-52

Tornatore, K.M., Kanarkowski, R., McCarthy, T.L., Gardner, M.J., Yurchak, A.M. & Jusko, W.J. (1982) Effect of chronic oral contraceptive steroids on theophylline disposition. *Eur. J. clin. Pharmacol.*, 23, 129-134

Tse, F.L.S. & Szeto, D.W. (1982) Theophylline bioavailability in the dog. *J. pharm. Sci., 71*, 1301-1303

Tsuboi, M. & Yanagishima, N. (1975) Comparative studies on sporulation-promotive actions of cyclic AMP, theophylline and caffeine in *Saccharomyces cerevisiae. Arch. Microbiol., 105*, 83-86

Tucci, S.M. & Skalko, R.G. (1978) The teratogenic effects of theophylline in mice. *Toxicol. Lett., 1*, 337-341

US Bureau of the Census (1989) *US Imports for Consumption*, Washington DC, US Government Printing Office, pp. 1585, 2985-2986

US Pharmacopeial Convention (1990) *US Pharmacopeia — The National Formulary*, 22nd ed., Rockville, MD, pp. 1348-1354

Walton, H.F., Eiceman, G.A. & Otto, J.L. (1979) Chromatography of xanthines on ion-exchange resins. *J. Chromatogr., 180*, 145-156

Weinberger, M. (1978) Theophylline for treatment of asthma. *J. Pediatr., 92*, 1-7

Weinberger, M. & Ginchansky, E. (1977) Dose-dependent kinetics of theophylline disposition in asthmatic children. *J. Pediatr., 91*, 820-824

Weinstein, D., Mauer, I., Katz, M.L. & Kazmer, S. (1973) The effect of caffeine on chromosomes of human lymphocytes: a search for the mechanism of action. *Mutat. Res., 20*, 115-125

Weinstein, D., Mauer, I., Katz, M.L. & Kazmer, S. (1975) The effect of methylxanthines on chromosomes of human lymphocytes in culture. *Mutat. Res., 31*, 57-61

Welling, P.G., Lyons, L.L., Craig, W.A. & Trochta, G.A. (1975) Influence of diet and fluid on bioavailability of theophylline. *Clin. Pharmacol. Ther., 17*, 475-480

Windholz, M., ed. (1983) *The Merck Index*, 10th ed., Rahway, NJ, Merck & Co., p. 1328

Winek, C.L., Bricker, J.D., Collom, W.D. & Fochtman, F.W. (1980) Theophylline fatalities. *Forens. Sci. int., 15*, 233-236

Woo, O.F., Koup, J.R., Kraemer, M. & Robertson, W.O. (1980) Acute intoxication with theophylline while on chronic therapy. *Vet. hum. Toxicol., 22* (Suppl. 2), 48-51

Woodcock, A.A., Johnson, M.A. & Geddes, D.M. (1983) Theophylline prescribing, serum concentrations, and toxicity. *Lancet, ii*, 610-612

Yurchak, A.M. & Jusko, W.J. (1976) Theophylline secretion into breast milk. *Pediatrics, 57*, 518-520

Zajdela, F. & Latarjet, R. (1973) Inhibition by caffeine of induction of skin tumours with ultraviolet light in the mouse (Fr.). *C.R. Acad. Sci. (Paris), 277*, Serie D, 1073-1076

Zajdela, F. & Latarjet, R. (1974) The inhibitory effect of caffeine on the induction of cutaneous tumors in mice by ultraviolet rays. *Excerpta med. int. Congr. Ser., 351*, 120-123

Zajdela, F. & Latarjet, R. (1978a) Ultraviolet light induction of skin carcinoma in the mouse; influence of cAMP modifying agents. *Bull. Cancer, 65*, 305-314

Zajdela, F. & Latarjet, R. (1978b) Inhibition of skin carcinogenesis *in vivo* by caffeine and other agents. *Natl Cancer Inst. Monogr., 50*, 133-140

THEOBROMINE

1. Chemical and Physical Data

1.1 Synonyms

Chem. Abstr. Services Reg. No.: 83-67-0

Chem. Abstr. Name: 3,7-Dihydro-3,7-dimethyl-1*H*-purine-2,6-dione
Synonym: 3,7-Dimethylxanthine

1.2 Structural and molecular formulae and molecular weight

$C_7H_8N_4O_2$ Mol. wt: 180.17

1.3 Chemical and physical properties of the pure substance

(a) *Description*: White crystalline powder (Moffat, 1986)
(b) *Sublimation-point*: 290-295°C (Windholz, 1983)
(c) *Melting-point*: 357°C (Windholz, 1983)
(d) *Spectroscopy data*: Ultraviolet spectra: aqueous acid-272 nm (A_1^1 = 563a); aqueous alkali-274 nm; infrared spectra: principal peaks at wave numbers 1690, 1665, 1221, 1550, 1595, 680 nm (potassium bromide disc); mass spectra: principal peaks at *m/z* 180, 55, 67, 109, 82, 42, 137, 70; 3-methylxanthine, 166, 68, 95, 41, 53, 123; 7-methylxanthine, 166, 68, 123, 53, 42, 41, 95 (Moffat, 1986)
(e) *Solubility*: Soluble in water (1.0 g/2 l), boiling water (1.0 g/0.15 l) and 95% ethanol (1.0 g/2.2 l) (Windholz, 1983); slightly soluble in chloroform (1.0 g/6 l; Moffat, 1986); almost insoluble in benzene, diethyl ether and carbon tetrachloride (Windholz, 1983)

(f) *Equilibrium constants*: acidic (Ka) 0.9×10^{-10} and basic (Kb) 1.3×10^{-14} at 18°C (Windholz, 1983)

(g) *Reactivity*: Forms salts, which are decomposed by water, and compounds with bases, which are more stable (Windholz, 1983)

(h) *Octanol/water partition coefficient (P)*: log P -0.8 (Moffat, 1986)

1.4 Technical products and impurities

Theobromine should contain not less than 99.0% and not more than 101.0% of the product calculated on a dry basis (Anon., 1988).

Trade names: Riddospas; Riddovydrin; Santheose; Seominal; Theobrominum; Theoguardenal; Theominal; Théoxalvose

2. Production, Use, Occurrence and Analysis

2.1 Production and use

(a) *Production*

Theobromine is the principal alkaloid (1.5-3%) of the cacao bean (*Theobroma cacao*); it is usually extracted from the husks of cacao beans, which contain 0.7-1.2% theobromine. It has been synthesized from 3-methyluric acid (Windholz, 1983), but is not known to be produced commercially. Annual production of theobromine in the mid-1970s was over 33 000 tonnes (Cordell, 1978). In 1980, 607 million pounds (276 million kg) of cocoa were imported into the USA, which represents 9.11 million pounds (4.1 million kg) of theobromine (Hirsh, 1984).

(b) *Use*

Theobromine is used principally to make caffeine (McCutheon, 1969). Formerly, theobromine and its derivatives were used in diuretics, myocardial stimulants, vasodilators and smooth muscle relaxants (Windholz, 1983). Theobromine salts (calcium salicylate, sodium salicylate and sodium acetate) were used previously to dilate coronary arteries (Tarka, 1982; Gennaro, 1985) at doses of 300 to 600 mg per day (Moffat, 1986). There is no current therapeutic use of theobromine (Tarka, 1982).

2.2 Occurrence

(a) *Natural occurrence*

Theobromine is found in chocolate, tea and cocoa products (Graham, 1984a; Shively & Tarka, 1984; Stavric, 1988). Cacao is the major natural source of theobromine; the concentration in whole cacao beans and nibs (cotyledon) increases during the first day of fermentation and that in the shells increases subsequently (Timbie *et al.*, 1978; Shively & Tarka, 1984).

Theobromine has been reported in cacao husks and beans at 0.7-1.2% and 1.5-3% (15-30 g/kg) (Windholz, 1983). Levels have been reported to be 20 mg/kg in green coffee beans (Spiller, 1984), 0.15-0.20% in manufactured tea (Jalal & Collin, 1976; Graham, 1984a) and 0.3% in dried mate (Michl & Haberler, 1954; Graham, 1984b).

(b)   Occupational exposure

No data were available to the Working Group.

(c)   Water and sediments

Theobromine has not been found in US industrial effluents (Perry *et al.*, 1979) or drinking-water (National Research Council, 1977).

(d)   Foods and beverages (see also the monograph on caffeine, pp. 296 *et seq.*)

Theobromine is a component of the cocoa solids, or nonlipid portion, of chocolate liquor (Shively & Tarka, 1984). An average theobromine level of 1.89% was found in eight commercial brands of cocoa powder (not calculated on a dry basis; Zoumas *et al.*, 1980; Shively & Tarka, 1984). A level of 2% was reported in one cocoa powder (Sontag & Kral, 1980) and 2.5-3.3% in bulk unsweetened cocoa (Martinek & Wolman, 1955; Shively & Tarka, 1984). Hot chocolate beverages had average levels of 65 mg/5-oz serving (Zoumas *et al.*, 1980); chocolate milk samples prepared from instant, cold, sweetened cocoa powders had an average level of 58 mg theobromine per serving (Zoumas *et al.*, 1980; Shively & Tarka, 1984), and hot cocoa prepared from nine commercial instant mixes had an average of 62 mg theobromine per serving (Blauch & Tarka, 1983; Shively & Tarka, 1984). The mean concentration of theobromine in 12 varieties of cocoa powder was 0.26% (Craig & Nguyen, 1984).

Dark chocolate contains the largest amount of theobromine per serving of any type of eating chocolate; concentrations vary widely (0.36-0.63%) owing to the initial large difference in the theobromine content in chocolate liquors, but one 1-oz bar of dark chocolate contained 130 mg theobromine, and one 1-oz bar of milk chocolate contained 44 mg theobromine. The theobromine content of chocolate foods prepared from home recipes using standard chocolate sources (i.e., cocoa and baking chocolate) varies widely (24 mg per serving in chocolate brownies to 724 mg in chocolate frostings); chocolate frostings have relatively higher theobromine levels (0.055-0.213%) than chocolate cakes. The methylxanthine (theobromine and caffeine) content of manufactured chocolate foods and beverages varies according to food source and within different brands of the same item (Shively & Tarka, 1984).

Theobromine has been found in blended black tea beverage at a level of 0.69% of dry extractable solids present (Graham, 1984a).

In the USA in 1980, the daily per-caput intake of theobromine from food and beverages was estimated to be 39.05 mg; daily per-caput consumption of theobromine from cocoa was calculated to be 38.3 mg on the basis of the 276 million kg of cocoa imported (Hirsh, 1984).

2.3 Analysis

Analytical procedures for the determination of methylxanthines (including theobromine) in biological fluids (Schack & Waxler, 1949; Christensen & Whitsett, 1979; Tang-Liu & Riegelman, 1982; Klassen & Stavric, 1983; Christensen & Neims, 1984; Hurst *et al.*, 1984) and in foods (Hurst *et al.*, 1984) include ultraviolet spectroscopy, thin-layer chromatography, gas chromatography and high-performance liquid chromatography.

Modern methods for the determination of theobromine in foods and beverages (cocoa beans, cocoa and chocolate products) usually rely on high-performance liquid chromatography (Wildanger, 1975; Kreiser & Martin, 1978; Timbie *et al.*, 1978; Hatfull *et al.*, 1980; Horwitz, 1980; Kreiser & Martin, 1980; Sontag & Kral, 1980; Zoumas *et al.*, 1980; De Vries *et al.*, 1981; Reid & Good, 1982; Woollard, 1982; Blauch & Tarka, 1983; Craig & Nguyen, 1984; Vergnes & Alary, 1986) and, to a lesser extent, on thin-layer chromatography (Senanayake & Wijesekera, 1968a,b, 1971). These methods replaced the traditional titrimetric procedure using silver nitrate (Gerritsma & Koers, 1953), paper chromatography (Jalal & Collin, 1976), gravimetry and ultraviolet spectroscopy (Hurst *et al.*, 1984).

3. Biological Data Relevant to the Evaluation of Carcinogenic Risk to Humans

3.1 Carcinogenicity studies in animals

No data were available from studies on the carcinogenicity of theobromine.

Modifying effects on the activity of known carcinogens

Urethane

Groups of female ICR/Jcl *mice* [initial numbers unspecified], 25 days of age, received a single subcutaneous injection of 0.1 mg/g bw urethane followed immediately by seven intraperitoneal injections (0.05 μmol/g bw) of theobromine [purity unspecified] at 6-h intervals up to 36 h after urethane treatment, to give a total dose of 63 μg/g theobromine. Mice were killed five months after urethane treatment. The number of mice with lung tumours was significantly reduced in groups that received post-treatment with theobromine (11/56 versus 31/59; $p < 0.001$). The number of tumours/lung was also reduced (0.28 versus 1.07 in controls) (Nomura, 1983). [The Working Group noted that the effective numbers of mice varied considerably among the different groups.]

3.2 Other relevant data

(a) *Experimental systems*

(i) *Absorption, distribution, metabolism and excretion*

The pharmacokinetics and toxicity of theobromine have been reviewed extensively (Tarka, 1982; Arnaud, 1984, 1987; Tarka & Shively, 1987). As a metabolite of caffeine, theobromine has been detected in variable amounts in plasma and urine of humans and different animal species (Arnaud, 1984).

When theobromine was given as a single oral dose of 15-50 mg/kg bw to male dogs, peak plasma concentrations, with considerable individual variations, were observed within 3 h. With a higher dose (150 mg/kg bw), the peak plasma concentrations were attained 14-16 h later, showing delayed intestinal absorption (Gans *et al.*, 1980). In rats, plasma protein binding was very low (8-17%) after oral administration of 1-100 mg/kg bw theobromine (Bonati *et al.*, 1984).

Similar kinetic parameters were observed in male and female rabbits when theobromine was administered intravenously or orally at doses of 1 and 5 mg/kg bw, with complete gastrointestinal absorption. A reduction in the absorption rate constant was seen in rabbits when the dose was increased from 10 to 100 mg/kg bw. In spite of delayed gastrointestinal absorption at high doses, probably due to the low solubility of the compound, the absolute bioavailability of theobromine approached 100% (Latini *et al.*, 1984). Labelled theobromine was almost completely absorbed after oral administration (1-6 mg/kg; Arnaud & Welsch, 1979); the peak blood level tended to appear later with larger doses (100 mg/kg; Shively & Tarka, 1983).

Theobromine is absorbed and distributed rapidly after oral administration to rats (Shively & Tarka, 1983) and equilibrates freely between plasma and testicular fluid (Shively *et al.*, 1984).

The ratio of brain:blood theobromine concentrations decreased continuously from 0.96 at birth to 0.60 in 30-day-old rats (Arnaud & Getaz, 1982). After 24 h, no organ accumulation of theobromine or its metabolites could be seen in adult animals (Arnaud & Welsch, 1979).

In dogs, an average plasma half-time of 17.5 h was reported after single oral doses of theobromine ranging from 15 to 150 mg/kg bw (Gans et al., 1980). In rabbits, the mean elimination half-time was 4.3-5.6 h for doses ranging from 1 to 100 mg/kg bw (Latini et al., 1984). From these data, it was concluded that the pharmacokinetics of theobromine in rabbits are linear and not dose-dependent up to 100 mg/kg (Traina & Bonati, 1985). Linear pharmacokinetics were also observed in rats up to a dose of 100 mg/kg. No significant first-pass effect or sex difference were observed (Shively & Tarka, 1983; Bonati et al., 1984). Repeated administration of theobromine to dogs, rabbits or rats did not alter its kinetics or metabolism (Gans et al., 1980; Bonati et al., 1984; Latini et al., 1984). Pretreatment of rats with 3-methylcholanthrene in vivo markedly increased theobromine elimination, while phenobarbital had no effect (Shively & Vesell, 1987).

The kinetic parameters in rats on day 19 of gestation were similar to those of non-pregnant rats at doses ranging from 5 to 100 mg/kg bw (Shively & Tarka, 1983). A decrease in the elimination rate constant was observed in pregnant rabbits at a dose of 50 mg/kg bw, suggesting saturation (Latini et al., 1984).

The metabolic pathway of theobromine reported in rats and several other animal species is shown in Figure 1. 6-Amino-5-[N-methylformylamino]-1-methyluracil is quantitatively the most important theobromine metabolite in rats, accounting for 20-35% of urinary metabolites (Arnaud & Welsch, 1979; Shively & Tarka, 1983; Bonati et al., 1984). The majority of theobromine-derived radioactivity in the faeces of rats could be accounted for by 3,7-dimethyluric acid (Shively & Vesell, 1987). The most extensive metabolism of theobromine was observed in rabbits and mice; male mice converted theobromine more extensively into this metabolite than did female mice. In contrast, oxidation of theobromine to 3,7-dimethyluric acid was significantly greater in female than in male rats. Rabbits and dogs metabolized theobromine primarily to 7-methylxanthine and 3-methylxanthine, respectively, and dogs excreted small quantities of an unidentified metabolite (Miller et al., 1984).

The compounds identified in bile of phenobarbital-treated rats were 3,7-dimethyluric acid (64-76% of biliary radioactivity), dimethylallantoin (5-8%), 6-amino-5-[N-methylformylamino]-1-methyluracil (10-17%) and theobromine (8-10%). In 3-methylcholanthrene-treated rats, urinary elimination of unchanged theobromine was reduced from 23-27% to only 2%, while excretion of 6-amino-5-[N-methylformylamino]-1-methyluracil was significantly increased. Only 3,7-dimethyluric acid was produced by liver microsomal incubation in control rats while phenobarbital and 3-methylcholanthrene pretreatment enhanced the biotransformation resulting in the production of all metabolites found in vivo as well as unknown polar compounds (Shively & Vesell, 1987).

Figure 1. Metabolism of theobromine[a]

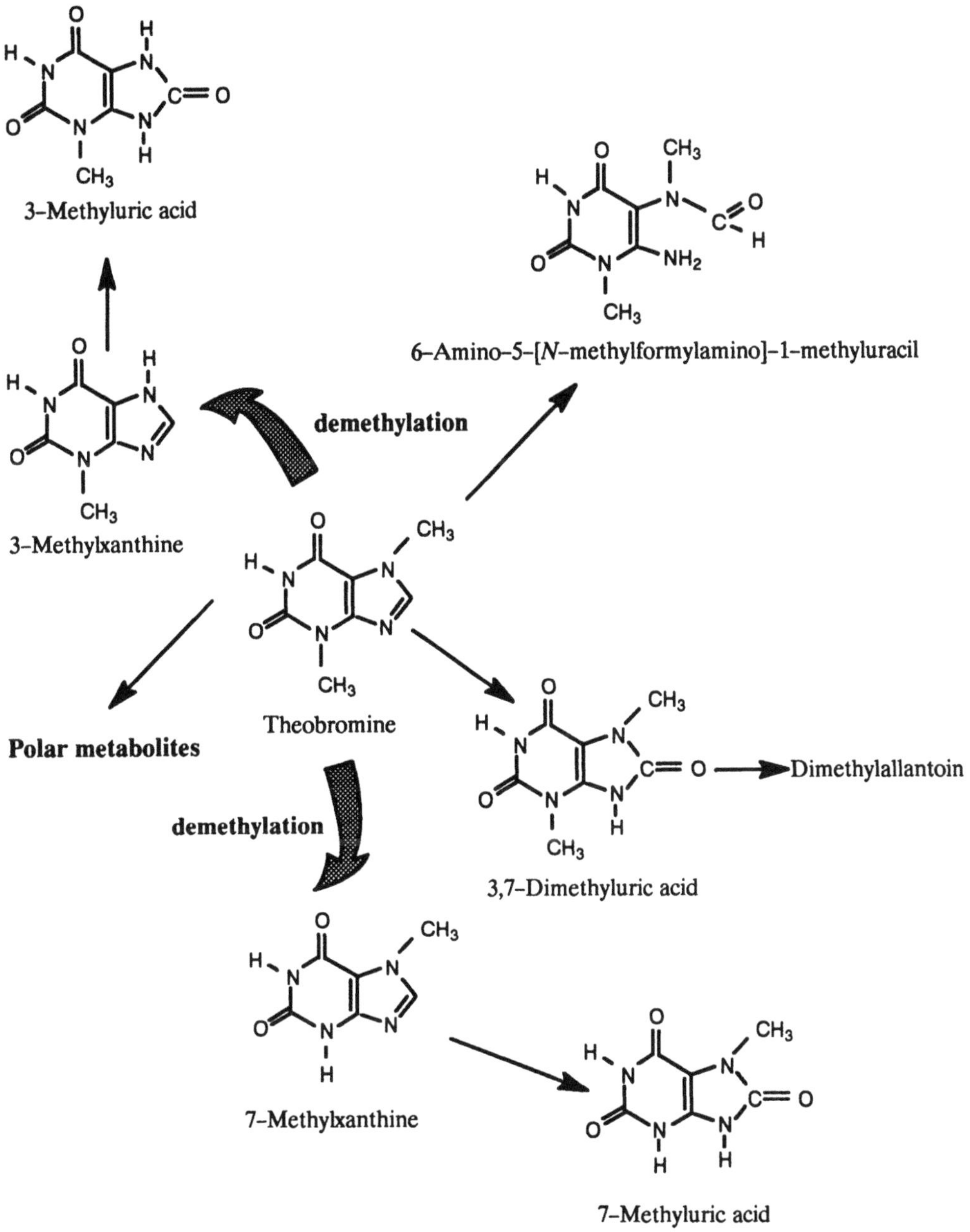
3-Methyluric acid
6-Amino-5-[N-methylformylamino]-1-methyluracil
demethylation
3-Methylxanthine
Theobromine
Polar metabolites
Dimethylallantoin
demethylation
3,7-Dimethyluric acid
7-Methylxanthine
7-Methyluric acid

[a]From Arnaud & Welsch (1979)

Pregnancy and increased doses of theobromine were shown to modify theobromine metabolism. At a dose of 50 mg/kg bw, pregnant rabbits excreted more unchanged theobromine in the urine (51% versus 35%; Latini et al., 1984). Pregnant rats excreted a higher percentage of a 5 mg/kg dose as unchanged theobromine (53%) than non-pregnant rats (39%); this difference disappeared at the saturation dose (100 mg/kg), when unchanged theobromine corresponded to about 60% of the dose in the urine of both pregnant and non-pregnant animals (Shively & Tarka, 1983). Rats given 100 mg/kg excreted more unchanged theobromine than those given 1 mg/kg (73% versus 51%), and showed a corresponding relative decrease in excretion of its uracil metabolite, 6-amino-5-[N-methylformylamino]-1-methyluracil (16% versus 28%) (Bonati et al., 1984).

About 60% of orally administered labelled theobromine was recovered unchanged in rat urine; 94-106% total urine radioactivity was recovered (Shively & Tarka, 1983). Large variations in faecal excretion (2-38% of the dose) were reported in metabolic experiments performed in rats, mice, hamsters, rabbits and dogs (Miller et al., 1984). Theobromine was excreted into the bile of dogs fed theobromine (Gans et al., 1980). Biliary secretion accounted for 5-10% of the administered [8-^{14}C]theobromine dose in phenobarbital-induced rats (Shively & Vesell, 1987).

Urinary excretion of theobromine metabolites and theobromine clearance were increased in rats on a commercial diet compared to those on a semipurified diet (Shively et al., 1986).

(ii) *Toxic effects*

The toxicity of theobromine as compared to other methylxanthines has been reviewed by Tarka (1982). The acute oral LD_{50} in rats was 950 mg/kg bw, whereas in mice it was 1356 mg/kg (for the sodium acetate). While the toxicity of theobromine in domestic animals has been indirectly attributed to excessive consumption of cocoa and chocolate products, there are few direct studies where theobromine was evaluated, because of its extremely low solubility in aqueous media. The oral LD_{50} of theobromine in dogs appears to be about 300 mg/kg bw (Gans et al., 1980).

The effects of theobromine on rodent and dog testis are reviewed below; the other target organ identified in rodents is the thymus gland. High doses — 250-300 mg/kg bw (mature animals) and 500 mg/kg bw (immature animals) — have been shown to cause complete thymic atrophy in male and female rats. This effect was seen in hamsters only at a level of 850 mg/kg bw and in mice at levels of 1840-1880 mg/kg bw (Tarka et al., 1979).

The only study of non-rodent species is that of Gans et al. (1980), who fed male dogs 100-150 mg/kg bw theobromine for periods of 21-28 days as well as various doses over a one-year period. They reported a degenerative and fibrotic lesion in the right atrial appendage of the heart. This finding appears to be unique to the dog since no such appendage exists in man. The study is further confounded by administration of varying doses in early treatment groups, with adjustments at several points in the one-year study.

A subchronic toxicity study performed in male and female Sprague-Dawley rats was reported in an abstract (Tarka & Zoumas, 1983). Theobromine was fed at levels of 0, 0.02, 0.1 and 0.2% of a chow diet for 90 days [corresponding to 25, 125 and 250 mg/kg bw/day]. The only changes noted were a reduction in body weight gain and testicular weight in males at the high dose. No pathological lesion was observed and there was no haematological change.

(iii) *Effects on reproduction and prenatal toxicity*

Reproductive toxicity: Feeding theobromine to male Osborne-Mendel rats at a dietary level of 0.5% for 64 weeks resulted in severe testicular atrophy in 94% of animals, with aspermatogenesis in 82% (Friedman *et al.*, 1979). The results were confirmed in another strain of rats (Holtzman); following 19 weeks of feeding theobromine, all rats showed atrophy, and 79% had aspermatogenesis.

Tarka *et al.* (1979) found that feeding theobromine at levels of 0.2-1.0% in the diet (90-140 to 500-600 mg/kg bw per day) for a period of 28 days to rats produced severe testicular atrophy at the 0.8% level and seminiferous tubular-cell degeneration at the 0.6% level. Rats were found to be most sensitive, while mice (doses, 0.2-1.2%; 300-1850 mg/kg bw per day) were more resistant, and testicular changes were seen only at concentrations that caused considerable mortality. Hamsters (doses, 0.2-1.0%; 182-1027 mg/kg bw per day) were almost totally resistant to testicular changes. These authors also studied the potential reversibility of this phenomenon by feeding proven breeder male Sprague-Dawley rats 0.2, 0.6 or 0.8% theobromine (88, 244 or 334 mg/kg bw per day, respectively) for 49 days, performing unilateral orchiectomy at that time and allowing rats to recover on a theobromine-free diet for an additional 49 days. Histologically, the effects at the two highest dose levels were largely irreversible (Tarka *et al.*, 1981). Daily administration of 500 mg/kg bw theobromine to Fü albino rats for three or five days interfered with germ cell kinetics but did not cause significant damage to spermatogonia. The release of late spermatids into the tubular lumen was retarded and generally occurred two weeks after treatment (Ettlin *et al.*, 1986).

Subsequent studies (Gans, 1982, 1984) substantiated these observations. Significantly higher serum theobromine concentrations were achieved with a semisynthetic diet, resulting in more advanced morphological changes in the testes in rats, than with a chow diet. Shively *et al.* (1986) demonstrated that rats fed 0.6% theobromine in a certified chow diet for 28 days did not develop the testicular atrophy induced by addition of theobromine to a semisynthetic diet, due to induction of theobromine metabolism in animals on the chow diet.

Gans *et al.* (1980) studied the effects of short-term and long-term theobromine administration to male dogs; no testicular atrophy was seen at doses of 25, 50, 100 or 150 mg/kg per day over a one-year period.

Male and female Sprague-Dawley rats were given cocoa powder containing 2.50-2.58% theobromine and 0.19% caffeine in the diet at concentrations of 0, 1.5, 3.5 and 5.0% for three generations. Males and females were given diets containing cocoa powder for 12 and 2 weeks, respectively, prior to mating. The average methylxanthine doses for males/females were 30/36, 72/86 and 104/126 mg/kg bw per day in the 1.5, 3.5 and 5.0% cocoa powder groups, respectively. No consistent dose-related effect was observed in any reproductive index; nonreproductive toxicity was observed at the two highest dose levels (Hostetler *et al.*, 1990).

Developmental toxicity: ICR-JCL mice received a single intraperitoneal injection of 500 or 600 mg/kg bw theobromine on day 12 of gestation. Maternal deaths occurred in 40% of the higher-dose group but not in the lower-dose group. The incidence of resorptions was significantly increased with the higher dose; at both dose levels, fetal body weight was decreased and the incidence of malformations and subcutaneous haematomas was increased (Fujii & Nishimura, 1969).

In Sprague-Dawley rats fed diets containing theobromine (daily doses, 53 or 99 mg/kg bw) on gestation days 6-19, no maternal toxicity was observed. Although no malformation occurred, slight decreases in fetal body weight were observed with the high dose, and a significant increase was seen in the frequency of skeletal variations. Serum concentrations of theobromine in the high-dose group were 15-20 µl/ml (Tarka *et al.*, 1986a).

New Zealand white rabbits were administered up to 200 mg/kg bw theobromine by gavage on gestation days 6-29. Maternal deaths occurred in 40% of the group receiving the highest dose level, but little or no maternal toxicity was observed with 25, 75 or 125 mg/kg bw per day. Decreased fetal body weight and malformations were seen at doses of 125 or 200 mg/kg; the incidence of skeletal variations was increased with 75 mg/kg and over. With 75 mg/kg per day — the lowest dose at which developmental toxicity was observed — serum concentrations of theobromine were 24-86 µl/ml. In other groups of New Zealand rabbits fed diets containing theobromine (daily doses, 21, 41 or 63 mg/kg bw), little or no maternal toxicity was observed at any dose level. Fetal body weight was decreased at 41 and 63 mg/kg bw, and there were significant increases in the frequency of skeletal variations. Average serum concentrations at the lowest effective concentrations were 12-15 µl/ml (Tarka *et al.*, 1986b). [The Working Group noted that serum concentrations of theobromine following administration of the lowest effective dose were proportionally higher in rabbits than in rats.]

(iv) *Genetic and related effects*

The genetic effects of theobromine have been reviewed (Timson, 1975, 1977; Tarka, 1982; Grice, 1987; Rosenkranz & Ennever, 1987a,b).

The results described below are listed in Table 1 on p. 433, with the evaluation of the Working Group, as positive, negative or inconclusive, as defined in the footnotes. The results are tabulated separately for the presence and absence of an exogenous metabolic system. The lowest effective dose (LED), in the case of positive results, or the highest ineffective dose (HID), in the case of negative results, are shown, together with the appropriate reference. The studies are summarized briefly below.

Theobromine has only a very weak capacity to displace acridine orange from DNA *in vitro* (Richardson *et al.*, 1981). In extracts of *Escherichia coli*, it selectively inhibited some purine nucleoside phosphorylases (Koch & Lamont, 1956). Theobromine was not incorporated to 'any great extent' into the DNA of *E. coli*, which possibly cannot demethylate this substance (Koch, 1956). The effects of theobromine on relevant targets other than DNA are discussed in the monograph on caffeine (p. 332).

Theobromine was mutagenic to *E. coli* under conditions in which a constant growth rate and cell population density were maintained, but it was not mutagenic to *Salmonella typhimurium*. Theobromine induced mutations in a lower eukaryote, *Euglena gracilis*.

Theobromine did not induce chromosomal aberrations in plants (*Vicia faba*). It was reported in an abstract that chromosomal aberrations were not observed in *Drosophila melanogaster* treated with 0.45% theobromine in feeding experiments (Mittler & Mittler, 1968).

Theobromine increased the frequency of mutant *tk* colonies in mouse lymphoma cells, but only at extremely cytotoxic doses. Significant increases in the frequency of sister chromatid exchange were induced in Chinese hamster CHO cells in the absence of an exogenous metabolic system; in the presence of an exogenous metabolic system the results were equivocal and not dose-related (Brusick *et al.*, 1986). Chromosomal aberrations were not induced by theobromine in Chinese hamster cells. BALB/c 3T3 cells were not morphologically transformed by treatment with theobromine, and, unlike theophylline but like caffeine, theobromine did not reduce the expression of parameters associated with morphological transformation (Rajaraman & Faulkner, 1984).

In human lymphocyte cultures, theobromine did not significantly increase the number of sister chromatid exchanges per cell, but, in another experiment using higher doses, the numbers of sister chromatid exchanges per cell were increased in the absence of an exogenous metabolic system. The induction of sister chromatid exchange is not necessarily due to a directly damaging effect upon DNA, since theobromine can have indirect effects (Levi *et al.*, 1978) which are associated with the induction of sister chromatid exchange (Morgan & Cleaver, 1982) and may even give rise to false-positive effects, the primary effect upon DNA being due to bromodeoxyuridine (Natarajan *et al.*, 1981). Theobromine did, however, induce breaks in human lymphocytes in culture, contrary to the results with rodent cells (see above).

Theobromine induced sister chromatid exchange and micronuclei, but not chromosomal aberrations, in the bone marrow of Chinese hamsters treated *in vivo*. No dominant lethal effect (increases in either preimplantation loss or dead implants) was observed in either CD-1 mice or in male Sprague-Dawley rats. The negative result in rats was not due to pharmacokinetic limitations, as demonstrated above.

(b) *Humans*

(i) *Absorption, distribution, excretion and metabolism*

Theobromine is readily absorbed from food and evenly distributed in body fluids; the half-times in plasma and saliva are highly correlated (Drouillard *et al.*, 1978). Theobromine has been reported to pass into the breast milk of nursing mothers (Resman *et al.*, 1977).

The mean half-time of theobromine in human serum ranged from 6.1 to 10 h (Drouillard *et al.*, 1978; Tarka *et al.*, 1983; Shively *et al.*, 1985); the apparent volumes of distribution and clearance were estimated to be 0.76 l/kg bw and 0.88 ml/min/kg bw, respectively (Shively *et al.*, 1985).

The major metabolite of theobromine in human urine is 7-methylxanthine (34-48%), followed by 3-methylxanthine (20%) and 7-methyluric acid (7-12%), 6-amino-5-[*N*-methylformylamino]-1-methyluracil (6-9%) and 3,7-dimethyluric acid (1%). Of the dose, 1-18% is recovered in the urine as unchanged theobromine (Tarka *et al.*, 1983; Birkett *et al.*, 1985). Theobromine metabolites were not found in the plasma of human subjects (Tarka *et al.*, 1983). Theobromine has a low protein binding capacity in both serum (15-21%) and breast milk (12%) (Resman *et al.*, 1977; Birkett *et al.*, 1985).

(ii) *Toxic effects*

It has been stated that 'in large doses' theobromine may cause nausea and anorexia (Reynolds, 1982) and that daily intake of 50-100 g cocoa (0.8-1.5 g theobromine) by humans has been associated with sweating, trembling and severe headache (Czok, 1974). In a study of 13 volunteers who consumed 200 mg

Table 1. Genetic and related effects of theobromine

Test system		Results		Dose LED/HID	Reference
		Without exogenous metabolic activation	With exogenous metabolic activation		
SA0,	Salmonella typhimurium TA100, reverse mutation	–	–	2500.0000	Renner & Münzer (1982)
SA0,	Salmonella typhimurium TA100, reverse mutation	–	–	2500.0000	Brusick et al. (1986)
SA5,	Salmonella typhimurium TA1535, reverse mutation	–	–	2500.0000	Renner & Münzer (1982)
SA5,	Salmonella typhimurium TA1535, reverse mutation	–	–	500.0000	Brusick et al. (1986)
SA7,	Salmonella typhimurium TA1537, reverse mutation	–	–	2500.0000	Renner & Münzer (1982)
SA7,	Salmonella typhimurium TA1537, reverse mutation	–	–	500.0000	Brusick et al. (1986)
SA8,	Salmonella typhimurium TA1538, reverse mutation	–	–	2500.0000	Renner & Münzer (1982)
SA8,	Salmonella typhimurium TA1538, reverse mutation	–	–	500.0000	Brusick et al. (1986)
SA9,	Salmonella typhimurium TA98, reverse mutation	–	–	2500.0000	Renner & Münzer (1982)
SA9,	Salmonella typhimurium TA98, reverse mutation	–	–	2500.0000	Brusick et al. (1986)
ECR,	Escherichia coli, phage T5-resistance	+	0	150.0000	Novick & Szilard (1951)
ECR,	Escherichia coli, phage T5-resistance	+	0	150.0000	Novick & Szilard (1952)
???,	Euglena gracilis, auxotrophic mutations	–	0	0.0000	Come & Travis (1969)
G5T,	Gene mutation, mouse lymphoma L5178Y cells, tk locus	(+)	(+)	2000.0000	Brusick et al. (1986)
SIC,	Sister chromatid exchange, Chinese hamster CHO cells	+	0	100.0000	Brusick et al. (1986)
CIC,	Chromosomal aberrations, Chinese hamster CHO cells	–	0	1000.0000	Brusick et al. (1986)
TBM,	Cell transformation, BALB/c 3T3 cells	–	0	5000.0000	Brusick et al. (1986)
SHL,	Sister chromatid exchange, human lymphocytes	+	0	100.0000	Mourelatos et al. (1982)
SHL,	Sister chromatid exchange, human lymphocytes	–	0	120.0000	Mourelatos et al. (1983)
CHL,	Chromosomal aberrations, human lymphocytes	+	0	250.0000	Weinstein et al. (1973)
CHL,	Chromosomal aberrations, human lymphocytes	+	0	500.0000	Weinstein et al. (1975)
SVA,	Sister chromatid exchanges, Chinese hamster bone marrow	+	0	150.0000 oral	Renner (1982)
SVA,	Sister chromatid exchanges, Chinese hamster bone marrow	+	0	200.0000 oral	Renner & Münzer (1982)
MVC,	Micronucleus test, Chinese hamster bone marrow	–	0	1300.0000 oral	Renner & Münzer (1982)
CBA,	Chromosomal aberrations, Chinese hamster bone-marrow	–	0	1300.0000 oral	Renner & Münzer (1982)
DLM,	Dominant lethal test, male Swiss CD-1 mice	–	0	380.0000 i.p.	Epstein & Shafer (1968)
DLM,	Dominant lethal test, male Swiss CD-1 mice	–	0	380.0000 i.p.	Epstein et al. (1972)
DLR,	Dominant lethal test, male Sprague-Dawley rats	–	0	450.0000 oral x 5 d	Shively et al. (1984)

i.p., intraperitoneal; oral, by gavage; d, days

theobromine orally three times during a 24-h period, no clinical symptom or other pharmacological activity was observed (Birkett *et al.*, 1985). Ingestion of theobromine in sweet chocolate at a dose of 6 mg/kg bw per day had no effect on clinical parameters in 12 human subjects (Shively *et al.*, 1985).

Studies on a possible association between consumption of methylxanthines and benign breast disease are summarized on pp. 347-350.

(iii) *Effects on reproduction and prenatal toxicity*

No data were available to the Working Group.

(iv) *Genetic and related effects*

No data were available to the Working Group.

3.3 Epidemiological studies of carcinogenicity to humans

Studies on methylxanthines are summarized in the monograph on caffeine.

4. Summary of Data Reported and Evaluation

4.1 Exposure data

Theobromine is the principal alkaloid of the cacao bean. It is extracted from the bean husks and used in the synthesis of caffeine. It has been used in various pharmaceutical products. Theobromine is consumed in cocoa and chocolate beverages and in various forms of chocolate-based foods. Theobromine is also present in small amounts in green coffee beans, tea and mate.

Daily per-caput consumption of theobromine in the USA in 1980 from food and beverages was estimated to be 39 mg.

4.2 Experimental carcinogenicity data

No data on the carcinogenicity of theobromine were available.

4.3 Human carcinogenicity data

No data were available to the Working Group to evaluate the carcinogenicity of theobromine *per se*.

For descriptions of studies on methylxanthines, see the monograph on caffeine.

4.4 Other relevant data

Oral administration of high doses of theobromine to rats caused severe testicular atrophy, which was largely irreversible. Administration of lower levels for prolonged periods had no significant adverse effect on the testis. Mice, hamsters and dogs were less sensitive than rats or were resistant to the effect of theobromine in causing testicular changes. No adverse reproductive effect was observed in a three-generation study in rats given cocoa powder containing theobromine in their diet. Teratogenic effects were observed in rabbits after gavage but not after dietary administration of theobromine. The signs of developmental toxicity observed at the lowest dose level included decreased fetal body weight and increased skeletal variations in rabbits. No teratogenic effect was seen in rats.

In vivo, theobromine did not induce dominant lethal effects in mice or rats. It induced sister chromatid exchange and micronuclei but not chromosomal aberrations in the bone marrow of Chinese hamsters. In human cells *in vitro*, theobromine induced sister chromatid exchange and chromosomal breaks. In cultured mammalian cells, it induced gene mutations and sister chromatid exchange but not chromosomal aberrations or cell transformation. In plants, theobromine did not induce chromosomal aberrations. It induced gene mutations in lower eukaryotes and bacteria but gave negative results in the *Salmonella*/mammalian microsome assay.

4.5 Evaluation[1]

There is *inadequate evidence* for the carcinogenicity in humans of theobromine.

There are no data on the carcinogenicity of theobromine in experimental animals.

Overall evaluation

Theobromine is *not classifiable as to its carcinogenicity to humans (Group 3)*.

---

[1]For descriptions of the italicized terms, see Preamble, pp. 27-31.

5. References

Anon. (1988) *British Pharmacopoeia*, Vol. 1, London, Her Majesty's Stationery Office, p. 564

Arnaud, M.J. (1984) Products of metabolism of caffeine. In: Dews, P.B., ed., *Caffeine. Perspectives from Recent Research*, Berlin, Springer, pp. 3-38

Arnaud, M.J. (1987) The pharmacology of caffeine. *Progr. Drug Res.*, *31*, 273-313

Arnaud, M.J. & Getaz, F. (1982) Postnatal establishment of a blood-brain barrier for theobromine in the rat (Abstract). *Experientia*, *38*, 752

Arnaud, M.J. & Welsch, C. (1979) Metabolic pathway of theobromine in the rat and identification of two new metabolites in human urine. *J. agric. Food Chem.*, *27*, 524-527

Birkett, D.J., Dahlqvist, R., Miners, J.O., Lelo, A. & Billing, B. (1985) Comparison of theophylline and theobromine metabolism in man. *Drug Metab. Disposition*, *13*, 725-728

Blauch, J.L. & Tarka, S.M., Jr (1983) HPLC determination of caffeine and theobromine in coffee, tea and instant hot cocoa mixes. *J. Food Sci.*, *48*, 745-750

Bonati, M., Latini, R., Sadurska, B., Riva, E., Galletti, F., Borzelleca, J.F., Tarka, S.M., Arnaud, M.J. & Garattini, S. (1984) I. Kinetics and metabolism of theobromine in male rats. *Toxicology*, *30*, 327-341

Brusick, D., Myhr, B., Galloway, S., Rundell, J., Jagannath, D.R. & Tarka, S. (1986) Genotoxicity of theobromine in a series of short-term assays. *Mutat. Res.*, *169*, 105-114

Christensen, H.D. & Neims, A.H. (1984) Measurement of caffeine and its metabolites in biological fluids. In: Dews, P.B., ed., *Caffeine. Perspectives from Recent Research*, Berlin, Springer, pp. 39-47

Christensen, H.D. & Whitsett, T.L. (1979) Measurement of xanthines and their metabolites by means of high pressure liquid chromatography. In: Hawk, G.L., ed., *Biological/Biomedical Applications of Liquid Chromatography* (Chromatogr. Ser. 10), New York, Marcel Dekker, pp. 507-537

Come, T.V. & Travis, D.M. (1969) Induction of auxotrophic mutations in *Euglena gracilis*. *J. Hered.*, *60*, 39-41

Cordell, G.A. (1978) Alkaloids. In: Mark, H.F., Othmer, D.F., Overberger, C.G., Seaborg, G.T. & Grayson, M., eds, *Kirk-Othmer Encyclopedia of Chemical Technology*, 3rd ed., Vol. 1, New York, John Wiley & Sons, pp. 923-925

Craig, W.J. & Nguyen, T.T. (1984) Caffeine and theobromine levels in cocoa and carob products. *J. Food Sci.*, *49*, 302-305

Czok, G. (1974) Concerning the question of the biological effectiveness of methylxanthines in cocoa products (Ger.). *Z. Ernahrungswiss.*, *13*, 165-171

De Vries, J.W., Johnson, K.D. & Heroff, J.C. (1981) HPLC determination of caffeine and theobromine content of various natural and red dutched cocoas. *J. Food Sci.*, *46*, 1968-1969

Drouillard, D.D., Vesell, E.S. & Dvorchik, B.H. (1978) Studies on theobromine disposition in normal subjects. Alterations induced by dietary abstention or exposure to methylxanthines. *Clin. pharmacol. Ther.*, *23*, 296-302

Epstein, S.S. & Shafner, H. (1968) Chemical mutagens in the human environment. *Nature*, *219*, 385-387

Epstein, S.S., Arnold, E., Andrea, J., Bass, W. & Bishop, Y. (1972) Detection of chemical mutagens by the dominant lethal assay in the mouse. *Toxicol. appl. Pharmacol.*, *23*, 288-325

Ettlin, R.A., Armstrong, J.M., Buser, S. & Hennes, U. (1986) Retardation of spermiation following short-term treatment of rats with theobromine. *Arch. Toxicol., Suppl. 9*, 441-446

Friedman, L., Weinberger, M.A., Farber, T.M., Moreland, F.M., Peters, E.L., Gilmore, C.E. & Khan, M.A. (1979) Testicular atrophy and impaired spermatogenesis in rats fed high levels of the methylxanthines caffeine, theobromine, or theophylline. *J. environ. Pathol. Toxicol.*, *2*, 687-706

Fujii, T. & Nishimura, H. (1969) Teratogenic actions of some methylated xanthines in mice. *Okajimas Folia anat. jpn.*, *46*, 167-175

Gans, J.H. (1982) Dietary influences on theobromine-induced toxicity in rats. *Toxicol. appl. Pharmacol.*, *63*, 312-320

Gans, J.H. (1984) Comparative toxicities of dietary caffeine and theobromine in the rat. *Food chem. Toxicol.*, *22*, 365-369

Gans, J.H., Korson, R., Cater, M.R. & Ackerly, C.C. (1980) Effects of short-term and long-term theobromine administration to male dogs. *Toxicol. appl. Pharmacol.*, *53*, 481-496

Gennaro, A.R., ed. (1985) *Remington's Pharmaceutical Sciences*, 17th ed., Easton, PA, Mack Publishing, pp. 944, 1070, 1135

Gerritsma, K.W. & Koers, J. (1953) Determination of theobromine in cocoa residues. *Analyst*, *78*, 201-205

Graham, H.N. (1984a) Tea: the plant and its manufacture: chemistry and conception of the beverage. In: Spiller, G.A., ed., *The Methylxanthine Beverages and Foods: Chemistry, Consumption, and Health Effects*, New York, Alan R. Liss, pp. 29-74

Graham, H.N. (1984b) Mate. In: Spiller, G.A., ed., *The Methylxanthine Beverages and Foods: Chemistry, Consumption, and Health Effects*, New York, Alan R. Liss, pp. 179-183

Grice, H.C. (1987) Genotoxicity and carcinogenicity assessment of caffeine and theobromine (Letter to the Editor). *Food chem. Toxicol.*, *25*, 295-296

Hatfull, R.S., Milner, I. & Stanway, V. (1980) Determination of theobromine in animal feeding stuffs. *J. Assoc. public Analysts*, *18*, 19-22

Hirsh, K. (1984) Central nervous system pharmacology of the dietary methylxanthines. In: Spiller, G.A., ed., *The Methylxanthine Beverages and Foods: Chemistry, Consumption, and Health Effects*, New York, Alan R. Liss, pp. 235-301

Horwitz, W., ed. (1980) *Official Methods of Analysis of the Association of Official Analytical Chemists*, 13th ed., Washington DC, Association of Official Analytical Chemists

Hostetler, K.A., Morrissey, R.B., Tarka, S.M., Jr, Apgar, J.L. & Shively, C.A. (1990) Three generations reproductive study of cocoa powder in rats. *Food chem. Toxicol.*, *28*, 483-490

Hurst, W.J., Martin, R.A. & Tarka, S.M., Jr (1984) Analytical methods for quantitation of methylxanthines. In: Spiller, G.A., ed., *The Methylxanthine Beverages and Foods: Chemistry, Consumption and Health Effects*, New York, Alan R. Liss, pp. 17-28

Jalal, M.A.F. & Collin, H.A. (1976) Estimation of caffeine, theophylline and theobromine in plant material. *New Phytol.*, 76, 277-281

Klassen, R. & Stavric, B. (1983) HPLC separation of theophylline, paraxanthine, theobromine, caffeine and other metabolites in biological fluids. *J. liquid Chromatogr.*, 6, 895-906

Koch, A.L. (1956) The metabolism of methylpurines by *Escherichia coli*. I. Tracer studies. *J. biol. Chem.*, 219, 181-188

Koch, A.L. & Lamont, W.A. (1956) The metabolism of methylpurines by *Escherichia coli*. II. Enzymatic studies. *J. biol. Chem.*, 219, 189-201

Kreiser, W.R. & Martin, R.A., Jr (1978) High pressure liquid chromatographic determination of theobromine and caffeine in cocoa and chocolate products. *J. Assoc. off. anal. Chem.*, 61, 1424-1427

Kreiser, W.R. & Martin, R.A., Jr (1980) High pressure liquid chromatographic determination of theobromine and caffeine in cocoa and chocolate products: collaborative study. *J. Assoc. off. anal. Chem.*, 63, 591-594

Latini, R., Bonati, M., Gaspari, F., Traina, G.L., Jiritano, L., Bortolotti, A., Borzelleca, J.F., Tarka, S.M., Arnaud, M.J. & Garattini, S. (1984) II. Kinetics and metabolism of theobromine in male and female non-pregnant and pregnant rabbits. *Toxicology*, 30, 343-354

Levi, V., Jacobson, E.L. & Jacobson, M.K. (1978) Inhibition of poly(ADP-ribose)polymerase by methylated xanthines and cytokinins. *FEBS Lett.*, 88, 144-146

Martinek, R.G. & Wolman, W. (1955) Xanthines, tannins and sodium in coffee, tea and cocoa. *J. Am. med. Assoc.*, 158, 1030-1031

McCutheon, G.F. (1969) Caffeine. In: Snell, F.D. & Ettre, L.S., eds, *Encyclopedia of Industrial Chemical Analysis*, Vol. 8, New York, Interscience, pp. 55-71

Michl, H. & Haberler, F. (1954) Determination of purines in caffeine-containing drugs (Ger.). *Monatshefte Chem.*, 85, 779-795

Miller, G.E., Radulovic, L.L., Dewit, R.H., Brabec, M.J., Tarka, S.M. & Cornish, H.H. (1984) Comparative theobromine metabolism in five mammalian species. *Drug Metab. Disposition*, 12, 154-160

Mittler, S. & Mittler, J.E. (1968) Theobromine and theophylline and chromosome aberrations in *Drosophila melanogaster* (Abstract). *Genetics*, 60, 205

Moffat, A.C., ed. (1986) *Clarke's Isolation and Identification of Drugs*, 2nd ed., London, The Pharmaceutical Press, pp. 1010-1011

Morgan, W.F. & Cleaver, J.E. (1982) 3-Aminobenzamide synergistically increases sister-chromatid exchanges in cells exposed to methyl methanesulfonate but not to ultraviolet light. *Mutat. Res.*, 104, 361-366

Mourelatos, D., Dozi-Vassiliades, J. & Granitsas, A. (1982) Anti-tumour alkylating agents act synergistically with methylxanthines on induction of sister-chromatid exchange in human lymphocytes. *Mutat. Res.*, 104, 243-247

Mourelatos, D., Dozi-Vassiliades, J., Tsigalidou-Balla & Granitsas, A. (1983) Enhancement by methylxanthines of sister-chromatid exchange frequency induced by cytostatics in normal and leukemic human lymphocytes. *Mutat. Res.*, *121*, 147-152

Natarajan, A.T., Csukás, I. & van Zeeland, A.A. (1981) Contribution of incorporated 5-bromodeoxyuridine in DNA to the frequencies of sister-chromatid exchanges induced by inhibitors of poly-(ADP-ribose)-polymerase. *Mutat. Res.*, *84*, 125-132

National Research Council (1977) *Drinking Water and Health*, Washington DC, National Academy of Sciences

Nomura, T. (1983) Comparative inhibiting effects of methylxanthines on urethan-induced tumors, malformations, and presumed somatic mutations in mice. *Cancer Res.*, *43*, 1342-1346

Novick, A. (1956) Mutagens and antimutagens. *Brookhaven Symp. Biol.*, *8*, 201-214

Novick, A. & Szilard, L. (1951) Experiments in spontaneous and chemically induced mutations of bacteria growing in the chemostat. *Cold Spring Harbor Symp. quant. Biol.*, *16*, 337-343

Novick, A. & Szilard, L. (1952) Anti-mutagens. *Nature*, *170*, 926-927

Perry, D.L., Chuang, C.C., Jungclaus, G.A. & Warner, J.S. (1979) *Identification of Organic Compounds in Industrial Effluent Discharges* (EPA-600/4-79-016), Athens, GA, US Environmental Protection Agency

Rajaraman, R. & Faulkner, G. (1984) Reverse transformation of Chinese hamster ovary cells by methyl xanthines. *Exp. Cell Res.*, *154*, 342-356

Reid, S.J. & Good, T.J. (1982) Use of chromatographic mode sequencing for sample preparation in the analysis of caffeine and theobromine from beverages. *J. agric. Food Chem.*, *30*, 775-778

Renner, H.W. (1982) Sister chromatid exchanges induced by methylxanthines contained in coffee, tea and cocoa. *Experientia*, *38*, 600

Renner, H.W. & Münzner, R. (1982) Genotoxicity of cocoa examined by microbial and mammalian systems. *Mutat. Res.*, *103*, 275-281

Resman, B.H., Blumenthal, H.P. & Jusko, W.J. (1977) Breast milk distribution of theobromine from chocolate. *J. Pediatr.*, *91*, 477-480

Reynolds, J.E.F., ed. (1982) *Martindale. The Extra Pharmacopoeia*, 28th ed., London, The Pharmaceutical Press, pp. 348-349

Richardson, C.L., Grant, A.D. & Schulman, G.E. (1981) The interaction of caffeine and other xanthine analogs with DNA as measured by competitive fluorescence polarization (Abstract No. Ac-5). *Environ. Mutagenesis*, *3*, 343

Rosenkranz, H.S. & Ennever, F.K. (1987a) Evaluation of the genotoxicity of theobromine and caffeine. *Food chem. Toxicol.*, *25*, 247-251

Rosenkranz, H.S. & Ennever, F.K. (1987b) Genotoxicity and carcinogenicity assessment of caffeine and theobromine (Letter to the Editor). *Food chem. Toxicol.*, *25*, 795-796

Schack, J.A. & Waxler, S.H. (1949) An ultraviolet spectrophotometric method for the determination of theophylline and theobromine in blood and tissues. *J. Pharmacol. exp. Ther.*, *97*, 283-291

Senanayake, U.M. & Wijesekera, R.O.B. (1968a) Determination of the fat-free cocoa mass in chocolate products based on the theobromine and caffeine content. *Int. Chocolate Rev.*, 23, 214-217

Senanayake, U.M. & Wijesekera, R.O.B. (1968b) A rapid micro-method for the separation, identification and estimation of the purine bases: caffeine, theobromine and theophylline. *J. Chromatogr.*, 32, 75-86

Senanayake, U.M. & Wijesekera, R.O.B. (1971) Theobromine and caffeine content of the cocoa bean during its growth. *J. Sci. Food Agric.*, 22, 262-263

Shively, C.A. & Tarka, S.M., Jr (1983) Theobromine metabolism and pharmacokinetics in pregnant and nonpregnant Sprague-Dawley rats. *Toxicol. appl. Pharmacol.*, 67, 376-382

Shively, C.A. & Tarka, S.M., Jr (1984) Methylxanthine composition and consumption patterns of cocoa and chocolate products. In: Spiller, G.A., ed., *The Methylxanthine Beverages and Foods: Chemistry, Consumption, and Health Effects*, New York, Alan R. Liss, pp. 149-178

Shively, C.A. & Vesell, E.S. (1987) In vivo and in vitro biotransformation of theobromine by phenobarbital- and 3-methylcholanthrene-inducible cytochrome P-450 monooxygeneses in rat liver. Role of thiol compounds. *Drug Metab. Disposition*, 15, 217-224

Shively, C.A., White, D.M., Blauch, J.L. & Tarka, S.M., Jr (1984) Dominant lethal testing of theobromine in rats. *Toxicol. Lett.*, 20, 325-329

Shively, C.A., Tarka, S.M., Jr, Arnaud, M.J., Dvorchik, B.H., Passananti, G.T. & Vesell, E.S. (1985) High levels of methylxanthines in chocolate do not alter theobromine disposition. *Clin. pharmacol. Ther.*, 37, 415-424

Shively, C.A., White, D.M. & Tarka, S.M., Jr (1986) Diet-induced alterations in theobromine disposition and toxicity in the rat. *Toxicol. appl. Pharmacol.*, 84, 593-598

Sontag, G. & Kral, K. (1980) Determination of caffeine, theobromine and theophylline in tea, coffee, cocoa and beverages by HPLC with electrochemical detector (Ger.). *Mikrochim. Acta (Wien)*, II, 39-52

Spiller, M.A. (1984) The chemical components of coffee. In: Spiller, G.A., ed., *The Methylxanthine Beverages and Foods: Chemistry, Consumption, and Health Effects*, New York, Alan R. Liss, pp. 91-147

Stavric, B. (1988) Methyl xanthines: toxicity to humans. 3. Theobromine, paraxanthine and the combined effects of methylxanthines. *Food chem. Toxicol.*, 26, 725-733

Sturelid, S. & Kihlman, B.A. (1975) Enhancement by methylated oxypurines of the frequency of induced chromosomal aberrations. I. The dependence of the effect on the molecular structure of the potentiating agent. *Hereditas*, 79, 29-42

Tang-Liu, D.D.-S. & Riegelman, S. (1982) An automated HPLC assay for simultaneous quantitation of methylated xanthines and uric acids in urine. *J. chromatogr. Sci.*, 20, 155-159

Tarka, S.M., Jr (1982) The toxicology of cocoa and methylxanthines: a review of the literature. *Crit. Rev. Toxicol.*, 9, 275-312

Tarka, S.M., Jr & Shively, C.A. (1987) Methylxanthines. In: Miller, K., ed., *Toxicological Aspects of Food*, Amsterdam, Elsevier, pp. 373-423

Tarka, S.M., Jr & Zoumas, B.L. (1983) Subchronic and oral toxicity evaluation of cocoa powder and theobromine in Sprague-Dawley rat (Abstract). *Toxicologist*, *3*, 4

Tarka, S.M., Jr, Zoumas, B.L. & Gans, J.H. (1979) Short-term effects of graded levels of theobromine in laboratory rodents. *Toxicol. appl. Pharmacol.*, *49*, 127-149

Tarka, S.M., Jr, Zoumas, B.L. & Gans, J.H. (1981) Effects of continuous administration of dietary theobromine on rat testicular weight and morphology. *Toxicol. appl. Pharmacol.*, *58*, 76-82

Tarka, S.M., Jr, Arnaud, M.J., Dvorchik, B.H. & Vesell, E.S. (1983) Theobromine kinetics and metabolic disposition. *Clin. pharmacol. Ther.*, *34*, 546-555

Tarka, S.M., Jr, Applebaum, R.S. & Borzelleca, J.F. (1986a) Evaluation of the perinatal, postnatal and teratogenic effects of cocoa powder and theobromine in Sprague-Dawley/CD rats. *Food chem. Toxicol.*, *24*, 375-382

Tarka, S.M., Jr, Applebaum, R.S. & Borzelleca, J.F. (1986b) Evaluation of the teratogenic potential of cocoa powder and theobromine in New Zealand white rabbits. *Food chem. Toxicol.*, *24*, 363-374

Timbie, D.J., Sechrist, L. & Keeney, P.G. (1978) Application of high-pressure liquid chromatography to the study of variables affecting theobromine and caffeine concentrations in cocoa beans. *J. Food Sci.*, *43*, 560-565

Timson, J. (1975) Theobromine and theophylline. *Mutat. Res.*, *32*, 169-178

Timson, J. (1977) Caffeine. *Mutat. Res.*, *47*, 1-52

Traina, G.L. & Bonati, M. (1985) Pharmacokinetics of theobromine and its metabolites in rabbits. *J. Pharmacokinet. Biopharmacol.*, *13*, 41-53

Vergnes, M.F. & Alary, J. (1986) Determination of natural xanthines by HPLC (Fr.). *Talanta*, *33*, 997-1000

Weinstein, D., Mauer, I., Katz, M.L. & Kazmer, S. (1973) The effect of caffeine on chromosomes of human lymphocytes: a search for the mechanism of action. *Mutat. Res.*, *20*, 115-125

Weinstein, D., Mauer, I., Katz, M.L. & Kazmer, S. (1975) The effect of methylxanthines on chromosomes of human lymphocytes in culture. *Mutat. Res.*, *31*, 57-61

Wildanger, W. (1975) Separation of caffeine, theophylline and theobromine using high-pressure liquid chromatography (Ger.). *J. Chromatogr.*, *114*, 480-482

Windholz, M., ed. (1983) *The Merck Index*, 10th ed., Rahway, NJ, Merck & Co., p. 1327

Woollard, D.C. (1982) The determination of cocoa solids in milkpowder products using high performance liquid chromatography. *N.Z. J. Dairy Sci. Technol.*, *17*, 63-68

Zoumas, B.L., Kreiser, W.R. & Martin, R.A. (1980) Theobromine and caffeine content of chocolate products. *J. Food Sci.*, *45*, 314-316

METHYLGLYOXAL

1. Chemical and Physical Data

1.1 Synonyms

Chem. Abstr. Services Reg. No.: 78-98-8
Chem. Abstr. Name: 2-Oxopropanal
Synonyms: Acetylformaldehyde; 2-ketopropionaldehyde; pyruvaldehyde

1.2 Structural and molecular formulae and molecular weight

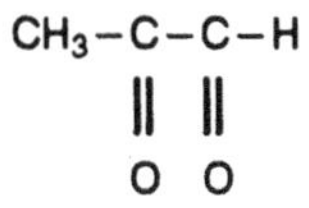

$$CH_3-\underset{\underset{O}{\|}}{C}-\underset{\underset{O}{\|}}{C}-H$$

$C_3H_4O_2$ Mol. wt: 72.06

1.3 Chemical and physical properties of the pure substance

From Windholz (1983)

(a) *Description*: Yellow liquid with pungent odour
(b) *Boiling-point*: 72°C
(c) *Density*: d^{24} 1.0455
(d) *Solubility*: Soluble in water, ethanol, diethyl ether and benzene
(e) *Reactivity*: Polymerizes very readily; hygroscopic

1.4 Technical products and impurities

No data were available to the Working Group.

2. Production, Use, Occurrence and Analysis

2.1 Production and use

(a) Production

Methylglyoxal is not produced commercially. It can be obtained by warming isonitrosoacetone with dilute sulfuric acid; by distilling a dilute solution of dihydroxyacetone from calcium carbonate (Windholz, 1983); by the catalytic dehydrogenation of glycerol (Baltes & Leupold, 1981); and by the oxidation of acetone with selenium dioxide (Musashino Chemical Research Institute Ltd, 1981).

(b) Use

No commercial use of methylglyoxal has been reported.

2.2 Occurrence

(a) Natural occurrence

Methylglyoxal has been identified as a metabolite during glycolysis (Kasai *et al.*, 1982) and as a sugar fragmentation product. It is one of the most highly reactive compounds in a browning reaction (Hodge, 1953). It is also formed by several bacteria of the human intestine (Baskaran *et al.*, 1989).

(b) Occupational exposure

No data on exposure levels were available to the Working Group.

(c) Air

Methylglyoxal has been reported to be a degradation product of toluene under simulated atmospheric conditions (Dumdei & O'Brien, 1984). It has been found in cigarette smoke at levels ranging from 5 to 60 µg per cigarette (Moree-Testa & Saint-Jalm, 1981).

(d) Water and sediments

Methylglyoxal has not been detected in US industrial effluents (Perry *et al.*, 1979) or in drinking-water (National Research Council, 1977).

(e) Food and beverages

Methylglyoxal has been detected in a broad range of commercial food products and beverages, including bread (Wiseblatt & Kohn, 1960; Nagao *et al.*, 1986a), toast

(Nagao et al., 1986a), tomatoes (Schormüller & Grosch, 1964), boiled potatoes (Kajita & Senda, 1972), caramelized sucrose (Lukesch, 1956), soya sauce and soya bean paste (Hayashi & Shibamato, 1985; Nagao et al., 1986a), roast turkey (Hrdlicka & Kuca, 1965), alcohol from sugar cane (Matsubara & Tamura, 1970), wine, saké, apple brandy and bourbon whiskey (Nagao et al., 1986a), apple, orange and tomato juices, maple syrup, beer, root-beer and cola, non-fat dry milk (Hayashi & Shibamato, 1985), instant, brewed and decaffeinated coffees (Kasai et al., 1982; Hayashi & Shibamato, 1985; Nagao et al., 1986a; Shane et al., 1988), and cocoa and instant tea (Hayashi & Shibamato, 1985). Table 1 summarizes the amounts of methylglyoxal determined in various foods and beverages (Nagao et al., 1986a) and Table 2 gives the amounts in foods and the calculated intake.

Table 1. Amounts of methylglyoxal found in various beverages and foods[a]

Beverage or food	Methylglyoxal (μg/ml)
Bourbon whiskey	1.5
Apple brandy	0.32
Wine	0.57
Japanese saké	0.26
Instant coffee[b]	1.6
Brewed coffee[c]	7.0
Black tea[d]	0.05
Green tea[e]	Trace
Soft drink	1.4
Bread	0.79 μg/g
Toast	2.5 μg/g
Soya sauce	8.7
Soya bean paste	5.1 μg/g

[a] From Nagao et al. (1986a)
[b] Prepared by dissolving 1.5 g coffee powder in 100 ml water
[c] Prepared from 10 g ground coffee beans and 150 ml boiling water
[d] Prepared from 4 g tea leaves and 100 ml boiling water
[e] Prepared from 5 g tea leaves and 20 ml hot water

Table 2. Methylglyoxal in foods and calculated amounts of methylglyoxal intake for each food when consumed[a]

Beverage or food	Amount of item per serving	Methylglyoxal (μg/g)	Methylglyoxal intake per serving (μg)
Brewed coffee	3 g/180 ml	25	75.6
Decaffeinated brewed coffee	3 g/180 ml	47	140.4
Instant coffee	1 g/180 ml	23	22.7
Cocoa	4 g/180 ml	1.2	4.9
Instant tea	0.3 g/180 ml	2.4	0.7
Nonfat dry milk	22.7 g/240 ml	1.4	31.2
Soya sauce A	Not calculated	3-7.6	-
Soya bean paste (Miso)	Not calculated	0.7	-
Cola	354 ml/can	0.23	81.4
Root beer	354 ml/can	0.76	269.0
Beer	355 ml/can	0.08	29.7
Wine (white)	100 ml/glass	0.11	11.0
Apple juice	300 ml/glass	0.26	78.0
Orange juice	354 ml/can	0.04	14.2
Tomato juice	177 ml/can	0.06	11.3
Maple syrup	Not calculated	2.5	-

[a]From Hayashi & Shibamato (1985)

Among the various beverages, coffee contains the largest amount of methylglyoxal (Hayashi & Shibamato, 1985; Nagao et al., 1986a), with a daily intake resulting from the consumption of two to three cups of coffee per day calculated as 1 mg. The content of methylglyoxal in soya sauce (8.7 μg/ml) was comparable to that of brewed coffee (7.0 μg/ml), but the average daily per-caput intake of soya sauce in Japan is 30 ml (Nagao et al., 1986a). In an examination of nine brands of coffee, the concentration of methylglyoxal was highest in roasted instant coffees compared to filtered and to decaffeinated instant and filtered coffees. The mean concentration of methylglyoxal in filtered coffees was 319 μg/g, whereas that in instant coffees was 731 μg/g (Shane et al., 1988). These results are at variance with those of earlier studies in which one cup of instant coffee (1 g/100 ml) contained 100-150 μg methylglyoxal, whereas one cup of coffee prepared from ground coffee beans (8 g/100 ml) contained 470-730 μg methylglyoxal (Kasai et al., 1982). Aeschbacher et al. (1989) also determined the amounts of methylglyoxal in brewed coffee and instant coffees (Table 3).

Table 3. Contents of methylglyoxal in coffee

Reference	Methylglyoxal	
	In roasted coffee	In brewed coffee
Kasai et al. (1982)	[58-75 μg/g]	470-730 μg/cup[a]
Hayashi & Shibamato (1985)	25 μg/g	76 μg/cup[b]
Nagao et al. (1986a)	NA	7 μg/ml[c]
Shane et al. (1988)	NA	273-341 μg/g (filtered)[d]
Aeschbacher et al. (1989)	[21-39 μg/g][e]	106-197 μg/g[f]

[a] In a brew using 8 g roasted coffee per 100 ml water
[b] In a brew using 3 g roasted coffee per 180 ml water
[c] In a brew using 10 g roasted coffee per 150 ml water
[d] In a brew containing 25 g roasted coffee per 250 ml water
[e] Calculated assuming extraction yield of 20% of dry soluble solids in the brew
[f] μg/g dried product (brew, 1 g roasted coffee per 10 ml water)
NA, not available

Methylgyoxal has been determined in bread at 0.5 ppm (mg/kg) (Borovikova & Reuter, 1971) and in beer at 0.03-11 ppm (mg/l) (Palamand et al., 1970; Wheeler et al., 1971).

2.3 Analysis

Trace quantities of methylglyoxal have been determined by derivatization with cysteamine to yield 2-acetylthiazolidine in a food or beverage sample at pH 6, then extraction with dichloromethane and analysis by gas chromatography (Hayashi & Shibamato, 1985). Methylglyoxal has been determined in coffee (Kasai et al., 1982; Shane et al., 1988) and in cigarette smoke (Moree-Testa & Saint-Jalm, 1981) as the 2-methylquinoxaline derivative by gas chromatography (Kasai et al., 1982), gas chromatography-mass spectrometry (Shane et al., 1988) or high-performance liquid chromatography (Moree-Testa & Saint-Jalm, 1981) following its initial reaction with ortho-phenylenediamine. Methylglyoxal was determined in biological tissues with the fluorescent 2-(2-benzimidiazolyl)-3-methylquinoxaline following separation by high-performance liquid chromatography; the detection limit was 48.4 pmol per 30-μl sample (Matsuura et al., 1985).

3. Biological Data Relevant to the Evaluation of Carcinogenic Risk to Humans

3.1 Carcinogenicity studies in animals

(a) *Oral administration*

Rat: In a study reported as an abstract, 40 male Fischer 344 rats were administered 0.5% methylglyoxal in deionized water as drinking-water for life (854 days; average daily intake, 7.7 mg per rat); 40 controls received deionized water alone. The average body weight of the treated rats was 15% lower than that of the controls. No tumour was found that could be ascribed to administration of methylglyoxal (Fujita *et al.*, 1986).

(b) *Subcutaneous administration*

Rat: Groups of ten male and ten female Fischer 344 rats, eight weeks of age, received subcutaneous injections of 0 or 1.3 mg methylglyoxal solution neutralized with sodium hydroxide (purity, 65.6%; the impurity 'might have been' pyruvic acid) in 0.2 ml saline twice a week for ten weeks. A group of 20 controls received saline solution for ten weeks. After 70 weeks, subcutaneous tumours [type unspecified] were found in two treated animals, but none were seen in controls (Takayama *et al.*, 1984). [The Working Group noted the impurity of the test solution and the limited reporting of the experiment.]

Groups of eight male and ten female Fischer 344 rats [age unspecified] received subcutaneous injections of 2 mg methylglyoxal (unpurified) in 0.2 ml saline twice a week for ten weeks. A control group of 21 males and 19 females received saline only. After 20 months, four of the treated rats (three males and one female) developed malignant tumours (fibrosarcomas) at the injection site, whereas no tumour was seen in controls (Nagao *et al.*, 1986a,b). [The Working Group noted the impurity of the test solution].

(c) *Modifying effects on the activity of known carcinogens*

N-*Methyl*-N'-*nitro*-N-*nitrosoguanidine*: Groups of 30 male Wistar *rats*, seven weeks of age, were administered 100 mg/l N-methyl-N'-nitro-N-nitrosoguanidine in the drinking-water and were simultaneously fed a diet supplemented with 10% sodium chloride for eight weeks; they were then returned to basal diet and maintained on drinking-water containing no additive (controls) or 0.25%

methylglyoxal [purity unspecified] for 32 weeks. Animals were killed at week 40. Methylglyoxal caused a significant increase in the incidence of hyperplasia induced by the nitrosamine but did not enhance the incidence of gastric adenocarcinomas (Takahashi *et al.*, 1989).

3.2 Other relevant data

(a) Experimental systems

(i) *Absorption, distribution, excretion and metabolism*

No experiment on the metabolism or tissue distribution of methylglyoxal after oral ingestion in animals or man has been reported (Arnaud, 1988). The biosynthesis and degradation of methylglyoxal in animals has been reviewed (Ohmori *et al.*, 1989). There is still uncertainty about the biochemistry of methylglyoxal in animals, owing to the difficulty of determining it in biological tissues, which is due to the active glyoxalase system (Brandt & Siegel, 1979).

Facultative, strictly anaerobic bacteria present in the human gut were shown to produce (and may be one of the most important sources of) methylglyoxal. Several groups of bacteria from human faeces produced methylglyoxal *in vitro* (Baskaran *et al.*, 1989).

Methylglyoxal can be formed from acetoacetate and carbohydrates in glycolysing tissues and from triose phosphates by nonenzymatic processes (Ohmori *et al.*, 1989). An enzyme fraction that specifically catalyses the formation of methylglyoxal from dihydroxyacetone phosphate has been isolated from goat liver (Ray & Ray, 1981). Amine oxidase from goat plasma was shown to catalyse the oxidation of aminoacetone to methylglyoxal (Ray & Ray, 1983). Methylglyoxal has been measured at levels of micrograms per gram in the liver and skeletal muscle of normal and diabetic rats (Ohmori *et al.*, 1989). Methylglyoxal was shown to be present in liver noncovalently bound to protein (Fodor *et al.*, 1978). The biosynthetic routes of methylglyoxal are shown in Figure 1 (Ohmori *et al.*, 1989).

Methylglyoxal can be detoxified by the glyoxalase system present in mammalian intestinal mucosa (Baskaran & Balasubramanian, 1987), and it is converted into D-lactic acid (Neuberg, 1913). Hepatocytes convert methylglyoxal to pyruvate (Ray & Ray, 1982) and to glucose and L-lactate (Sáez *et al.*, 1985).

(ii) *Toxic effects*

The average acute oral LD_{50}s of methylglyoxal in rats were 531 mg/kg bw in newborn, between 1165 and 1623 mg/kg bw in females depending on age and/or stage of pregnancy and 1990 mg/kg bw in adult males (Peters *et al.*, 1978).

The effects of pre- (initiation) and post-treatment (promotion) with methylglyoxal (0.05 or 0.2% in drinking-water) on the induction of γ-glutamyl-

450   IARC MONOGRAPHS VOLUME 51

Fig. 1. Biosynthesis of methylglyoxal

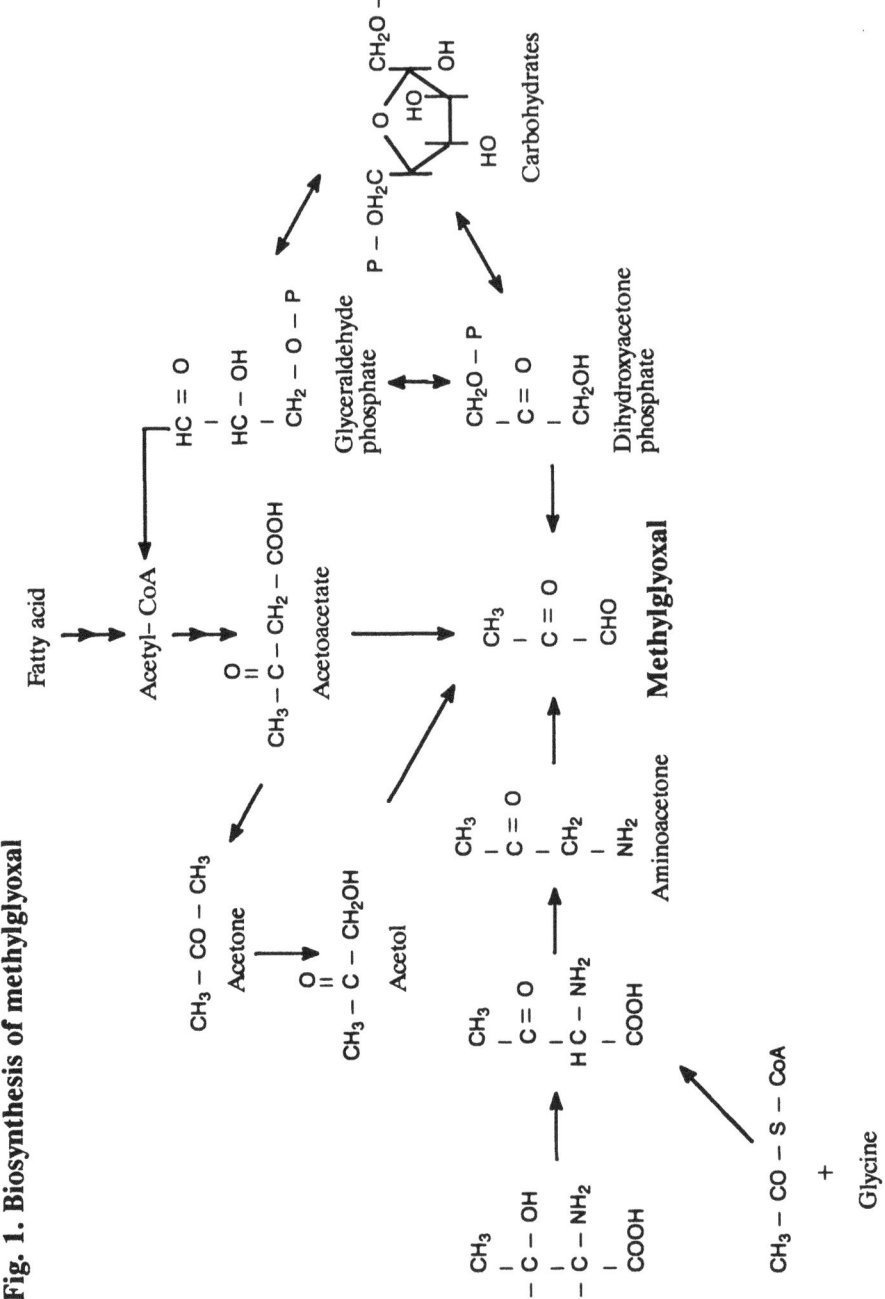

transpeptidase-positive foci in the livers were studied in Fischer 344 rats (weighing 150-200 g; five to six animals per group). Foci were induced in dose-related amounts both in the absence and presence of initiation with 0.02% 2-acetylaminofluorene in the diet (Martelli *et al.*, 1988). [The Working Group noted the limited number of animals used.]

Intraperitoneal treatment of mice with methylglyoxal at 600 mg/kg bw enhanced aminopyrine *N*-demethylase and *para*-nitroanisole-*O*-demethylase activities, while ethoxycoumarin -*O*-deethylase activity and total cytochrome P450 content was only weakly increased (Bronzetti *et al.*, 1987). Administration of 300-600 mg/kg bw by gastric intubation to male Fisher 344 rats induced a 100-fold increase in ornithine decarboxylase activity within 7 h, a 26-fold increase in DNA synthesis within 16 h and a 16-fold increase in the labelling index of S-phase cells within 16 h in the glandular stomach mucosa (Furihata *et al.*, 1985).

(iii) *Effects on reproduction and prenatal toxicity*

While no data on reproductive or developmental toxicity were available to the Working Group, available information on acute toxicity suggests that neonates are more sensitive to methylglyoxal than adult male rats (Peters *et al.*, 1978).

(iv) *Genetic and related effects*

The results described below are listed in Table 4 on p. 453, with the evaluation of the Working Group, as positive, negative or inconclusive, as defined in the footnotes. The results are tabulated separately for the presence and absence of an exogenous metabolic system. The lowest effective dose (LED), in the case of positive results, or the highest ineffective dose (HID), in the case of negative results, are shown, together with the appropriate reference. The studies are summarized briefly below.

Methylglyoxal induced mutations in *Salmonella typhimurium* strains containing the pKM101 plasmid and in *Escherichia coli* WP2 *uvrA* and WP2 *uvrA* (pKM101). Mutagenicity in *S. typhimurium* was partially dependent upon the pKM101 plasmid and *uvrB* deletion, as shown by comparing the responses between TA104 and TA2659 and between TA104 and TA2638, respectively (Marnett *et al.*, 1985). Methylglyoxal was also active in the forward mutation ara^R test in *S. typhimurium*. Mutagenicity in *S. typhimurium* reversion tests was suppressed by sulfite, glutathione, dithiothreitol (Nagao *et al.*, 1984, 1986b) and cysteine, but not by catalase (Fujita *et al.*, 1985). There is no evidence for the formation of a stable conjugate of methylglyoxal with cysteine, the most active of the thiol inhibitors of mutagenic activity (Nagao *et al.*, 1986b).

In *Saccharomyces cerevisiae* (strain D7), methylglyoxal induced gene conversions and reverse mutations. An exogenous metabolic system reduced the effects (Bronzetti *et al.*, 1987).

In cultured mammalian cells, methylglyoxal induced mutations, sister chromatid exchange and (on the basis of alkaline elution and sensitivity to proteinase K) reparable DNA-protein cross-links (Brambilla *et al.*, 1985).

In cultured human lymphocytes, methylglyoxal induced sister chromatid exchange, chromosomal aberrations and micronuclei.

Unscheduled DNA synthesis appeared to be induced in the pyloric mucosa of rats, but only a small proportion of the tritiated thymidine incorporation was not inhibited by hydroxyurea during simultaneous S-phase stimulation by methylglyoxal, making interpretation difficult (Furihata *et al.*, 1985).

A single oral administration of methylgloxal induced neither sister chromatid exchange nor chromosomal aberrations in the ileum of mice.

Combined with hydrogen peroxide in the quantities typically found in a solution of 15 mg instant coffee, methylglyoxal was significantly mutagenic, whereas the individual components (5 μg hydrogen peroxide, 1.5 μg methylglyoxal) had only minor effects (Nagao *et al.*, 1986a). Synergism with hydrogen peroxide was also demonstrated in the ara^R test (Ariza *et al.*, 1988), which the authors suggested was due to inefficient detoxification of methylglyoxal in cells depleted of reduced glutathione (Meister & Anderson, 1983; Alonso-Moraga *et al.*, 1987) by hydrogen peroxide (Smith *et al.*, 1984). This explanation is in agreement with the fact that the addition of glyoxalase I and II together with reduced glutathione abolished the mutagenic activity of methylglyoxal and reduced the mutagenicity of instant coffee (20 mg/plate) by approximately 80% in the Ames test (Friederich *et al.*, 1985). Antimutagenic activity of methylglyoxal was seen against heterocyclic amines, such as Trp-P-1, Trp-P-2, Glu-P-1, Glu-P-2 and IQ, in *S. typhimurium* TA98 (Kim *et al.*, 1987).

In *E. coli*, methylglyoxal inhibited protein synthesis and interfered with cell population growth (Fraval & McBrien, 1980). Interaction of methylglyoxal with guanosine triphosphate (Krymkiewicz *et al.*, 1971) and with DNA and RNA has been reported (Krymkiewicz, 1973). An N^2-alkylguanine has been identified from the reaction of methylglyoxal with guanine; glyoxal undergoes a similar reaction (Shapiro *et al.*, 1969).

(*b*) *Humans*

No data were available to the Working Group.

3.3 Case reports and epidemiological studies of carcinogenicity to humans

No data were available to the Working Group.

Table 4. Genetic and related effects of methylglyoxal

Test system	Results without exogenous metabolic activation	Results with exogenous metabolic activation	Dose LED/HID	Reference
SAF, Salmonella typhimurium BA13, forward mutation (ara^R)	+	0	140.0000	Ariza et al. (1988)
SA0, Salmonella typhimurium TA100, reverse mutation	+	(+)	5.0000	Kasai et al. (1982)
SA0, Salmonella typhimurium TA100, reverse mutation	+	0	5.0000	Yamaguchi (1982)
SA0, Salmonella typhimurium TA100, reverse mutation	+	0	5.0000	Fujita et al. (1985)
SA0, Salmonella typhimurium TA100, reverse mutation	+	0	40.0000	Kim et al. (1987)
SA2, Salmonella typhimurium TA102, reverse mutation	+	0	0.0000	Nagao et al. (1986b)
SA2, Salmonella typhimurium TA102, reverse mutation	+	+	30.0000	Bronzetti et al. (1987)
SA2, Salmonella typhimurium TA102, reverse mutation	+	+	2.2500	Migliore et al. (1990)
SA4, Salmonella typhimurium TA104, reverse mutation	+	0	5.0000	Marnett et al. (1985)
SA4, Salmonella typhimurium TA104, reverse mutation	+	0	0.0000	Nagao et al. (1986b)
SA4, Salmonella typhimurium TA104, reverse mutation	+	0	1.2500	Migliore et al. (1990)
SA5, Salmonella typhimurium TA1535, reverse mutation	–	0	0.0000	Nagao et al. (1986a)
SA8, Salmonella typhimurium TA1538, reverse mutation	+	0	0.0000	Nagao et al. (1986a)
SA9, Salmonella typhimurium TA98, reverse mutation	(+)	0	0.0000	Nagao et al. (1986b)
SAS, Salmonella typhimurium TA2638, reverse mutation	+	0	25.0000	Marnett et al. (1985)
SAS, Salmonella typhimurium TA2659, reverse mutation	+	0	25.0000	Marnett et al. (1985)
SAS, Salmonella typhimurium TA97, reverse mutation	+	+	115.0000	Bronzetti et al. (1987)
ECW, Escherichia coli WP2 uvrA, reverse mutation	+	0	0.0000	Kasai et al. (1982)
ECR, Escherichia coli WP2 uvrA pKM101, reverse mutation	+	0	0.0000	Kasai et al. (1982)
SCG, Saccharomyces cerevisiae, mitotic gene conversion	+	0	1000.0000	Nagao et al. (1986b)
SCG, Saccharomyces cerevisiae, mitotic gene conversion	+	(+)	1100.0000	Bronzetti et al. (1987)
SCR, Saccharomyces cerevisiae, reverse mutation	+	–	1100.0000	Bronzetti et al. (1987)
GCL, Gene mutation, Chinese hamster lung (CHL) cells, DTr	+	0	30.0000	Nakasato et al. (1984)
G9H, Gene mutation, Chinese hamster V79 cells, 6-thioguanine resistance	+	+	36.0000	Cajelli et al. (1987)
SIC, Sister chromatid exchange, Chinese hamster ovary cells	+	0	7.0000	Faggin et al. (1985)
SHL, Sister chromatid exchange, human lymphocytes in vitro	+	–	110.0000	Migliore et al. (1990)
MIH, Micronucleus test, human lymphocytes in vitro	+	–	110.0000	Migliore et al. (1990)
CHL, Chromosomal aberrations, human lymphocytes in vitro	+	0	110.0000	Migliore et al. (1990)
SVA, Sister chromatid exchange, Swiss mouse ileum	–	0	600.0000 oral	Migliore et al. (1990)
CVA, Chromosomal aberrations, Swiss mouse ileum	–	0	600.0000 oral	Migliore et al. (1990)
DIA, DNA cross-links, Chinese hamster ovary cells	+	–	100.0000	Brambilla et al. (1985)

oral, by gavage

4. Summary of Data Reported and Evaluation

4.1 Exposure data

Methylglyoxal is present in many foods and drinks, including coffee, and is produced during glycolysis and sugar fermentation. It is produced by many strains of bacteria present in the intestinal tract. It is also present in tobacco smoke.

4.2 Experimental carcinogenicity data

No adequate study was available for the evaluation of methylglyoxal.

4.3 Human carcinogenicity data

No data were available to the Working Group.

4.4 Other relevant data

Methylglyoxal induced sister chromatid exchange, chromosomal aberrations and micronuclei in cultured human cells. It induced sister chromatid exchange and gene mutations in cultured mammalian cells. In yeast, it increased the frequencies of reverse mutations and of mitotic gene conversion. In prokaryotes, methylglyoxal was mutagenic in the absence of an exogenous metabolic system. Methylglyoxal forms adducts with guanine bases and nucleic acids.

4.5 Evaluation[1]

There are no data on the carcinogenicity in humans of methylglyoxal.

There is *inadequate evidence* in experimental animals for the carcinogenicity of methylglyoxal.

Overall evaluation

Methylglyoxal is *not classifiable as to its carcinogenicity to humans (Group 3)*.

5. References

Aeschbacher, H.U., Wolleb, U., Löliger, J., Spadone, J.C. & Liardon, R. (1989) Contribution of coffee aroma constituents to the mutagenicity of coffee. *Food chem. Toxicol.*, 27, 227-232

---

[1]For definition of the italicized terms, see Preamble, pp. 27-31.

Alonso-Moraga, A., Bocanegra, A., Torres, J.M., López-Barea, J. & Pueyo, C. (1987) Glutathione status and sensitivity to GSH-reacting compounds of *Escherichia coli* strains deficient in glutathione metabolism and/or catalase activity. *Mol. cell. Biochem.*, 73, 61-68

Ariza, R.R., Dorado, G., Barbancho, M. & Pueyo, C. (1988) Study of the causes of direct-acting mutagenicity in coffee and tea using the Ara test in *Salmonella typhimurium*. *Mutat. Res.*, 201, 89-96

Arnaud, M.J. (1988) The metabolism of coffee constituents. In Clarke, R.J. & Macrae, R., eds, *Coffee*, Vol. 3, *Physiology*, London, Elsevier Applied Science, pp. 33-55

Baltes, H. & Leupold, E.I. (1981) *Methylglyoxal*, German Patent 2,927,524 (Hoechst A.-G.) [*Chem. Abstr.*, 94, 139222h]

Baskaran, S. & Balasubramanian, K.A. (1987) Purification and active site modification studies on glyoxalase-I from monkey intestinal mucosa. *Biochim. biophys. Acta*, 913, 377-385

Baskaran, S., Prasanna Rajan, D. & Balasubramanian, K.A. (1989) Formation of methylglyoxal by bacteria isolated from human faeces. *J. med. Microbiol.*, 28, 211-215

Borovikova, L.A. & Reuter, I.M. (1971) Influence of duration of cooking on content of carbonic compounds in bread (Russ.). *Chlebopekarnaja Konditersk. Prom.*, 15, 5-7

Brambilla, G., Sciabà, L., Faggin, P., Finollo, R., Bassi, A.M., Ferro, M. & Marinari, U.M. (1985) Methylglyoxal-induced DNA-protein cross-links and cytotoxicity in Chinese hamster ovary cells. *Carcinogenesis*, 5, 683-686

Brandt, R.B. & Siegel, S.A. (1979) Methylglyoxal production in human blood. *Ciba Found. Symp.*, 67, 211-223

Bronzetti, G., Corsi, C., Del Chiaro, D., Boccardo, P., Vellosi, R., Rossi, F., Paolini, M. & Cantelli Forti, G. (1987) Methylglyoxal: genotoxicity studies and its effect *in vivo* on the hepatic microsomal mono-oxygenase system of the mouse. *Mutagenesis*, 2, 275-277

Cajelli, E., Canonero, R., Martelli, A. & Brambilla, G. (1987) Methylglyoxal-induced mutation to 6-thioguanine resistance in V79 cells. *Mutat. Res.*, 190, 47-50

Dumdei, B.E. & O'Brien, R.J. (1984) Toluene degradation products in simulated atmospheric conditions. *Nature*, 311, 248-250

Faggin, P., Bassi, A.M., Finollo, R. & Brambilla, G. (1985) Induction of sister-chromatid exchanges in Chinese hamster ovary cells by the biotic ketoaldehyde methylglyoxal. *Mutat. Res.*, 144, 189-191

Fodor, G., Mujumdar, R. & Szent-Gyorgyi, A. (1978) Isolation of methylglyoxal from liver. *Proc. natl Acad. Sci. USA*, 75, 4317-4319

Fraval, H.N.A. & McBrien, D.C.H. (1980) The effect of methylglyoxal on cell division and the synthesis of protein and DNA in synchronous and asynchronous cultures of *Escherichia coli* B/r. *J. gen. Microbiol.*, 117, 127-134

Friederich, U., Hann, D., Albertini, S., Schlatter, C. & Würgler, F.E. (1985) Mutagenicity studies on coffee. The influence of different factors on the mutagenic activity in the *Salmonella*/mammalian microsome assay. *Mutat. Res.*, 156, 39-52

Fujita, Y., Wakabayashi, K., Nagao, M. & Sugimura, T. (1985) Characteristics of major mutagenicity of instant coffee. *Mutat. Res.*, 142, 145-148

Fujita, Y., Wakabayashi, K., Ohgaki, H., Nagao, M. & Sugimura, T. (1986) Absence of carcinogenicity of methylglyoxal in F344 rats by oral administration (Abstract). *Proc. ann. Mtg Jpn. Cancer Assoc.*, *45*, 64

Furihata, C., Sato, Y., Matsushima, T. & Tatematsu, M. (1985) Induction of ornithine decarboxylase and DNA synthesis in rat stomach mucosa by methylglyoxal. *Carcinogenesis*, *6*, 91-94

Hayashi, T. & Shibamato, T. (1985) Analysis of methylglyoxal in foods and beverages. *J. agric. Food Chem.*, *33*, 1090-1093

Hodge, J.E. (1953) Dehydrated foods. Chemistry of browning reactions in model systems. *J. agric. Food Chem.*, *1*, 928-943

Hrdlicka, J. & Kuca, J. (1965) The changes of carbonyl compounds in the heat-processing of meat. 2. Turkey meat. *Poult. Sci.*, *44*, 27-31

Kajita, T. & Senda, M. (1972) Simultaneous determination of L-ascorbic acid, triose reductone and their related compounds in foods by polarographic method (Jpn.). *Nippon Nogei Kagaku Kaishi*, *972*, 137-145

Kasai, H., Kumeno, K., Yamaizumi, Z., Nishimura, S., Nagao, M., Fujita, Y., Sugimura, T., Nukaya, H. & Kosuge, T. (1982) Mutagenicity of methylglyoxal in coffee. *Gann*, *73*, 681-683

Kim, S.B., Hayase, F. & Kato, H. (1987) Desmutagenic effects of alpha-dicarbonyl and alpha-hydroxycarbonyl compounds against mutagenic heterocyclic amines. *Mutat. Res.*, *177*, 9-15

Krymkiewicz, N. (1973) Reactions of methylglyoxal with nucleic acids. *FEBS Lett.*, *29*, 51-54

Krymkiewicz, N., Diéguez, E., Rekarte, U.D. & Zwaig, N. (1971) Properties and mode of action of a bactericidal compound (= methylglyoxal) produced by a mutant of *Escherichia coli*. *J. Bacteriol.*, *108*, 1338-1347

Lukesch, H. (1956) Decomposition products of caramelized saccharose (Ger.). *Naturwissenschaften*, *43*, 108-109

Marnett, L.J., Hurd, H.K., Hollstein, M.C., Levin, D.E., Esterbauer, H. & Ames, B.N. (1985) Naturally occurring carbonyl compounds are mutagens in *Salmonella* tester strain TA104. *Mutat. Res.*, *148*, 25-34

Martelli, A., Ghia, M., Mereto, E., Marinari, U.M. & Brambilla, G. (1988) Induction and promotion of γ-glutamyltranspeptidase-positive foci in the rat liver by methylglyoxal. *Jpn. J. Cancer Res. (Gann)*, *79*, 666-669

Matsubara, I. & Tamura, K. (1970) Trace constituents in alcohol. III. Identification of low boiling point carbonyl compounds (Jpn.). *Hakko Kyokaishi*, *28*, 89-94

Matsuura, T., Yoshino, K., Ooki, E., Saito, S., Ooishi, E. & Tomita, I. (1985) Studies on methylglyoxal. 1. Fluorometric determination of methylglyoxal using high-performance liquid chromatography. *Chem. pharm. Bull.*, *33*, 3567-3570

Meister, A. & Anderson, M.E. (1983) Glutathione. *Ann. Rev. Biochem.*, *52*, 711-760

Migliori, L., Barale, R., Basco, E., Giorgelli, F., Minunni, M., Scarpato, R. & Loprieno, N. (1990) Genotoxicity of methylglyoxal: cytogenetic damage in human lymphocytes *in vitro* and in intestinal cells of mice. *Carcinogenesis*, *11*, 1503-1507

Moree-Testa, P. & Saint-Jalm, Y. (1981) Determination of α-dicarbonyl compounds in cigarette smoke. *J. Chromatogr.*, *217*, 197-208

Musashino Chemical Research Institute Ltd (1981) *Methylgloxal*, Japanese Patent 81 40632, 16 April 1981, Appl. 79/116,065

Nagao, M., Suwa, Y., Yoshizumi, H. & Sugimura, T. (1984) Mutagens in coffee. In: MacMahon, B. & Sugimura, T., eds, *Coffee and Health* (Banbury Report 17), Cold Spring Harbor, NY, CSH Press, pp. 69-77

Nagao, M., Fujita, Y., Wakabayashi, K., Nukaya, H., Kosuge, T. & Sugimura, T. (1986a) Mutagens in coffee and other beverages. *Environ. Health Perspect.*, *67*, 89-91

Nagao, M., Fujita, Y., Sugimura, T. & Kosuge, T. (1986b) Methylglyoxal in beverages and foods: its mutagenicity and carcinogenicity. In: Singer, B. & Bartsch, H., eds, *The Role of Cyclic Nucleic Acid Adducts in Carcinogenesis and Mutagenesis* (IARC Scientific Publications No. 70), Lyon, IARC, pp. 283-291

Nakasato, F., Nakayasu, M., Fujita, Y., Nagao, M., Terada, M. & Sugimura, T. (1984) Mutagenicity of instant coffee on cultured Chinese hamster lung cells. *Mutat. Res.*, *141*, 109-112

National Research Council (1977) *Drinking Water and Health*, Washington DC, National Academy of Sciences

Neuberg, C. (1913) New studies on biochemical transformation of methylglyoxal in lactic acid as well as observations on the formation of various lactic acids in nature (Ger.). *Biochem. Z.*, *51*, 484-508

Ohmori, S., Mori, M., Shiraha, K. & Kawase, M. (1989) Biosynthesis and degradation of methylglyoxal in animals. *Progr. clin. biol. Res.*, *290*, 397-412

Palamand, S.R., Nelson, G.D. & Hardwich, W.A. (1970) Some vicinal dicarbonyl compounds in beer and their influence on beer flavor. *Tech. Q. Master Brew. Assoc. Am.*, *7*, 111-115

Perry, D.L., Chuang, C.C., Jungclaus, G.A. & Warner, J.S. (1979) *Identification of Organic Compounds in Industrial Effluent Discharges* (EPA-600/4-79-016), Athens, GA, US Environmental Protection Agency, Environmental Research Laboratory

Peters, M.A., Hudson, P.M. & Jurgelske, W., Jr (1978) The acute toxicity of methylglyoxal in rats: the influence of age, sex, and pregnancy. *Ecotoxicol. environ. Saf.*, *2*, 369-374

Ray, S. & Ray, M. (1981) Isolation of methylglyoxal synthase from goat liver. *J. biol. Chem.*, *256*, 6230-6233

Ray, S. & Ray, M. (1982) Purification and characterization of NAD and NADP-linked α-ketoaldehyde dehydrogenases involved in catalyzing the oxidation of methylglyoxal to pyruvate. *J. biol. Chem.*, *257*, 10566-10570

Ray, S. & Ray, M. (1983) Formation of methylglyoxal from aminoacetone by amine oxidase from goat plasma. *J. biol. Chem.*, *258*, 3461-3462

Sáez, G.T., Blay, P., Viña, J.R. & Viña, J. (1985) Glucose formation from methylglyoxal in rat hepatocytes. *Biochem. Soc. Trans.*, *13*, 945-946

Schormüller, J. & Grosch, W. (1964) Study of aromatic compounds in foodstuffs. II. Occurrence of new carbonyl compounds in tomatoes (Ger.). *Lebensmittel. Untersuch-Forsch.*, *126*, 38-49

Shane, B.S., Troxclair, A.M., McMillin, D.J. & Henry, C.B. (1988) Comparative mutagenicity of nine brands of coffee to *Salmonella typhimurium* TA100, TA102 and TA104. *Environ. mol. Mutagenesis*, *11*, 195-206 (corrigendum, p. 553)

Shapiro, R., Cohen, B.I., Shiuey, S. & Maurer, H. (1969) On the reaction of guanine with glyoxal, pyruvaldehyde, and kethoxal, and the structure of acylguanines. A new synthesis of N2-alkylguanines. *Biochemistry*, *8*, 238-245

Smith, I.K., Kendall, A.C., Keys, A.J., Turner, J.C. & Lea, P.J. (1984) Increased level of glutathione in a catalase-deficient mutant of barley (*Hordeum vulgare* L.). *Plant Sci. Lett.*, *37*, 29-33

Takahashi, M., Okamiya, H., Furukawa, F., Toyoda, K., Sato, H., Imaida, K. & Hayashi, Y. (1989) Effects of glyoxal and methylglyoxal administration on gastric carcinogenesis in Wistar rats after initiation with N-methyl-N'-nitro-N-nitrosoguanidine. *Carcinogenesis*, *10*, 1925-1927

Takayama, S., Nagao, M., Suwa, Y. & Sugimura, T. (1984) Long-term carcinogenicity studies on caffeine, instant coffee, and methylglyoxal in rats. In: MacMahon, B. & Sugimura, T., eds, *Coffee and Health* (Banbury Report 17), Cold Spring Harbor, NY, CSH Press, pp. 99-106

Wheeler, R.E., Pragnell, M.J. & Pierce, J.S. (1971) The identification of factors affecting flavour stability in beer. *Eur. Brew. Conv.*, *13*, 423-436

Windholz, M., ed. (1983) *The Merck Index*, 10th ed., Rahway, NJ, Merck & Co., pp. 1157

Wiseblatt, L. & Kohn, F.E. (1960) Some volatile aromatic compounds in fresh bread. *Cereal Chem.*, *37*, 55-66

Yamaguchi, T. (1982) Mutagenicity of trioses and methylglyoxal on *Salmonella typhimurium*. *Agric. biol. Chem.*, *46*, 849-851

GLOSSARY

Baking chocolate	See *chocolate liquor*
Bittersweet chocolate	See *sweet chocolate*
Boiled coffee	Brewed prepared by boiling coarsely ground, lightly roasted coffee (50-70 g/l) in water (for 10 min or more); the infusion is consumed without separation of grounds (1 cup = 150-190 ml). Drunk particularly in the northern part of the Nordic countries
Cacao	The terms *cacao* and *cocoa* are often used interchangeably; the term *cacao* is generally reserved for botanical contexts
Chocolate liquor	Also called *chocolate mass* (in Europe); a solid or semi-plastic food prepared by finely grinding the nib of the cacao bean; also called *baking* or *cooking chocolate*; the initial material from which all chocolate products are produced
Chocolate mass	See *chocolate liquor*
Cocoa	The tropical tree from which *cocoa powder* and chocolate are derived. Cocoa trees are of the family Sterculiaceae, generally *Theobroma cacao*, rarely *T. pentagona* or *T. spherocarpa*.
Cocoa butter	Pure fat extracted by pressure from ground and crushed cocoa beans
Cocoa powder	Prepared by pulverizing the material remaining after a portion of the fat (*cocoa butter*) has been removed from the *liquor*
Cooking chocolate	See *chocolate liquor*
Dark chocolate	See *sweet chocolate*
Drip coffee	Brew prepared by pouring boiling water over finely ground, light (North America (28-40 g/l), northern Europe), medium (UK, Switzerland) or dark roasted coffee (France, Belgium) in a filter paper (50-70 g/l; 1 cup = 150-190 ml) or in a cloth (Brazil; 1 cup = 80 g/l)

Espresso	Brew prepared by extracting 6-8 g of finely ground, medium-to-dark roasted coffee with water at 8-12 bar and 92-95 °C for 15-25 sec (Italy; 25-50-ml cup) or longer (France, Switzerland; 150-ml cup)
Infusion	Brew prepared by infusing with boiling water in a pot for a few minutes coarsely ground, light-to-medium roasted coffee (northern Europe and Australia; 55-65 g/l) or very light roasted coffee (North America; 28-40 g/l) and separating the brew from the grounds by pouring through a metal screen strainer (1 cup = 150-190 ml)
Milk chocolate	Produced from *chocolate liquor*, sugar, *cocoa butter* and milk solids
Mocca coffee	Brew prepared in a 'Neapolitan' coffee maker by forcing just overheated water through a bed of finely ground, medium-to-very dark roasted coffee (Italy, Spain; 6-10 g/50-ml cup)
Nib	Cotyledon
Percolated coffee	Brew prepared by extracting coarsely ground, light (North America; 28-40 g/l) or medium roasted (UK; 60 g/l) coffee with recirculating boiling water until the desired brew strength is reached (1 cup = 150-190 ml)
Semisweet chocolate	See *sweet chocolate*
Soluble coffee	Brew prepared by dissolving 1.5-3.0 g of instant coffee powder in 150-190 ml of hot water (worldwide)
Sweet chocolate	Produced from *chocolate liquor* by addition of sugar and *cocoa butter*; also called *dark chocolate*, *bittersweet chocolate* and *semisweet chocolate*
Turkish/Greek coffee	Brew prepared by bringing to a gentle boil until a foam is formed very finely ground, medium-to-dark roasted coffee (~5 g) in water (60 ml), usually with sugar (5-10 g) (Middle East; 1 cup = 40-60 ml)

SUMMARY OF FINAL EVALUATIONS

Agent	Degree of evidence for carcinogenicity[a]		Overall evaluation of carcinogenicity to humans
	Human	Animal	
Coffee	L (urinary bladder)	I	2B (urinary bladder)[b]
	ESL (female breast, large bowel)		
	I (pancreas, ovary, other sites)		
Tea	I	I	3
Mate		ND	3
Hot mate drinking	L		2A
Caffeine	I	I	3
Theophylline	I	I	3
Theobromine	I	ND	3
Methylglyoxal	ND	I	3

[a]L, limited evidence; I, inadequate evidence; ESL, evidence suggesting lack of carcinogenicity; 2B, possibly carcinogenic to humans; 3, unclassifiable as to carcinogenicity to humans; 2A, probably carcinogenic to humans; ND, no data

[b]There is some evidence of an inverse relationship between coffee drinking and cancer of the large bowel; coffee drinking could not be classified as to its carcinogenicity to other organs.

Appendix 2. Summary table of genetic and related effects

Nonmammalian systems														Mammalian systems																			
Prokaryotes	Lower eukaryotes					Plants				Insects				In vitro															In vivo					
														Animal cells								Human cells								Animals						Humans				
D	G	D	R	G	A	A	D	G	C	C	R	G	A	D	G	S	M	C	A	T	I	D	G	S	M	C	A	T	I	D	G	S	M	C	DL	A	D	S	M	C	A

Coffee

Brewed coffee
| +¹ | | | | | | | | | | ?¹ | −¹ | −¹ | −¹ | | | +¹ | | | | | | | | +¹ | | +¹ | | | | | | | | | | | | | +¹ | | |

Instant coffee
| +¹ | | | | | | | | | | ?¹ | −¹ | −¹ | −¹ | +¹ | +¹ | | | | | | | | | +¹ | | | | | | | | | | | | | | | | | |

Decaffeinated coffee
| +¹ | | | | | | | | | | | | −¹ | −¹ | | | +¹ | | | | | | | | +¹ | | | | | | | | | −¹ | − | | | | | | | |

Tea
| + | | | | | | | | | | | | | | | | | | | | −¹ᵇ | | | | | | | | | | | | | | | | | | | | | |

Caffeineᶜ
| + | ? | +¹ | −ᵈ | +¹ | + | +¹ | + | + | ? | − | + | ? | − | ? | − | + | −¹ | + | + | + | | − | −¹ | + | ? | + | | + | | +¹ | − | + | +¹ | + | ? | ? | − | − | | +¹ | −¹ |

Theophylline
| −¹ | ? | + | | | | | | ? | | | −¹ | | | | −¹ | + | + | +¹ | ? | | | | | + | −¹ | ? | | + | | | | | +¹ | | −¹ | −¹ | | | | | |

Theobromine
| ? | +¹ | | | | | | | | | −¹ | −¹ | | | +¹ | +¹ | +¹ | | | −¹ | −¹ | | | | ? | | + | | | | | | | + | +¹ | −¹ | − | | | | | |

Methylglyoxal
| + | +¹ | | | | | | | | | | | | | + | +¹ | +¹ | | | | | | +¹ | +¹ | +¹ | | +¹ | | | | | | −¹ | | −¹ | | | | | | | |

A, aneuploidy; C, chromosomal aberrations; D, DNA damage; DL, dominant lethal mutation; G, gene mutation; I, inhibition of intercellular communication; M, micronuclei; R, mitotic recombination and gene conversion; S, sister chromatid exchange; T, cell transformation

In completing the tables, the following symbols indicate the consensus of the Working Group with regard to the results for each endpoint:

+   considered to be positive for the specific endpoint and level of biological complexity
+¹ considered to be positive, but only one valid study was available to the Working Group
−   considered to be negative
−¹ considered to be negative, but only one valid study was available to the Working Group
?   (e.g., there were contradictory results from different laboratories; there were confounding exposures; the results were equivocal)
?¹ considered to be equivocal or inconclusive; only one study was available to the Working Group

ᵃTest for sex-linked recessive lethal mutation gave negative results, but there was a weak positive trend for somatic mutation
ᵇGreen tea only
ᶜSperm morphology in animals, −¹
ᵈIncludes sister chromatid exchange

APPENDIX 3

ACTIVITY PROFILES
FOR GENETIC AND RELATED EFFECTS

Methods

The x-axis of the activity profile (Waters *et al.*, 1987, 1988) represents the bioassays in phylogenetic sequence by endpoint, and the values on the y-axis represent the logarithmically transformed lowest effective doses (LED) and highest ineffective doses (HID) tested. The term 'dose', as used in this report, does not take into consideration length of treatment or exposure and may therefore be considered synonymous with concentration. In practice, the concentrations used in all the in-vitro tests were converted to µg/ml, and those for in-vivo tests were expressed as mg/kg bw. Because dose units are plotted on a log scale, differences in molecular weights of compounds do not, in most cases, greatly influence comparisons of their activity profiles. Conventions for dose conversions are given below.

Profile-line height (the magnitude of each bar) is a function of the LED or HID, which is associated with the characteristics of each individual test system – such as population size, cell-cycle kinetics and metabolic competence. Thus, the detection limit of each test system is different, and, across a given activity profile, responses will vary substantially. No attempt is made to adjust or relate responses in one test system to those of another.

Line heights are derived as follows: for negative test results, the highest dose tested without appreciable toxicity is defined as the HID. If there was evidence of extreme toxicity, the next highest dose is used. A single dose tested with a negative result is considered to be equivalent to the HID. Similarly, for positive results, the LED is recorded. If the original data were analysed statistically by the author, the dose recorded is that at which the response was significant ($p < 0.05$). If the available data were not analysed statistically, the dose required to produce an effect is estimated as follows: when a dose-related positive response is observed with two or more doses, the lower of the doses is taken as the LED; a single dose resulting in a positive response is considered to be equivalent to the LED.

In order to accommodate both the wide range of doses encountered and positive and negative responses on a continuous scale, doses are transformed logarithmically, so that effective (LED) and ineffective (HID) doses are represented by positive and negative numbers, respectively. The response, or logarithmic dose unit (LDU_{ij}), for a given test system i and chemical j is represented by the expressions

$LDU_{ij} = -\log_{10}$ (dose), for HID values; $LDU \leq 0$
and (1)
$LDU_{ij} = -\log_{10}$ (dose x 10^{-5}), for LED values; $LDU \geq 0$.

These simple relationships define a dose range of 0 to −5 logarithmic units for ineffective doses (1–100 000 μg/ml or mg/kg bw) and 0 to +8 logarithmic units for effective doses (100 000–0.001 μg/ml or mg/kg bw). A scale illustrating the LDU values is shown in Figure 1. Negative responses at doses less than 1 μg/ml (mg/kg bw) are set equal to 1. Effectively, an LED value $\geq$100 000 or an HID value $\leq$1 produces an LDU = 0; no quantitative information is gained from such extreme values. The dotted lines at the levels of log dose units 1 and −1 define a 'zone of uncertainty' in which positive results are reported at such high doses (between 10 000 and 100 000 μg/ml or mg/kg bw) or negative results are reported at such low dose levels (1 to 10 μg/ml or mg/kg bw) as to call into question the adequacy of the test.

Fig. 1. Scale of log dose units used on the y-axis of activity profiles

Positive (μg/ml or mg/kg bw)		Log dose units	
0.001		8	—
0.01		7	—
0.1		6	—
1.0		5	—
10		4	—
100		3	—
1000		2	—
10 000		1	—
100 000	1	0	—
	10	−1	—
	100	−2	—
	1000	−3	—
	10 000	−4	—
	100 000	−5	—
	Negative (μg/ml or mg/kg bw)		

LED and HID are expressed as μg/ml or mg/kg bw.

In practice, an activity profile is computer generated. A data entry programme is used to store abstracted data from published reports. A sequential file (in ASCII) is created for each compound, and a record within that file consists of the name and Chemical Abstracts Service number of the compound, a three-letter code for the test system (see below), the qualitative test result (with and without an exogenous metabolic system), dose (LED or HID), citation number and additional source information. An abbreviated citation for each publication is stored in a segment of a record accessing both the test data file and the citation file. During processing of the data file, an average of the logarithmic values of the data subset is calculated, and the length of the profile line represents this average value. All dose values are plotted for each profile line, regardless of whether results are positive or negative. Results obtained in the absence of an exogenous metabolic system are indicated by a bar (-), and results obtained in the presence of an exogenous metabolic system are indicated by an upward-directed arrow (↑). When all results for a given assay are either positive or negative, the mean of the LDU values is plotted as a solid line; when conflicting data are reported for the same assay (i.e., both positive and negative results), the majority data are shown by a solid line and the minority data by a dashed line (drawn to the extreme conflicting response). In the few cases in which the numbers of positive and negative results are equal, the solid line is drawn in the positive direction and the maximal negative response is indicated with a dashed line.

Profile lines are identified by three-letter code words representing the commonly used tests. Code words for most of the test systems in current use in genetic toxicology were defined for the US Environmental Protection Agency's GENE-TOX Program (Waters, 1979; Waters & Auletta, 1981). For IARC Monographs Supplement 6, Volume 44 and subsequent volumes, including this publication, codes were redefined in a manner that should facilitate inclusion of additional tests. Naming conventions are described below.

Data listings are presented in the text and include endpoint and test codes, a short test code definition, results [either with (M) or without (NM) an exogenous activation system], the associated LED or HID value and a short citation. Test codes are organized phylogenetically and by endpoint from left to right across each activity profile and from top to bottom of the corresponding data listing. Endpoints are defined as follows: A, aneuploidy; C, chromosomal aberrations; D, DNA damage; F, assays of body fluids; G, gene mutation; H, host-mediated assays; I, inhibition of intercellular communication; M, micronuclei; P, sperm morphology; R, mitotic recombination or gene conversion; S, sister chromatid exchange; and T, cell transformation.

Dose conversions for activity profiles

Doses are converted to μg/ml for in-vitro tests and to mg/kg bw per day for in-vivo experiments.

1. In-vitro test systems

    (a) Weight/volume converts directly to μg/ml.

    (b) Molar (M) concentration × molecular weight = mg/ml = 10^3 μg/ml; mM concentration × molecular weight = μg/ml.

    (c) Soluble solids expressed as % concentration are assumed to be in units of mass per volume (i.e., 1% = 0.01 g/ml = 10 000 μg/ml; also, 1 ppm = 1 μg/ml).

    (d) Liquids and gases expressed as % concentration are assumed to be given in units of volume per volume. Liquids are converted to weight per volume using the density (D) of the solution (D = g/ml). Gases are converted from volume to mass using the ideal gas law, PV = nRT. For exposure at 20–37°C at standard atmospheric pressure, 1% (v/v) = 0.4 μg/ml × molecular weight of the gas. Also, 1 ppm (v/v) = 4×10^{-5} μg/ml × molecular weight.

    (e) In microbial plate tests, it is usual for the doses to be reported as weight/plate, whereas concentrations are required to enter data on the activity profile chart. While remaining cognisant of the errors involved in the process, it is assumed that a 2-ml volume of top agar is delivered to each plate and that the test substance remains in solution within it; concentrations are derived from the reported weight/plate values by dividing by this arbitrary volume. For spot tests, a 1-ml volume is used in the calculation.

    (f) Conversion of particulate concentrations given in μg/cm^2 are based on the area (A) of the dish and the volume of medium per dish; i.e., for a 100-mm dish: A = πR^2 = $\pi \times (5 \text{ cm})^2$ = 78.5 cm^2. If the volume of medium is 10 ml, then 78.5 cm^2 = 10 ml and 1 cm^2 = 0.13 ml.

2. In-vitro systems using in-vivo activation

    For the body fluid–urine (BF–) test, the concentration used is the dose (in mg/kg bw) of the compound administered to test animals or patients.

3. In-vivo test systems

    (a) Doses are converted to mg/kg bw per day of exposure, assuming 100% absorption. Standard values are used for each sex and species of rodent, including body weight and average intake per day, as reported by Gold *et al.* (1984). For example, in a test using male mice fed 50 ppm of the agent in the diet, the standard food intake per day is 12% of body weight, and the conversion is dose = 50 ppm × 12% = 6 mg/kg bw per day.

Standard values used for humans are: weight – males, 70 kg; females, 55 kg; surface area, 1.7 m^2; inhalation rate, 20 l/min for light work, 30 l/min for mild exercise.

(b) When reported, the dose at the target site is used. For example, doses given in studies of lymphocytes of humans exposed *in vivo* are the measured blood concentrations in μg/ml.

Codes for test systems

For specific nonmammalian test systems, the first two letters of the three-symbol code word define the test organism (e.g., SA- for *Salmonella typhimurium*, EC- for *Escherichia coli*). If the species is not known, the convention used is -S-. The third symbol may be used to define the tester strain (e.g., SA8 for *S. typhimurium* TA1538, ECW for *E. coli* WP2*uvr*A). When strain designation is not indicated, the third letter is used to define the specific genetic endpoint under investigation (e.g., —D for differential toxicity, —F for forward mutation, —G for gene conversion or genetic crossing-over, —N for aneuploidy, —R for reverse mutation, —U for unscheduled DNA synthesis). The third letter may also be used to define the general endpoint under investigation when a more complete definition is not possible or relevant (e.g., —M for mutation, —C for chromosomal aberration).

For mammalian test systems, the first letter of the three-letter code word defines the genetic endpoint under investigation: A— for aneuploidy, B— for binding, C— for chromosomal aberration, D— for DNA strand breaks, G— for gene mutation, I— for inhibition of intercellular communication, M— for micronucleus formation, R— for DNA repair, S— for sister chromatid exchange, T— for cell transformation and U— for unscheduled DNA synthesis.

For animal (i.e., non-human) test systems *in vitro*, when the cell type is not specified, the code letters -IA are used. For such assays *in vivo*, when the animal species is not specified, the code letters -VA are used. Commonly used animal species are identified by the third letter (e.g., —C for Chinese hamster, —M for mouse, —R for rat, —S for Syrian hamster).

For test systems using human cells *in vitro*, when the cell type is not specified, the code letters -IH are used. For assays on humans *in vivo*, when the cell type is not specified, the code letters -VH are used. Otherwise, the second letter specifies the cell type under investigation (e.g., -BH for bone marrow, -LH for lymphocytes).

Some other specific coding conventions used for mammalian systems are as follows: BF- for body fluids, HM- for host-mediated, —L for leucocytes or lymphocytes *in vitro* (-AL, animals; -HL, humans), -L- for leucocytes *in vivo* (-LA, animals; -LH, humans), —T for transformed cells.

Note that these are examples of major conventions used to define the assay code words. The alphabetized listing of codes must be examined to confirm a specific code word. As might be expected from the limitation to three symbols, some codes do not fit the naming conventions precisely. In a few cases, test systems are defined by first-letter code words, for example: MST, mouse spot test; SLP, mouse specific locus test, postspermatogonia; SLO, mouse specific locus test, other stages; DLM, dominant lethal test in mice; DLR, dominant lethal test in rats; MHT, mouse heritable translocation test.

The genetic activity profiles and listings that follow were prepared in collaboration with Environmental Health Research and Testing Inc. (EHRT) under contract to the US Environmental Protection Agency; EHRT also determined the doses used. The references cited in each genetic activity profile listing can be found in the list of references in the appropriate monograph.

References

Garrett, N.E., Stack, H.F., Gross, M.R. & Waters, M.D. (1984) An analysis of the spectra of genetic activity produced by known or suspected human carcinogens. *Mutat. Res.,* 134, 89-111

Gold, L.S., Sawyer, C.B., Magaw, R., Backman, G.M., de Veciana, M., Levinson, R., Hooper, N.K., Havender, W.R., Bernstein, L., Peto, R., Pike, M.C. & Ames, B.N. (1984) A carcinogenic potency database of the standardized results of animal bioassays. *Environ. Health Perspect.,* 58, 9-319

Waters, M.D. (1979) *The GENE-TOX program.* In: Hsie, A.W., O'Neill, J.P. & McElheny, V.K., eds, *Mammalian Cell Mutagenesis: The Maturation of Test Systems* (Banbury Report 2), Cold Spring Harbor, NY, CHS Press, pp. 449-467

Waters, M.D. & Auletta, A. (1981) The GENE-TOX program: genetic activity evaluation. *J. chem. Inf. comput. Sci.,* 21, 35-38

Waters, M.D., Stack, H.F., Brady, A.L., Lohman, P.H.M., Haroun, L. & Vainio, H. (1987) Appendix 1: Activity profiles for genetic and related tests. In: *IARC Monographs on the Evaluation of the Carcinogenic Risk of Chemicals to Humans,* Suppl. 6, *Genetic and Related Effects: An Update of Selected* IARC Monographs *from Volumes 1 to 42*, Lyon, IARC, pp. 687-696

Waters, M.D., Stack, H.F., Brady, A.L., Lohman, P.H.M., Haroun, L. & Vainio, H. (1988) Use of computerized data listings and activity profiles of genetic and related effects in the review of 195 compounds. *Mutat. Res.,* 205, 295-312

APPENDIX 3

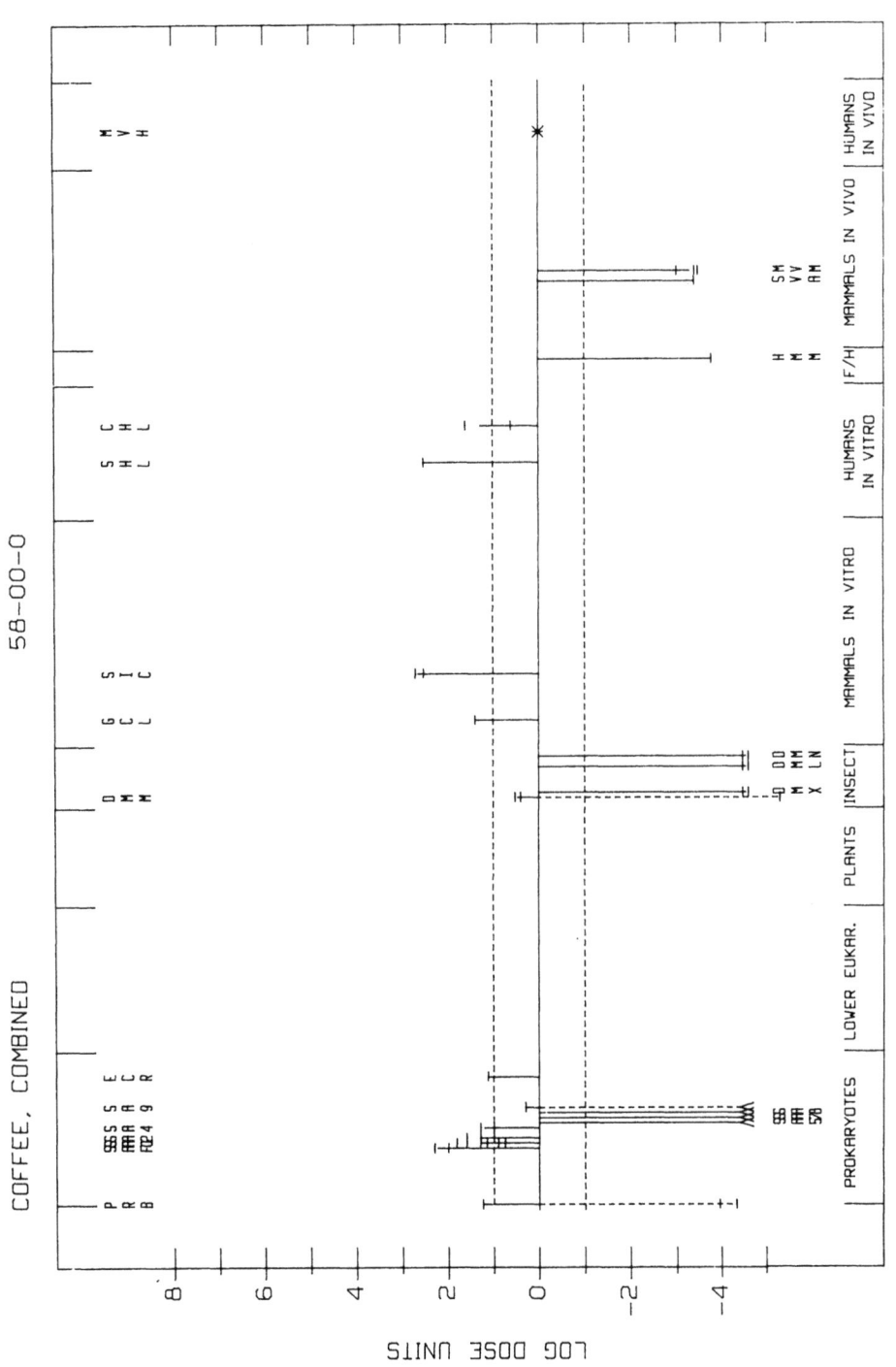

472

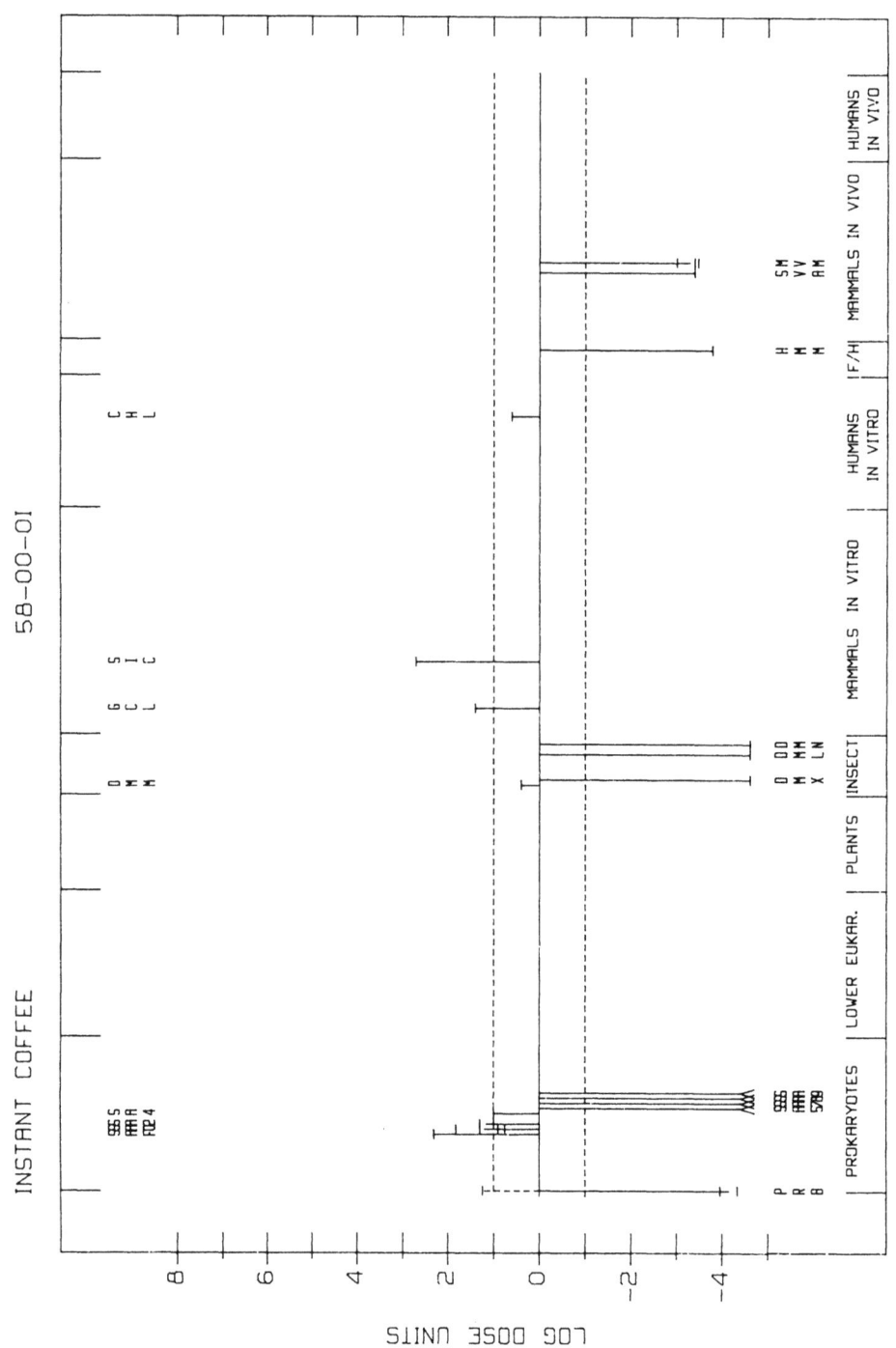

APPENDIX 3

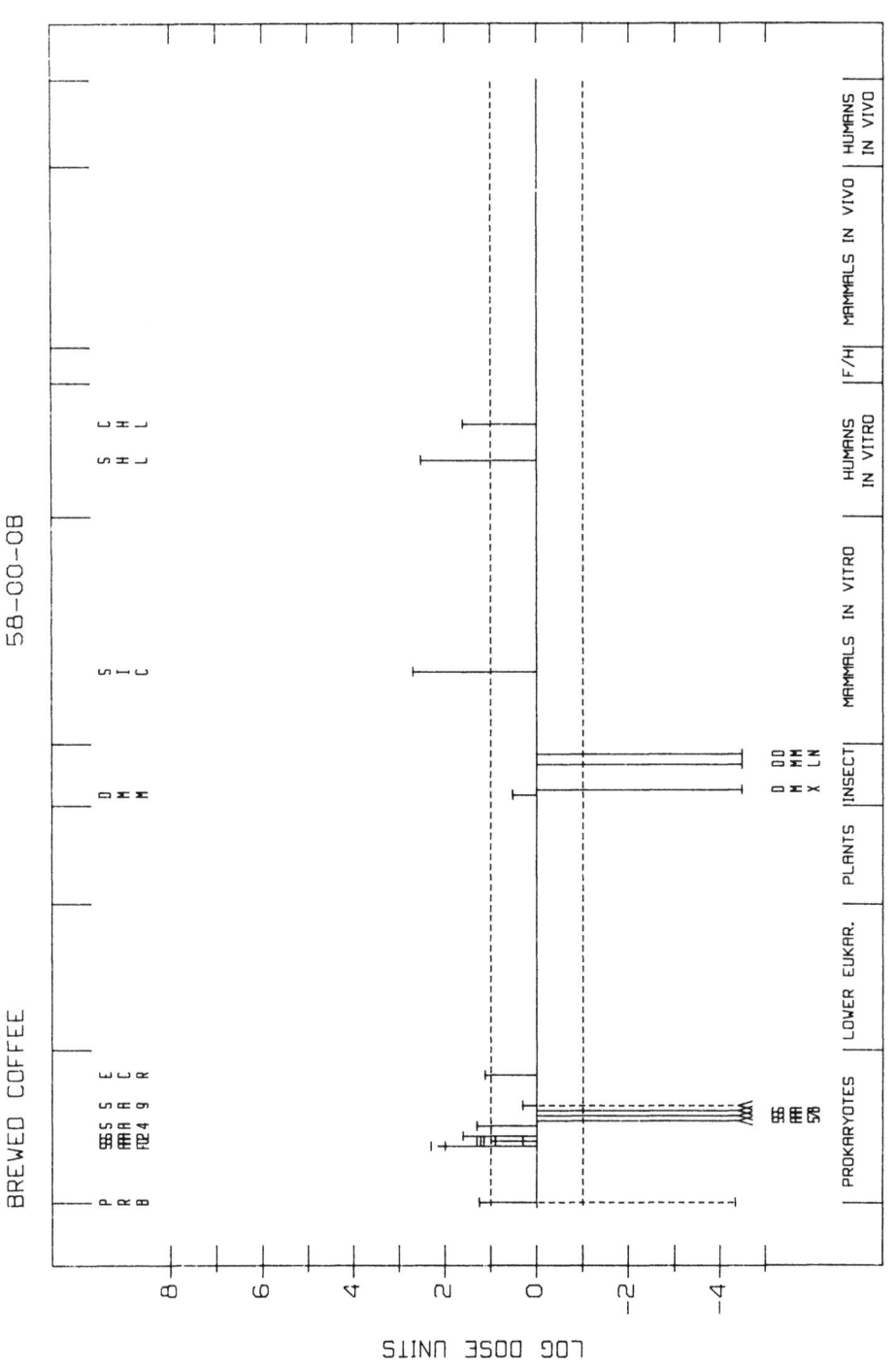

474 IARC MONOGRAPHS VOLUME 51

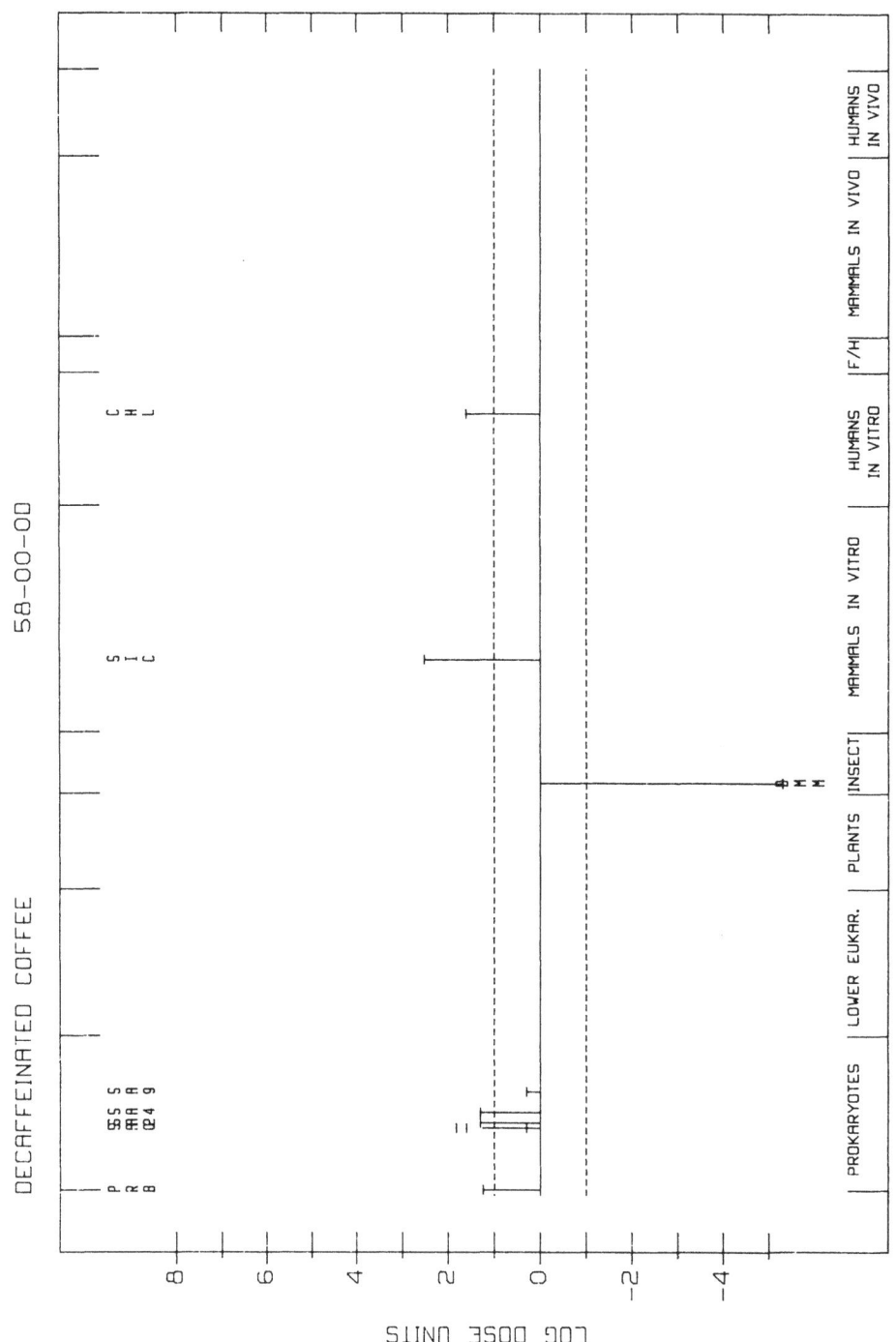

APPENDIX 3

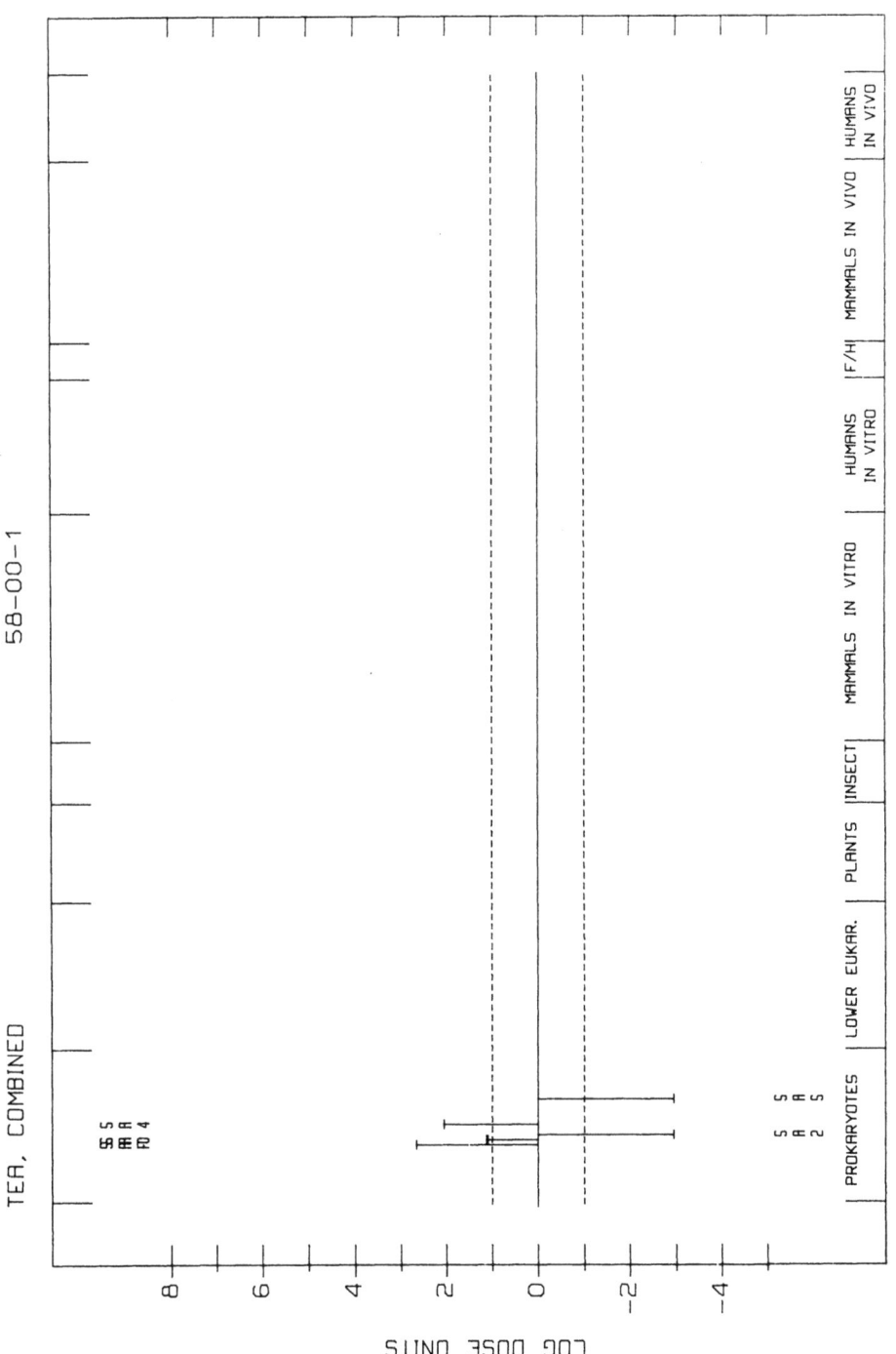

476 IARC MONOGRAPHS VOLUME 51

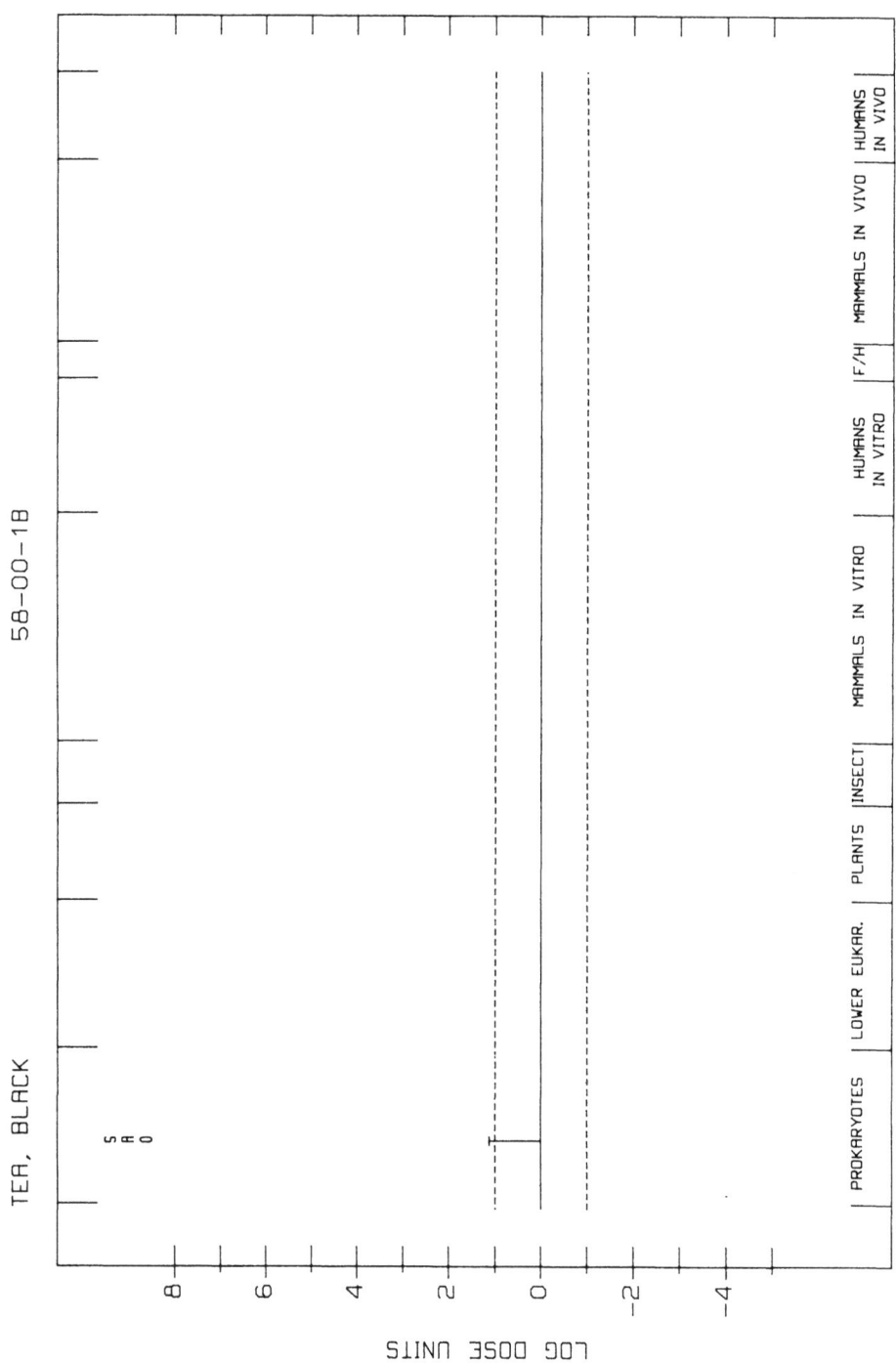

APPENDIX 3

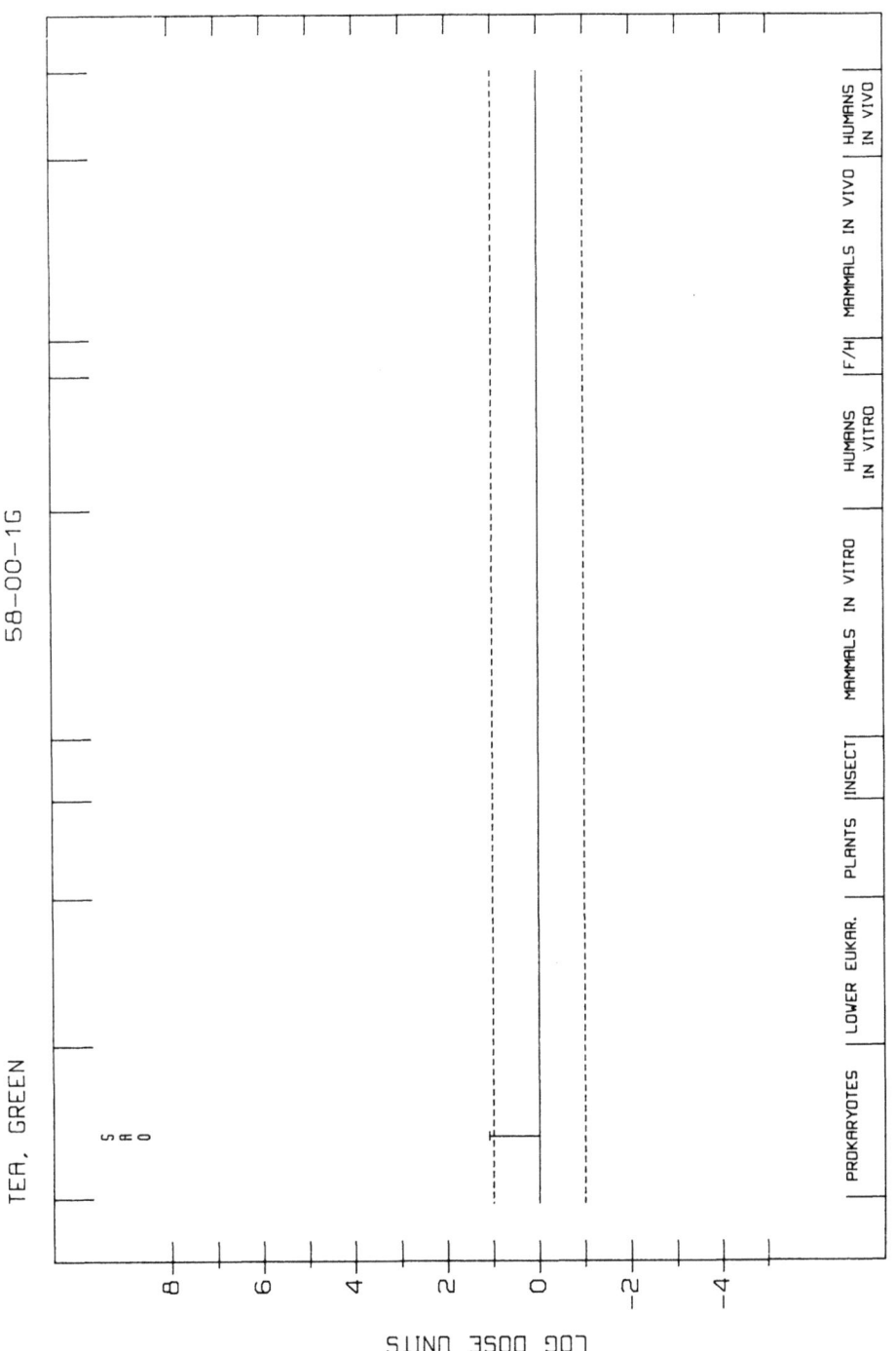

478 IARC MONOGRAPHS VOLUME 51

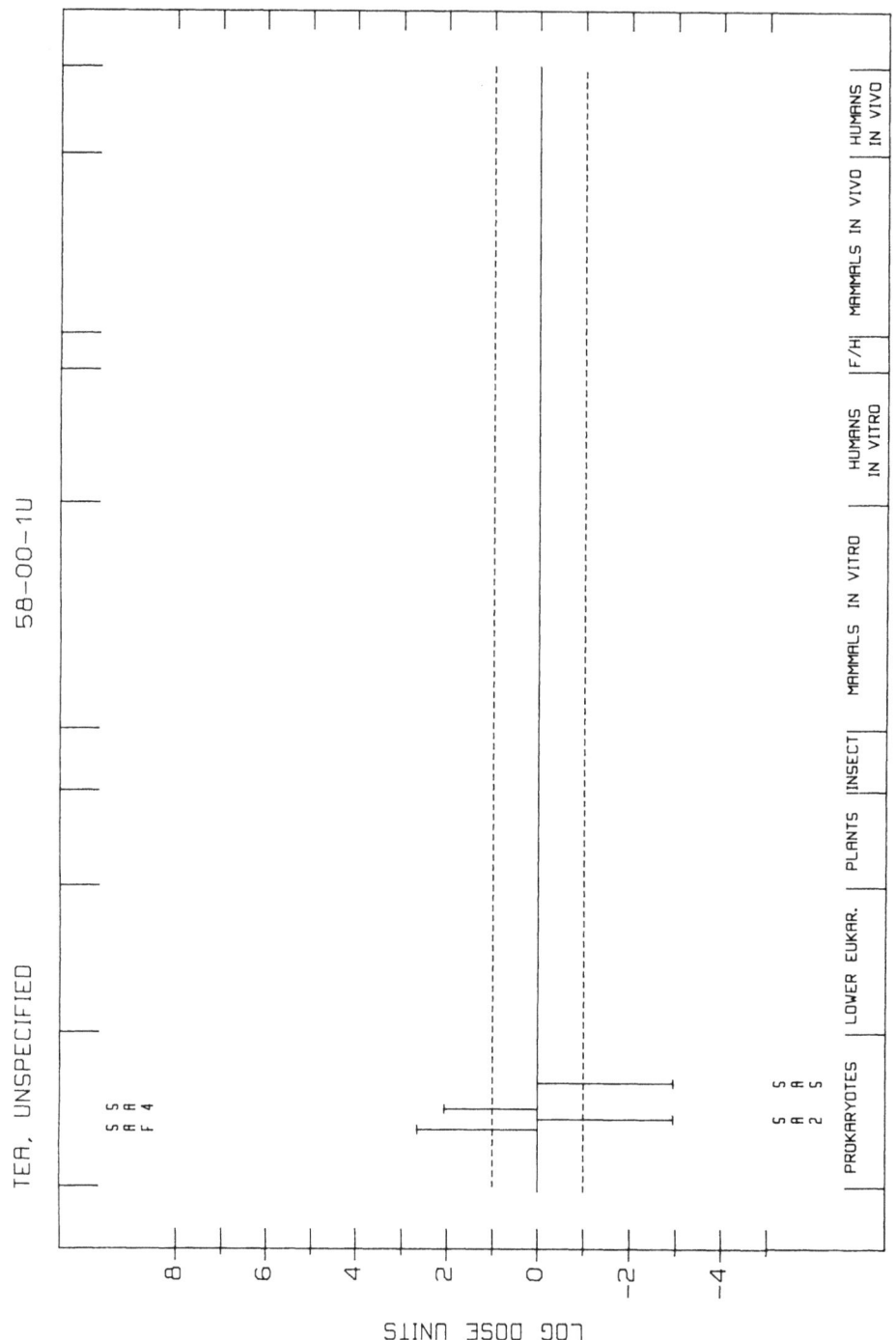

APPENDIX 3

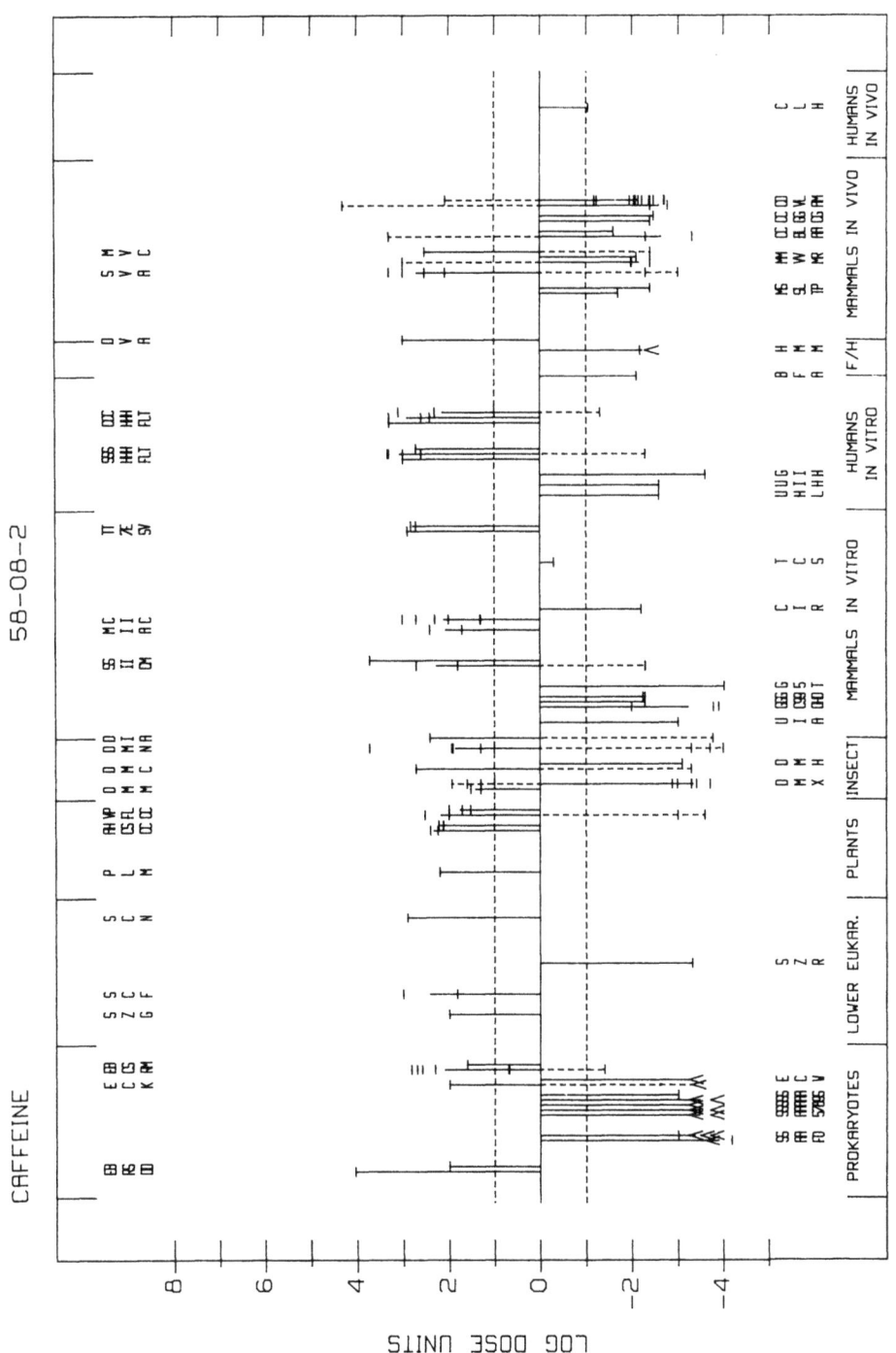

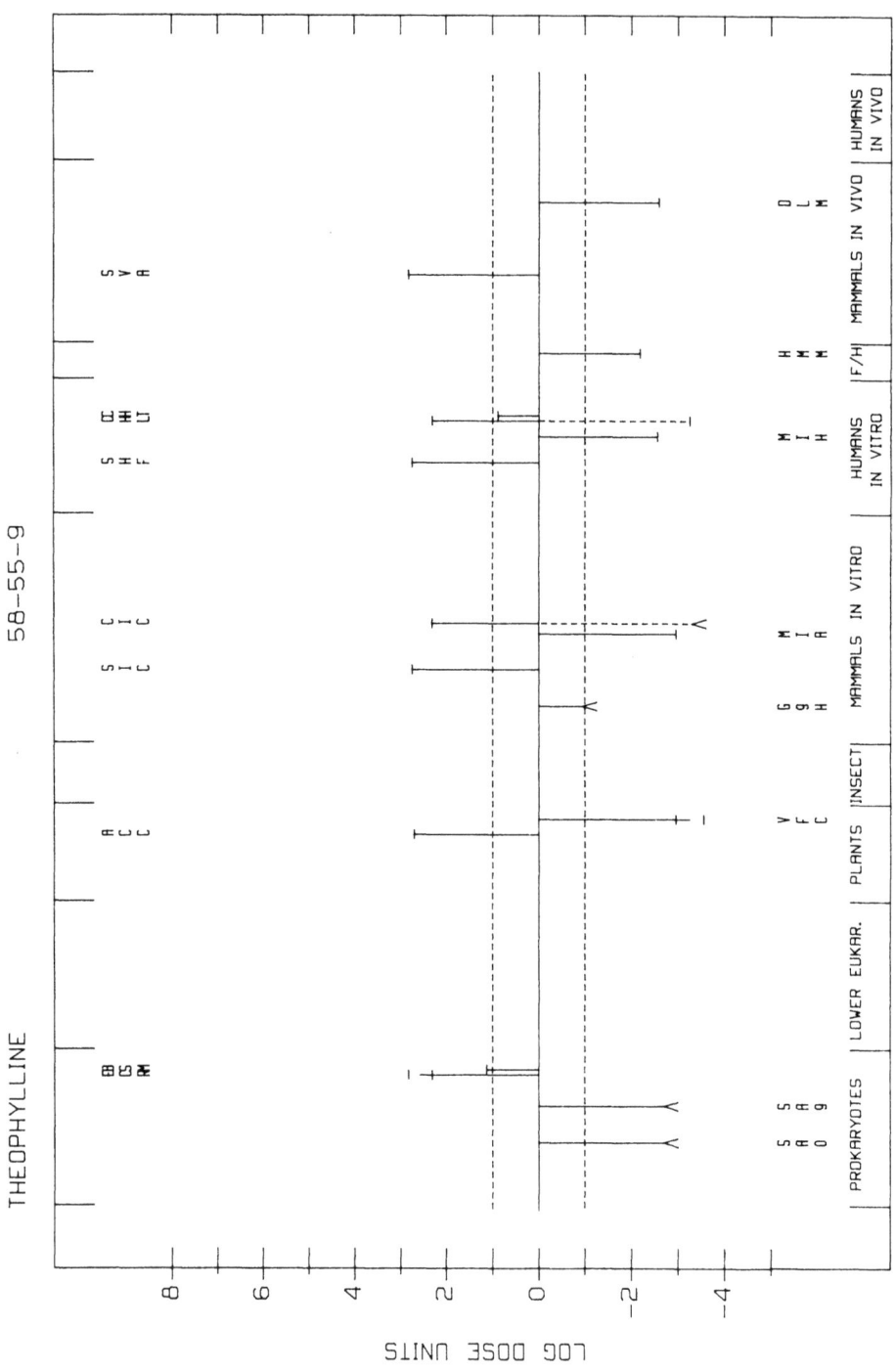

APPENDIX 3

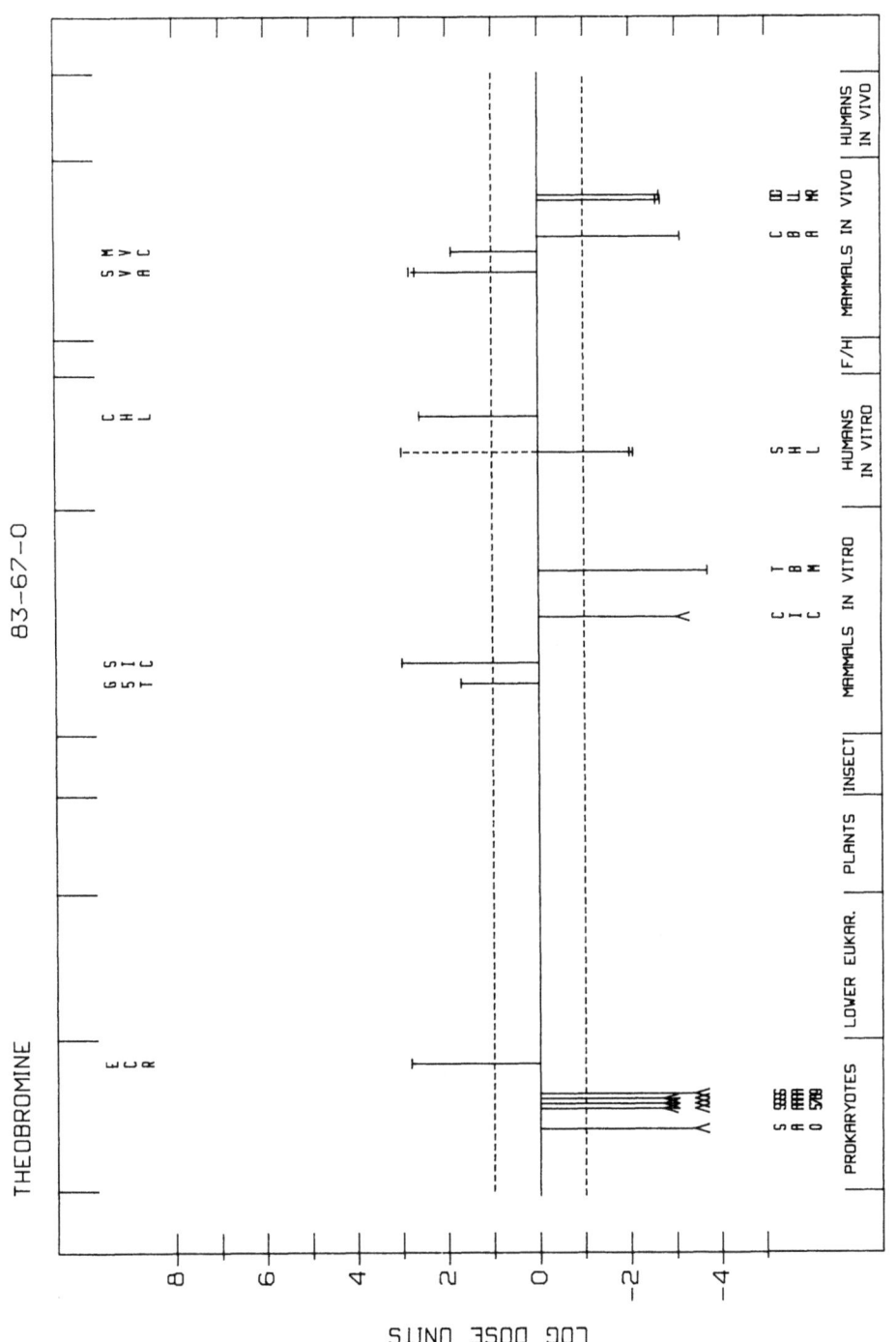

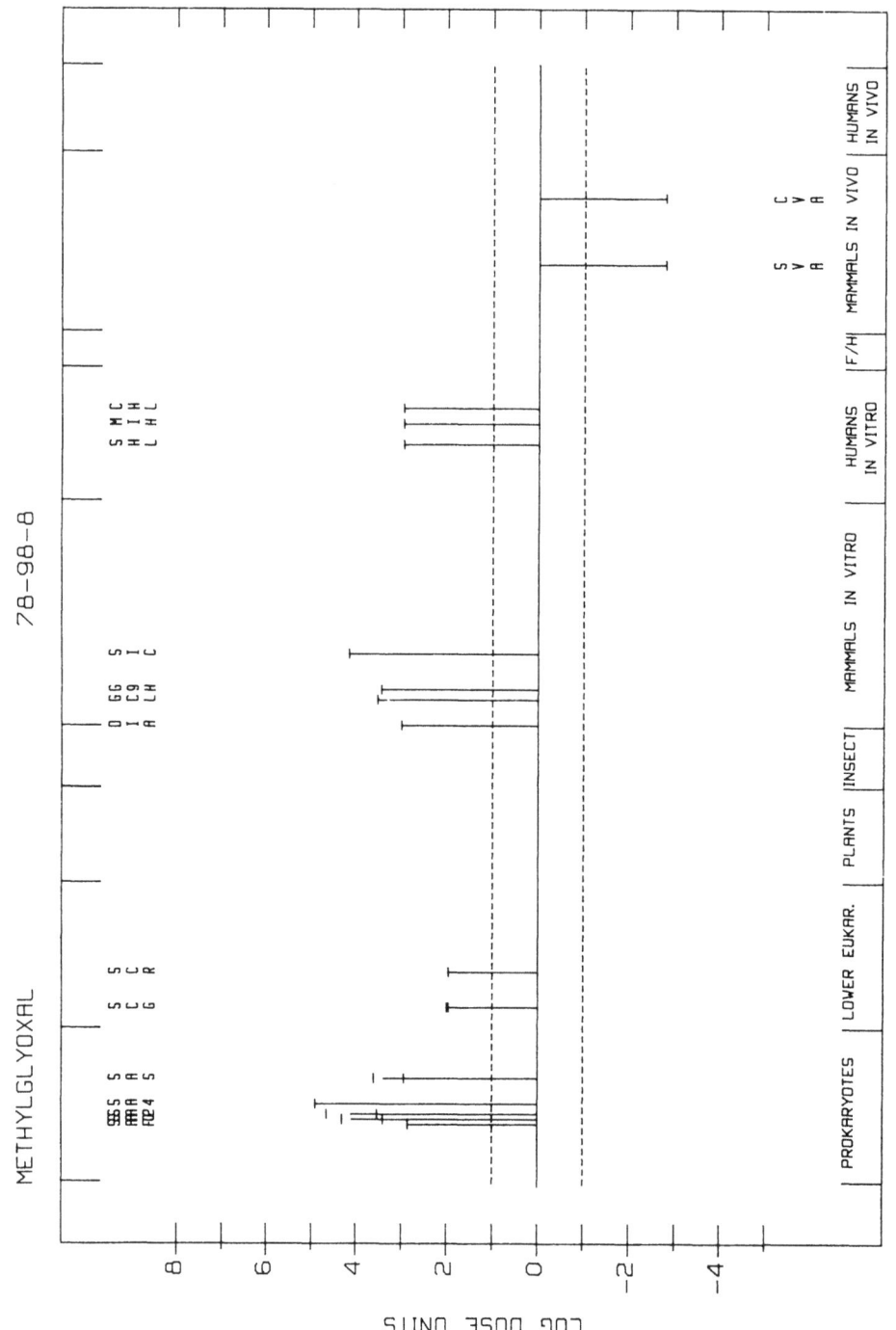

SUPPLEMENTARY CORRIGENDA TO VOLUMES 1–50

Volume 41 p. 241 last line, *replace* 1.3 ppb (4.6 µg/m^3) *by* 0.17 ppb (0.6 µg/m^3)

Volume 48 p. 218 *Replace* (a) Fibre production *by* (a) Fabrics production

   p. 275 Nousiainen, P. & Sundquist, J. (1979) *Replace present title* by Kemialliset Haittatekijät Tekstiiliteollisuudessa. Työilman Epäpuhtaudet

Volume 49 p. 137 Table 22 (contd)
Replace Calcium chromate   Intraperitoneal
by   Calcium chromate   Intrapleural
(three times)

CUMULATIVE CROSS INDEX TO *IARC MONOGRAPHS ON THE EVALUATION OF CARCINOGENIC RISKS TO HUMANS*

The volume, page and year are given. References to corrigenda are given in parentheses.

A

A-α-C	*40*, 245 (1986); *Suppl. 7*, 56 (1987)
Acetaldehyde	*36*, 101 (1985) (*corr. 42*, 263); *Suppl. 7*, 77 (1987)
Acetaldehyde formylmethylhydrazone (*see* Gyromitrin)	
Acetamide	*7*, 197 (1974); *Suppl. 7*, 389 (1987)
Acetaminophen (*see* Paracetamol)	
Acridine orange	*16*, 145 (1978); *Suppl. 7*, 56 (1987)
Acriflavinium chloride	*13*, 31 (1977); *Suppl. 7*, 56 (1987)
Acrolein	*19*, 479 (1979); *36*, 133 (1985); *Suppl. 7*, 78 (1987);
Acrylamide	*39*, 41 (1986); *Suppl. 7*, 56 (1987)
Acrylic acid	*19*, 47 (1979); *Suppl. 7*, 56 (1987)
Acrylic fibres	*19*, 86 (1979); *Suppl. 7*, 56 (1987)
Acrylonitrile	*19*, 73 (1979); *Suppl. 7*, 79 (1987)
Acrylonitrile-butadiene-styrene copolymers	*19*, 91 (1979); *Suppl. 7*, 56 (1987)
Actinolite (*see* Asbestos)	
Actinomycins	*10*, 29 (1976) (*corr. 42*, 255); *Suppl. 7*, 80 (1987)
Adriamycin	*10*, 43 (1976); *Suppl. 7*, 82 (1987)
AF-2	*31*, 47 (1983); *Suppl. 7*, 56 (1987)
Aflatoxins	*1*, 145 (1972) (*corr. 42*, 251); *10*, 51 (1976); *Suppl. 7*, 83 (1987)
Aflatoxin B_1 (*see* Aflatoxins)	
Aflatoxin B_2 (*see* Aflatoxins)	
Aflatoxin G_1 (*see* Aflatoxins)	
Aflatoxin G_2 (*see* Aflatoxins)	
Aflatoxin M_1 (*see* Aflatoxins)	
Agaritine	*31*, 63 (1983); *Suppl. 7*, 56 (1987)

Alcohol drinking	*44*
Aldrin	*5*, 25 (1974); *Suppl. 7*, 88 (1987)
Allyl chloride	*36*, 39 (1985); *Suppl. 7*, 56 (1987)
Allyl isothiocyanate	*36*, 55 (1985); *Suppl. 7*, 56 (1987)
Allyl isovalerate	*36*, 69 (1985); *Suppl. 7*, 56 (1987)
Aluminium production	*34*, 37 (1984); *Suppl. 7*, 89 (1987)
Amaranth	*8*, 41 (1975); *Suppl. 7*, 56 (1987)
5-Aminoacenaphthene	*16*, 243 (1978); *Suppl. 7*, 56 (1987)
2-Aminoanthraquinone	*27*, 191 (1982); *Suppl. 7*, 56 (1987)
para-Aminoazobenzene	*8*, 53 (1975); *Suppl. 7*, 390 (1987)
ortho-Aminoazotoluene	*8*, 61 (1975) (*corr. 42*, 254);. *Suppl. 7*, 56 (1987)
para-Aminobenzoic acid	*16*, 249 (1978); *Suppl. 7*, 56 (1987)
4-Aminobiphenyl	*1*, 74 (1972) (*corr. 42*, 251); *Suppl. 7*, 91 (1987)
2-Amino-3,4-dimethylimidazo[4,5-*f*]quinoline (*see* MeIQ)	
2-Amino-3,8-dimethylimidazo[4,5-*f*]quinoxaline (*see* MeIQx)	
3-Amino-1,4-dimethyl-5*H*-pyrido[4,3-*b*]indole (*see* Trp-P-1)	
2-Aminodipyrido[1,2-*a*:3',2'-*d*]imidazole (*see* Glu-P-2)	
1-Amino-2-methylanthraquinone	*27*, 199 (1982); *Suppl. 7*, 57 (1987)
2-Amino-3-methylimidazo[4,5-*f*]quinoline (*see* IQ)	
2-Amino-6-methyldipyrido[1,2-*a*:3',2'-*d*]-imidazole (*see* Glu-P-1)	
2-Amino-3-methyl-9*H*-pyrido[2,3-*b*]indole (*see* MeA-α-C)	
3-Amino-1-methyl-5*H*-pyrido[4,3-*b*]indole (*see* Trp-P-2)	
2-Amino-5-(5-nitro-2-furyl)-1,3,4-thiadiazole	*7*, 143 (1974); *Suppl. 7*, 57 (1987)
4-Amino-2-nitrophenol	*16*, 43 (1978); *Suppl.7*, 57 (1987)
2-Amino-5-nitrothiazole	*31*, 71 (1983); *Suppl. 7*, 57 (1987)
2-Amino-9*H*-pyrido[2,3-*b*]indole [*see* A-α-C]	
11-Aminoundecanoic acid	*39*, 239 (1986); *Suppl. 7*, 57 (1987)
Amitrole	*7*, 31 (1974); *41*, 293 (1986) *Suppl. 7*, 92 (1987)
Ammonium potassium selenide (*see* Selenium and selenium compounds)	
Amorphous silica (*see also* Silica)	*Suppl. 7*, 341 (1987)
Amosite (*see* Asbestos)	
Ampicillin	*50*, 153 (1990)
Anabolic steroids (*see* Androgenic (anabolic) steroids)	
Anaesthetics, volatile	*11*, 285 (1976); *Suppl. 7*, 93 (1987)
Analgesic mixtures containing phenacetin (*see also* Phenacetin)	*Suppl. 7*, 310 (1987)
Androgenic (anabolic) steroids	*Suppl. 7*, 96 (1987)
Angelicin and some synthetic derivatives (*see also* Angelicins)	*40*, 291 (1986)
Angelicin plus ultraviolet radiation (*see also* Angelicin and some synthetic derivatives)	*Suppl. 7*, 57 (1987)
Angelicins	*Suppl. 7*, 57 (1987)

Aniline	4, 27 (1974) (corr. 42, 252); 27, 39 (1982); Suppl. 7, 99 (1987)
ortho-Anisidine	27, 63 (1982); Suppl. 7, 57 (1987)
para-Anisidine	27, 65 (1982); Suppl. 7, 57 (1987)
Anthanthrene	32, 95 (1983); Suppl. 7, 57 (1987)
Anthophyllite (*see* Asbestos)	
Anthracene	32, 105 (1983); Suppl. 7, 57 (1987)
Anthranilic acid	16, 265 (1978); Suppl. 7, 57 (1987)
Antimony trioxide	47, 291 (1989)
Antimony trisulfide	47, 291 (1989)
ANTU (*see* 1-Naphthylthiourea)	
Apholate	9, 31 (1975); Suppl. 7, 57 (1987)
Aramite®	5, 39 (1974); Suppl. 7, 57 (1987)
Areca nut (*see* Betel quid)	
Arsanilic acid (*see* Arsenic and arsenic compounds)	
Arsenic and arsenic compounds	1, 41 (1972); 2, 48 (1973); 23, 39 (1980); Suppl. 7, 100 (1987)
Arsenic pentoxide (*see* Arsenic and arsenic compounds)	
Arsenic sulphide (*see* Arsenic and arsenic compounds)	
Arsenic trioxide (*see* Arsenic and arsenic compounds)	
Arsine (*see* Arsenic and arsenic compounds)	
Asbestos	2, 17 (1973) (corr. 42, 252); 14 (1977) (corr. 42, 256); Suppl. 7, 106 (1987) (corr. 45, 283)
Attapulgite	42, 159 (1987); Suppl. 7, 117 (1987)
Auramine (technical-grade)	1, 69 (1972) (corr. 42, 251); Suppl. 7, 118 (1987)
Auramine, manufacture of (*see also* Auramine, technical-grade)	Suppl. 7, 118 (1987)
Aurothioglucose	13, 39 (1977); Suppl. 7, 57 (1987)
Azacitidine	26, 37 (1981); Suppl. 7, 57 (1987); 50, 47 (1990)
5-Azacytidine (*see* Azacitidine)	
Azaserine	10, 73 (1976) (corr. 42, 255); Suppl. 7, 57 (1987)
Azathioprine	26, 47 (1981); Suppl. 7, 119 (1987)
Aziridine	9, 37 (1975); Suppl. 7, 58 (1987)
2-(1-Aziridinyl)ethanol	9, 47 (1975); Suppl. 7, 58 (1987)
Aziridyl benzoquinone	9, 51 (1975); Suppl. 7, 58 (1987)
Azobenzene	8, 75 (1975); Suppl. 7, 58 (1987)

B

Barium chromate (*see* Chromium and chromium compounds)
Basic chromic sulphate (*see* Chromium and chromium compounds)
BCNU (*see* Bischloroethyl nitrosourea)

Benz[a]acridine	32, 123 (1983); Suppl. 7, 58 (1987)
Benz[c]acridine	3, 241 (1973); 32, 129 (1983); Suppl. 7, 58 (1987)
Benzal chloride (see also α-Chlorinated toluenes)	29, 65 (1982); Suppl. 7, 148 (1987)
Benz[a]anthracene	3, 45 (1973); 32, 135 (1983); Suppl. 7, 58 (1987)
Benzene	7, 203 (1974) (corr. 42, 254); 29, 93, 391 (1982); Suppl. 7, 120 (1987)
Benzidine	1, 80 (1972); 29, 149, 391 (1982); Suppl. 7, 123 (1987)
Benzidine-based dyes	Suppl. 7, 125 (1987)
Benzo[b]fluoranthene	3, 69 (1973); 32, 147 (1983); Suppl. 7, 58 (1987)
Benzo[j]fluoranthene	3, 82 (1973); 32, 155 (1983); Suppl. 7, 58 (1987)
Benzo[k]fluoranthene	32, 163 (1983); Suppl. 7, 58 (1987)
Benzo[ghi]fluoranthene	32, 171 (1983); Suppl. 7, 58 (1987)
Benzo[a]fluorene	32, 177 (1983); Suppl. 7, 58 (1987)
Benzo[b]fluorene	32, 183 (1983); Suppl. 7, 58 (1987)
Benzo[c]fluorene	32, 189 (1983); Suppl. 7, 58 (1987)
Benzo[ghi]perylene	32, 195 (1983); Suppl. 7, 58 (1987)
Benzo[c]phenanthrene	32, 205 (1983); Suppl. 7, 58 (1987)
Benzo[a]pyrene	3, 91 (1973); 32, 211 (1983); Suppl. 7, 58 (1987)
Benzo[e]pyrene	3, 137 (1973); 32, 225 (1983); Suppl. 7, 58 (1987)
para-Benzoquinone dioxime	29, 185 (1982); Suppl. 7, 58 (1987)
Benzotrichloride (see also α-Chlorinated toluenes)	29, 73 (1982); Suppl. 7, 148 (1987)
Benzoyl chloride	29, 83 (1982) (corr. 42, 261); Suppl. 7, 126 (1987)
Benzoyl peroxide	36, 267 (1985); Suppl. 7, 58 (1987)
Benzyl acetate	40, 109 (1986); Suppl. 7, 58 (1987)
Benzyl chloride (see also α-Chlorinated toluenes)	11, 217 (1976) (corr. 42, 256); 29, 49 (1982); Suppl. 7, 148 (1987)
Benzyl violet 4B	16, 153 (1978); Suppl. 7, 58 (1987)
Bertrandite (see Beryllium and beryllium compounds)	
Beryllium and beryllium compounds	1, 17 (1972); 23, 143 (1980) (corr. 42, 260); Suppl. 7, 127 (1987)
Beryllium acetate (see Beryllium and beryllium compounds)	
Beryllium acetate, basic (see Beryllium and beryllium compounds)	
Beryllium–aluminium alloy (see Beryllium and beryllium compounds)	
Beryllium carbonate (see Beryllium and beryllium compounds)	
Beryllium chloride (see Beryllium and beryllium compounds)	
Beryllium–copper alloy (see Beryllium and beryllium compounds)	

Beryllium–copper–cobalt alloy (*see* Beryllium and beryllium compounds)
Beryllium fluoride (*see* Beryllium and beryllium compounds)
Beryllium hydroxide (*see* Beryllium and beryllium compounds)
Beryllium–nickel alloy (*see* Beryllium and beryllium compounds)
Beryllium oxide (*see* Beryllium and beryllium compounds)
Beryllium phosphate (*see* Beryllium and beryllium compounds)
Beryllium silicate (*see* Beryllium and beryllium compounds)
Beryllium sulphate (*see* Beryllium and beryllium compounds)
Beryl ore (*see* Beryllium and beryllium compounds)

Betel quid	*37*, 141 (1985); *Suppl. 7*, 128 (1987)
Betel-quid chewing (*see* Betel quid)	
BHA (*see* Butylated hydroxyanisole)	
BHT (*see* Butylated hydroxytoluene)	
Bis(1-aziridinyl)morpholinophosphine sulphide	*9*, 55 (1975); *Suppl. 7*, 58 (1987)
Bis(2-chloroethyl)ether	*9*, 117 (1975); *Suppl. 7*, 58 (1987)
N,N-Bis(2-chloroethyl)-2-naphthylamine	*4*, 119 (1974) (*corr. 42*, 253); *Suppl. 7*, 130 (1987)
Bischloroethyl nitrosourea (*see also* Chloroethyl nitrosoureas)	*26*, 79 (1981); *Suppl. 7*, 150 (1987)
1,2-Bis(chloromethoxy)ethane	*15*, 31 (1977); *Suppl. 7*, 58 (1987)
1,4-Bis(chloromethoxymethyl)benzene	*15*, 37 (1977); *Suppl. 7*, 58 (1987)
Bis(chloromethyl)ether	*4*, 231 (1974) (*corr. 42*, 253); *Suppl. 7*, 131 (1987)
Bis(2-chloro-1-methylethyl)ether	*41*, 149 (1986); *Suppl. 7*, 59 (1987)
Bis(2,3-epoxycyclopentyl)ether	*47*, 231 (1989)
Bitumens	*35*, 39 (1985); *Suppl. 7*, 133 (1987)
Bleomycins	*26*, 97 (1981); *Suppl. 7*, 134 (1987)
Blue VRS	*16*, 163 (1978); *Suppl. 7*, 59 (1987)
Boot and shoe manufacture and repair	*25*, 249 (1981); *Suppl. 7*, 232 (1987)
Bracken fern	*40*, 47 (1986); *Suppl. 7*, 135 (1987)
Brilliant Blue FCF	*16*, 171 (1978) (*corr. 42*, 257); *Suppl. 7*, 59 (1987)
1,3-Butadiene	*39*, 155 (1986) (*corr. 42*, 264); *Suppl. 7*, 136 (1987)
1,4-Butanediol dimethanesulphonate	*4*, 247 (1974); *Suppl. 7*, 137 (1987)
n-Butyl acrylate	*39*, 67 (1986); *Suppl. 7*, 59 (1987)
Butylated hydroxyanisole	*40*, 123 (1986); *Suppl. 7*, 59 (1987)
Butylated hydroxytoluene	*40*, 161 (1986); *Suppl. 7*, 59 (1987)
Butyl benzyl phthalate	*29*, 193 (1982) (*corr. 42*, 261); *Suppl. 7*, 59 (1987)
β-Butyrolactone	*11*, 225 (1976); *Suppl. 7*, 59 (1987)
γ-Butyrolactone	*11*, 231 (1976); *Suppl. 7*, 59 (1987)

C

Cabinet-making (*see* Furniture and cabinet-making)

Cadmium acetate (*see* Cadmium and cadmium compounds)
Cadmium and cadmium compounds 2, 74 (1973); *11*, 39 (1976) (*corr.* 42, 255); *Suppl.* 7, 139 (1987)

Cadmium chloride (*see* Cadmium and cadmium compounds)
Cadmium oxide (*see* Cadmium and cadmium compounds)
Cadmium sulphate (*see* Cadmium and cadmium compounds)
Cadmium sulphide (*see* Cadmium and cadmium compounds)
Caffeine *51*, 291 (1991)
Calcium arsenate (*see* Arsenic and arsenic compounds)
Calcium chromate (*see* Chromium and chromium compounds)
Calcium cyclamate (*see* Cyclamates)
Calcium saccharin (*see* Saccharin)
Cantharidin *10*, 79 (1976); *Suppl.* 7, 59 (1987)
Caprolactam *19*, 115 (1979) (*corr.* 42, 258); *39*, 247 (1986) (*corr.* 42, 264); *Suppl.* 7, 390 (1987)
Captan *30*, 295 (1983); *Suppl.* 7, 59 (1987)
Carbaryl *12*, 37 (1976); *Suppl.* 7, 59 (1987)
Carbazole *32*, 239 (1983); *Suppl.* 7, 59 (1987)
3-Carbethoxypsoralen *40*, 317 (1986); *Suppl.* 7, 59 (1987)
Carbon blacks *3*, 22 (1973); *33*, 35 (1984); *Suppl.* 7, 142 (1987)
Carbon tetrachloride *1*, 53 (1972); *20*, 371 (1979); *Suppl.* 7, 143 (1987)
Carmoisine *8*, 83 (1975); *Suppl.* 7, 59 (1987)
Carpentry and joinery *25*, 139 (1981); *Suppl.* 7, 378 (1987)
Carrageenan *10*, 181 (1976) (*corr.* 42, 255); *31*, 79 (1983); *Suppl.* 7, 59 (1987)
Catechol *15*, 155 (1977); *Suppl.* 7, 59 (1987)
CCNU (*see* 1-(2-Chloroethyl)-3-cyclohexyl-1-nitrosourea)
Ceramic fibres (*see* Man-made mineral fibres)
Chemotherapy, combined, including alkylating agents
 (*see* MOPP and other combined chemotherapy including alkylating agents)
Chlorambucil *9*, 125 (1975); *26*, 115 (1981); *Suppl.* 7, 144 (1987)
Chloramphenicol *10*, 85 (1976); *Suppl.* 7, 145 (1987); *50*, 169 (1990)
Chlorendic acid *48*, 45 (1990)
Chlordane (*see also* Chlordane/Heptachlor) *20*, 45 (1979) (*corr.* 42, 258)
Chlordane/Heptachlor *Suppl.* 7, 146 (1987)
Chlordecone *20*, 67 (1979); *Suppl.* 7, 59 (1987)
Chlordimeform *30*, 61 (1983); *Suppl.* 7, 59 (1987)
Chlorinated dibenzodioxins (other than TCDD) *15*, 41 (1977); *Suppl.* 7, 59 (1987)
Chlorinated paraffins *48*, 55 (1990)

α-Chlorinated toluenes — *Suppl. 7*, 148 (1987)
Chlormadinone acetate (*see also* Progestins; Combined oral contraceptives) — *6*, 149 (1974); *21*, 365 (1979)
Chlornaphazine (*see N,N*-Bis(2-chloroethyl)-2-naphthylamine)
Chlorobenzilate — *5*, 75 (1974); *30*, 73 (1983); *Suppl. 7*, 60 (1987)
Chlorodifluoromethane — *41*, 237 (1986); *Suppl. 7*, 149 (1987)
1-(2-Chloroethyl)-3-cyclohexyl-1-nitrosourea (*see also* Chloroethyl nitrosoureas) — *26*, 137 (1981) (*corr. 42*, 260); *Suppl. 7*, 150 (1987)
1-(2-Chloroethyl)-3-(4-methylcyclohexyl)-1-nitrosourea (*see also* Chloroethyl nitrosoureas) — *Suppl. 7*, 150 (1987)
Chloroethyl nitrosoureas — *Suppl. 7*, 150 (1987)
Chlorofluoromethane — *41*, 229 (1986); *Suppl. 7*, 60 (1987)
Chloroform — *1*, 61 (1972); *20*, 401 (1979); *Suppl. 7*, 152 (1987)
Chloromethyl methyl ether (technical-grade) (*see also* Bis(chloromethyl)ether) — *4*, 239 (1974)
(4-Chloro-2-methylphenoxy)acetic acid (*see* MCPA)
Chlorophenols — *Suppl. 7*, 154 (1987)
Chlorophenols (occupational exposures to) — *41*, 319 (1986)
Chlorophenoxy herbicides — *Suppl. 7*, 156 (1987)
Chlorophenoxy herbicides (occupational exposures to) — *41*, 357 (1986)
4-Chloro-*ortho*-phenylenediamine — *27*, 81 (1982); *Suppl. 7*, 60 (1987)
4-Chloro-*meta*-phenylenediamine — *27*, 82 (1982); *Suppl. 7*, 60 (1987)
Chloroprene — *19*, 131 (1979); *Suppl. 7*, 160 (1987)
Chloropropham — *12*, 55 (1976); *Suppl. 7*, 60 (1987)
Chloroquine — *13*, 47 (1977); *Suppl. 7*, 60 (1987)
Chlorothalonil — *30*, 319 (1983); *Suppl. 7*, 60 (1987)
para-Chloro-*ortho*-toluidine and its strong acid salts (*see also* Chlordimeform) — *16*, 277 (1978); *30*, 65 (1983); *Suppl. 7*, 60 (1987); *48*, 123 (1990)
Chlorotrianisene (*see also* Nonsteroidal oestrogens) — *21*, 139 (1979)
2-Chloro-1,1,1-trifluoroethane — *41*, 253 (1986); *Suppl. 7*, 60 (1987)
Chlorozotocin — *50*, 65 (1990)
Cholesterol — *10*, 99 (1976); *31*, 95 (1983); *Suppl. 7*, 161 (1987)

Chromic acetate (*see* Chromium and chromium compounds)
Chromic chloride (*see* Chromium and chromium compounds)
Chromic oxide (*see* Chromium and chromium compounds)
Chromic phosphate (*see* Chromium and chromium compounds)
Chromite ore (*see* Chromium and chromium compounds)
Chromium and chromium compounds — *2*, 100 (1973); *23*, 205 (1980); *Suppl. 7*, 165 (1987); *49*, 49 (1990)

Chromium carbonyl (*see* Chromium and chromium compounds)
Chromium potassium sulphate (*see* Chromium and chromium compounds)
Chromium sulphate (*see* Chromium and chromium compounds)

Chromium trioxide (see Chromium and chromium compounds)
Chrysazin (see Dantron)
Chrysene   3, 159 (1973); 32, 247 (1983);
                                                        Suppl. 7, 60 (1987)
Chrysoidine   8, 91 (1975); Suppl. 7, 169 (1987)
Chrysotile (see Asbestos)
Ciclosporin   50, 77 (1990)
CI Disperse Yellow 3   8, 97 (1975); Suppl. 7, 60 (1987)
Cimetidine   50, 235 (1990)
Cinnamyl anthranilate   16, 287 (1978); 31, 133 (1983);
                                                        Suppl. 7, 60 (1987)
Cisplatin   26, 151 (1981); Suppl. 7, 170 (1987)
Citrinin   40, 67 (1986); Suppl. 7, 60 (1987)
Citrus Red No. 2   8, 101 (1975) (corr. 42, 254);
                                                        Suppl. 7, 60 (1987)
Clofibrate   24, 39 (1980); Suppl. 7, 171 (1987)
Clomiphene citrate   21, 551 (1979); Suppl. 7, 172 (1987)
Coal gasification   34, 65 (1984); Suppl. 7, 173 (1987)
Coal-tar pitches (see also Coal-tars)   Suppl. 7, 174 (1987)
Coal-tars   35, 83 (1985); Suppl. 7, 175 (1987)
Cobalt–chromium alloy (see Chromium and chromium
    compounds)
Coffee   51, 41 (1991)
Coke production   34, 101 (1984); Suppl. 7, 176 (1987)
Combined oral contraceptives (see also Oestrogens, progestins   Suppl. 7, 297 (1987)
    and combinations)
Conjugated oestrogens (see also Steroidal oestrogens)   21, 147 (1979)
Contraceptives, oral (see Combined oral contraceptives;
    Sequential oral contraceptives)
Copper 8-hydroxyquinoline   15, 103 (1977); Suppl. 7, 61 (1987)
Coronene   32, 263 (1983); Suppl. 7, 61 (1987)
Coumarin   10, 113 (1976); Suppl. 7, 61 (1987)
Creosotes (see also Coal-tars)   Suppl. 7, 177 (1987)
meta-Cresidine   27, 91 (1982); Suppl. 7, 61 (1987)
para-Cresidine   27, 92 (1982); Suppl. 7, 61 (1987)
Crocidolite (see Asbestos)
Crude oil   45, 119 (1989)
Crystalline silica (see also Silica)   Suppl. 7, 341 (1987)
Cycasin   1, 157 (1972) (corr. 42, 251); 10,
                                                        121 (1976); Suppl. 7, 61 (1987)
Cyclamates   22, 55 (1980); Suppl. 7, 178 (1987)
Cyclamic acid (see Cyclamates)
Cyclochlorotine   10, 139 (1976); Suppl. 7, 61 (1987)
Cyclohexanone   47, 157 (1989)
Cyclohexylamine (see Cyclamates)

Cyclopenta[*cd*]pyrene	*32*, 269 (1983); *Suppl. 7*, 61 (1987)
Cyclopropane (*see* Anaesthetics, volatile)	
Cyclophosphamide	*9*, 135 (1975); *26*, 165 (1981); *Suppl. 7*, 182 (1987)

D

2,4-D (*see also* Chlorophenoxy herbicides; Chlorophenoxy herbicides, occupational exposures to)	*15*, 111 (1977)
Dacarbazine	*26*, 203 (1981); *Suppl. 7*, 184 (1987)
Dantron	*50*, 265 (1990)
D & C Red No. 9	*8*, 107 (1975); *Suppl. 7*, 61 (1987)
Dapsone	*24*, 59 (1980); *Suppl. 7*, 185 (1987)
Daunomycin	*10*, 145 (1976); *Suppl. 7*, 61 (1987)
DDD (*see* DDT)	
DDE (*see* DDT)	
DDT	*5*, 83 (1974) (*corr. 42*, 253); *Suppl. 7*, 186 (1987)
Decabromodiphenyl oxide	*48*, 73 (1990)
Diacetylaminoazotoluene	*8*, 113 (1975); *Suppl. 7*, 61 (1987)
N,N'-Diacetylbenzidine	*16*, 293 (1978); *Suppl. 7*, 61 (1987)
Diallate	*12*, 69 (1976); *30*, 235 (1983); *Suppl. 7*, 61 (1987)
2,4-Diaminoanisole	*16*, 51 (1978); *27*, 103 (1982); *Suppl. 7*, 61 (1987)
4,4'-Diaminodiphenyl ether	*16*, 301 (1978); *29*, 203 (1982); *Suppl. 7*, 61 (1987)
1,2-Diamino-4-nitrobenzene	*16*, 63 (1978); *Suppl. 7*, 61 (1987)
1,4-Diamino-2-nitrobenzene	*16*, 73 (1978); *Suppl. 7*, 61 (1987)
2,6-Diamino-3-(phenylazo)pyridine (*see* Phenazopyridine hydrochloride)	
2,4-Diaminotoluene (*see also* Toluene diisocyanates)	*16*, 83 (1978); *Suppl. 7*, 61 (1987)
2,5-Diaminotoluene (*see also* Toluene diisocyanates)	*16*, 97 (1978); *Suppl. 7*, 61 (1987)
ortho-Dianisidine (*see* 3,3'-Dimethoxybenzidine)	
Diazepam	*13*, 57 (1977); *Suppl. 7*, 189 (1987)
Diazomethane	*7*, 223 (1974); *Suppl. 7*, 61 (1987)
Dibenz[*a,h*]acridine	*3*, 247 (1973); *32*, 277 (1983); *Suppl. 7*, 61 (1987)
Dibenz[*a,j*]acridine	*3*, 254 (1973); *32*, 283 (1983); *Suppl. 7*, 61 (1987)
Dibenz[*a,c*]anthracene	*32*, 289 (1983) (*corr. 42*, 262); *Suppl. 7*, 61 (1987)
Dibenz[*a,h*]anthracene	*3*, 178 (1973) (*corr. 43*, 261); *32*, 299 (1983); *Suppl. 7*, 61 (1987)
Dibenz[*a,j*]anthracene	*32*, 309 (1983); *Suppl. 7*, 61 (1987)

7H-Dibenzo[c,g]carbazole — 3, 260 (1973); 32, 315 (1983); Suppl. 7, 61 (1987)

Dibenzodioxins, chlorinated (other than TCDD) (see Chlorinated dibenzodioxins (other than TCDD))

Dibenzo[a,e]fluoranthene — 32, 321 (1983); Suppl. 7, 61 (1987)

Dibenzo[h,rst]pentaphene — 3, 197 (1973); Suppl. 7, 62 (1987)

Dibenzo[a,e]pyrene — 3, 201 (1973); 32, 327 (1983); Suppl. 7, 62 (1987)

Dibenzo[a,h]pyrene — 3, 207 (1973); 32, 331 (1983); Suppl. 7, 62 (1987)

Dibenzo[a,i]pyrene — 3, 215 (1973); 32, 337 (1983); Suppl. 7, 62 (1987)

Dibenzo[a,l]pyrene — 3, 224 (1973); 32, 343 (1983); Suppl. 7, 62 (1987)

1,2-Dibromo-3-chloropropane — 15, 139 (1977); 20, 83 (1979); Suppl. 7, 191 (1987)

Dichloroacetylene — 39, 369 (1986); Suppl. 7, 62 (1987)

ortho-Dichlorobenzene — 7, 231 (1974); 29, 213 (1982); Suppl. 7, 192 (1987)

para-Dichlorobenzene — 7, 231 (1974); 29, 215 (1982); Suppl. 7, 192 (1987)

3,3'-Dichlorobenzidine — 4, 49 (1974); 29, 239 (1982); Suppl. 7, 193 (1987)

trans-1,4-Dichlorobutene — 15, 149 (1977); Suppl. 7, 62 (1987)

3,3'-Dichloro-4,4'-diaminodiphenyl ether — 16, 309 (1978); Suppl. 7, 62 (1987)

1,2-Dichloroethane — 20, 429 (1979); Suppl. 7, 62 (1987)

Dichloromethane — 20, 449 (1979); 41, 43 (1986); Suppl. 7, 194 (1987)

2,4-Dichlorophenol (see Chlorophenols; Chlorophenols, occupational exposures to)

(2,4-Dichlorophenoxy)acetic acid (see 2,4-D)

2,6-Dichloro-para-phenylenediamine — 39, 325 (1986); Suppl. 7, 62 (1987)

1,2-Dichloropropane — 41, 131 (1986); Suppl. 7, 62 (1987)

1,3-Dichloropropene (technical-grade) — 41, 113 (1986); Suppl. 7, 195 (1987)

Dichlorvos — 20, 97 (1979); Suppl. 7, 62 (1987)

Dicofol — 30, 87 (1983); Suppl. 7, 62 (1987)

Dicyclohexylamine (see Cyclamates)

Dieldrin — 5, 125 (1974); Suppl. 7, 196 (1987)

Dienoestrol (see also Nonsteroidal oestrogens) — 21, 161 (1979)

Diepoxybutane — 11, 115 (1976) (corr. 42, 255); Suppl. 7, 62 (1987)

Diesel and gasoline engine exhausts — 46, 41 (1989)

Diesel fuels — 45, 219 (1989) (corr. 47, 505)

Diethyl ether (see Anaesthetics, volatile)

Di(2-ethylhexyl)adipate — 29, 257 (1982); Suppl. 7, 62 (1987)

Di(2-ethylhexyl)phthalate	29, 269 (1982) (corr. 42, 261); Suppl. 7, 62 (1987)
1,2-Diethylhydrazine	4, 153 (1974); Suppl. 7, 62 (1987)
Diethylstilboestrol	6, 55 (1974); 21, 173 (1979) (corr. 42, 259); Suppl. 7, 273 (1987)
Diethylstilboestrol dipropionate (see Diethylstilboestrol)	
Diethyl sulphate	4, 277 (1974); Suppl. 7, 198 (1987)
Diglycidyl resorcinol ether	11, 125 (1976); 36, 181 (1985); Suppl. 7, 62 (1987)
Dihydrosafrole	1, 170 (1972); 10, 233 (1976); Suppl. 7, 62 (1987)
1,8-Dihydroxyanthraquinone (see Dantron)	
Dihydroxybenzenes (see Catechol; Hydroquinone; Resorcinol)	
Dihydroxymethylfuratrizine	24, 77 (1980); Suppl. 7, 62 (1987)
Dimethisterone (see also Progestins; Sequential oral contraceptives)	6, 167 (1974); 21, 377 (1979)
Dimethoxane	15, 177 (1977); Suppl. 7, 62 (1987)
3,3'-Dimethoxybenzidine	4, 41 (1974); Suppl. 7, 198 (1987)
3,3'-Dimethoxybenzidine-4,4'-diisocyanate	39, 279 (1986); Suppl. 7, 62 (1987)
para-Dimethylaminoazobenzene	8, 125 (1975); Suppl. 7, 62 (1987)
para-Dimethylaminoazobenzenediazo sodium sulphonate	8, 147 (1975); Suppl. 7, 62 (1987)
trans-2-[(Dimethylamino)methylimino]-5-[2-(5-nitro-2-furyl)-vinyl]-1,3,4-oxadiazole	7, 147 (1974) (corr. 42, 253); Suppl. 7, 62 (1987)
4,4'-Dimethylangelicin plus ultraviolet radiation (see also Angelicin and some synthetic derivatives)	Suppl. 7, 57 (1987)
4,5'-Dimethylangelicin plus ultraviolet radiation (see also Angelicin and some synthetic derivatives)	Suppl. 7, 57 (1987)
Dimethylarsinic acid (see Arsenic and arsenic compounds)	
3,3'-Dimethylbenzidine	1, 87 (1972); Suppl. 7, 62 (1987)
Dimethylcarbamoyl chloride	12, 77 (1976); Suppl. 7, 199 (1987)
Dimethylformamide	47, 171 (1989)
1,1-Dimethylhydrazine	4, 137 (1974); Suppl.7, 62 (1987)
1,2-Dimethylhydrazine	4, 145 (1974) (corr. 42, 253); Suppl. 7, 62 (1987)
Dimethyl hydrogen phosphite	48, 85 (1990)
1,4-Dimethylphenanthrene	32, 349 (1983); Suppl. 7, 62 (1987)
Dimethyl sulphate	4, 271 (1974); Suppl. 7, 200 (1987)
3,7-Dinitrofluoranthene	46, 189 (1989)
3,9-Dinitrofluoranthene	46, 195 (1989)
1,3-Dinitropyrene	46, 201 (1989)
1,6-Dinitropyrene	46, 215 (1989)
1,8-Dinitropyrene	33, 171 (1984); Suppl. 7, 63 (1987); 46, 231 (1989)
Dinitrosopentamethylenetetramine	11, 241 (1976); Suppl. 7, 63 (1987)
1,4-Dioxane	11, 247 (1976); Suppl. 7, 201 (1987)

2,4'-Diphenyldiamine	*16*, 313 (1978); *Suppl. 7*, 63 (1987)
Direct Black 38 (*see also* Benzidine-based dyes)	*29*, 295 (1982) (*corr. 42*, 261)
Direct Blue 6 (*see also* Benzidine-based dyes)	*29*, 311 (1982)
Direct Brown 95 (*see also* Benzidine-based dyes)	*29*, 321 (1982)
Disperse Blue 1	*48*, 139 (1990)
Disperse Yellow 3	*48*, 149 (1990)
Disulfiram	*12*, 85 (1976); *Suppl. 7*, 63 (1987)
Dithranol	*13*, 75 (1977); *Suppl. 7*, 63 (1987)
Divinyl ether (*see* Anaesthetics, volatile)	
Dulcin	*12*, 97 (1976); *Suppl. 7*, 63 (1987)

E

Endrin	*5*, 157 (1974); *Suppl. 7*, 63 (1987)
Enflurane (*see* Anaesthetics, volatile)	
Eosin	*15*, 183 (1977); *Suppl. 7*, 63 (1987)
Epichlorohydrin	*11*, 131 (1976) (*corr. 42*, 256); *Suppl. 7*, 202 (1987)
1,2-Epoxybutane	*47*, 217 (1989)
1-Epoxyethyl-3,4-epoxycyclohexane	*11*, 141 (1976); *Suppl. 7*, 63 (1987)
3,4-Epoxy-6-methylcyclohexylmethyl-3,4-epoxy-6-methyl-cyclohexane carboxylate	*11*, 147 (1976); *Suppl. 7*, 63 (1987)
cis-9,10-Epoxystearic acid	*11*, 153 (1976); *Suppl. 7*, 63 (1987)
Erionite	*42*, 225 (1987); *Suppl. 7*, 203 (1987)
Ethinyloestradiol (*see also* Steroidal oestrogens)	*6*, 77 (1974); *21*, 233 (1979)
Ethionamide	*13*, 83 (1977); *Suppl. 7*, 63 (1987)
Ethyl acrylate	*19*, 57 (1979); *39*, 81 (1986); *Suppl. 7*, 63 (1987)
Ethylene	*19*, 157 (1979); *Suppl. 7*, 63 (1987)
Ethylene dibromide	*15*, 195 (1977); *Suppl. 7*, 204 (1987)
Ethylene oxide	*11*, 157 (1976); *36*, 189 (1985) (*corr. 42*, 263); *Suppl. 7*, 205 (1987)
Ethylene sulphide	*11*, 257 (1976); *Suppl. 7*, 63 (1987)
Ethylene thiourea	*7*, 45 (1974); *Suppl. 7*, 207 (1987)
Ethyl methanesulphonate	*7*, 245 (1974); *Suppl. 7*, 63 (1987)
N-Ethyl-*N*-nitrosourea	*1*, 135 (1972); *17*, 191 (1978); *Suppl. 7*, 63 (1987)
Ethyl selenac (*see also* Selenium and selenium compounds)	*12*, 107 (1976); *Suppl. 7*, 63 (1987)
Ethyl tellurac	*12*, 115 (1976); *Suppl. 7*, 63 (1987)
Ethynodiol diacetate (*see also* Progestins; Combined oral contraceptives)	*6*, 173 (1974); *21*, 387 (1979)
Eugenol	*36*, 75 (1985); *Suppl. 7*, 63 (1987)
Evans blue	*8*, 151 (1975); *Suppl. 7*, 63 (1987)

F

Fast Green FCF	*16*, 187 (1978); *Suppl. 7*, 63 (1987)
Ferbam	*12*, 121 (1976) (*corr. 42*, 256); *Suppl. 7*, 63 (1987)
Ferric oxide	*1*, 29 (1972); *Suppl. 7*, 216 (1987)
Ferrochromium (*see* Chromium and chromium compounds)	
Fluometuron	*30*, 245 (1983); *Suppl. 7*, 63 (1987)
Fluoranthene	*32*, 355 (1983); *Suppl. 7*, 63 (1987)
Fluorene	*32*, 365 (1983); *Suppl. 7*, 63 (1987)
Fluorides (inorganic, used in drinking-water)	*27*, 237 (1982); *Suppl. 7*, 208 (1987)
5-Fluorouracil	*26*, 217 (1981); *Suppl. 7*, 210 (1987)
Fluorspar (*see* Fluorides)	
Fluosilicic acid (*see* Fluorides)	
Fluroxene (*see* Anaesthetics, volatile)	
Formaldehyde	*29*, 345 (1982); *Suppl. 7*, 211 (1987)
2-(2-Formylhydrazino)-4-(5-nitro-2-furyl)thiazole	*7*, 151 (1974) (*corr. 42*, 253); *Suppl. 7*, 63 (1987)
Frusemide (*see* Furosemide)	
Fuel oils (heating oils)	*45*, 239 (1989) (*corr. 47*, 505)
Furazolidone	*31*, 141 (1983); *Suppl. 7*, 63 (1987)
Furniture and cabinet-making	*25*, 99 (1981); *Suppl. 7*, 380 (1987)
Furosemide	*50*, 277 (1990)
2-(2-Furyl)-3-(5-nitro-2-furyl)acrylamide (*see* AF-2)	
Fusarenon-X	*11*, 169 (1976); *31*, 153 (1983); *Suppl. 7*, 64 (1987)

G

Gasoline	*45*, 159 (1989) (*corr. 47*, 505)
Gasoline engine exhaust (*see* Diesel and gasoline engine exhausts)	
Glass fibres (*see* Man-made mineral fibres)	
Glasswool (*see* Man-made mineral fibres)	
Glass filaments (*see* Man-made mineral fibres)	
Glu-P-1	*40*, 223 (1986); *Suppl. 7*, 64 (1987)
Glu-P-2	*40*, 235 (1986); *Suppl. 7*, 64 (1987)
L-Glutamic acid, 5-[2-(4-hydroxymethyl)phenylhydrazide] (*see* Agaratine)	
Glycidaldehyde	*11*, 175 (1976); *Suppl. 7*, 64 (1987)
Some glycidyl ethers	*47*, 237 (1989)
Glycidyl oleate	*11*, 183 (1976); *Suppl. 7*, 64 (1987)
Glycidyl stearate	*11*, 187 (1976); *Suppl. 7*, 64 (1987)
Griseofulvin	*10*, 153 (1976); *Suppl. 7*, 391 (1987)
Guinea Green B	*16*, 199 (1978); *Suppl. 7*, 64 (1987)
Gyromitrin	*31*, 163 (1983); *Suppl. 7*, 391 (1987)

H

Haematite	*1*, 29 (1972); *Suppl. 7*, 216 (1987)
Haematite and ferric oxide	*Suppl. 7*, 216 (1987)
Haematite mining, underground, with exposure to radon	*1*, 29 (1972); *Suppl. 7*, 216 (1987)
Hair dyes, epidemiology of	*16*, 29 (1978); *27*, 307 (1982)
Halothane (*see* Anaesthetics, volatile)	
α-HCH (*see* Hexachlorocyclohexanes)	
β-HCH (*see* Hexachlorocyclohexanes)	
γ-HCH (*see* Hexachlorocyclohexanes)	
Heating oils (*see* Fuel oils)	
Heptachlor (*see also* Chlordane/Heptachlor)	*5*, 173 (1974); *20*, 129 (1979)
Hexachlorobenzene	*20*, 155 (1979); *Suppl. 7*, 219 (1987)
Hexachlorobutadiene	*20*, 179 (1979); *Suppl. 7*, 64 (1987)
Hexachlorocyclohexanes	*5*, 47 (1974); *20*, 195 (1979) (*corr.* *42*, 258); *Suppl. 7*, 220 (1987)
Hexachlorocyclohexane, technical-grade (*see* Hexachlorocyclohexanes)	
Hexachloroethane	*20*, 467 (1979); *Suppl. 7*, 64 (1987)
Hexachlorophene	*20*, 241 (1979); *Suppl. 7*, 64 (1987)
Hexamethylphosphoramide	*15*, 211 (1977); *Suppl. 7*, 64 (1987)
Hexoestrol (*see* Nonsteroidal oestrogens)	
Hycanthone mesylate	*13*, 91 (1977); *Suppl. 7*, 64 (1987)
Hydralazine	*24*, 85 (1980); *Suppl. 7*, 222 (1987)
Hydrazine	*4*, 127 (1974); *Suppl. 7*, 223 (1987)
Hydrochlorothiazide	*50*, 293 (1990)
Hydrogen peroxide	*36*, 285 (1985); *Suppl. 7*, 64 (1987)
Hydroquinone	*15*, 155 (1977); *Suppl. 7*, 64 (1987)
4-Hydroxyazobenzene	*8*, 157 (1975); *Suppl. 7*, 64 (1987)
17α-Hydroxyprogesterone caproate (*see also* Progestins)	*21*, 399 (1979) (*corr.* *42*, 259)
8-Hydroxyquinoline	*13*, 101 (1977); *Suppl. 7*, 64 (1987)
8-Hydroxysenkirkine	*10*, 265 (1976); *Suppl. 7*, 64 (1987)

I

Indeno[1,2,3-*cd*]pyrene	*3*, 229 (1973); *32*, 373 (1983); *Suppl. 7*, 64 (1987)
IQ	*40*, 261 (1986); *Suppl. 7*, 64 (1987)
Iron and steel founding	*34*, 133 (1984); *Suppl. 7*, 224 (1987)
Iron–dextran complex	*2*, 161 (1973); *Suppl. 7*, 226 (1987)
Iron–dextrin complex	*2*, 161 (1973) (*corr.* *42*, 252); *Suppl. 7*, 64 (1987)
Iron oxide (*see* Ferric oxide)	
Iron oxide, saccharated (*see* Saccharated iron oxide)	
Iron sorbitol–citric acid complex	*2*, 161 (1973); *Suppl. 7*, 64 (1987)

Isatidine	*10*, 269 (1976); *Suppl. 7*, 65 (1987)
Isoflurane (*see* Anaesthetics, volatile)	
Isoniazid (*see* Isonicotinic acid hydrazide)	
Isonicotinic acid hydrazide	*4*, 159 (1974); *Suppl. 7*, 227 (1987)
Isophosphamide	*26*, 237 (1981); *Suppl. 7*, 65 (1987)
Isopropyl alcohol	*15*, 223 (1977); *Suppl. 7*, 229 (1987)
Isopropyl alcohol manufacture (strong-acid process) (*see also* Isopropyl alcohol)	*Suppl. 7*, 229 (1987)
Isopropyl oils	*15*, 223 (1977); *Suppl. 7*, 229 (1987)
Isosafrole	*1*, 169 (1972); *10*, 232 (1976); *Suppl. 7*, 65 (1987)

J

Jacobine	*10*, 275 (1976); *Suppl. 7*, 65 (1987)
Jet fuel	*45*, 203 (1989)
Joinery (*see* Carpentry and joinery)	

K

Kaempferol	31, 171 (1983); *Suppl. 7*, 65 (1987)
Kepone (*see* Chlordecone)	

L

Lasiocarpine	*10*, 281 (1976); *Suppl. 7*, 65 (1987)
Lauroyl peroxide	*36*, 315 (1985); Suppl. 7, 65 (1987)
Lead acetate (*see* Lead and lead compounds)	
Lead and lead compounds	*1*, 40 (1972) (*corr. 42*, 251); *2*, 52, 150 (1973); *12*, 131 (1976); *23*, 40, 208, 209, 325 (1980); *Suppl. 7*, 230 (1987)
Lead arsenate (*see* Arsenic and arsenic compounds)	
Lead carbonate (*see* Lead and lead compounds)	
Lead chloride (*see* Lead and lead compounds)	
Lead chromate (*see* Chromium and chromium compounds)	
Lead chromate oxide (*see* Chromium and chromium compounds)	
Lead naphthenate (*see* Lead and lead compounds)	
Lead nitrate (*see* Lead and lead compounds)	
Lead oxide (*see* Lead and lead compounds)	
Lead phosphate (*see* Lead and lead compounds)	
Lead subacetate (*see* Lead and lead compounds)	
Lead tetroxide (*see* Lead and lead compounds)	
Leather goods manufacture	*25*, 279 (1981); *Suppl. 7*, 235 (1987)
Leather industries	*25*, 199 (1981); *Suppl. 7*, 232 (1987)

Leather tanning and processing	25, 201 (1981); *Suppl. 7*, 236 (1987)
Ledate (*see also* Lead and lead compounds)	12, 131 (1976)
Light Green SF	16, 209 (1978); *Suppl. 7*, 65 (1987)
Lindane (*see* Hexachlorocyclohexanes)	
The lumber and sawmill industries (including logging)	25, 49 (1981); *Suppl. 7*, 383 (1987)
Luteoskyrin	10, 163 (1976); *Suppl. 7*, 65 (1987)
Lynoestrenol (*see also* Progestins; Combined oral contraceptives)	21, 407 (1979)

M

Magenta	4, 57 (1974) (*corr.* 42, 252); *Suppl. 7*, 238 (1987)
Magenta, manufacture of (*see also* Magenta)	*Suppl. 7*, 238 (1987)
Malathion	30, 103 (1983); *Suppl. 7*, 65 (1987)
Maleic hydrazide	4, 173 (1974) (*corr.* 42, 253); *Suppl. 7*, 65 (1987)
Malonaldehyde	36, 163 (1985); *Suppl. 7*, 65 (1987)
Maneb	12, 137 (1976); *Suppl. 7*, 65 (1987)
Man-made mineral fibres	43, 39 (1988)
Mannomustine	9, 157 (1975); *Suppl. 7*, 65 (1987)
Mate	51, 273 (1991)
MCPA (*see also* Chlorophenoxy herbicides; Chlorophenoxy herbicides, occupational exposures to)	30, 255 (1983)
MeA-α-C	40, 253 (1986); *Suppl. 7*, 65 (1987)
Medphalan	9, 168 (1975); *Suppl. 7*, 65 (1987)
Medroxyprogesterone acetate	6, 157 (1974); 21, 417 (1979) (*corr.* 42, 259); *Suppl. 7*, 289 (1987)
Megestrol acetate (*see* also Progestins; Combined oral contraceptives)	
MeIQ	40, 275 (1986); *Suppl. 7*, 65 (1987)
MeIQx	40, 283 (1986); *Suppl. 7*, 65 (1987)
Melamine	39, 333 (1986); *Suppl. 7*, 65 (1987)
Melphalan	9, 167 (1975); *Suppl. 7*, 239 (1987)
6-Mercaptopurine	26, 249 (1981); *Suppl. 7*, 240 (1987)
Merphalan	9, 169 (1975); *Suppl. 7*, 65 (1987)
Mestranol (*see also* Steroidal oestrogens)	6, 87 (1974); 21, 257 (1979) (*corr.* 42, 259)
Methanearsonic acid, disodium salt (*see* Arsenic and arsenic compounds)	
Methanearsonic acid, monosodium salt (*see* Arsenic and arsenic compounds	
Methotrexate	26, 267 (1981); *Suppl. 7*, 241 (1987)
Methoxsalen (*see* 8-Methoxypsoralen)	
Methoxychlor	5, 193 (1974); 20, 259 (1979); *Suppl. 7*, 66 (1987)

Methoxyflurane (see Anaesthetics, volatile)	
5-Methoxypsoralen	*40*, 327 (1986); *Suppl. 7*, 242 (1987)
8-Methoxypsoralen (see also 8-Methoxypsoralen plus ultraviolet radiation)	*24*, 101 (1980)
8-Methoxypsoralen plus ultraviolet radiation	*Suppl. 7*, 243 (1987)
Methyl acrylate	*19*, 52 (1979); *39*, 99 (1986); *Suppl. 7*, 66 (1987)
5-Methylangelicin plus ultraviolet radiation (see also Angelicin and some synthetic derivatives)	*Suppl. 7*, 57 (1987)
2-Methylaziridine	*9*, 61 (1975); *Suppl. 7*, 66 (1987)
Methylazoxymethanol acetate	*1*, 164 (1972); *10*, 131 (1976); *Suppl. 7*, 66 (1987)
Methyl bromide	*41*, 187 (1986) (corr. *45*, 283); *Suppl. 7*, 245 (1987)
Methyl carbamate	*12*, 151 (1976); *Suppl. 7*, 66 (1987)
Methyl-CCNU [see 1-(2-Chloroethyl)-3-(4-methylcyclohexyl)-1-nitrosourea]	
Methyl chloride	*41*, 161 (1986); *Suppl. 7*, 246 (1987)
1-, 2-, 3-, 4-, 5- and 6-Methylchrysenes	*32*, 379 (1983); *Suppl. 7*, 66 (1987)
N-Methyl-N,4-dinitrosoaniline	*1*, 141 (1972); *Suppl. 7*, 66 (1987)
4,4'-Methylene bis(2-chloroaniline)	*4*, 65 (1974) (corr. *42*, 252); *Suppl. 7*, 246 (1987)
4,4'-Methylene bis(N,N-dimethyl)benzenamine	*27*, 119 (1982); *Suppl. 7*, 66 (1987)
4,4'-Methylene bis(2-methylaniline)	*4*, 73 (1974); *Suppl. 7*, 248 (1987)
4,4'-Methylenedianiline	*4*, 79 (1974) (corr. *42*, 252); *39*, 347 (1986); *Suppl. 7*, 66 (1987)
4,4'-Methylenediphenyl diisocyanate	*19*, 314 (1979); *Suppl. 7*, 66 (1987)
2-Methylfluoranthene	*32*, 399 (1983); *Suppl. 7*, 66 (1987)
3-Methylfluoranthene	*32*, 399 (1983); *Suppl. 7*, 66 (1987)
Methylglyoxal	*51*, 443 (1991)
Methyl iodide	*15*, 245 (1977); *41*, 213 (1986); *Suppl. 7*, 66 (1987)
Methyl methacrylate	*19*, 187 (1979); *Suppl. 7*, 66 (1987)
Methyl methanesulphonate	*7*, 253 (1974); *Suppl. 7*, 66 (1987)
2-Methyl-1-nitroanthraquinone	*27*, 205 (1982); *Suppl. 7*, 66 (1987)
N-Methyl-N'-nitro-N-nitrosoguanidine	*4*, 183 (1974); *Suppl. 7*, 248 (1987)
3-Methylnitrosaminopropionaldehyde (see 3-(N-Nitrosomethylamino)propionaldehyde)	
3-Methylnitrosaminopropionitrile (see 3-(N-Nitrosomethylamino)propionitrile)	
4-(Methylnitrosamino)-4-(3-pyridyl)-1-butanal (see 4-(N-Nitrosomethylamino)-4-(3-pyridyl)-1-butanal)	
4-(Methylnitrosamino)-1-(3-pyridyl)-1-butanone (see 4-(N-Nitrosomethylamino)-1-(3-pyridyl)-1-butanone)	

N-Methyl-N-nitrosourea	1, 125 (1972); 17, 227 (1978); Suppl. 7, 66 (1987)
N-Methyl-N-nitrosourethane	4, 211 (1974); Suppl. 7, 66 (1987)
Methyl parathion	30, 131 (1983); Suppl. 7, 392 (1987)
1-Methylphenanthrene	32, 405 (1983); Suppl. 7, 66 (1987)
7-Methylpyrido[3,4-c]psoralen	40, 349 (1986); Suppl. 7, 71 (1987)
Methyl red	8, 161 (1975); Suppl. 7, 66 (1987)
Methyl selenac (see also Selenium and selenium compounds)	12, 161 (1976); Suppl. 7, 66 (1987)
Methylthiouracil	7, 53 (1974); Suppl. 7, 66 (1987)
Metronidazole	13, 113 (1977); Suppl. 7, 250 (1987)
Mineral oils	3, 30 (1973); 33, 87 (1984) (corr. 42, 262); Suppl. 7, 252 (1987)
Mirex	5, 203 (1974); 20, 283 (1979) (corr. 42, 258); Suppl. 7, 66 (1987)
Mitomycin C	10, 171 (1976); Suppl. 7, 67 (1987)
MNNG (see N-Methyl-N'-nitro-N-nitrosoguanidine)	
MOCA (see 4,4'-Methylene bis(2-chloroaniline))	
Modacrylic fibres	19, 86 (1979); Suppl. 7, 67 (1987)
Monocrotaline	10, 291 (1976); Suppl. 7, 67 (1987)
Monuron	12, 167 (1976); Suppl. 7, 67 (1987)
MOPP and other combined chemotherapy including alkylating agents	Suppl. 7, 254 (1987)
Morpholine	47, 199 (1989)
5-(Morpholinomethyl)-3-[(5-nitrofurfurylidene)amino]-2-oxazolidinone	7, 161 (1974); Suppl. 7, 67 (1987)
Mustard gas	9, 181 (1975) (corr. 42, 254); Suppl. 7, 259 (1987)
Myleran (see 1,4-Butanediol dimethanesulphonate)	

N

Nafenopin	24, 125 (1980); Suppl. 7, 67 (1987)
1,5-Naphthalenediamine	27, 127 (1982); Suppl. 7, 67 (1987)
1,5-Naphthalene diisocyanate	19, 311 (1979); Suppl. 7, 67 (1987)
1-Naphthylamine	4, 87 (1974) (corr. 42, 253); Suppl. 7, 260 (1987)
2-Naphthylamine	4, 97 (1974); Suppl. 7, 261 (1987)
1-Naphthylthiourea	30, 347 (1983); Suppl. 7, 263 (1987)
Nickel acetate (see Nickel and nickel compounds)	
Nickel ammonium sulphate (see Nickel and nickel compounds)	
Nickel and nickel compounds	2, 126 (1973) (corr. 42, 252); 11, 75 (1976); Suppl. 7, 264 (1987) (corr. 45, 283); 49, 257 (1990)
Nickel carbonate (see Nickel and nickel compounds)	
Nickel carbonyl (see Nickel and nickel compounds)	

Nickel chloride (*see* Nickel and nickel compounds)
Nickel-gallium alloy (*see* Nickel and nickel compounds)
Nickel hydroxide (*see* Nickel and nickel compounds)
Nickelocene (*see* Nickel and nickel compounds)
Nickel oxide (*see* Nickel and nickel compounds)
Nickel subsulphide (*see* Nickel and nickel compounds)
Nickel sulphate (*see* Nickel and nickel compounds)

Niridazole	*13*, 123 (1977); *Suppl. 7*, 67 (1987)
Nithiazide	*31*, 179 (1983); *Suppl. 7*, 67 (1987)
Nitrilotriacetic acid and its salts	*48*, 181 (1990)
5-Nitroacenaphthene	*16*, 319 (1978); *Suppl. 7*, 67 (1987)
5-Nitro-*ortho*-anisidine	*27*, 133 (1982); *Suppl. 7*, 67 (1987)
9-Nitroanthracene	*33*, 179 (1984); *Suppl. 7*, 67 (1987)
7-Nitrobenz[*a*]anthracene	*46*, 247 (1989)
6-Nitrobenzo[*a*]pyrene	*33*, 187 (1984); *Suppl. 7*, 67 (1987); *46*, 255 (1989)
4-Nitrobiphenyl	*4*, 113 (1974); *Suppl. 7*, 67 (1987)
6-Nitrochrysene	*33*, 195 (1984); *Suppl. 7*, 67 (1987); *46*, 267 (1989)
Nitrofen (technical-grade)	*30*, 271 (1983); *Suppl. 7*, 67 (1987)
3-Nitrofluoranthene	*33*, 201 (1984); *Suppl. 7*, 67 (1987)
2-Nitrofluorene	*46*, 277 (1989)
Nitrofural	*7*, 171 (1974); *Suppl. 7*, 67 (1987); *50*, 195 (1990)

5-Nitro-2-furaldehyde semicarbazone (*see* Nitrofural)

Nitrofurantoin	*50*, 211 (1990)

Nitrofurazone (*see* Nitrofural)

1-[(5-Nitrofurfurylidene)amino]-2-imidazolidinone	*7*, 181 (1974); *Suppl. 7*, 67 (1987)
N-[4-(5-Nitro-2-furyl)-2-thiazolyl]acetamide	*1*, 181 (1972); *7*, 185 (1974); *Suppl. 7*, 67 (1987)
Nitrogen mustard	*9*, 193 (1975); *Suppl. 7*, 269 (1987)
Nitrogen mustard *N*-oxide	*9*, 209 (1975); *Suppl. 7*, 67 (1987)
1-Nitronaphthalene	*46*, 291 (1989)
2-Nitronaphthalene	*46*, 303 (1989)
3-Nitroperylene	*46*, 313 (1989)
2-Nitropropane	*29*, 331 (1982); *Suppl. 7*, 67 (1987)
1-Nitropyrene	*33*, 209 (1984); *Suppl. 7*, 67 (1987); *46*, 321 (1989)
2-Nitropyrene	*46*, 359 (1989)
4-Nitropyrene	*46*, 367 (1989)
N-Nitrosatable drugs	*24*, 297 (1980) (*corr. 42*, 260)
N-Nitrosatable pesticides	*30*, 359 (1983)
N'-Nitrosoanabasine	*37*, 225 (1985); *Suppl. 7*, 67 (1987)
N'-Nitrosoanatabine	*37*, 233 (1985); *Suppl. 7*, 67 (1987)

N-Nitrosodi-n-butylamine	4, 197 (1974); 17, 51 (1978); Suppl. 7, 67 (1987)
N-Nitrosodiethanolamine	17, 77 (1978); Suppl. 7, 67 (1987)
N-Nitrosodiethylamine	1, 107 (1972) (corr. 42, 251); 17, 83 (1978) (corr. 42, 257); Suppl. 7, 67 (1987)
N-Nitrosodimethylamine	1, 95 (1972); 17, 125 (1978) (corr. 42, 257); Suppl. 7, 67 (1987)
N-Nitrosodiphenylamine	27, 213 (1982); Suppl. 7, 67 (1987)
para-Nitrosodiphenylamine	27, 227 (1982) (corr. 42, 261); Suppl. 7, 68 (1987)
N-Nitrosodi-n-propylamine	17, 177 (1978); Suppl. 7, 68 (1987)
N-Nitroso-N-ethylurea (see N-Ethyl-N-nitrosourea)	
N-Nitrosofolic acid	17, 217 (1978); Suppl. 7, 68 (1987)
N-Nitrosoguvacine	37, 263 (1985); Suppl. 7, 68 (1987)
N-Nitrosoguvacoline	37, 263 (1985); Suppl. 7, 68 (1987)
N-Nitrosohydroxyproline	17, 304 (1978); Suppl. 7, 68 (1987)
3-(N-Nitrosomethylamino)propionaldehyde	37, 263 (1985); Suppl. 7, 68 (1987)
3-(N-Nitrosomethylamino)propionitrile	37, 263 (1985); Suppl. 7, 68 (1987)
4-(N-Nitrosomethylamino)-4-(3-pyridyl)-1-butanal	37, 205 (1985); Suppl. 7, 68 (1987)
4-(N-Nitrosomethylamino)-1-(3-pyridyl)-1-butanone	37, 209 (1985); Suppl. 7, 68 (1987)
N-Nitrosomethylethylamine	17, 221 (1978); Suppl. 7, 68 (1987)
N-Nitroso-N-methylurea (see N-Methyl-N-nitrosourea)	
N-Nitroso-N-methylurethane (see N-Methyl-N-methylurethane)	
N-Nitrosomethylvinylamine	17, 257 (1978); Suppl. 7, 68 (1987)
N-Nitrosomorpholine	17, 263 (1978); Suppl. 7, 68 (1987)
N'-Nitrosonornicotine	17, 281 (1978); 37, 241 (1985); Suppl. 7, 68 (1987)
N-Nitrosopiperidine	17, 287 (1978); Suppl. 7, 68 (1987)
N-Nitrosoproline	17, 303 (1978); Suppl. 7, 68 (1987)
N-Nitrosopyrrolidine	17, 313 (1978); Suppl. 7, 68 (1987)
N-Nitrososarcosine	17, 327 (1978); Suppl. 7, 68 (1987)
Nitrosoureas, chloroethyl (see Chloroethyl nitrosoureas)	
5-Nitro-ortho-toluidine	48, 169 (1990)
Nitrous oxide (see Anaesthetics, volatile)	
Nitrovin	31, 185 (1983); Suppl. 7, 68 (1987)
NNA (see 4-(N-Nitrosomethylamino)-4-(3-pyridyl)-1-butanal)	
NNK (see 4-(N-Nitrosomethylamino)-1-(3-pyridyl)-1-butanone)	
Nonsteroidal oestrogens (see also Oestrogens, progestins and combinations)	Suppl. 7, 272 (1987)
Norethisterone (see also Progestins; Combined oral contraceptives)	6, 179 (1974); 21, 461 (1979)
Norethynodrel (see also Progestins; Combined oral contraceptives	6, 191 (1974); 21, 461 (1979) (corr. 42, 259)
Norgestrel (see also Progestins, Combined oral contraceptives)	6, 201 (1974); 21, 479 (1979)

Nylon 6	*19*, 120 (1979); *Suppl. 7*, 68 (1987)

O

Ochratoxin A	*10*, 191 (1976); *31*, 191 (1983) (*corr. 42*, 262); *Suppl. 7*, 271 (1987)
Oestradiol-17β (*see also* Steroidal oestrogens)	*6*, 99 (1974); *21*, 279 (1979)
Oestradiol 3-benzoate (*see* Oestradiol-17β)	
Oestradiol dipropionate (*see* Oestradiol-17β)	
Oestradiol mustard	*9*, 217 (1975)
Oestradiol-17β-valerate (*see* Oestradiol-17β)	
Oestriol (*see also* Steroidal oestrogens)	*6*, 117 (1974); *21*, 327 (1979)
Oestrogen-progestin combinations (*see* Oestrogens, progestins and combinations)	
Oestrogen-progestin replacement therapy (*see also* Oestrogens, progestins and combinations)	*Suppl. 7*, 308 (1987)
Oestrogen replacement therapy (*see also* Oestrogens, progestins and combinations)	*Suppl. 7*, 280 (1987)
Oestrogens (*see* Oestrogens, progestins and combinations)	
Oestrogens, conjugated (*see* Conjugated oestrogens)	
Oestrogens, nonsteroidal (*see* Nonsteroidal oestrogens)	
Oestrogens, progestins and combinations	*6* (1974); *21* (1979); *Suppl. 7*, 272 (1987)
Oestrogens, steroidal (*see* Steroidal oestrogens)	
Oestrone (*see also* Steroidal oestrogens)	*6*, 123 (1974); *21*, 343 (1979) (*corr. 42*, 259)
Oestrone benzoate (*see* Oestrone)	
Oil Orange SS	*8*, 165 (1975); *Suppl. 7*, 69 (1987)
Oral contraceptives, combined (*see* Combined oral contraceptives)	
Oral contraceptives, investigational (*see* Combined oral contraceptives)	
Oral contraceptives, sequential (*see* Sequential oral contraceptives)	
Orange I	*8*, 173 (1975); *Suppl. 7*, 69 (1987)
Orange G	*8*, 181 (1975); *Suppl. 7*, 69 (1987)
Organolead compounds (*see also* Lead and lead compounds)	*Suppl. 7*, 230 (1987)
Oxazepam	*13*, 58 (1977); *Suppl. 7*, 69 (1987)
Oxymetholone (*see also* Androgenic (anabolic) steroids)	*13*, 131 (1977)
Oxyphenbutazone	*13*, 185 (1977); *Suppl. 7*, 69 (1987)

P

Paint manufacture and painting (occupational exposures in)	*47*, 329 (1989)
Panfuran S (*see also* Dihydroxymethylfuratrizine)	*24*, 77 (1980); *Suppl. 7*, 69 (1987)
Paper manufacture (*see* Pulp and paper manufacture)	
Paracetamol	*50*, 307 (1990)

Parasorbic acid	10, 199 (1976) (corr. 42, 255); Suppl. 7, 69 (1987)
Parathion	30, 153 (1983); Suppl. 7, 69 (1987)
Patulin	10, 205 (1976); 40, 83 (1986); Suppl. 7, 69 (1987)
Penicillic acid	10, 211 (1976); Suppl. 7, 69 (1987)
Pentachloroethane	41, 99 (1986); Suppl. 7, 69 (1987)
Pentachloronitrobenzene (see Quintozene)	
Pentachlorophenol (see also Chlorophenols; Chlorophenols, occupational exposures to)	20, 303 (1979)
Perylene	32, 411 (1983); Suppl. 7, 69 (1987)
Petasitenine	31, 207 (1983); Suppl. 7, 69 (1987)
Petasites japonicus (see Pyrrolizidine alkaloids)	
Petroleum refining (occupational exposures in)	45, 39 (1989)
Some petroleum solvents	47, 43 (1989)
Phenacetin	13, 141 (1977); 24, 135 (1980); Suppl. 7, 310 (1987)
Phenanthrene	32, 419 (1983); Suppl. 7, 69 (1987)
Phenazopyridine hydrochloride	8, 117 (1975); 24, 163 (1980) (corr. 42, 260); Suppl. 7, 312 (1987)
Phenelzine sulphate	24, 175 (1980); Suppl. 7, 312 (1987)
Phenicarbazide	12, 177 (1976); Suppl. 7, 70 (1987)
Phenobarbital	13, 157 (1977); Suppl. 7, 313 (1987)
Phenol	47, 263 (1989)
Phenoxyacetic acid herbicides (see Chlorophenoxy herbicides)	
Phenoxybenzamine hydrochloride	9, 223 (1975); 24, 185 (1980); Suppl. 7, 70 (1987)
Phenylbutazone	13, 183 (1977); Suppl. 7, 316 (1987)
meta-Phenylenediamine	16, 111 (1978); Suppl. 7, 70 (1987)
para-Phenylenediamine	16, 125 (1978); Suppl. 7, 70 (1987)
N-Phenyl-2-naphthylamine	16, 325 (1978) (corr. 42, 257); Suppl. 7, 318 (1987)
ortho-Phenylphenol	30, 329 (1983); Suppl. 7, 70 (1987)
Phenytoin	13, 201 (1977); Suppl. 7, 319 (1987)
Piperazine oestrone sulphate (see Conjugated oestrogens)	
Piperonyl butoxide	30, 183 (1983); Suppl. 7, 70 (1987)
Pitches, coal-tar (see Coal-tar pitches)	
Polyacrylic acid	19, 62 (1979); Suppl. 7, 70 (1987)
Polybrominated biphenyls	18, 107 (1978); 41, 261 (1986); Suppl. 7, 321 (1987)
Polychlorinated biphenyls	7, 261 (1974); 18, 43 (1978) (corr. 42, 258); Suppl. 7, 322 (1987)
Polychlorinated camphenes (see Toxaphene)	
Polychloroprene	19, 141 (1979); Suppl. 7, 70 (1987)
Polyethylene	19, 164 (1979); Suppl. 7, 70 (1987)

Polymethylene polyphenyl isocyanate	*19*, 314 (1979); *Suppl. 7*, 70 (1987)
Polymethyl methacrylate	*19*, 195 (1979); *Suppl. 7*, 70 (1987)
Polyoestradiol phosphate (*see* Oestradiol-17β)	
Polypropylene	*19*, 218 (1979); *Suppl. 7*, 70 (1987)
Polystyrene	*19*, 245 (1979); *Suppl. 7*, 70 (1987)
Polytetrafluoroethylene	*19*, 288 (1979); *Suppl. 7*, 70 (1987)
Polyurethane foams	*19*, 320 (1979); *Suppl. 7*, 70 (1987)
Polyvinyl acetate	*19*, 346 (1979); *Suppl. 7*, 70 (1987)
Polyvinyl alcohol	*19*, 351 (1979); *Suppl. 7*, 70 (1987)
Polyvinyl chloride	*7*, 306 (1974); *19*, 402 (1979); *Suppl. 7*, 70 (1987)
Polyvinyl pyrrolidone	*19*, 463 (1979); *Suppl. 7*, 70 (1987)
Ponceau MX	*8*, 189 (1975); *Suppl. 7*, 70 (1987)
Ponceau 3R	*8*, 199 (1975); *Suppl. 7*, 70 (1987)
Ponceau SX	*8*, 207 (1975); *Suppl. 7*, 70 (1987)
Potassium arsenate (*see* Arsenic and arsenic compounds)	
Potassium arsenite (*see* Arsenic and arsenic compounds)	
Potassium bis(2-hydroxyethyl)dithiocarbamate	*12*, 183 (1976); *Suppl. 7*, 70 (1987)
Potassium bromate	*40*, 207 (1986); *Suppl. 7*, 70 (1987)
Potassium chromate (*see* Chromium and chromium compounds)	
Potassium dichromate (*see* Chromium and chromium compounds)	
Prednimustine	*50*, 115 (1990)
Prednisone	*26*, 293 (1981); *Suppl. 7*, 326 (1987)
Procarbazine hydrochloride	*26*, 311 (1981); *Suppl. 7*, 327 (1987)
Proflavine salts	*24*, 195 (1980); *Suppl. 7*, 70 (1987)
Progesterone (*see also* Progestins; Combined oral contraceptives)	*6*, 135 (1974); *21*, 491 (1979) (*corr. 42*, 259)
Progestins (*see also* Oestrogens, progestins and combinations)	*Suppl. 7*, 289 (1987)
Pronetalol hydrochloride	*13*, 227 (1977) (*corr. 42*, 256); *Suppl. 7*, 70 (1987)
1,3-Propane sultone	*4*, 253 (1974) (*corr. 42*, 253); *Suppl. 7*, 70 (1987)
Propham	*12*, 189 (1976); *Suppl. 7*, 70 (1987)
β-Propiolactone	*4*, 259 (1974) (*corr. 42*, 253); *Suppl. 7*, 70 (1987)
n-Propyl carbamate	*12*, 201 (1976); *Suppl. 7*, 70 (1987)
Propylene	*19*, 213 (1979); *Suppl. 7*, 71 (1987)
Propylene oxide	*11*, 191 (1976); *36*, 227 (1985) (*corr. 42*, 263); *Suppl. 7*, 328 (1987)
Propylthiouracil	*7*, 67 (1974); *Suppl. 7*, 329 (1987)
Ptaquiloside (*see also* Bracken fern)	*40*, 55 (1986); *Suppl. 7*, 71 (1987)
Pulp and paper manufacture	*25*, 157 (1981); *Suppl. 7*, 385 (1987)
Pyrene	*32*, 431 (1983); *Suppl. 7*, 71 (1987)
Pyrido[3,4-*c*]psoralen	*40*, 349 (1986); *Suppl. 7*, 71 (1987)
Pyrimethamine	*13*, 233 (1977); *Suppl. 7*, 71 (1987)

Pyrrolizidine alkaloids (see Hydroxysenkirkine; Isatidine;
  Jacobine; Lasiocarpine; Monocrotaline; Retrorsine; Riddelliine;
  Seneciphylline; Senkirkine)

Q

Quercetin (see also Bracken fern)	*31*, 213 (1983); *Suppl. 7*, 71 (1987)
para-Quinone	*15*, 255 (1977); *Suppl. 7*, 71 (1987)
Quintozene	*5*, 211 (1974); *Suppl. 7*, 71 (1987)

R

Radon	*43*, 173 (1988) (corr. *45*, 283)
Reserpine	*10*, 217 (1976); *24*, 211 (1980) (corr. *42*, 260); *Suppl. 7*, 330 (1987)
Resorcinol	*15*, 155 (1977); *Suppl. 7*, 71 (1987)
Retrorsine	*10*, 303 (1976); *Suppl. 7*, 71 (1987)
Rhodamine B	*16*, 221 (1978); *Suppl. 7*, 71 (1987)
Rhodamine 6G	*16*, 233 (1978); *Suppl. 7*, 71 (1987)
Riddelliine	*10*, 313 (1976); *Suppl. 7*, 71 (1987)
Rifampicin	*24*, 243 (1980); *Suppl. 7*, 71 (1987)
Rockwool (see Man-made mineral fibres)	
The rubber industry	*28* (1982) (corr. *42*, 261); *Suppl. 7*, 332 (1987)
Rugulosin	*40*, 99 (1986); *Suppl. 7*, 71 (1987)

S

Saccharated iron oxide	*2*, 161 (1973); *Suppl. 7*, 71 (1987)
Saccharin	*22*, 111 (1980) (corr. *42*, 259); *Suppl. 7*, 334 (1987)
Safrole	*1*, 169 (1972); *10*, 231 (1976); *Suppl. 7*, 71 (1987)
The sawmill industry (including logging) (see The lumber and sawmill industry (including logging))	
Scarlet Red	*8*, 217 (1975); *Suppl. 7*, 71 (1987)
Selenium and selenium compounds	*9*, 245 (1975) (corr. *42*, 255); *Suppl. 7*, 71 (1987)
Selenium dioxide (see Selenium and selenium compounds)	
Selenium oxide (see Selenium and selenium compounds)	
Semicarbazide hydrochloride	*12*, 209 (1976) (corr. *42*, 256); *Suppl. 7*, 71 (1987)
Senecio jacobaea L. (see Pyrrolizidine alkaloids)	
Senecio longilobus (see Pyrrolizidine alkaloids)	
Seneciphylline	*10*, 319, 335 (1976); *Suppl. 7*, 71 (1987)

Senkirkine	*10*, 327 (1976); *31*, 231 (1983); Suppl. 7, 71 (1987)
Sepiolite	*42*, 175 (1987); Suppl. 7, 71 (1987)
Sequential oral contraceptives (*see also* Oestrogens, progestins and combinations)	Suppl. 7, 296 (1987)
Shale-oils	*35*, 161 (1985); Suppl. 7, 339 (1987)
Shikimic acid (*see also* Bracken fern)	*40*, 55 (1986); Suppl. 7, 71 (1987)
Shoe manufacture and repair (*see* Boot and shoe manufacture and repair)	
Silica (*see also* Amorphous silica; Crystalline silica)	*42*, 39 (1987)
Slagwool (*see* Man-made mineral fibres)	
Sodium arsenate (*see* Arsenic and arsenic compounds)	
Sodium arsenite (*see* Arsenic and arsenic compounds)	
Sodium cacodylate (*see* Arsenic and arsenic compounds)	
Sodium chromate (*see* Chromium and chromium compounds)	
Sodium cyclamate (*see* Cyclamates)	
Sodium dichromate (*see* Chromium and chromium compounds)	
Sodium diethyldithiocarbamate	*12*, 217 (1976); Suppl. 7, 71 (1987)
Sodium equilin sulphate (*see* Conjugated oestrogens)	
Sodium fluoride (*see* Fluorides)	
Sodium monofluorophosphate (*see* Fluorides)	
Sodium oestrone sulphate (*see* Conjugated oestrogens)	
Sodium *ortho*-phenylphenate (*see also ortho*-Phenylphenol)	*30*, 329 (1983); Suppl. 7, 392 (1987)
Sodium saccharin (*see* Saccharin)	
Sodium selenate (*see* Selenium and selenium compounds)	
Sodium selenite (*see* Selenium and selenium compounds)	
Sodium silicofluoride (*see* Fluorides)	
Soots	*3*, 22 (1973); *35*, 219 (1985); Suppl. 7, 343 (1987)
Spironolactone	*24*, 259 (1980); Suppl. 7, 344 (1987)
Stannous fluoride (*see* Fluorides)	
Steel founding (*see* Iron and steel founding)	
Sterigmatocystin	*1*, 175 (1972); *10*, 245 (1976); Suppl. 7, 72 (1987)
Steroidal oestrogens (*see also* Oestrogens, progestins and combinations)	Suppl. 7, 280 (1987)
Streptozotocin	*4*, 221 (1974); *17*, 337 (1978); Suppl. 7, 72 (1987)
Strobane® (*see* Terpene polychlorinates)	
Strontium chromate (*see* Chromium and chromium compounds)	
Styrene	*19*, 231 (1979) (*corr. 42*, 258); Suppl. 7, 345 (1987)
Styrene-acrylonitrile copolymers	*19*, 97 (1979); Suppl. 7, 72 (1987)
Styrene-butadiene copolymers	*19*, 252 (1979); Suppl. 7, 72 (1987)

Styrene oxide	*11*, 201 (1976); *19*, 275 (1979); *36*, 245 (1985); *Suppl. 7*, 72 (1987)
Succinic anhydride	*15*, 265 (1977); *Suppl. 7*, 72 (1987)
Sudan I	*8*, 225 (1975); *Suppl. 7*, 72 (1987)
Sudan II	*8*, 233 (1975); *Suppl. 7*, 72 (1987)
Sudan III	*8*, 241 (1975); *Suppl. 7*, 72 (1987)
Sudan Brown RR	*8*, 249 (1975); *Suppl. 7*, 72 (1987)
Sudan Red 7B	*8*, 253 (1975); *Suppl. 7*, 72 (1987)
Sulfafurazole	*24*, 275 (1980); *Suppl. 7*, 347 (1987)
Sulfallate	*30*, 283 (1983); *Suppl. 7*, 72 (1987)
Sulfamethoxazole	*24*, 285 (1980); *Suppl. 7*, 348 (1987)
Sulphisoxazole (*see* Sulfafurazole)	
Sulphur mustard (*see* Mustard gas)	
Sunset Yellow FCF	*8*, 257 (1975); *Suppl. 7*, 72 (1987)
Symphytine	*31*, 239 (1983); *Suppl. 7*, 72 (1987)

T

2,4,5-T (*see also* Chlorophenoxy herbicides; Chlorophenoxy herbicides, occupational exposures to)	*15*, 273 (1977)
Talc	*42*, 185 (1987); *Suppl. 7*, 349 (1987)
Tannic acid	*10*, 253 (1976) (*corr. 42*, 255); *Suppl. 7*, 72 (1987)
Tannins (*see also* Tannic acid)	*10*, 254 (1976); *Suppl. 7*, 72 (1987)
TCDD (*see* 2,3,7,8-Tetrachlorodibenzo-*para*-dioxin)	
TDE (*see* DDT)	
Tea	*51*, 207 (1991)
Terpene polychlorinates	*5*, 219 (1974); *Suppl. 7*, 72 (1987)
Testosterone (*see also* Androgenic (anabolic) steroids)	*6*, 209 (1974); *21*, 519 (1979)
Testosterone oenanthate (*see* Testosterone)	
Testosterone propionate (*see* Testosterone)	
2,2',5,5'-Tetrachlorobenzidine	*27*, 141 (1982); *Suppl. 7*, 72 (1987)
2,3,7,8-Tetrachlorodibenzo-*para*-dioxin	*15*, 41 (1977); *Suppl. 7*, 350 (1987)
1,1,1,2-Tetrachloroethane	*41*, 87 (1986); *Suppl. 7*, 72 (1987)
1,1,2,2-Tetrachloroethane	*20*, 477 (1979); *Suppl. 7*, 354 (1987)
Tetrachloroethylene	*20*, 491 (1979); *Suppl. 7*, 355 (1987)
2,3,4,6-Tetrachlorophenol (*see* Chlorophenols; Chlorophenols, occupational exposures to)	
Tetrachlorvinphos	*30*, 197 (1983); *Suppl. 7*, 72 (1987)
Tetraethyllead (*see* Lead and lead compounds)	
Tetrafluoroethylene	*19*, 285 (1979); *Suppl. 7*, 72 (1987)
Tetrakis(hydroxymethyl) phosphonium salts	*48*, 95 (1990)
Tetramethyllead (*see* Lead and lead compounds)	
Textile manufacturing industry, exposures in	*48*, 215 (1990)
Theobromine	*51*, 421 (1991)

Theophylline	*51*, 391 (1991)
Thioacetamide	*7*, 77 (1974); *Suppl. 7*, 72 (1987)
4,4'-Thiodianiline	*16*, 343 (1978); *27*, 147 (1982); *Suppl. 7*, 72 (1987)
Thiotepa	*9*, 85 (1975); *Suppl. 7*, 368 (1987); *50*, 123 (1990)
Thiouracil	*7*, 85 (1974); *Suppl. 7*, 72 (1987)
Thiourea	*7*, 95 (1974); *Suppl. 7*, 72 (1987)
Thiram	*12*, 225 (1976); *Suppl. 7*, 72 (1987)
Titanium dioxide	*47*, 307 (1989)
Tobacco habits other than smoking (*see* Tobacco products, smokeless)	
Tobacco products, smokeless	*37* (1985) (*corr. 42*, 263); *Suppl. 7*, 357 (1987)
Tobacco smoke	*38* (1986) (*corr. 42*, 263); *Suppl. 7*, 357 (1987)
Tobacco smoking (*see* Tobacco smoke)	
ortho-Tolidine (*see* 3,3'-Dimethylbenzidine)	
2,4-Toluene diisocyanate (*see also* Toluene diisocyanates)	*19*, 303 (1979); *39*, 287 (1986)
2,6-Toluene diisocyanate (*see also* Toluene diisocyanates)	*19*, 303 (1979); *39*, 289 (1986)
Toluene	*47*, 79 (1989)
Toluene diisocyanates	*39*, 287 (1986) (*corr. 42*, 264); *Suppl. 7*, 72 (1987)
Toluenes, α-chlorinated (*see* α-Chlorinated toluenes)	
ortho-Toluenesulphonamide (*see* Saccharin)	
ortho-Toluidine	*16*, 349 (1978); *27*, 155 (1982); *Suppl. 7*, 362 (1987)
Toxaphene	*20*, 327 (1979); *Suppl. 7*, 72 (1987)
Tremolite (*see* Asbestos)	
Treosulphan	*26*, 341 (1981); *Suppl. 7*, 363 (1987)
Triaziquone (*see* Tris(aziridinyl)-*para*-benzoquinone)	
Trichlorfon	*30*, 207 (1983); *Suppl. 7*, 73 (1987)
Trichlormethine	*9*, 229 (1975); *Suppl. 7*, 73 (1987); *50*, 143 (1990)
1,1,1-Trichloroethane	*20*, 515 (1979); *Suppl. 7*, 73 (1987)
1,1,2-Trichloroethane	*20*, 533 (1979); *Suppl. 7*, 73 (1987)
Trichloroethylene	*11*, 263 (1976); *20*, 545 (1979); *Suppl. 7*, 364 (1987)
2,4,5-Trichlorophenol (*see also* Chlorophenols; Chlorophenols occupational exposures to)	*20*, 349 (1979)
2,4,6-Trichlorophenol (*see also* Chlorophenols; Chlorophenols, occupational exposures to)	*20*, 349 (1979)
(2,4,5-Trichlorophenoxy)acetic acid (*see* 2,4,5-T)	
Trichlorotriethylamine hydrochloride (*see* Trichlormethine)	
T_2-Trichothecene	*31*, 265 (1983); *Suppl. 7*, 73 (1987)

Triethylene glycol diglycidyl ether   *11*, 209 (1976); *Suppl. 7*, 73 (1987)
4,4',6-Trimethylangelicin plus ultraviolet radiation (*see also*   *Suppl. 7*, 57 (1987)
   Angelicin and some synthetic derivatives)
2,4,5-Trimethylaniline   *27*, 177 (1982); *Suppl. 7*, 73 (1987)
2,4,6-Trimethylaniline   *27*, 178 (1982); *Suppl. 7*, 73 (1'987)
4,5',8-Trimethylpsoralen   *40*, 357 (1986); *Suppl. 7*, 366 (1987)
Trimustine hydrochloride (*see* Trichlormethine)
Triphenylene   *32*, 447 (1983); *Suppl. 7*, 73 (1987)
Tris(aziridinyl)-*para*-benzoquinone   *9*, 67 (1975); *Suppl. 7*, 367 (1987)
Tris(1-aziridinyl)phosphine oxide   *9*, 75 (1975); *Suppl. 7*, 73 (1987)
Tris(1-aziridinyl)phosphine sulphide (*see* Thiotepa)
2,4,6-Tris(1-aziridinyl)-*s*-triazine   *9*, 95 (1975); *Suppl. 7*, 73 (1987)
Tris(2-chloroethyl) phosphate   *48*, 109 (1990)
1,2,3-Tris(chloromethoxy)propane   *15*, 301 (1977); *Suppl. 7*, 73 (1987)
Tris(2,3-dibromopropyl)phosphate   *20*, 575 (1979); *Suppl. 7*, 369 (1987)
Tris(2-methyl-1-aziridinyl)phosphine oxide   *9*, 107 (1975); *Suppl. 7*, 73 (1987)
Trp-P-1   *31*, 247 (1983); *Suppl. 7*, 73 (1987)
Trp-P-2   *31*, 255 (1983); *Suppl. 7*, 73 (1987)
Trypan blue   *8*, 267 (1975); *Suppl. 7*, 73 (1987)
Tussilago farfara L. (*see* Pyrrolizidine alkaloids)

U

Ultraviolet radiation   *40*, 379 (1986)
Underground haematite mining with exposure to radon   *1*, 29 (1972); *Suppl. 7*, 216 (1987)
Uracil mustard   *9*, 235 (1975); *Suppl. 7*, 370 (1987)
Urethane   *7*, 111 (1974); *Suppl. 7*, 73 (1987)

V

Vat Yellow 4   *48*, 161 (1990)
Vinblastine sulphate   *26*, 349 (1981) (*corr. 42*, 261);
                                                                         Suppl. 7, 371 (1987)
Vincristine sulphate   *26*, 365 (1981); *Suppl. 7*, 372 (1987)
Vinyl acetate   *19*, 341 (1979); *39*, 113 (1986);
                                                                         Suppl. 7, 73 (1987)
Vinyl bromide   *19*, 367 (1979); *39*, 133 (1986);
                                                                         Suppl. 7, 73 (1987)
Vinyl chloride   *7*, 291 (1974); *19*, 377 (1979)
                                                                         (*corr. 42*, 258); *Suppl. 7*, 373 (1987)
Vinyl chloride-vinyl acetate copolymers   *7*, 311 (1976); *19*, 412 (1979) (*corr.
                                                                         42*, 258); *Suppl. 7*, 73 (1987)
4-Vinylcyclohexene   *11*, 277 (1976); *39*, 181 (1986);
                                                                         Suppl. 7, 73 (1987)
Vinyl fluoride   *39*, 147 (1986); *Suppl. 7*, 73 (1987)

Vinylidene chloride	*19*, 439 (1979); *39*, 195 (1986); *Suppl. 7*, 376 (1987)
Vinylidene chloride–vinyl chloride copolymers	*19*, 448 (1979) (*corr. 42*, 258); *Suppl. 7*, 73 (1987)
Vinylidene fluoride	*39*, 227 (1986); *Suppl. 7*, 73 (1987)
N-Vinyl-2-pyrrolidone	*19*, 461 (1979); *Suppl. 7*, 73 (1987)

W

Welding	*49*, 447 (1990)
Wollastonite	*42*, 145 (1987); *Suppl. 7*, 377 (1987)
Wood industries	*25* (1981); *Suppl. 7*, 378 (1987)

X

Xylene	*47*, 125 (1989)
2,4-Xylidine	*16*, 367 (1978); *Suppl. 7*, 74 (1987)
2,5-Xylidine	*16*, 377 (1978); *Suppl. 7*, 74 (1987)

Y

Yellow AB	*8*, 279 (1975); *Suppl. 7*, 74 (1987)
Yellow OB	*8*, 287 (1975); *Suppl. 7*, 74 (1987)

Z

Zearalenone	*31*, 279 (1983); *Suppl. 7*, 74 (1987)
Zectran	*12*, 237 (1976); *Suppl. 7*, 74 (1987)
Zinc beryllium silicate (*see* Beryllium and beryllium compounds)	
Zinc chromate (*see* Chromium and chromium compounds)	
Zinc chromate hydroxide (*see* Chromium and chromium compounds)	
Zinc potassium chromate (*see* Chromium and chromium compounds)	
Zinc yellow (*see* Chromium and chromium compounds)	
Zineb	*12*, 245 (1976); *Suppl. 7*, 74 (1987)
Ziram	*12*, 259 (1976); *Suppl. 7*, 74 (1987)

PUBLICATIONS OF THE INTERNATIONAL AGENCY FOR RESEARCH ON CANCER
Scientific Publications Series
(Available from Oxford University Press through local bookshops)

No. 1 Liver Cancer
1971; 176 pages (*out of print*)

No. 2 Oncogenesis and Herpesviruses
Edited by P.M. Biggs, G. de-Thé and L.N. Payne
1972; 515 pages (*out of print*)

No. 3 N-Nitroso Compounds: Analysis and Formation
Edited by P. Bogovski, R. Preussman and E.A. Walker
1972; 140 pages (*out of print*)

No. 4 Transplacental Carcinogenesis
Edited by L. Tomatis and U. Mohr
1973; 181 pages (*out of print*)

No. 5/6 Pathology of Tumours in Laboratory Animals, Volume 1, Tumours of the Rat
Edited by V.S. Turusov
1973/1976; 533 pages; £50.00

No. 7 Host Environment Interactions in the Etiology of Cancer in Man
Edited by R. Doll and I. Vodopija
1973; 464 pages; £32.50

No. 8 Biological Effects of Asbestos
Edited by P. Bogovski, J.C. Gilson, V. Timbrell and J.C. Wagner
1973; 346 pages (*out of print*)

No. 9 N-Nitroso Compounds in the Environment
Edited by P. Bogovski and E.A. Walker
1974; 243 pages; £21.00

No. 10 Chemical Carcinogenesis Essays
Edited by R. Montesano and L. Tomatis
1974; 230 pages (*out of print*)

No. 11 Oncogenesis and Herpesviruses II
Edited by G. de-Thé, M.A. Epstein and H. zur Hausen
1975; Part I: 511 pages
Part II: 403 pages; £65.00

No. 12 Screening Tests in Chemical Carcinogenesis
Edited by R. Montesano, H. Bartsch and L. Tomatis
1976; 666 pages; £45.00

No. 13 Environmental Pollution and Carcinogenic Risks
Edited by C. Rosenfeld and W. Davis
1975; 441 pages (*out of print*)

No. 14 Environmental N-Nitroso Compounds. Analysis and Formation
Edited by E.A. Walker, P. Bogovski and L. Griciute
1976; 512 pages; £37.50

No. 15 Cancer Incidence in Five Continents, Volume III
Edited by J.A.H. Waterhouse, C. Muir, P. Correa and J. Powell
1976; 584 pages; (*out of print*)

No. 16 Air Pollution and Cancer in Man
Edited by U. Mohr, D. Schmähl and L. Tomatis
1977; 328 pages (*out of print*)

No. 17 Directory of On-going Research in Cancer Epidemiology 1977
Edited by C.S. Muir and G. Wagner
1977; 599 pages (*out of print*)

No. 18 Environmental Carcinogens. Selected Methods of Analysis. Volume 1: Analysis of Volatile Nitrosamines in Food
Editor-in-Chief: H. Egan
1978; 212 pages (*out of print*)

No. 19 Environmental Aspects of N-Nitroso Compounds
Edited by E.A. Walker, M. Castegnaro, L. Griciute and R.E. Lyle
1978; 561 pages (*out of print*)

No. 20 Nasopharyngeal Carcinoma: Etiology and Control
Edited by G. de-Thé and Y. Ito
1978; 606 pages (*out of print*)

No. 21 Cancer Registration and its Techniques
Edited by R. MacLennan, C. Muir, R. Steinitz and A. Winkler
1978; 235 pages; £35.00

No. 22 Environmental Carcinogens. Selected Methods of Analysis. Volume 2: Methods for the Measurement of Vinyl Chloride in Poly(vinyl chloride), Air, Water and Foodstuffs
Editor-in-Chief: H. Egan
1978; 142 pages (*out of print*)

No. 23 Pathology of Tumours in Laboratory Animals. Volume II: Tumours of the Mouse
Editor-in-Chief: V.S. Turusov
1979; 669 pages (*out of print*)

No. 24 Oncogenesis and Herpesviruses III
Edited by G. de-Thé, W. Henle and F. Rapp
1978; Part I: 580 pages, Part II: 512 pages (*out of print*)

Prices, valid for January 1990, are subject to change without notice

List of IARC Publications

No. 25 Carcinogenic Risk. Strategies for Intervention
Edited by W. Davis and C. Rosenfeld
1979; 280 pages (*out of print*)

No. 26 Directory of On-going Research in Cancer Epidemiology 1978
Edited by C.S. Muir and G. Wagner
1978; 550 pages (*out of print*)

No. 27 Molecular and Cellular Aspects of Carcinogen Screening Tests
Edited by R. Montesano, H. Bartsch and L. Tomatis
1980; 372 pages; £29.00

No. 28 Directory of On-going Research in Cancer Epidemiology 1979
Edited by C.S. Muir and G. Wagner
1979; 672 pages (*out of print*)

No. 29 Environmental Carcinogens. Selected Methods of Analysis. Volume 3: Analysis of Polycyclic Aromatic Hydrocarbons in Environmental Samples
Editor-in-Chief: H. Egan
1979; 240 pages (*out of print*)

No. 30 Biological Effects of Mineral Fibres
Editor-in-Chief: J.C. Wagner
1980; Volume 1: 494 pages; Volume 2: 513 pages; £65.00

No. 31 N-Nitroso Compounds: Analysis, Formation and Occurrence
Edited by E.A. Walker, L. Griciute, M. Castegnaro and M. Börzsönyi
1980; 835 pages (*out of print*)

No. 32 Statistical Methods in Cancer Research. Volume 1. The Analysis of Case-control Studies
By N.E. Breslow and N.E. Day
1980; 338 pages; £20.00

No. 33 Handling Chemical Carcinogens in the Laboratory
Edited by R. Montesano *et al.*
1979; 32 pages (*out of print*)

No. 34 Pathology of Tumours in Laboratory Animals. Volume III. Tumours of the Hamster
Editor-in-Chief: V.S. Turusov
1982; 461 pages; £39.00

No. 35 Directory of On-going Research in Cancer Epidemiology 1980
Edited by C.S. Muir and G. Wagner
1980; 660 pages (*out of print*)

No. 36 Cancer Mortality by Occupation and Social Class 1851-1971
Edited by W.P.D. Logan
1982; 253 pages; £22.50

No. 37 Laboratory Decontamination and Destruction of Aflatoxins B_1, B_2, G_1, G_2 in Laboratory Wastes
Edited by M. Castegnaro *et al.*
1980; 56 pages; £6.50

No. 38 Directory of On-going Research in Cancer Epidemiology 1981
Edited by C.S. Muir and G. Wagner
1981; 696 pages (*out of print*)

No. 39 Host Factors in Human Carcinogenesis
Edited by H. Bartsch and B. Armstrong
1982; 583 pages; £46.00

No. 40 Environmental Carcinogens. Selected Methods of Analysis. Volume 4: Some Aromatic Amines and Azo Dyes in the General and Industrial Environment
Edited by L. Fishbein, M. Castegnaro, I.K. O'Neill and H. Bartsch
1981; 347 pages; £29.00

No. 41 N-Nitroso Compounds: Occurrence and Biological Effects
Edited by H. Bartsch, I.K. O'Neill, M. Castegnaro and M. Okada
1982; 755 pages; £48.00

No. 42 Cancer Incidence in Five Continents, Volume IV
Edited by J. Waterhouse, C. Muir, K. Shanmugaratnam and J. Powell
1982; 811 pages (*out of print*)

No. 43 Laboratory Decontamination and Destruction of Carcinogens in Laboratory Wastes: Some N-Nitrosamines
Edited by M. Castegnaro *et al.*
1982; 73 pages; £7.50

No. 44 Environmental Carcinogens. Selected Methods of Analysis. Volume 5: Some Mycotoxins
Edited by L. Stoloff, M. Castegnaro, P. Scott, I.K. O'Neill and H. Bartsch
1983; 455 pages; £29.00

No. 45 Environmental Carcinogens. Selected Methods of Analysis. Volume 6: N-Nitroso Compounds
Edited by R. Preussmann, I.K. O'Neill, G. Eisenbrand, B. Spiegelhalder and H. Bartsch
1983; 508 pages; £29.00

No. 46 Directory of On-going Research in Cancer Epidemiology 1982
Edited by C.S. Muir and G. Wagner
1982; 722 pages (*out of print*)

No. 47 Cancer Incidence in Singapore 1968-1977
Edited by K. Shanmugaratnam, H.P. Lee and N.E. Day
1983; 171 pages (*out of print*)

No. 48 Cancer Incidence in the USSR (2nd Revised Edition)
Edited by N.P. Napalkov, G.F. Tserkovny, V.M. Merabishvili, D.M. Parkin, M. Smans and C.S. Muir
1983; 75 pages; £12.00

No. 49 Laboratory Decontamination and Destruction of Carcinogens in Laboratory Wastes: Some Polycyclic Aromatic Hydrocarbons
Edited by M. Castegnaro, *et al.*
1983; 87 pages; £9.00

No. 50 Directory of On-going Research in Cancer Epidemiology 1983
Edited by C.S. Muir and G. Wagner
1983; 731 pages (*out of print*)

No. 51 Modulators of Experimental Carcinogenesis
Edited by V. Turusov and R. Montesano
1983; 307 pages; £22.50

List of IARC Publications

No. 52 Second Cancers in Relation to Radiation Treatment for Cervical Cancer: Results of a Cancer Registry Collaboration
Edited by N.E. Day and J.C. Boice, Jr
1984; 207 pages; £20.00

No. 53 Nickel in the Human Environment
Editor-in-Chief: F.W. Sunderman, Jr
1984; 529 pages; £41.00

No. 54 Laboratory Decontamination and Destruction of Carcinogens in Laboratory Wastes: Some Hydrazines
Edited by M. Castegnaro, et al.
1983; 87 pages; £9.00

No. 55 Laboratory Decontamination and Destruction of Carcinogens in Laboratory Wastes: Some N-Nitrosamides
Edited by M. Castegnaro et al.
1984; 66 pages; £7.50

No. 56 Models, Mechanisms and Etiology of Tumour Promotion
Edited by M. Börzsönyi, N.E. Day, K. Lapis and H. Yamasaki
1984; 532 pages; £42.00

No. 57 N-Nitroso Compounds: Occurrence, Biological Effects and Relevance to Human Cancer
Edited by I.K. O'Neill, R.C. von Borstel, C.T. Miller, J. Long and H. Bartsch
1984; 1013 pages; £80.00

No. 58 Age-related Factors in Carcinogenesis
Edited by A. Likhachev, V. Anisimov and R. Montesano
1985; 288 pages; £20.00

No. 59 Monitoring Human Exposure to Carcinogenic and Mutagenic Agents
Edited by A. Berlin, M. Draper, K. Hemminki and H. Vainio
1984; 457 pages; £27.50

No. 60 Burkitt's Lymphoma: A Human Cancer Model
Edited by G. Lenoir, G. O'Conor and C.L.M. Olweny
1985; 484 pages; £29.00

No. 61 Laboratory Decontamination and Destruction of Carcinogens in Laboratory Wastes: Some Haloethers
Edited by M. Castegnaro et al.
1985; 55 pages; £7.50

No. 62 Directory of On-going Research in Cancer Epidemiology 1984
Edited by C.S. Muir and G. Wagner
1984; 717 pages (*out of print*)

No. 63 Virus-associated Cancers in Africa
Edited by A.O. Williams, G.T. O'Conor, G.B. de-Thé and C.A. Johnson
1984; 773 pages; £22.00

No. 64 Laboratory Decontamination and Destruction of Carcinogens in Laboratory Wastes: Some Aromatic Amines and 4-Nitrobiphenyl
Edited by M. Castegnaro et al.
1985; 84 pages; £6.95

No. 65 Interpretation of Negative Epidemiological Evidence for Carcinogenicity
Edited by N.J. Wald and R. Doll
1985; 232 pages; £20.00

No. 66 The Role of the Registry in Cancer Control
Edited by D.M. Parkin, G. Wagner and C.S. Muir
1985; 152 pages; £10.00

No. 67 Transformation Assay of Established Cell Lines: Mechanisms and Application
Edited by T. Kakunaga and H. Yamasaki
1985; 225 pages; £20.00

No. 68 Environmental Carcinogens. Selected Methods of Analysis. Volume 7. Some Volatile Halogenated Hydrocarbons
Edited by L. Fishbein and I.K. O'Neill
1985; 479 pages; £42.00

No. 69 Directory of On-going Research in Cancer Epidemiology 1985
Edited by C.S. Muir and G. Wagner
1985; 745 pages; £22.00

No. 70 The Role of Cyclic Nucleic Acid Adducts in Carcinogenesis and Mutagenesis
Edited by B. Singer and H. Bartsch
1986; 467 pages; £40.00

No. 71 Environmental Carcinogens. Selected Methods of Analysis. Volume 8: Some Metals: As, Be, Cd, Cr, Ni, Pb, Se Zn
Edited by I.K. O'Neill, P. Schuller and L. Fishbein
1986; 485 pages; £42.00

No. 72 Atlas of Cancer in Scotland, 1975–1980. Incidence and Epidemiological Perspective
Edited by I. Kemp, P. Boyle, M. Smans and C.S. Muir
1985; 285 pages; £35.00

No. 73 Laboratory Decontamination and Destruction of Carcinogens in Laboratory Wastes: Some Antineoplastic Agents
Edited by M. Castegnaro et al.
1985; 163 pages; £10.00

No. 74 Tobacco: A Major International Health Hazard
Edited by D. Zaridze and R. Peto
1986; 324 pages; £20.00

No. 75 Cancer Occurrence in Developing Countries
Edited by D.M. Parkin
1986; 339 pages; £20.00

No. 76 Screening for Cancer of the Uterine Cervix
Edited by M. Hakama, A.B. Miller and N.E. Day
1986; 315 pages; £25.00

No. 77 Hexachlorobenzene: Proceedings of an International Symposium
Edited by C.R. Morris and J.R.P. Cabral
1986; 668 pages; £50.00

List of IARC Publications

No. 78 Carcinogenicity of Alkylating Cytostatic Drugs
Edited by D. Schmähl and J.M. Kaldor
1986; 337 pages; £25.00

No. 79 Statistical Methods in Cancer Research. Volume III: The Design and Analysis of Long-term Animal Experiments
By J.J. Gart, D. Krewski, P.N. Lee, R.E. Tarone and J. Wahrendorf
1986; 213 pages; £20.00

No. 80 Directory of On-going Research in Cancer Epidemiology 1986
Edited by C.S. Muir and G. Wagner
1986; 805 pages; £22.00

No. 81 Environmental Carcinogens: Methods of Analysis and Exposure Measurement. Volume 9: Passive Smoking
Edited by I.K. O'Neill, K.D. Brunnemann, B. Dodet and D. Hoffmann
1987; 383 pages; £35.00

No. 82 Statistical Methods in Cancer Research. Volume II: The Design and Analysis of Cohort Studies
By N.E. Breslow and N.E. Day
1987; 404 pages; £30.00

No. 83 Long-term and Short-term Assays for Carcinogens: A Critical Appraisal
Edited by R. Montesano, H. Bartsch, H. Vainio, J. Wilbourn and H. Yamasaki
1986; 575 pages; £48.00

No. 84 The Relevance of N-Nitroso Compounds to Human Cancer: Exposure and Mechanisms
Edited by H. Bartsch, I.K. O'Neill and R. Schulte-Hermann
1987; 671 pages; £50.00

No. 85 Environmental Carcinogens: Methods of Analysis and Exposure Measurement. Volume 10: Benzene and Alkylated Benzenes
Edited by L. Fishbein and I.K. O'Neill
1988; 327 pages; £35.00

No. 86 Directory of On-going Research in Cancer Epidemiology 1987
Edited by D.M. Parkin and J. Wahrendorf
1987; 676 pages; £22.00

No. 87 International Incidence of Childhood Cancer
Edited by D.M. Parkin, C.A. Stiller, C.A. Bieber, G.J. Draper, B. Terracini and J.L. Young
1988; 401 pages; £35.00

No. 88 Cancer Incidence in Five Continents Volume V
Edited by C. Muir, J. Waterhouse, T. Mack, J. Powell and S. Whelan
1987; 1004 pages; £50.00

No. 89 Method for Detecting DNA Damaging Agents in Humans: Applications in Cancer Epidemiology and Prevention
Edited by H. Bartsch, K. Hemminki and I.K. O'Neill
1988; 518 pages; £45.00

No. 90 Non-occupational Exposure to Mineral Fibres
Edited by J. Bignon, J. Peto and R. Saracci
1989; 500 pages; £45.00

No. 91 Trends in Cancer Incidence in Singapore 1968–1982
Edited by H.P. Lee, N.E. Day and K. Shanmugaratnam
1988; 160 pages; £25.00

No. 92 Cell Differentiation, Genes and Cancer
Edited by T. Kakunaga, T. Sugimura, L. Tomatis and H. Yamasaki
1988; 204 pages; £25.00

No. 93 Directory of On-going Research in Cancer Epidemiology 1988
Edited by M. Coleman and J. Wahrendorf
1988; 662 pages (*out of print*)

No. 94 Human Papillomavirus and Cervical Cancer
Edited by N. Muñoz, F.X. Bosch and O.M. Jensen
1989; 154 pages; £19.00

No. 95 Cancer Registration: Principles and Methods
Edited by O.M. Jensen, D.M. Parkin, R. MacLennan, C.S. Muir and R. Skeet
Publ. due 1991; approx. 300 pages £28.00

No. 96 Perinatal and Multigeneration Carcinogenesis
Edited by N.P. Napalkov, J.M. Rice, L. Tomatis and H. Yamasaki
1989; 436 pages; £48.00

No. 97 Occupational Exposure to Silica and Cancer Risk
Edited by L. Simonato, A.C. Fletcher, R. Saracci and T. Thomas
1990; 124 pages; £19.00

No. 98 Cancer Incidence in Jewish Migrants to Israel, 1961–1981
Edited by R. Steinitz, D.M. Parkin, J.L. Young, C.A. Bieber and L. Katz
1989; 320 pages; £30.00

No. 99 Pathology of Tumours in Laboratory Animals, Second Edition, Volume 1, Tumours of the Rat
Edited by V.S. Turusov and U. Mohr
740 pages; £85.00

No. 100 Cancer: Causes, Occurrence and Control
Editor-in-Chief L. Tomatis
1990; 352 pages; £24.00

List of IARC Publications

No. 101 **Directory of On-going Research in Cancer Epidemiology 1989/90**
Edited by M. Coleman and J. Wahrendorf
1989; 818 pages; £36.00

No. 102 **Patterns of Cancer in Five Continents**
Edited by S.L. Whelan and D.M. Parkin
1990; 162 pages; £25.00

No. 103 **Evaluating Effectiveness of Primary Prevention of Cancer**
Edited by M. Hakama, V. Beral, J.W. Cullen and D.M. Parkin
1990; 250 pages; £32.00

No. 104 **Complex Mixtures and Cancer Risk**
Edited by H. Vainio, M. Sorsa and A.J. McMichael
1990; 442 pages; £38.00

No. 105 **Relevance to Human Cancer of N-Nitroso Compounds, Tobacco Smoke and Mycotoxins**
Edited by I.K. O'Neill, J. Chen and H. Bartsch
Publ. due 1991; approx. 600 pages £70.00

No. 108 **Environmental Carcinogens: Methods of Analysis and Exposure Measurement. Volume 11: Polychlorinated Dioxins and Dibenzofurans**
Edited by C. Rappe, H.R. Buser, B. Dodet and I.K. O'Neill
Publ. due 1991; approx. 400 pages; £45.00

No. 109 **Environmental Carcinogens: Methods of Analysis and Exposure Measurement. Volume 12: Indoor Air Contaminants**
Edited by B. Seifert, B. Dodet and I.K. O'Neill
Publ. due 1991; approx. 400 pages

No. 110 **Directory of On-going Research in Cancer Epidemiology 1991**
Edited by M. Coleman and J. Wahrendorf
1991; approx. 720 pages; £38.00

No. 112 **Autopsy in Epidemiology and Medical Research**
Edited by E. Riboli and m. Delendi
1991; approx 250 pages; **£25.00**

List of IARC Publications

IARC MONOGRAPHS ON THE EVALUATION OF CARCINOGENIC RISKS TO HUMANS

(Available from booksellers through the network of WHO Sales Agents*)

Volume 1 **Some Inorganic Substances, Chlorinated Hydrocarbons, Aromatic Amines, *N*-Nitroso Compounds, and Natural Products**
1972; 184 pages (*out of print*)

Volume 2 **Some Inorganic and Organometallic Compounds**
1973; 181 pages (out of print)

Volume 3 **Certain Polycyclic Aromatic Hydrocarbons and Heterocyclic Compounds**
1973; 271 pages (*out of print*)

Volume 4 **Some Aromatic Amines, Hydrazine and Related Substances, *N*-Nitroso Compounds and Miscellaneous Alkylating Agents**
1974; 286 pages;
Sw. fr. 18.-/US $14.40

Volume 5 **Some Organochlorine Pesticides**
1974; 241 pages (*out of print*)

Volume 6 **Sex Hormones** 1974;
243 pages (*out of print*)

Volume 7 **Some Anti-Thyroid and Related Substances, Nitrofurans and Industrial Chemicals**
1974; 326 pages (*out of print*)

Volume 8 **Some Aromatic Azo Compounds**
1975; 375 pages;
Sw. fr. 36.-/US $28.80

Volume 9 **Some Aziridines, *N*-, *S*- and *O*-Mustards and Selenium**
1975; 268 pages;
Sw.fr. 27.-/US $21.60

Volume 10 **Some Naturally Occurring Substances**
1976; 353 pages (*out of print*)

Volume 11 **Cadmium, Nickel, Some Epoxides, Miscellaneous Industrial Chemicals and General Considerations on Volatile Anaesthetics**
1976; 306 pages (*out of print*)

Volume 12 **Some Carbamates, Thiocarbamates and Carbazides**
1976; 282 pages;
Sw. fr. 34.-/US $27.20

Volume 13 **Some Miscellaneous Pharmaceutical Substances** 1977;
255 pages;
Sw. fr. 30.-/US$ 24.00

Volume 14 **Asbestos**
1977; 106 pages (*out of print*)

Volume 15 **Some Fumigants, The Herbicides 2,4-D and 2,4,5-T, Chlorinated Dibenzodioxins and Miscellaneous Industrial Chemicals**
1977; 354 pages;
Sw. fr. 50.-/US $40.00

Volume 16 **Some Aromatic Amines and Related Nitro Compounds - Hair Dyes, Colouring Agents and Miscellaneous Industrial Chemicals**
1978; 400 pages;
Sw. fr. 50.-/US $40.00

Volume 17 **Some *N*-Nitroso Compounds**
1987; 365 pages;
Sw. fr. 50.-/US $40.00

Volume 18 **Polychlorinated Biphenyls and Polybrominated Biphenyls**
1978; 140 pages;
Sw. fr. 20.-/US $16.00

Volume 19 **Some Monomers, Plastics and Synthetic Elastomers, and Acrolein**
1979; 513 pages;
Sw. fr. 60.-/US $48.00

Volume 20 **Some Halogenated Hydrocarbons**
1979; 609 pages (*out of print*)

Volume 21 **Sex Hormones (II)**
1979; 583 pages;
Sw. fr. 60.-/US $48.00

Volume 22 **Some Non-Nutritive Sweetening Agents**
1980; 208 pages;
Sw. fr. 25.-/US $20.00

Volume 23 **Some Metals and Metallic Compounds**
1980; 438 pages (*out of print*)

Volume 24 **Some Pharmaceutical Drugs**
1980; 337 pages;
Sw. fr. 40.-/US $32.00

Volume 25 **Wood, Leather and Some Associated Industries**
1981; 412 pages;
Sw. fr. 60-/US $48.00

Volume 26 **Some Antineoplastic and Immunosuppressive Agents**
1981; 411 pages;
Sw. fr. 62.-/US $49.60

Volume 27 **Some Aromatic Amines, Anthraquinones and Nitroso Compounds, and Inorganic Fluorides Used in Drinking Water and Dental Preparations**
1982; 341 pages;
Sw. fr. 40.-/US $32.00

Volume 28 **The Rubber Industry**
1982; 486 pages;
Sw. fr. 70.-/US $56.00

Volume 29 **Some Industrial Chemicals and Dyestuffs**
1982; 416 pages;
Sw. fr. 60.-/US $48.00

Volume 30 **Miscellaneous Pesticides**
1983; 424 pages;
Sw. fr. 60.-/US $48.00

Volume 31 **Some Food Additives, Feed Additives and Naturally Occurring Substances**
1983; 314 pages;
Sw. fr. 60-/US $48.00

List of IARC Publications

Volume 32 **Polynuclear Aromatic Compounds, Part 1: Chemical, Environmental and Experimental Data**
1984; 477 pages;
Sw. fr. 60.-/US $48.00

Volume 33 **Polynuclear Aromatic Compounds, Part 2: Carbon Blacks, Mineral Oils and Some Nitroarenes**
1984; 245 pages;
Sw. fr. 50.-/US $40.00

Volume 34 **Polynuclear Aromatic Compounds, Part 3: Industrial Exposures in Aluminium Production, Coal Gasification, Coke Production, and Iron and Steel Founding**
1984; 219 pages;
Sw. fr. 48.-/US $38.40

Volume 35 **Polynuclear Aromatic Compounds, Part 4: Bitumens, Coal-tars and Derived Products, Shale-oils and Soots**
1985; 271 pages;
Sw. fr. 70.-/US $56.00

Volume 37 **Tobacco Habits Other than Smoking: Betel-quid and Areca-nut Chewing; and some Related Nitrosamines**
1985; 291 pages;
Sw. fr. 70.-/US $56.00

Volume 38 **Tobacco Smoking**
1986; 421 pages;
Sw. fr. 75.-/US $60.00

Volume 39 **Some Chemicals Used in Plastics and Elastomers**
1986; 403 pages;
Sw. fr. 60.-/US $48.00

Volume 40 **Some Naturally Occurring and Synthetic Food Components, Furocoumarins and Ultraviolet Radiation**
1986; 444 pages;
Sw. fr. 65.-/US $52.00

Volume 41 **Some Halogenated Hydrocarbons and Pesticide Exposures**
1986; 434 pages;
Sw. fr. 65.-/US $52.00

Volume 42 **Silica and Some Silicates**
1987; 289 pages;
Sw. fr. 65.-/US $52.00

Volume 43 **Man-Made Mineral Fibres and Radon**
1988; 300 pages;
Sw. fr. 65.-/US $52.00

Volume 44 **Alcohol Drinking**
1988; 416 pages;
Sw. fr. 65.-/US $52.00

Volume 45 **Occupational Exposures in Petroleum Refining; Crude Oil and Major Petroleum Fuels**
1989; 322 pages;
Sw. fr. 65.-/US $52.00

Volume 46 **Diesel and Gasoline Engine Exhausts and Some Nitroarenes**
1989; 458 pages;
Sw. fr. 65.-/US $52.00

Volume 47 **Some Organic Solvents, Resin Monomers and Related Compounds, Pigments and Occupational Exposures in Paint Manufacture and Painting**
1990; 536 pages;
Sw. fr. 85.-/US $68.00

Volume 48 **Some Flame Retardants and Textile Chemicals, and Exposures in the Textile Manufacturing Industry**
1990; 345 pages;
Sw. fr. 65.-/US $52.00

Volume 49 **Chromium, Nickel and Welding**
1990; 677 pages;
Sw. fr. 95.-/US$76.00

Volume 50 **Pharmaceutical Drugs**
1990; 415 pages;
Sw. fr. 65.-/US$52.00

Volume 51 **Coffee, Tea, Mate, Methylxanthines and Methylglyoxal**
1991; 513 pages;
Sw. fr. 80.-/US$64.00

Supplement No. 1
Chemicals and Industrial Processes Associated with Cancer in Humans (IARC Monographs, Volumes 1 to 20)
1979; 71 pages; (*out of print*)

Supplement No. 2
Long-term and Short-term Screening Assays for Carcinogens: A Critical Appraisal
1980; 426 pages;
Sw. fr. 40.-/US $32.00

Supplement No. 3
Cross Index of Synonyms and Trade Names in Volumes 1 to 26
1982; 199 pages (*out of print*)

Supplement No. 4
Chemicals, Industrial Processes and Industries Associated with Cancer in Humans (IARC Monographs, Volumes 1 to 29)
1982; 292 pages (*out of print*)

Supplement No. 5
Cross Index of Synonyms and Trade Names in Volumes 1 to 36
1985; 259 pages;
Sw. fr. 46.-/US $36.80

Supplement No. 6
Genetic and Related Effects: An Updating of Selected IARC Monographs from Volumes 1 to 42
1987; 729 pages;
Sw. fr. 80.-/US $64.00

Supplement No. 7
Overall Evaluations of Carcinogenicity: An Updating of IARC Monographs Volumes 1-42
1987; 434 pages;
Sw. fr. 65.-/US $52.00

Supplement No. 8
Cross Index of Synonyms and Trade Names in Volumes 1 to 46 of the IARC Monographs
1990; 260 pages;
Sw. fr. 60.-/US $48.00

List of IARC Publications

IARC TECHNICAL REPORTS*

No. 1 Cancer in Costa Rica
Edited by R. Sierra,
R. Barrantes, G. Muñoz Leiva,
D.M. Parkin, C.A. Bieber and
N. Muñoz Calero
1988; 124 pages;
Sw. fr. 30.-/US $24.00

No. 2 SEARCH: A Computer Package to Assist the Statistical Analysis of Case-control Studies
Edited by G.J. Macfarlane,
P. Boyle and P. Maisonneuve (in press)

No. 3 Cancer Registration in the European Economic Community
Edited by M.P. Coleman and
E. Démaret
1988; 188 pages;
Sw. fr. 30.-/US $24.00

No. 4 Diet, Hormones and Cancer: Methodological Issues for Prospective Studies
Edited by E. Riboli and
R. Saracci
1988; 156 pages;
Sw. fr. 30.-/US $24.00

No. 5 Cancer in the Philippines
Edited by A.V. Laudico,
D. Esteban and D.M. Parkin
1989; 186 pages;
Sw. fr. 30.-/US $24.00

No. 6 La genèse du Centre International de Recherche sur le Cancer
Par R. Sohier et A.G.B. Sutherland
1990; 104 pages
Sw. fr. 30.-/US $24.00

No. 7 Epidémiologie du cancer dans les pays de langue latine
1990; 310 pages
Sw. fr. 30.-/US $24.00

No. 8 Comparative Study of Anti-smoking Legislation in Countries of the European Economic Community
Edited by A. Sasco
1990; c. 80 pages
Sw. fr. 30.-/US $24.00
(English and French editions available) (in press)

DIRECTORY OF AGENTS BEING TESTED FOR CARCINOGENICITY (Until Vol. 13 Information Bulletin on the Survey of Chemicals Being Tested for Carcinogenicity)*

No. 8 Edited by M.-J. Ghess,
H. Bartsch and L. Tomatis
1979; 604 pages; Sw. fr. 40.-

No. 9 Edited by M.-J. Ghess,
J.D. Wilbourn, H. Bartsch and
L. Tomatis
1981; 294 pages; Sw. fr. 41.-

No. 10 Edited by M.-J. Ghess,
J.D. Wilbourn and H. Bartsch
1982; 362 pages; Sw. fr. 42.-

No. 11 Edited by M.-J. Ghess,
J.D. Wilbourn, H. Vainio and
H. Bartsch
1984; 362 pages; Sw. fr. 50.-

No. 12 Edited by M.-J. Ghess,
J.D. Wilbourn, A. Tossavainen and
H. Vainio
1986; 385 pages; Sw. fr. 50.-

No. 13 Edited by M.-J. Ghess,
J.D. Wilbourn and A. Aitio 1988;
404 pages; Sw. fr. 43.-

No. 14 Edited by M.-J. Ghess,
J.D. Wilbourn and H. Vainio
1990; c. 370 pages; Sw. fr. 45.-

NON-SERIAL PUBLICATIONS †

Alcool et Cancer
By A. Tuyns (in French only)
1978; 42 pages; Fr. fr. 35.-

Cancer Morbidity and Causes of Death Among Danish Brewery Workers
By O.M. Jensen 1980;
143 pages; Fr. fr. 75.-

Directory of Computer Systems Used in Cancer Registries
By H.R. Menck and D.M. Parkin
1986; 236 pages;
Fr. fr. 50.-

---

* Available from booksellers through the network of WHO sales agents.

†Available directly from IARC

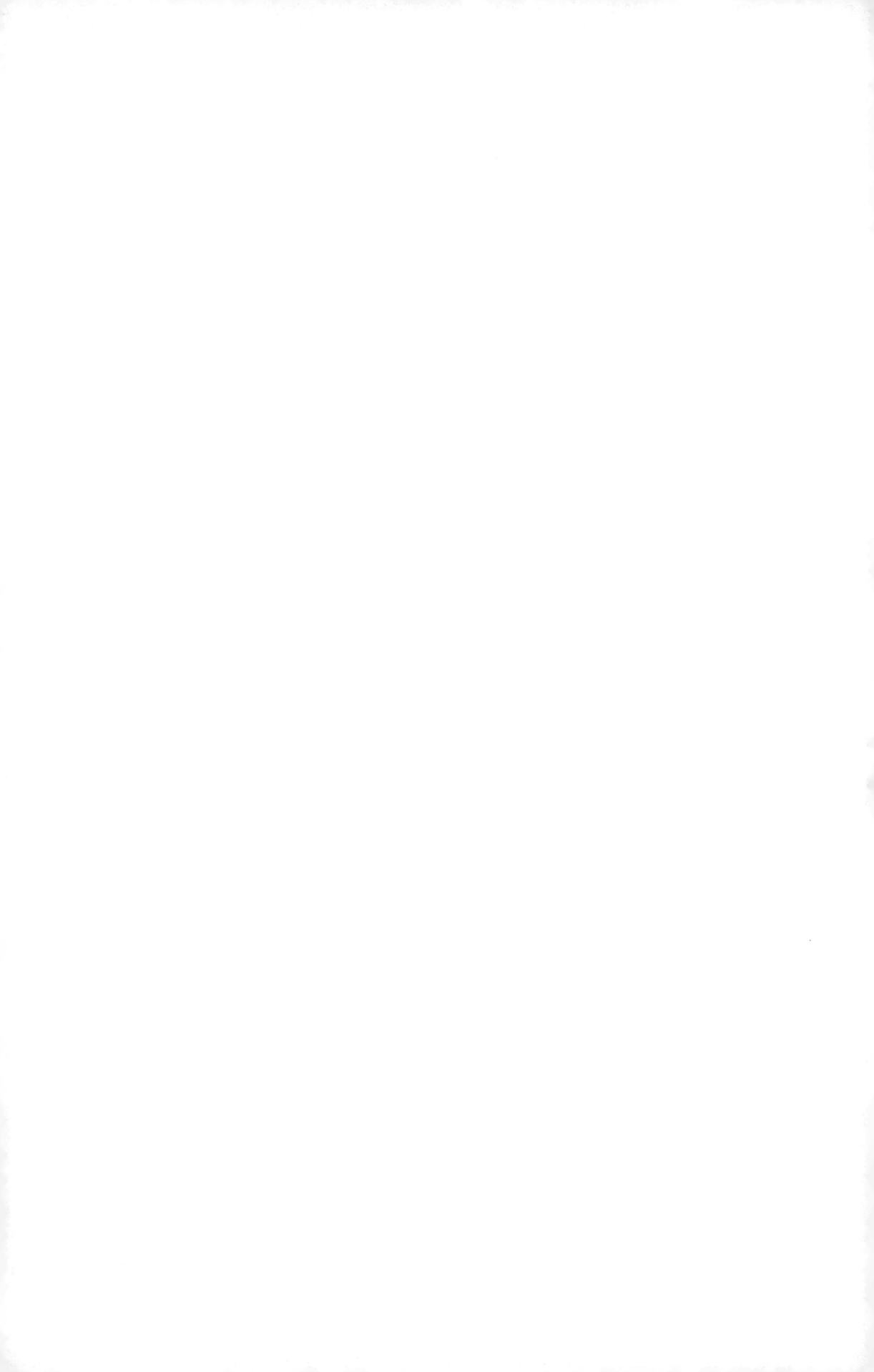

www.ingramcontent.com/pod-product-compliance
Ingram Content Group UK Ltd.
Pitfield, Milton Keynes, MK11 3LW, UK
UKHW051258180426
11947UKWH00020B/1771